Eating and Mental Health Disorders

Eating and Mental Health Disorders

Guest Editor

Hubertus Himmerich

MDPI

Basel • Beijing • Wuhan • Barcelona • Belgrade • Novi Sad • Cluj • Manchester

Guest Editor
Hubertus Himmerich
Department of Psychological
Medicine
King's College London
London
UK

Editorial Office
MDPI AG
Grosspeteranlage 5
4052 Basel, Switzerland

This is a reprint of the Special Issue, published open access by the journal *Nutrients* (ISSN 2072-6643), freely accessible at: https://www.mdpi.com/journal/nutrients/special_issues/1GT7736K88.

For citation purposes, cite each article independently as indicated on the article page online and as indicated below:

Lastname, A.A.; Lastname, B.B. Article Title. *Journal Name* **Year**, *Volume Number*, Page Range.

ISBN 978-3-7258-7801-7 (Hbk)
ISBN 978-3-7258-7802-4 (PDF)
https://doi.org/10.3390/books978-3-7258-7802-4

Cover image courtesy of Ella Frith and Hubertus Himmerich

Contents

About the Editor

Hubertus Himmerich

Hubertus Himmerich is a Reader in Eating Disorders at King's College London and a consultant psychiatrist on an inpatient ward for patients with eating disorders at the Bethlem Royal Hospital in London. His scientific and clinical interests include eating and weight disorders, psychopharmacology, psychoimmunology, and the therapeutic use of music. He has led and performed national and international scientific projects with researchers from Africa, Asia, Australia, America, and Europe.

Preface

This Special Issue invites readers to deepen their understanding of psychosocial determinants contributing to eating disorders and obesity such as food insecurity, educational pressures, a diminished quality of life and adverse psychological factors like increased harm avoidance, a disturbed sense of self, and low body appreciation.

It addresses comorbid conditions that complicate the clinical picture, such as personality disorders, depression, attention-deficit/hyperactivity disorder (ADHD), and orthorexia nervosa, and it explores complex behaviors like emotional eating, binge eating, and pro-inflammatory dietary patterns.

The Special Issue provides practical advice for effective clinical management of eating disorders and obesity including integrated care for comorbidities, nutritional support, as well as innovative and complementary therapeutics.

My thanks go to all the contributing authors, and to Ella Frith for designing the cover. Her piece, titled 'Ed,' references the common abbreviation for eating disorders.

Hubertus Himmerich
Guest Editor

nutrients

MDPI

Editorial

Eating and Mental Health Disorders

Hubertus Himmerich [1,2]

[1] Centre for Research in Eating and Weight Disorders (CREW), Department of Psychological Medicine, Institute of Psychiatry, Psychology & Neuroscience, King's College London, London SE5 8AF, UK; hubertus.himmerich@kcl.ac.uk

[2] South London and Maudsley NHS Foundation Trust, London SE5 8AZ, UK

Recent studies on eating disorders (EDs) and obesity have made substantial progress, leading to an improved understanding of diagnostic entities as well as the psychological, nutritional and biological factors associated with these diseases.

Such innovative scientific and clinical insights have led to the inclusion of avoidant restrictive food intake disorder (ARFID), pica and rumination disorder into the 5th edition of the Diagnostic and Statistical Manual of Mental Disorders (DSM-5) [1], the recognition of the importance of biological factors associated with EDs [2] and awareness of the significance of neurodevelopmental disorders, such as autism spectrum disorder (ASD) and attention deficit hyperactivity disorder (ADHD), for the treatment of EDs [3,4].

However, disturbed eating behavior is not restricted to EDs. A change in food intake can be a symptom of other mental health disorders such as depression [5], or a consequence of psychopharmacological treatment [6]. Obesity is often associated with depression, and a calorie-restricted diet can reduce depressive symptoms in people with obesity [7]. These examples indicate the close association between eating and mental health disorders.

This Special Issue covers psychological, clinical, nutritional, biological and pharmacological aspects of disordered eating, EDs and obesity. The articles build upon advancements in the field and further elucidate the association between eating and mental health disorders.

Psychological and clinical aspects: Four articles of this Special Issue address the topic of depression [8–11]. Depression is a key mental health problem in people with EDs or obesity, as well as their families. It appears to be closely associated with emotional eating, obesity and food insecurity (FI). In a cross-sectional study, which included more than 700 Peruvian adolescents, Calizaya-Milla et al. found that emotional eating was significantly associated with having depressive symptoms [8]. Bludau et al. reported data on almost 2600 multimorbid patients aged 65 years and older from a prospective multicenter observational cohort study and found a significant prevalence of depression across all body mass index (BMI) classes, with obesity class III showing the highest frequency of cases [9]. Kilpela et al. investigated 295 midlife and older women utilizing a food bank and found that women with FI and binge eating reported significantly worsened anxiety, depression and quality of life compared to women with FI alone [10]. Amianto et al. found that mothers of daughters with anorexia nervosa (AN) exhibited greater harm avoidance and lower self-directedness compared to mothers of daughters without AN, and maternal depressive symptoms were specifically linked to earlier AN onset. These findings suggest that treating maternal depression could be a beneficial preventive strategy [11].

Two articles address eating-related problems associated with neurodiversity [12,13]: In a descriptive qualitative study, Chen et al. conducted focus groups with 12 parents in Hong Kong to explore the eating challenges of their school-age children with ADHD and the parental coping strategies employed. The findings revealed that children's eating difficulties were linked to ADHD symptoms and educational pressures [12]. Makin et al. provided a review of the literature on autism and ADHD in adults with obesity. They found a potential overrepresentation of ADHD in obese people and ascertained that patients with ADHD and obesity often exhibit increased impulsivity, more psychopathological symptoms and show poorer response to behavioral weight loss programs [13].

Four further articles on psychological aspects report results on identity, personality, body appreciation, cognitive function and FI [14–17]: A study by Claes et al. investigated the relationship between three identity dimensions and personality disorder (PD) symptoms in 176 female inpatients with an ED. The findings showed that a disturbed identity was strongly associated with cluster B PDs and dependent PD, while a lack of identity predicted cluster A PDs and two cluster C PDs, suggesting that identity is a transdiagnostic feature and that identity-based interventions may benefit patients with co-occurring EDs and PDs [14]. Czepczor-Bernat et al. reported a study in 374 Polish men that investigated whether the combination of high body appreciation and healthy weight was associated with better psychological and motivational profiles compared to low body appreciation and excess weight. They showed that men with high body appreciation and healthy weight reported significantly lower muscle dysmorphia and non-adaptive body attitudes, alongside higher levels of pro-health and adaptive exercise motives [15]. Jowik-Krzemińska et al. compared cognitive function and laboratory parameters in 36 adolescent girls with AN, both during acute malnutrition and after nutritional rehabilitation, against 48 healthy controls. Unexpectedly, in their study, AN patients scored better at both time points than controls in terms of total cognition, attention, estimation, and spatial perception, suggesting the adolescent body maintains a high compensatory capacity for cognitive function despite severe malnutrition [16]. A study by Bryson et al. explored how FI impacted individuals with current or past EDs; the results suggest that FI may exacerbate eating- and food-related symptoms and hinder recovery. Participants reported that FI is associated with low rates of help-seeking due to shame [17].

Nutritional aspects: Three studies in this Special Issue cover the nutritional aspects of eating and mental health disorders [18–20]. Çıtar Dazıroğlu et al. reported a cross-sectional study based on data from 907 university students which found that a pro-inflammatory diet, as measured by a higher Dietary Inflammatory Index (DII), was associated with significantly higher depression scores and lower well-being scores. Conversely, a higher Dietary Antioxidant Index (DAI) was linked to significantly lower scores for anxiety, depression, and stress, suggesting that improving the anti-inflammatory potential of the diet may be a beneficial strategy for supporting student mental health [18]. A review paper by Szulc et al. highlighted the significant similarity between orthorexia nervosa (ON) and plant-based diets, noting that while a vegetarian diet may mask ON, rigid dietary adherence can also lead to the misperception of disorder [19]. Dhopatkar et al. wrote a scoping review of 37 studies, examining outcomes associated with Enteral Tube Nutrition (ETN) used for refeeding in AN. They found that ETN usage resulted in similar or higher weight gain compared to oral nutrition, with comparable risks of refeeding syndrome [20].

Biological and pharmacological aspects: Finally, three articles addressed biological and pharmacological aspects of eating- and weight-related disorders [21–23]. A study by Žák et al. compared plasma lipids, fatty acids (FAs), and bile acid (BA) profiles in 39 women with restrictive AN and 35 healthy controls. Women with restrictive AN exhibited elevated high density lipoprotein cholesterol (HDL-C), altered FA profiles including lower total polyunsaturated fatty acids (PUFAs) n-6 and increased Δ9-desaturase activity, and significantly decreased levels of tauroursodeoxycholic acid (TUDCA), suggesting TUDCA could potentially serve as a biomarker for AN [21]. A systematic review by Micoanski et al.

https://doi.org/10.3390/nu18071122

based on 44 case reports on potomania and beer potomania found that these disorders are rare causes of dilutional hyponatremia due to excessive fluid intake, and that patients often present with neurological symptoms like confusion and seizures [22]. A review by Ma et al. summarized the complex pharmacological and clinical effects of natural compounds and mixtures derived from Rosmarinus officinalis, Ginkgo biloba, Bupleurum chinense, and Berberis vulgaris (berberine-containing plants), all traditionally used for mental health and eating-related issues [23]. The information might offer inspiration for the development of novel pharmacological treatments, because approved psychopharmacological options are limited to fluoxetine for bulimia nervosa and lisdexamfetamine for binge eating disorder in some countries [24]. Even though there are case reports about novel ED medications like ketamine [25], randomized controlled trials are lacking.

Table 1 summarizes the psychological traits, psychiatric disorders, social factors, eating behaviors and nutrition-related factors, as well as the treatment strategies mentioned in this Special Issue.

Table 1. Psychological and nutritional risk factors as well as therapeutic strategies mentioned in this Special Issue.

Psychosocial Risk Factors	Eating and Nutrition	Treatment Strategies
Psychological traits - Increased harm avoidance - Low self-directedness - Disturbed/lack of identity - Low body appreciation Psychiatric disorders - Personality disorder - Depression - ADHD - Orthorexia nervosa Social factors - Food insecurity - Educational pressure - Low quality of life	Eating behaviors - Emotional eating - Binge eating - Excessive fluid intake - Pro-inflammatory diet Nutritional risk factors - Extreme body weight - HDL-C ↑ - Δ9-desaturase ↑ - PUFA n-6 ↓ - TUDCA ↓	Treatment of comorbidities - Depression - ADHD Nutritional strategies - Oral refeeding - Enteral Tube Nutrition Natural compounds - Rosmarinus officinalis - Ginkgo biloba - Bupleurum chinense - Berberis vulgaris

Abbreviations: Attention deficit hyperactivity disorder (ADHD), high-density lipoprotein cholesterol (HDL-C), polyunsaturated fatty acid (PUFA), tauroursodeoxycholic acid (TUDCA).

Biomarkers in EDs and obesity: The Special Issue touches on innovations in the field of EDs and obesity. For example, Žák et al. [21] and Micoanski et al. [22] included biological parameters that are associated with disturbed eating and EDs. Regarding biological, and particularly genetic markers, genome-wide association studies (GWASs) across EDs have identified ED-specific but also shared risk genes that suggest a biological vulnerability for EDs [26]. Genetic correlations have implicated both psychiatric and metabolic factors in the origin of EDs [27], and researchers using polygenic risk scores (PRSs) identified a shared genetic background between bipolar I and II disorders, schizophrenia, and AN [28]. Large-scale epigenome-wide association studies have found significant changes in the NR1H3, TNXB, SYNJ2, PRDM16 and HDAC4 genes [29–33]. These genes are relevant for cholesterol metabolism and lipid synthesis (NR1H3), for the structure and stability of connective tissues such as skin, muscles, and joints (TNXB), for membrane trafficking and cell motility (SYNJ2), brown fat differentiation and lipid metabolism (PRDM16) and gene transcription (HDAC4). These findings indicate that AN is closely related to severe mental health disorders like bipolar disorder and schizophrenia but also associated with disorders affecting metabolism and the connective tissue [2].

https://doi.org/10.3390/nu18071122

Structural neuroimaging reveals that AN is associated with white matter, grey matter and global volume loss [34–43] and changes in subcortical shape, cortical complexity and gyrification [44–47], whereas BN and BED often show localized changes in the orbitofrontal cortex, an area critical for decision-making and taste preference [48–56]. Investigations into functional connectivity indicate that in AN, there is excessive control over hunger, while in BED and BN, the brain's reward centers often override the cognitive control centers [57–61]. These findings corroborate the relevance of emotional eating and binge eating, as investigated by Calizaya-Milla et al. [8] and Kilpela et al. [10]; their results are included in this Special Issue.

These changes of structure and function in the brain are associated with molecular markers of brain plasticity and brain damage. Levels of leptin [62–66] and BDNF [67] have frequently been found altered in EDs, particularly in AN, suggesting that impaired neuroplasticity may lock patients into repetitive, compulsive behavioral loops. Additionally, fluctuations in Tau protein, neurofilament proteins, and glial fibrillary acidic protein (GFAP) have been studied as potential biomarkers in AN to monitor the neurotoxic effects of malnutrition and inflammatory processes [68–70].

Inflammation in eating and mental health disorders: Evidence for the role of inflammatory processes is derived from findings of a bidirectional and shared risk between autoimmune diseases (like type 1 diabetes, celiac disease, Crohn's disease, and psoriasis) and the development of EDs [71–74], changes in cytokine concentrations, e.g., tumor necrosis factor (TNF)-α, interleukin (IL)-6, IL-12 and IL-12 in people with EDs [75–78] and obesity [79,80], changes in white blood cell concentrations [81] and findings of antibody production against molecules and molecule receptors that are involved in appetite regulation and food intake, e.g., α-melanocyte-stimulating hormone (α-MSH) and ghrelin, in people with AN and obesity [82–90]. It was even suggested that anti-cytokine medication such as TNF-α and IL-6 blockers could play a future role in the treatment of restrictive EDs such as AN as they have been shown to influence body weight [91,92].

Against this backdrop, it makes sense that Çıtar Dazıroğlu et al. reported in this Special Issue that a pro-inflammatory diet was associated with higher depression scores, whereas an anti-inflammatory diet was linked to lower scores for mental health problems [18]. This finding aligns with previous research that found increased levels of pro-inflammatory cytokines in people with depression [93,94] and in animal models of stress-related [95] and depression-like behavior [96]. Such findings might become relevant in the future as etanercept, a blocker of the pro-inflammatory cytokine TNF-α, has been shown to have anti-depressant effects in animals [96] and to some degree in humans [97]. Chen et al. [12] and Makin et al. [13] linked eating and metabolic health issues to autism and ADHD [13]. Even though the role of inflammation for neurodevelopmental disorders needs to be elucidated further, a recent study suggests an association of neurodevelopmental disorders with prenatal maternal immune activation [98]. Thus, inflammation is likely to play a relevant role in EDs and obesity, depression and neurodevelopmental disorders like ADHD and autism.

Anti-inflammatory natural compounds for the treatment of eating and mental health disorders: Reflecting on the role of inflammation in these disorders, it makes sense that the natural compounds suggested for treatment of eating and mental health disorders by Ma et al. in this Special Issue [23]—Rosmarinus officinalis [99–104], Ginkgo biloba [105–108], Bupleurum chinense [109–111] and Berberis vulgaris [112–115]—have been reported to have anti-inflammatory properties.

Summary: The contributions of this Special Issue suggest that information on depression, maternal depression, autism and ADHD, identity, personality, body appreciation, cognition, FI and a person's diet and drinking habits should inform the individual psychiatric formulation for the treatment of a person with an eating or mental health disorder. Biomarkers like body weight, HDL-C, Δ9-desaturase, PUFA n-6 and TUDCA might help to assess nutritional health. In severe cases of restrictive EDs, ETN might be a time-limited clinical option. Rosmarinus officinalis, Ginkgo biloba, Bupleurum chinense, and Berberis vulgaris have been suggested as traditional remedies for the treatment of eating and mental health disorders.

Conflicts of Interest: The author declares no conflicts of interest.

References

1. American Psychiatric Association. *Diagnostic and Statistical Manual of Mental Disorders*, 5th ed.; American Psychiatric Association: Washington, DC, USA, 2022.
2. Himmerich, H.; Keeler, J.L.; King, J.A.; Ehrlich, S.; Kaufmann, L.K.; Bulik, C.M.; Cohen-Woods, S.; Wade, T.; Steiger, H.; Booij, L.; et al. World Federation of Societies of Biological Psychiatry (WFSBP) consensus statement on candidate biomarkers for anorexia nervosa. *World J. Biol. Psychiatry* **2026**, *Online ahead of print*. [CrossRef]
3. Tchanturia, K. What we can do about Autism and Eating Disorder comorbidity. *Eur. Eat. Disord. Rev.* **2022**, *30*, 437–441. [CrossRef]
4. Makin, L.; Zesch, E.; Meyer, A.; Mondelli, V.; Tchanturia, K. Autism, ADHD, and Their Traits in Adults with Bulimia Nervosa and Binge Eating Disorder: A Scoping Review. *Eur. Eat. Disord. Rev.* **2025**, *33*, 647–665. [CrossRef] [PubMed]
5. Puccio, F.; Fuller-Tyszkiewicz, M.; Ong, D.; Krug, I. A systematic review and meta-analysis on the longitudinal relationship between eating pathology and depression. *Int. J. Eat. Disord.* **2016**, *49*, 439–454. [CrossRef]
6. Himmerich, H.; Minkwitz, J.; Kirkby, K.C. Weight Gain and Metabolic Changes During Treatment with Antipsychotics and Antidepressants. *Endocr. Metab. Immune Disord. Drug Targets* **2015**, *15*, 252–260. [CrossRef]
7. Applewhite, B.; Penninx, B.W.J.H.; Young, A.H.; Schmidt, U.; Himmerich, H.; Keeler, J.L. The effect of a low-calorie diet on depressive symptoms in individuals with overweight or obesity: A systematic review and meta-analysis of interventional studies. *Psychol. Med.* **2024**, *54*, 1671–1683. [CrossRef]
8. Calizaya-Milla, Y.E.; Puente De La Vega-Fernández, I.; Javier-Aliaga, D.; Rodríguez-Vásquez, M.; Casas-Gálvez, C.; Valle-Chafloque, A.; Saintila, J. Relationships Between Consumption of High-Saturated-Fat Foods, Sleep Duration, BMI, Depression, Age and Sex, and Emotional Eating in Peruvian Adolescents: A Cross-Sectional Study. *Nutrients* **2025**, *17*, 2662. [CrossRef]
9. Bludau, D.C.; Pabst, A.; Bleck, F.; Weyerer, S.; Maier, W.; Gensichen, J.; Mergenthal, K.; Bickel, H.; Fuchs, A.; Schäfer, I.; et al. Overweight, Obesity, and Depression in Multimorbid Older Adults: Prevalence, Diagnostic Agreement, and Associated Factors in Primary Care—Results from a Multicenter Observational Study. *Nutrients* **2025**, *17*, 1394. [CrossRef]
10. Kilpela, L.S.; Loera, T.; Wilfred, S.A.; Salinas, J.; Cuauro, S.E.; Becker, C.B. The Additive Psychosocial Effects of Binge Eating and Food Insecurity Among Midlife and Older Women. *Nutrients* **2025**, *17*, 730. [CrossRef]
11. Amianto, F.; Dell'Oca, G.; Marcotulli, D.; Davico, C.; Martinuzzi, A. Parents of Adolescents with Anorexia Nervosa and Parents of Adult Women with Anorexia Nervosa. *Nutrients* **2025**, *17*, 1115. [CrossRef] [PubMed]
12. Chen, S.-C.; Wu, T.M.S.; Li, H.; Shou, J.-W.; Qin, J.; Wu, G.-T.; Cheng, W.-Y.; Yeung, W.-F. Parental Perspectives on Eating Disorders of Their School-Age Children with ADHD in Hong Kong: A Qualitative Study. *Nutrients* **2025**, *17*, 513. [CrossRef] [PubMed]
13. Makin, L.; Meyer, A.; Zesch, E.; Mondelli, V.; Tchanturia, K. Autism, ADHD, and Their Traits in Adults with Obesity: A Scoping Review. *Nutrients* **2025**, *17*, 787. [CrossRef] [PubMed]
14. Claes, L.; Bogaerts, A.; Bastiaens, T.; Kiekens, G.; Dierckx, E.; Schoevaerts, K.; Luyckx, K. The Association Between Identity Functioning and Personality Pathology in Female Patients with Eating Disorders. *Nutrients* **2025**, *17*, 2329. [CrossRef]
15. Czepczor-Bernat, K.; Modrzejewska, A.; Modrzejewska, J. #BodyPositivity: The Role of Body Appreciation and Body Mass Index for Muscle Dysmorphia, Body Attitudes and Exercise Motives Among Men. *Nutrients* **2025**, *17*, 1177. [CrossRef]
16. Jowik-Krzemińska, K.; Dylewska, D.; Pawlińska-Maćkowiak, A.; Słopień, A.; Tyszkiewicz-Nwafor, M. Cognitive Functions in Adolescent Girls with Anorexia Nervosa during Nutritional Rehabilitation. *Nutrients* **2024**, *16*, 3435. [CrossRef]
17. Bryson, C.; Wilkins, J.; İnce, B.; Hemmings, A.; Kuehne, C.; Douglas, D.; Phillips, M.; Sharpe, H.; Schmidt, U. Food Insecurity in Individuals with Eating Disorders: A UK-Wide Survey of Impact, Help-Seeking, and Suggestions for Guidance. *Nutrients* **2026**, *18*, 852. [CrossRef] [PubMed]
18. Çıtar Dazıroğlu, M.E.; Bilici, S.; Türker, P.F. Associations of Dietary Inflammatory and Antioxidant Indices with Mental Health Indicators Among University Students: A Cross-Sectional Study. *Nutrients* **2025**, *17*, 2442. [CrossRef]
19. Szulc, P.; Willich, K.; Gogga, P. Association Between Orthorexia and Plant-Based Diets—Is There a Vicious Cycle? *Nutrients* **2025**, *17*, 1337. [CrossRef]

https://doi.org/10.3390/nu18071122

20. Dhopatkar, N.; Keeler, J.L.; Gravina, D.; Gower, J.; Mutwalli, H.; Bektas, S.; Fuller, S.J.; Himmerich, H.; Treasure, J. Enteral Tube Nutrition in Anorexia Nervosa and Atypical Anorexia Nervosa and Outcomes: A Systematic Scoping Review. *Nutrients* **2025**, *17*, 425. [CrossRef] [PubMed]
21. Žák, A.; Vecka, M.; Szitanyi, P.; Floriánková, M.; Staňková, B.; Uhlíková, P.; Dostálová, V.; Burda, M. Dyslipidemia in Anorexia Nervosa Is Associated with Decreased Plasma Tauroursodeoxycholic Acid and a Specific Fatty Acid Pattern. *Nutrients* **2025**, *17*, 2347. [CrossRef]
22. Micoanski, K.S.; Soriano, J.M.; Gozalbo, M.M. Potomania and Beer Potomania: A Systematic Review of Published Case Reports. *Nutrients* **2025**, *17*, 2012. [CrossRef]
23. Ma, W.; Regenthal, R.; Krügel, U. Natural Compounds and Their Potential in Eating-Related Aspects of Mental Health Disorders. *Nutrients* **2025**, *17*, 2383. [CrossRef] [PubMed]
24. Himmerich, H.; Lewis, Y.D.; Conti, C.; Mutwalli, H.; Karwautz, A.; Sjögren, J.M.; Uribe Isaza, M.M.; Tyszkiewicz-Nwafor, M.; Aigner, M.; McElroy, S.L.; et al. World Federation of Societies of Biological Psychiatry (WFSBP) guidelines update 2023 on the pharmacological treatment of eating disorders. *World J. Biol. Psychiatry* **2023**, *24*, 643–706. [CrossRef]
25. Keeler, J.L.; Treasure, J.; Himmerich, H.; Brendle, M.; Moore, C.; Robison, R. Case report: Intramuscular ketamine or intranasal esketamine as a treatment in four patients with major depressive disorder and comorbid anorexia nervosa. *Front. Psychiatry* **2023**, *14*, 1181447. [CrossRef]
26. Termorshuizen, J.D.; Davies, H.L.; Lee, S.H.; Dennis, J.K.; Hübel, C.; Johnson, J.S.; Lu, Y.; Munn-Chernoff, M.A.; Peters, T.; Qi, B.; et al. Genome-wide association studies of binge eating behaviour and anorexia nervosa yield insights into the unique and shared biology of eating disorder phenotypes. *medRxiv* **2025**. [CrossRef]
27. Bulik, C.M.; Blake, L.; Austin, J. Genetics of Eating Disorders: What the Clinician Needs to Know. *Psychiatr. Clin. N. Am.* **2019**, *42*, 59–73. [CrossRef]
28. Ihm, H.K.; Kim, H.; Kim, J.; Park, W.Y.; Kang, H.S.; Park, J.; Won, H.H.; Myung, W. Genetic network structure of 13 psychiatric disorders in the general population. *Eur. Arch. Psychiatry Clin. Neurosci.* **2024**, *274*, 1231–1236. [CrossRef]
29. Booij, L.; Casey, K.F.; Antunes, J.M.; Szyf, M.; Joober, R.; Israël, M.; Steiger, H. DNA methylation in individuals with anorexia nervosa and in matched normal-eater controls: A genome-wide study. *Int. J. Eat. Disord.* **2015**, *48*, 874–882. [CrossRef]
30. Kesselmeier, M.; Pütter, C.; Volckmar, A.L.; Baurecht, H.; Grallert, H.; Illig, T.; Ismail, K.; Ollikainen, M.; Silén, Y.; Keski-Rahkonen, A.; et al. High-throughput DNA methylation analysis in anorexia nervosa confirms TNXB hypermethylation. *World J. Biol. Psychiatry* **2018**, *19*, 187–199. [CrossRef]
31. Steiger, H.; Booij, L.; Kahan, E.; McGregor, K.; Thaler, L.; Fletcher, E.; Labbe, A.; Joober, R.; Israël, M.; Szyf, M.; et al. A longitudinal, epigenome-wide study of DNA methylation in anorexia nervosa: Results in actively ill, partially weight-restored, long-term remitted and non-eating-disordered women. *J. Psychiatry Neurosci.* **2019**, *44*, 205–213. [CrossRef] [PubMed]
32. Iranzo-Tatay, C.; Hervas-Marin, D.; Rojo-Bofill, L.M.; Garcia, D.; Vaz-Leal, F.J.; Calabria, I.; Beato-Fernandez, L.; Oltra, S.; Sandoval, J.; Rojo-Moreno, L. Genome-wide DNA methylation profiling in anorexia nervosa discordant identical twins. *Transl. Psychiatry* **2022**, *12*, 15. [CrossRef] [PubMed]
33. Steiger, H.; Booij, L.; Thaler, L.; St-Hilaire, A.; Israël, M.; Casey, K.F.; Oliverio, S.; Crescenzi, O.; Lee, V.; Turecki, G.; et al. DNA methylation in people with anorexia nervosa: Epigenome-wide patterns in actively ill, long-term remitted, and healthy-eater women. *World J. Biol. Psychiatry* **2023**, *24*, 254–259. [CrossRef]
34. King, J.A.; Frank, G.K.; Thompson, P.M.; Ehrlich, S. Structural neuroimaging of anorexia nervosa: Future directions in the quest for mechanisms underlying dynamic alterations. *Biol. Psychiatry* **2018**, *83*, 224–234. [CrossRef]
35. Barona, M.; Brown, M.; Clark, C.; Frangou, S.; White, T.; Micali, N. White matter alterations in anorexia nervosa: Evidence from a voxel-based meta-analysis. *Neurosci. Biobehav. Rev.* **2019**, *100*, 285–295. [CrossRef]
36. Bracké, K.F.M.; Steegers, C.P.M.; van der Harst, T.; Dremmen, M.H.G.; Vernooij, M.W.; White, T.J.H.; Dieleman, G.C. Can neuroimaging measures differentiate the disease course of anorexia nervosa? A systematic review. *J. Psychiatr. Res.* **2023**, *163*, 337–349. [CrossRef]
37. Gaudio, S.; Carducci, F.; Piervincenzi, C.; Olivo, G.; Schiöth, H.B. Altered thalamo–cortical and occipital–parietal–temporal–frontal white matter connections in patients with anorexia and bulimia nervosa: A systematic review of diffusion tensor imaging studies. *J. Psychiatry Neurosci.* **2019**, *44*, 324–339. [CrossRef] [PubMed]
38. Kappou, K.; Ntougia, M.; Kourtesi, A.; Panagouli, E.; Vlachopapadopoulou, E.; Michalacos, S.; Gonidakis, F.; Mastorakos, G.; Psaltopoulou, T.; Tsolia, M.; et al. Neuroimaging findings in adolescents and young adults with anorexia nervosa: A systematic review. *Children* **2021**, *8*, 137. [CrossRef] [PubMed]
39. Meneguzzo, P.; Collantoni, E.; Solmi, M.; Tenconi, E.; Favaro, A. Anorexia nervosa and diffusion weighted imaging: An open methodological question raised by a systematic review and a fractional anisotropy anatomical likelihood estimation meta-analysis. *Int. J. Eat. Disord.* **2019**, *52*, 1237–1250. [CrossRef]

https://doi.org/10.3390/nu18071122

40. Martin Monzon, B.; Henderson, L.A.; Madden, S.; Macefield, V.G.; Touyz, S.; Kohn, M.R.; Clarke, S.; Foroughi, N.; Hay, P. Grey matter volume in adolescents with anorexia nervosa and associated eating disorder symptoms. *Eur. J. Neurosci.* **2017**, *46*, 2297–2307. [CrossRef] [PubMed]
41. Seitz, J.; Herpertz-Dahlmann, B.; Konrad, K. Brain morphological changes in adolescent and adult patients with anorexia nervosa. *J. Neural Transm.* **2016**, *123*, 949–959. [CrossRef]
42. Su, T.; Gong, J.; Tang, G.; Qiu, S.; Chen, P.; Chen, G.; Wang, J.; Huang, L.; Wang, Y. Structural and functional brain alterations in anorexia nervosa: A multimodal meta-analysis of neuroimaging studies. *Hum. Brain Mapp.* **2021**, *42*, 5154–5169. [CrossRef]
43. Walton, E.; Bernardoni, F.; Batury, V.L.; Bahnsen, K.; Larivière, S.; Abbate-Daga, G.; Andres-Perpiña, S.; Bang, L.; Bischoff-Grethe, A.; Brooks, S.J.; et al. Brain structure in acutely underweight and partially weight-restored individuals with anorexia nervosa: A coordinated analysis by the ENIGMA Eating Disorders Working Group. *Biol. Psychiatry* **2022**, *92*, 730–738. [CrossRef] [PubMed]
44. Bernardoni, F.; King, J.A.; Geisler, D.; Birkenstock, J.; Tam, F.I.; Weidner, K.; Roessner, V.; White, T.; Ehrlich, S. Nutritional status affects cortical folding: Lessons learned from anorexia nervosa. *Biol. Psychiatry* **2018**, *84*, 692–701. [CrossRef] [PubMed]
45. Collantoni, E.; Madan, C.R.; Meneguzzo, P.; Chiappini, I.; Tenconi, E.; Manara, R.; Favaro, A. Cortical complexity in anorexia nervosa: A fractal dimension analysis. *J. Clin. Med.* **2020**, *9*, 833. [CrossRef] [PubMed]
46. Collantoni, E.; Pessotto, G.; Meregalli, V.; Madan, C.R.; Miola, A.; Cascino, G.; Monteleone, A.M.; Favaro, A. Cortical complexity in eating disorders: A systematic review and qualitative synthesis. *Eur. Arch. Psychiatry Clin. Neurosci.* **2025**, *Online ahead of print*. [CrossRef]
47. Leppanen, J.; Sedgewick, F.; Cardi, V.; Treasure, J.; Tchanturia, K. Cortical morphometry in anorexia nervosa: An out-of-sample replication study. *Eur. Eat. Disord. Rev.* **2019**, *27*, 507–520. [CrossRef]
48. Murray, M.F.; Richson, B.N.; Forester, G.; Jones, N.P.; Dougherty, E.N.; Bottera, A.R.; Anderson, L.M.; Schaefer, L.M.; Forbes, E.E.; Wildes, J.E. Prefrontal and ventral striatal neural correlates of reversal learning in anorexia nervosa and bulimia nervosa. *Cogn. Affect. Behav. Neurosci.* **2025**. [CrossRef]
49. Wang, Y.; Tang, L.; Li, W.; Wang, M.; Chen, Q.; Yu, F.; Yang, Z.; Li, Z.; Wang, Z.; Wang, J.; et al. Multimodal quantitative magnetic resonance imaging alterations of the basal ganglia circuit underlie the severity of bulimia nervosa. *Int. J. Clin. Health Psychol.* **2025**, *25*, 100557. [CrossRef]
50. Yu, X.; Robinson, L.; Bobou, M.; Zhang, Z.; Banaschewski, T.; Barker, G.J.; Bokde, A.L.W.; Flor, H.; Grigis, A.; Garavan, H.; et al. Multimodal Investigations of Structural and Functional Brain Alterations in Anorexia and Bulimia Nervosa and Their Relationships to Psychopathology. *Biol. Psychiatry* **2025**, *98*, 237–248. [CrossRef]
51. Chen, X.; Ai, C.; Liu, Z.; Wang, G. Neuroimaging studies of resting-state functional magnetic resonance imaging in eating disorders. *BMC Med. Imaging* **2024**, *24*, 265. [CrossRef]
52. Luo, L.; Luo, Y.; Chen, X.; Xiao, M.; Bian, Z.; Leng, X.; Li, W.; Wang, J.; Yang, Y.; Liu, Y.; et al. Structural and functional neural patterns among sub-threshold bulimia nervosa: Abnormalities in dorsolateral prefrontal cortex and orbitofrontal cortex. *Psychiatry Res. Neuroimaging* **2024**, *342*, 111825. [CrossRef]
53. Li, W.; Chen, X.; Luo, Y.; Xiao, M.; Liu, Y.; Chen, H. Altered connectivity patterns of medial and lateral orbitofrontal cortex underlie the severity of bulimic symptoms. *Int. J. Clin. Health Psychol.* **2024**, *24*, 100439. [CrossRef]
54. Svaldi, J.; Schopp, B.; Schroeder, P.A.; Werle, D.; Ehlis, A.C. Prefrontal Cortex Recruitment to Food Stimuli Differs in Overweight/Obesity and Binge Eating Disorder. *Eur. Eat. Disord. Rev.* **2026**, *34*, 202–212. [CrossRef]
55. Stice, E.; Yokum, S.; Gau, J.; Shaw, H. Neural risk factors that predict the future onset of binge eating or compensatory weight control behaviors: A prospective 4-year fMRI study. *Psychol. Med.* **2025**, *55*, e48. [CrossRef]
56. Berner, L.A.; Marsh, R. Frontostriatal circuits and the development of bulimia nervosa. *Front. Behav. Neurosci.* **2014**, *8*, 395. [CrossRef]
57. Ehrlich, S.; Geisler, D.; Ritschel, F.; King, J.A.; Seidel, M.; Boehm, I.; Breier, M.; Clas, S.; Weiss, J.; Marxen, M.; et al. Elevated cognitive control over reward processing in recovered female patients with anorexia nervosa. *J. Psychiatry Neurosci.* **2015**, *40*, 307–315. [CrossRef]
58. Hartogsveld, B.; Quaedflieg, C.W.E.M.; van Ruitenbeek, P.; Smeets, T. Volume and connectivity differences in brain networks associated with cognitive constructs of binge eating. *eNeuro* **2022**, *9*, ENEURO.0080-21.2021. [CrossRef] [PubMed]
59. Steward, T.; Menchon, J.M.; Jiménez-Murcia, S.; Soriano-Mas, C.; Fernandez-Aranda, F. Neural network alterations across eating disorders: A narrative review of fMRI studies. *Curr. Neuropharmacol.* **2018**, *16*, 1150–1163. [CrossRef] [PubMed]
60. Stopyra, M.A.; Simon, J.J.; Skunde, M.; Walther, S.; Bendszus, M.; Herzog, W.; Friederich, H.C. Altered functional connectivity in binge eating disorder and bulimia nervosa: A resting-state fMRI study. *Brain Behav.* **2019**, *9*, e01207. [CrossRef]
61. Wierenga, C.E.; Bischoff-Grethe, A.; Melrose, A.J.; Irvine, Z.; Torres, L.; Bailer, U.F.; Simmons, A.; Fudge, J.L.; McClure, S.M.; Ely, A.; et al. Hunger does not motivate reward circuit response in women remitted from anorexia nervosa. *Biol. Psychiatry* **2015**, *77*, 642–652. [CrossRef] [PubMed]

https://doi.org/10.3390/nu18071122

62. Wronski, M.L.; Bernardoni, F.; Bahnsen, K.; Seidel, M.; Arold, D.; Doose, A.; Steinhäuser, J.L.; Borucki, K.; Breithaupt, L.; Lawson, E.A.; et al. Dynamic amygdala nuclei alterations in relation to weight status in anorexia nervosa are mediated by leptin. *J. Am. Acad. Child Adolesc. Psychiatry* **2024**, *63*, 624–639. [CrossRef]
63. Wronski, M.L.; Geisler, D.; Bernardoni, F.; Seidel, M.; Bahnsen, K.; Doose, A.; Steinhäuser, J.L.; Gronow, F.; Böldt, L.V.; Plessow, F.; et al. Differential alterations of amygdala nuclei volumes in acutely ill patients with anorexia nervosa and their associations with leptin levels. *Psychol. Med.* **2023**, *53*, 6288–6303. [CrossRef]
64. Wronski, M.L.; Hohnemann, C.; Bernardoni, F.; Bahnsen, K.; Doose, A.; Arold, D.; Borucki, K.; Holsen, L.M.; Lawson, E.A.; Plessow, F.; et al. Explicating the role of amygdala substructure alterations in the link between hypoleptinemia and rumination in anorexia nervosa. *Acta Psychiatr. Scand.* **2023**, *148*, 368–381. [CrossRef]
65. Hebebrand, J.; Plieger, M.; Milos, G.; Peters, T.; Hinney, A.; Antel, J. Does hypoleptinemia trigger entrapment in anorexia nervosa? Etiological and clinical considerations. *Eur. Eat. Disord. Rev.* **2024**, *32*, 557–574. [CrossRef]
66. Hebebrand, J.; Hildebrandt, T.; Schlögl, H.; Seitz, J.; Denecke, S.; Vieira, D.; Gradl-Dietsch, G.; Peters, T.; Antel, J.; Lau, D.; et al. The role of hypoleptinemia in the psychological and behavioral adaptation to starvation: Implications for anorexia nervosa. *Neurosci. Biobehav. Rev.* **2022**, *141*, 104807. [CrossRef]
67. Keeler, J.L.; Robinson, L.; Keeler-Schäffeler, R.; Dalton, B.; Treasure, J.; Himmerich, H. Growth factors in anorexia nervosa: A systematic review and meta-analysis of cross-sectional and longitudinal data. *World J. Biol. Psychiatry* **2022**, *23*, 582–600. [CrossRef]
68. Doose, A.; Hellerhoff, I.; Tam, F.I.; King, J.A.; Seidel, M.; Geisler, D.; Plähn, H.C.I.; Roessner, V.; Akgün, K.; Ziemssen, T.; et al. Neural and glial damage markers in women after long-term weight-recovery from anorexia nervosa. *Psychoneuroendocrinology* **2022**, *135*, 105576. [CrossRef] [PubMed]
69. Hellerhoff, I.; King, J.A.; Tam, F.I.; Pauligk, S.; Seidel, M.; Geisler, D.; Bahnsen, K.; Kretschmann, N.; Akgün, K.; Roessner, V.; et al. Differential longitudinal changes of neuronal and glial damage markers in anorexia nervosa after partial weight restoration. *Transl. Psychiatry* **2021**, *11*, 86. [CrossRef]
70. Nilsson, I.A.K.; Millischer, V.; Karrenbauer, V.D.; Juréus, A.; Salehi, A.M.; Norring, C.; von Hausswolff-Juhlin, Y.; Schalling, M.; Blennow, K.; Bulik, C.M.; et al. Plasma neurofilament light chain concentration is increased in anorexia nervosa. *Transl. Psychiatry* **2019**, *9*, 180. [CrossRef]
71. Raevuori, A.; Haukka, J.; Vaarala, O.; Suvisaari, J.M.; Gissler, M.; Grainger, M.; Linna, M.S.; Suokas, J.T. The increased risk for autoimmune diseases in patients with eating disorders. *PLoS ONE* **2014**, *9*, e104845. [CrossRef]
72. Hedman, A.; Breithaupt, L.; Hübel, C.; Thornton, L.M.; Tillander, A.; Norring, C.; Birgegård, A.; Larsson, H.; Ludvigsson, J.F.; Sävendahl, L.; et al. Bidirectional relationship between eating disorders and autoimmune diseases. *J. Child Psychol. Psychiatry* **2019**, *60*, 803–812. [CrossRef] [PubMed]
73. Wotton, C.J.; James, A.; Goldacre, M.J. Coexistence of eating disorders and autoimmune diseases: Record linkage cohort study, UK. *Int. J. Eat. Disord.* **2016**, *49*, 663–672. [CrossRef] [PubMed]
74. Shah, V.; Larson, A.; Jafferany, M. Exploring the psychological impact of childhood-onset psoriasis: A systematic review. *Clin. Exp. Dermatol.* **2024**, *50*, 29–37. [CrossRef]
75. Keeler, J.L.; Bovenberg, C.; Himmerich, H.; Treasure, J.; Carter, B.; Schmidt, U.; Dalton, B. Cytokine concentrations in people with eating disorders: A comprehensive updated systematic review and meta-analysis. *Commun. Med.* **2025**, *5*, 408. [CrossRef]
76. Dalton, B.; Bartholdy, S.; Robinson, L.; Solmi, M.; Ibrahim, M.A.A.; Breen, G.; Schmidt, U.; Himmerich, H. A meta-analysis of cytokine concentrations in eating disorders. *J. Psychiatr. Res.* **2018**, *103*, 252–264. [CrossRef]
77. Dalton, B.; Whitmore, V.; Patsalos, O.; Ibrahim, M.A.A.; Schmidt, U.; Himmerich, H. A systematic review of in vitro cytokine production in eating disorders. *Mol. Cell. Endocrinol.* **2019**, *497*, 110308. [CrossRef] [PubMed]
78. Keeler, J.L.; Patsalos, O.; Chung, R.; Schmidt, U.; Breen, G.; Treasure, J.; Himmerich, H.; Dalton, B. Reduced MIP-1beta as a Trait Marker and Reduced IL-7 and IL-12 as State Markers of Anorexia Nervosa. *J. Pers. Med.* **2021**, *11*, 814. [CrossRef] [PubMed]
79. Schmidt, F.M.; Weschenfelder, J.; Sander, C.; Minkwitz, J.; Thormann, J.; Chittka, T.; Mergl, R.; Kirkby, K.C.; Faßhauer, M.; Stumvoll, M.; et al. Inflammatory cytokines in general and central obesity and modulating effects of physical activity. *PLoS ONE* **2015**, *10*, e0121971. [CrossRef] [PubMed]
80. Himmerich, H.; Fulda, S.; Linseisen, J.; Seiler, H.; Wolfram, G.; Himmerich, S.; Gedrich, K.; Pollmächer, T. TNF-alpha, soluble TNF receptor and interleukin-6 plasma levels in the general population. *Eur. Cytokine Netw.* **2006**, *17*, 196–201. [CrossRef]
81. Keeler, J.L.; Xu, C.; Morris, R.; Hartland, H.; Treasure, J.; Himmerich, H. A systematic review and meta-analysis of routine white blood cell concentrations in people with eating disorders. *Neuroscience* **2025**, *Online ahead of print*. [CrossRef]
82. Fetissov, S.O.; Hallman, J.; Oreland, L.; Af Klinteberg, B.; Grenbäck, E.; Hulting, A.L.; Hökfelt, T. Autoantibodies against α-MSH, ACTH, and LHRH in anorexia and bulimia nervosa patients. *Proc. Natl. Acad. Sci. USA* **2002**, *99*, 17155–17160. [CrossRef]
83. Seitz, J.; Lahaye, E.; Andreani, N.A.; Thomas, B.; Takhlidjt, S.; Chartrel, N.; Herpertz-Dahlmann, B.; Baines, J.F.; Fetissov, S.O. Long-term dynamics of serum α-MSH and α-MSH-binding immunoglobulins with a link to gut microbiota composition in patients with anorexia nervosa. *Neuroendocrinology* **2024**, *114*, 907–920. [CrossRef]

84. Escelsior, A.; Cogorno, L.; Sukkar, S.G.; Amerio, A.; Donini, L.M.; Bellomo, M.; Iervasi, E.; Amore, M.; Saverino, D. Anti-hypothalamus autoantibodies in anorexia nervosa: A possible new mechanism in neuro-physiological derangement? *Eat. Weight Disord.* **2022**, *27*, 2481–2496. [CrossRef]
85. Roubalova, R.; Prochazkova, P.; Dvorak, J.; Hill, M.; Papezova, H.; Kreisinger, J.; Bulant, J.; Lambertova, A.; Holanova, P.; Bilej, M.; et al. Altered serum immunological and biochemical parameters and microbiota composition in patients with AN during realimentation. *Front. Nutr.* **2021**, *8*, 680870. [CrossRef]
86. Lucas, N.; Legrand, R.; Bôle-Feysot, C.; Breton, J.; Coëffier, M.; Akkermann, K.; Järv, A.; Harro, J.; Déchelotte, P.; Fetissov, S.O. Immunoglobulin G modulation of the melanocortin 4 receptor signaling in obesity and eating disorders. *Transl. Psychiatry* **2019**, *9*, 87. [CrossRef]
87. Fetissov, S.O.; Hökfelt, T. On the origin of eating disorders: Altered signaling between gut microbiota, adaptive immunity and the brain melanocortin system regulating feeding behavior. *Curr. Opin. Pharmacol.* **2019**, *48*, 82–91. [CrossRef]
88. Takagi, K.; Legrand, R.; Asakawa, A.; Amitani, H.; François, M.; Tennoune, N.; Coëffier, M.; Claeyssens, S.; do Rego, J.C.; Déchelotte, P.; et al. Anti-ghrelin immunoglobulins modulate ghrelin stability and its orexigenic effect in obese mice and humans. *Nat. Commun.* **2013**, *4*, 2685. [CrossRef]
89. Terashi, M.; Asakawa, A.; Harada, T.; Ushikai, M.; Coquerel, Q.; Sinno, M.H.; Déchelotte, P.; Inui, A.; Fetissov, S.O. Ghrelin reactive autoantibodies in restrictive anorexia nervosa. *Nutrition* **2011**, *27*, 407–413. [CrossRef]
90. Fetissov, S.O.; Lucas, N.; Legrand, R. Ghrelin-Reactive Immunoglobulins in Conditions of Altered Appetite and Energy Balance. *Front. Endocrinol.* **2017**, *8*, 10. [CrossRef]
91. Patsalos, O.; Dalton, B.; Leppanen, J.; Ibrahim, M.A.A.; Himmerich, H. Impact of TNF-alpha Inhibitors on Body Weight and BMI: A Systematic Review and Meta-Analysis. *Front. Pharmacol.* **2020**, *11*, 481. [CrossRef] [PubMed]
92. Patsalos, O.; Dalton, B.; Himmerich, H. Effects of IL-6 Signaling Pathway Inhibition on Weight and BMI: A Systematic Review and Meta-Analysis. *Int. J. Mol. Sci.* **2020**, *21*, 6290. [CrossRef]
93. Schmidt, F.M.; Lichtblau, N.; Minkwitz, J.; Chittka, T.; Thormann, J.; Kirkby, K.C.; Sander, C.; Mergl, R.; Faßhauer, M.; Stumvoll, M.; et al. Cytokine levels in depressed and non-depressed subjects, and masking effects of obesity. *J. Psychiatr. Res.* **2014**, *55*, 29–34. [CrossRef] [PubMed]
94. Himmerich, H.; Fulda, S.; Linseisen, J.; Seiler, H.; Wolfram, G.; Himmerich, S.; Gedrich, K.; Kloiber, S.; Lucae, S.; Ising, M.; et al. Depression, comorbidities and the TNF-alpha system. *Eur. Psychiatry* **2008**, *23*, 421–429. [CrossRef] [PubMed]
95. Himmerich, H.; Fischer, J.; Bauer, K.; Kirkby, K.C.; Sack, U.; Krügel, U. Stress-induced cytokine changes in rats. *Eur. Cytokine Netw.* **2013**, *24*, 97–103. [CrossRef] [PubMed]
96. Krügel, U.; Fischer, J.; Radicke, S.; Sack, U.; Himmerich, H. Antidepressant effects of TNF-alpha blockade in an animal model of depression. *J. Psychiatr. Res.* **2013**, *47*, 611–616. [CrossRef] [PubMed]
97. Schmidt, F.M.; Kirkby, K.C.; Himmerich, H. The TNF-alpha inhibitor etanercept as monotherapy in treatment-resistant depression—Report of two cases. *Psychiatr. Danub.* **2014**, *26*, 288–290.
98. Starr, A.; Qu, X.; Hong, X.; Safi, S.; Wang, X. Individual and Combined Associations of Maternal Fever, Placental Inflammation, and Prematurity with Autism and ADHD. *J. Autism Dev. Disord.* **2026**, *Online ahead of print*. [CrossRef]
99. de Oliveira, J.R.; Camargo, S.E.A.; de Oliveira, L.D. *Rosmarinus officinalis* L. (rosemary) as therapeutic and prophylactic agent. *J. Biomed. Sci.* **2019**, *26*, 5. [CrossRef]
100. Ghasemzadeh Rahbardar, M.; Amin, B.; Mehri, S.; Mirnajafi-Zadeh, S.J.; Hosseinzadeh, H. Anti-inflammatory effects of ethanolic extract of *Rosmarinus officinalis* L. and rosmarinic acid in a rat model of neuropathic pain. *Biomed. Pharmacother.* **2017**, *86*, 441–449. [CrossRef]
101. Luo, C.; Zou, L.; Sun, H.; Peng, J.; Gao, C.; Bao, L.; Ji, R.; Jin, Y.; Sun, S. A Review of the Anti-Inflammatory Effects of Rosmarinic Acid on Inflammatory Diseases. *Front. Pharmacol.* **2020**, *11*, 153. [CrossRef]
102. Oduncuoglu, G.; Şanlıtürk, G. Anti-inflammatory and Antibacterial Activity of *Rosmarinus officinalis* L. Essential Oil and Hydrosol against Methicillin-Resistant *Staphylococcus aureus* (MRSA). *EMU J. Pharm. Sci.* **2025**, *8*, 124–131. [CrossRef]
103. Veenstra, J.P.; Johnson, J. Rosemary (*Salvia rosmarinus*): Health-Promoting Benefits and Food Preservative Properties. *Int. J. Nutr.* **2021**, *6*, 1–10. [CrossRef]
104. Xu, J.; Li, T.; Li, F.; Qiang, H.; Wie, X.; Zhan, R.; Chen, Y. The applications and mechanisms of *Rosmarinus officinalis* L. in the management of different wounds and UV-irradiated skin. *Front. Pharmacol.* **2025**, *15*, 1461790. [CrossRef] [PubMed]
105. Al-Haddad, M.; Bairam, A.; Hussain, H.; Majeed, S.; Al-Jalehawi, A. Evaluation of clinical efficacy of *Ginkgo biloba* extract in the treatment of knee osteoarthritis: A randomized clinical trial. *F1000Research* **2023**, *11*, 1231. [CrossRef]
106. Kim, H.; Kang, S.; Go, G.W. Exploring the multifaceted role of ginkgolides and bilobalide from *Ginkgo biloba* in mitigating metabolic disorders. *Food Sci. Biotechnol.* **2024**, *33*, 2903–2917. [CrossRef]
107. Mousavi, S.N.; Hosseinikia, M.; Yousefi Rad, E.; Saboori, S. Beneficial effects of *Ginkgo biloba* leaf extract on inflammatory markers: A systematic review and meta-analysis of clinical trials. *Phytother. Res.* **2022**, *36*, 3459–3469. [CrossRef]

https://doi.org/10.3390/nu18071122

108. Sun, L.; Apweiler, M.; Tirkey, A.; Klett, D.; Normann, C.; Dietz, G.P.H.; Lehner, M.D.; Fiebich, B.L. Anti-Neuroinflammatory Effects of *Ginkgo biloba* Extract EGb 761 in LPS-Activated BV2 Microglial Cells. *Int. J. Mol. Sci.* **2024**, *25*, 8108. [CrossRef]
109. Jiang, H.; Yang, L.; Hou, A.; Zhang, J.; Wang, S.; Man, W.; Zheng, S.; Yu, H.; Wang, X.; Yang, B.; et al. Botany, traditional uses, phytochemistry, analytical methods, processing, pharmacology and pharmacokinetics of *Bupleuri Radix*: A systematic review. *Biomed. Pharmacother.* **2020**, *131*, 110679. [CrossRef] [PubMed]
110. Yu, X.; Miao, Z.; Zhang, L.; Zhu, L.; Sheng, H. Extraction, purification, structure characteristics, biological activities and pharmaceutical application of *Bupleuri Radix* Polysaccharide: A review. *Int. J. Biol. Macromol.* **2023**, *237*, 124146. [CrossRef] [PubMed]
111. Sun, P.; Li, Y.; Wie, S.; Zhao, T.; Wang, Y.; Song, C.; Xue, L.; Wang, F.; Xiao, L.; Wu, J.; et al. Pharmacological Effects and Chemical Constituents of Bupleurum. *Mini Rev. Med. Chem.* **2019**, *19*, 34–55. [CrossRef]
112. Imenshahidi, M.; Hosseinzadeh, H. Berberine and barberry (*Berberis vulgaris*): A comprehensive review of their biological activities and health benefits. *Phytother. Res.* **2024**, *38*, 112–135. [CrossRef]
113. Fatima Hashmi, S.; Saleem, H.; Khurshid, U.; Khursheed, A.; Tauquir Alam, M.; Imran, M.; Abida, A.; Nayeem, N.; Gill, M.S.A. Genus Berberis: A Comprehensive and Updated Review on Ethnobotanical Uses, Phytochemistry and Pharmacological Activities. *Chem. Biodivers.* **2024**, *21*, e202400911. [CrossRef]
114. Mohi-Ud-Din, R.; Mir, R.H.; Mir, P.A.; Farooq, S.; Raza, S.N.; Raja, W.Y.; Masoodi, M.H.; Singh, I.P.; Bhat, Z.A. Ethnomedicinal uses, Phytochemistry and Pharmacological Aspects of the Genus Berberis Linn: A Comprehensive Review. *Comb. Chem. High Throughput Screen.* **2021**, *24*, 624–644. [CrossRef]
115. Tabeshpour, J.; Imenshahidi, M.; Hosseinzadeh, H. A review of the effects of *Berberis vulgaris* and its major component, berberine, in metabolic syndrome. *Iran. J. Basic Med. Sci.* **2017**, *20*, 557–568. [CrossRef]

https://doi.org/10.3390/nu18071122

nutrients

MDPI

Article

Food Insecurity in Individuals with Eating Disorders: A UK-Wide Survey of Impact, Help-Seeking, and Suggestions for Guidance

Callum Bryson [1], Jessica Wilkins [1], Başak İnce [1], Amelia Hemmings [1], Carina Kuehne [1], Daire Douglas [1], Matthew Phillips [2], Helen Sharpe [3,†] and Ulrike Schmidt [1,4,*,†]

1 Centre for Research in Eating and Weight Disorders, Department of Psychological Medicine, Institute of Psychiatry, Psychology & Neuroscience, King's College London, London SE5 8AF, UK; callum.bryson@kcl.ac.uk (C.B.); jessica.wilkins@kcl.ac.uk (J.W.); basak.ince@kcl.ac.uk (B.İ.); amelia.1.hemmings@kcl.ac.uk (A.H.); carina.1.kuehne@kcl.ac.uk (C.K.); daire.douglas@kcl.ac.uk (D.D.)
2 Department of Psychology, School of Life Sciences and the Environment, Royal Holloway, University of London, London TW20 0EX, UK; matthew.phillips.2023@live.rhul.ac.uk
3 School of Health in Social Science, University of Edinburgh, Edinburgh EH1 1LE, UK; helen.sharpe@ed.ac.uk
4 South London and Maudsley NHS Foundation Trust, London SE5 8AZ, UK
* Correspondence: ulrike.schmidt@kcl.ac.uk
† These authors share joint senior authorship.

Abstract

Background/Objectives: Food insecurity (FI) is significant and increasing in the UK's general population. Previous research has linked FI to disordered eating and obesity, yet most of this research is conducted in non-clinical populations in the USA. As such, little is known about the perspectives of people with current or past eating disorders (PwEDs) on the effects of FI on their eating disorder symptoms and treatment in the UK. The current study explores these effects, as well as PwEDs' experiences of help-seeking for food insecurity and their suggestions for clinical guidance. **Methods**: Data were collected via an online survey (n = 337) which included both open-ended and fixed response questions. A mixed methods approach was used for analysis, with a thematic analysis being used for qualitative data. **Results**: Recent FI was related to higher frequency of food restriction and less comfort discussing FI in clinical contexts. Additionally, participants reported that FI exacerbated symptoms and worsened recovery efforts. Help-seeking was generally low among participants. Shame was a barrier for help-seeking, and suggestions for guidance included adaptations to screening and treatment, improving clinician knowledge, and providing practical solutions to alleviate FI. **Conclusions**: FI is a serious public health issue in the UK that has large ramifications for eating disorder maintenance and recovery. Guidance is needed to address FI in clinical practice and reduce shame around FI. Ultimately, however, FI is a systemic issue that will require policy change to be eliminated.

Keywords: food insecurity; eating disorders; treatment; recovery; help-seeking; clinical guidance

1. Introduction

Food insecurity (FI) is defined as the inadequate or unreliable access to a sufficient amount of nutritious food and is often related to poverty or other forms of resource scarcity (e.g., access to water) [1]. FI experiences exist on a continuum from complete food security to moderate (e.g., skipping a meal) and severe forms (e.g., going an entire day without eating) [2]. The recent COVID-19 pandemic has led to an increase in FI globally [3], across countries in both the Global North and South [4–7]. While rates of FI differ over national contexts, there appears to be a shared vulnerability in certain populations, such as households with low income and children, and individuals with periods of unemployment and mental health diagnoses or disabilities [7–10]. Post-pandemic rates of FI in the UK are estimated to be around 13.9%, or 7.3 million adults, with severe FI remaining 1.5 times higher now than at the start of the pandemic [11,12]. Importantly, the UK has struggled with exceptionally high FI for some time. The UN's Food and Agriculture Organization estimated that between 2015 and 2017, on average, 2.2 million people in the UK had at least one experience of severe FI [13], which accounted for around 20% of these cases in Europe [1]. The available evidence suggests that these elevated rates of FI are connected to a wider array of social inequalities and policy decisions [14]. For example, FI has been consistently linked to austerity measures employed by the UK government in response to the 2008 Financial Crisis [15]. Additionally, since late 2021, the cost of necessities in the UK (such as heating, food, and transport) has risen, leading to a so-called cost-of-living crisis where approximately 12% of adults have been struggling financially [16].

The health consequences of FI are wide reaching. Inadequate access to nutritious foods impacts a myriad of physical health conditions, such as anaemia [17], diabetes [18], osteoporosis [19], respiratory diseases [20], chronic pain [21], obesity [22], and malnutrition [23]. For mental health conditions, however, the link with FI is less well understood. Individuals with experiences of FI have significantly higher rates of depression (diagnoses and symptoms) [24,25], as well as an elevated risk of suicidal ideation compared with those without such experiences [26]. Stress and anxiety levels have also been shown to be higher in FI individuals relative to those who are food secure [22,24,25]. Even though it is difficult to make causal inferences about these relationships—as evidence mostly comes from cross-sectional studies—this relationship is likely bidirectional, with FI increasing susceptibility to, and being influenced by, experiences of poor mental health [27].

Attempts to understand how FI impacts eating disorders (EDs) are nascent. EDs are a set of severe psychiatric conditions characterized by pathological eating behaviours [28], such as restriction of food intake, little to no interest in food or eating, binge eating, and/or engaging in compensatory behaviours (e.g., over-exercise or self-induced vomiting) to control weight and shape [29,30]. Notably, EDs have some of the greatest mortality and morbidity rates of any mental health condition. This underscores the importance of understanding risk factors that affect their development, maintenance, and relapse [31]. The available evidence indicates that, relative to food secure adults, FI is associated with a higher prevalence of: eating, weight and shape concerns [32], ED behaviours (such as objective binge eating and compensatory fasting) [33,34], and EDs like binge eating disorder (BED) and bulimia nervosa (BN) [35–37].

There are a number of mechanisms that may drive disordered eating in individuals with FI. First, FI is known to create a stressful preoccupation with food (e.g., via anxiety around when food can next be accessed, around choosing between food and other necessities, or due to shame around how food is acquired) which is thought to lead to other ED behaviours [38]. Second, stress may exert an indirect impact on the relationship between FI and EDs via epigenetic influences on the expression of key genes in vulnerable populations [39]. Third, binge behaviours in FI populations may arise from the 'feast/famine' cycle of food availability [37]; in times of relative dearth, food intake may be restricted by necessity or with intention (a known risk factor of binge eating) [40]. Binges may then follow on from periods of restriction as an emotion regulation tool in response to stress experienced by FI [41] or due to the compounding effects of weight stigma and body shame for those in larger bodies [42]. There has been less focus on understanding the link between

https://doi.org/10.3390/nu18050852

restrictive ED behaviours and FI in the literature, and as a consequence, there is a less cogent explanation for how FI may lead to illnesses like anorexia nervosa (AN), other than the generic mechanisms of stress [37], guilt, and eating [43]. Moreover, most of the focus in this literature has been on how FI contributes to the aetiology of EDs, with there being a relative absence of research surrounding how FI experiences may contribute to their persistence and relapse risk.

Although evidence indicates that FI and EDs are related, most studies have been conducted in non-clinical samples in the USA, so their comparability to ED populations and other national contexts is unclear [44]. Emerging evidence suggests a similar relationship in a UK sample [45], and a comparison with other national contexts has found the association between FI and binge/purge symptoms to be similar across the UK, USA, Australia and Canada [46]. According to a recent survey, ED healthcare professionals in the UK perceive FI as a growing issue for their patients, but feel they lack practical guidance and knowledge to address FI challenges in their clinical practice [47]. Lived-experience perspectives are valuable for understanding the role of FI in the pathogenesis of EDs and its impact on treatment; however, they have been largely underutilized [37]. Qualitative research from the US has shown that FI is implicated in the maintenance of ED symptoms and impairs patients' ability to engage in treatments, but is largely unaddressed by clinicians [48]. Similarly, evidence from Canada suggests that FI (and other social determinants of health) impedes access to and engagement with first-line ED treatments [49]. However, it is unknown how applicable these findings are to the ED treatment and service context of the UK and the National Health Service (NHS) in light of the recent cost-of-living crisis.

The current study used a mixed methods approach via an online survey in the UK to (a) quantify the experiences of FI, cost-of-living issues, and help-seeking in people experiencing a diagnosed or suspected ED, and (b) qualitatively explore their perspectives of the role that FI plays in the aetiology, maintenance, and relapse risk of their illness, as well as their suggestions for future clinical guidance. To achieve this, the following research questions were devised:

1. To what extent do people with a past or present ED (PwEDs) experience FI and other cost-of-living issues in the UK? How do PwEDs view FI and the cost of living in relation to the development, maintenance, and treatment of their ED?
2. To what extent do PwEDs seek help from healthcare professionals regarding their FI experiences? What factors facilitate or impede this help-seeking?
3. What suggestions for guidance (if any) do PwEDs have for how FI can be managed in healthcare settings?

2. Materials and Methods

2.1. Participants and Procedure

Ethical approval for the study was attained via the King's College London Research Ethics Committee (Review Reference: HR-22/23-34804). Eligibility criteria included being at least 16 years of age, residing in the UK, and having current or past ED or disordered eating behaviours. Responses to the online, cross-sectional survey were collected between June 2023 to July 2024, and the survey was advertised online via the research team's website (https://edifyresearch.co.uk), a reputable ED charity in the UK (BEAT Eating Disorders, Norwich, UK; https://www.beateatingdisorders.org.uk/), and social media (e.g., X (formerly Twitter), Bastrop, TX, USA and Instagram, Menlo Park, CA, USA). These advertisements made clear the study's eligibility criteria, as well as the aim of the study to "explore the effects of rising living costs, food insecurity and poverty on eating disorder symptoms and treatment".

https://doi.org/10.3390/nu18050852

There were 451 total responses to the survey. Prior to analysis, the data were cleaned to remove responses rated as a high probability of being fraudulent by Qualtrics, as well as responses from ineligible participants or those who stopped the survey prior to answering any FI questions (Figure 1). After data cleaning, there were 337 respondents (92.6% female) between the ages of 16 and 67 who provided some analysable data. Within this sample, 263 had previous diagnoses of at least one ED, while 70 indicated that they experience(d) disordered eating behaviours, and 4 preferred to not report if they had received a diagnosis. As participants may have been diagnosed with multiple EDs over the course of their life, they were able to select all applicable diagnoses they had received.

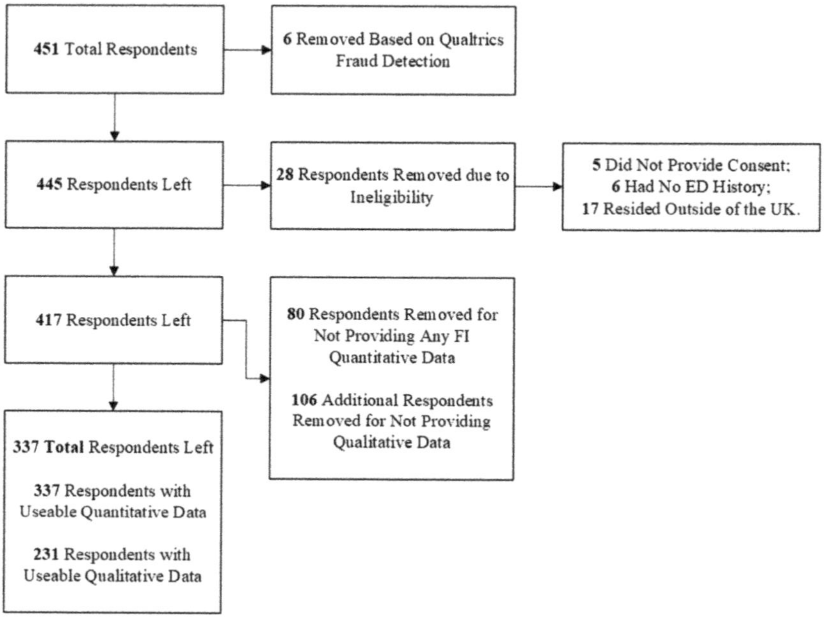

Figure 1. Flowchart of participants.

Participants self-selected to complete the survey after seeing the study advertisement online and clicking on a link to a Qualtrics survey (https://www.qualtrics.co.uk, Provo, UT, USA). At this point, they were also provided with the information sheet. After reviewing this, participants provided their consent and then filled out a brief screening question to check eligibility where, if eligible, they then went on to answer the survey questions. Data were retained from participants who provided partial responses to the survey. Lastly, previous research demonstrates that there are significant barriers to seeking help for an ED, with access to treatment for PwEDs being concerningly low [50,51]. As such, responses from all participants were included in the analyses, regardless of diagnostic status, to decrease the chances of replicating these biases.

2.2. Materials and Measures

2.2.1. Survey

Survey questions covered demographics, ED history, food insecurity experiences, other cost-of-living issues, food insecurity and EDs, ED symptoms, and additional thoughts or comments. Supplementary Materials File S1 contains the entire survey. For the sake of brevity, the full questions and responses are not replicated in this section. Definitions of FI at the beginning of the survey came from a 2019 report by the UK government's Environ-

https://doi.org/10.3390/nu18050852

mental Audit Committee [1]. Most of the survey questions were developed specifically by the authors based on their previous survey with ED clinicians [47]; questions adapted from established sources are listed below.

2.2.2. Food Insecurity Questions

Experiences of mild to severe food insecurity were measured using questions adapted from The Food Foundation's (a UK-based charity) Food Insecurity Tracking surveys [52] which are based on the US Department of Agriculture's Adult Food Security Survey [53]. Participants were asked to dichotomously select which of the following aspects of food insecurity they had experienced in the past month: "Been worried about accessing or affording enough nutritious food", "Had less nutritious or balanced meals because you couldn't afford or get access to food", "Had smaller meals than usual or skipped meals because you couldn't afford or get access to food", "Ever been hungry but not eaten because you couldn't afford or get access to food", "Not eaten for a whole day because you couldn't afford or get access to food", or "None of the above". Other FI questions exploring the relationship between FI and ED and recovery were created for the purposes of the survey. Respondents only answered these questions if they indicated an experience with FI.

2.2.3. Cost-of-Living Experiences

Participants were also asked about their wider cost-of-living experiences [47]. Participants rated the day-to-day impact of several cost-of-living experiences on a scale of 0–100 (0 being no impact). Cost-of-living experiences included (a) rising energy costs, (b) affordability of clothes, (c) rising transport costs, (d) reliance on zero/low hour contracts, (e) the ability to do other, non-food-related activities important for recovery/well-being, and (f) taking time off work to focus on recovery. Participants were also asked an open-ended question to assess the general impact of the cost-of-living crisis on their daily lives.

2.2.4. Eating Disorder Diagnostic Scale

The Eating Disorder Diagnostic Scale (EDDS) for the DSM-5 was included at the end of the survey [54,55]. Composite scores of ED symptoms were used to generate probable diagnoses for participants (i.e., AN, BN, BED, or other specified feeding or eating disorder (OSFED)) [55]. Atypical AN was subsumed under AN, while OSFED included purging disorder and night eating syndrome. A global score of ED symptoms was also derived using a previously established methodology to combine the raw scores of all relevant items [55,56]. Of the 337 total respondents, only 203 provided responses to all of the EDDS items, and thus the probable diagnosis was only computed for these participants. For 134 participants, the probable diagnosis was not computed due to missing responses to some/all EDDS items.

2.3. Statistical Analysis

2.3.1. Quantitative Analysis

Data were imported and analysed in SPSS Version 29.0.2.0 (IBM, Armonk, NY, USA). Descriptive statistics were computed for key variables and then participants were split into two groups: those with and without recent experiences of FI. Participants were placed in the former group if they self-reported at least one experience of FI in the past month, while the latter group was comprised of participants who self-reported no experience of the FI items. A liberal criterion was used here to encapsulate the most general experience of FI as possible due to the exploratory nature of the research. Analyses at different thresholds (e.g., reporting 3 or more FI items to be in the recent FI group) were not conducted. Inferential statistics (*t*-tests) were used to investigate whether recent experiences of FI were related to differences in confidence discussing FI in a clinical setting, the impact of cost-of-living

https://doi.org/10.3390/nu18050852

experiences, ED symptoms, and probable ED diagnosis. Non-parametric tests, like the Mann–Whitney U test, were used where assumptions for parametric tests were violated. A point-biserial correlation was also conducted to assess the strength of the relationship between FI experiences and ED symptoms. Due to the exploratory nature of the research, a priori power analyses were not conducted. Instead, post hoc power analyses and Cohen's d effect size were calculated in G*Power Version 3.1.9.7 (https://www.psychologie.hhu.de/arbeitsgruppen/allgemeine-psychologie-und-arbeitspsychologie/gpower; accessed on 22 August 2025, Heinrich Heine University Düsseldorf, Düsseldorf, Germany) using its manual. For Mann–Whitney U tests, the effect size r was calculated using the following formula:

$$r = \frac{Z}{\sqrt{N}}$$

where Z is the standardized difference between the two groups and N is total sample size. Partial responses were retained from participants and included in the analyses to maximise the power for each variable. Probable diagnosis was analysed dichotomously (No vs. Any diagnosis) using a chi-square test and categorically at five levels (No Current ED Diagnosis, Anorexia Nervosa, Bulimia Nervosa, Binge Eating Disorder, OSFED) using a Fisher–Freeman–Holton Exact test. Odds Ratios and Cramer's V were computed for the tests, respectively.

2.3.2. Qualitative Analysis

The qualitative data obtained from the online survey were analysed using Braun and Clarke's phases for inductive thematic analysis [57]. Two authors (Bİ, JW) independently coded 100% of the responses and the first author (CB) coded 50% from each question. Researchers (Bİ, JW, CB) then met to search the data for themes, refining them in an iterative process until all themes and subthemes expressed unique aspects of the data. Phase 3 saw the initial generation of 8 themes, which were later reduced to 6 in phases 4 and 5. The researchers then selected appropriate quotes to illustrate each theme/subtheme and created a thematic map to illustrate themes and subthemes.

3. Results

3.1. Quantitative Results

In the current sample, just over two-fifths (41.8%) of the participants reported experiencing at least one indicator of FI in the past month, with 46 participants (13.7%) endorsing three or more FI items, a marker of low food security. Only 11% of participants reported being asked about FI in healthcare appointments and just 7.7% ever sought help for their FI. Tables 1 and 2 summarise the sample demographics and descriptives, respectively.

Table 1. Participant demographics and clinical characteristics.

Demographic Variable	Total Sample (n = 337)
Age	16–67 years (Mean = 27.78)
Gender	312 Female; 9 Male; 14 Non-binary/third gender; 2 self-described [1]
Country of Residence	288 England; 37 Scotland; 11 Wales; 1 Northern Ireland
Employment Status [2]	187 In Full-/Part-time Employment; 117 In Education; 29 Unemployed; 13 Temporarily Unemployed; 6 Prefer Not to Say; 6 Parent/Informal Carer; 1 Retired
Ethnicity [3]	312 White; 12 Mixed or Multiple Ethnic Groups; 8 Asian; 3 Black; 2 Prefer Not to Say

https://doi.org/10.3390/nu18050852

Table 1. *Cont.*

Demographic Variable	Total Sample (n = 337)
Household Size [4]	1–17 [5] people (Mean = 2.91)
Number of Dependents	0–4 (Mean = 0.44)
Parents/Carers	11.28%
Receive Social Assistance	28.19%
Co-occurring Mental Health Diagnoses	244 Yes; 91 No; 2 Prefer Not to Say
Currently Experiencing ED Symptoms	282 Yes; 48 No; 7 Prefer Not to Say
Currently or Previously in ED Treatment	224 Yes; 39 No
Frequency of ED Diagnoses [6]	210 AN; 40 BN; 11 BED; 23 ARFID; 22 Other [7]

[1] Self-described as trans masc and neuroqueer; [2] Categories not discrete. "In Education" is inclusive of both school and university; [3] The full ethnic categories used in the survey are as follows: (1) Asian (e.g., Indian/Pakistani/Bangladeshi/Chinese/Asian British), (2) Black/African/Caribbean or Black British, (3) Mixed or multiple ethnic groups and (4) White (e.g., English/Welsh/Scottish/any other White background). Participants were given the option to specify their ethnicity if not included in this list; [4] Household size including participant; [5] Household size of 17 was reported by participant studying at university. This value may thus represent a university dorm; [6] Diagnoses are not discrete. 38 participants had multiple diagnoses. ARFID = Avoidant/Restrictive Food Intake Disorder; [7] Responses to "Other" include Eating Disorder Not Otherwise Specified (EDNOS), Other Specified Feeding or Eating Disorder (OSFED), and orthorexia nervosa.

Table 2. Descriptive statistics for dependent variables.

Dependent Variable	Mean (SD)
Food Insecurity Experience (n = 337) [1]	
Worry about Affording/Accessing Food	118 (35.01%)
Eaten Less Nutritious/Balanced Meals	67 (19.88%)
Had Smaller Meals/Skipped Meals	65 (19.29%)
Been Hungry but Not Eaten	35 (10.39%)
Not Eaten for an Entire Day	12 (3.56%)
Eating Disorder Symptoms (EDDS) [2]	
Fear of Weight Gain (n = 269)	5.14 (1.56)
Weight/Shape Concern (n = 269)	5.20 (1.38)
Frequency of Objective Binge Episodes (n = 269)	2.74 (4.22)
Frequency of Self-Induced Vomiting (n = 264)	2.02 (4.20)
Frequency of Laxative/Diuretic use (n = 265)	1.83 (4.15)
Frequency of Fasting (n = 265)	5.75 (5.76)
Frequency of Excessive Exercise (n = 264)	5.42 (5.66)
Global ED Symptoms (n = 205) [3]	40.42 (19.40)
Cost-of-Living Experiences	
Rising Energy Costs (n = 280)	54.62 (30.26)
Affordability of Clothing (n = 286)	52.05 (32.52)
Rising Transport Costs (n = 284)	49.06 (32.08)
Reliance on Zero/Low Hour Contracts (n = 248)	20.14 (32.13)
Partake in Activities for Recovery (n = 289)	63.01 (29.85)
Time Off Work for Recovery (n = 277)	58.17 (38.21)

[1] Participants were able to select all options that applied. Values outside of the parentheses for this variable are the frequency of each response; [2] The first 7 variables of the EDDS are from singular items on the scale (questions 2, 3, 6, 13, 14, 15, 16 respectively). The n for each item is variable because some participants chose to end the survey early; [3] There are two extra participants with Global ED symptom scores when compared to the Probable Diagnosis variable. This is because these participants did not provide information about their weight and/or their height, which is not used when computing the Global score.

https://doi.org/10.3390/nu18050852

For ED symptoms and probable ED diagnosis, those with recent FI experiences reported engaging in significantly higher rates of fasting to maintain weight and shape, and excessive exercise. No differences emerged between the groups for any other ED symptoms, nor probable diagnosis (see Tables 3 and 4). Effect sizes were small, and only the finding for fasting had sufficient power. Further correlational analysis revealed no significant relationship between FI experiences and global ED symptoms ($r_{pb} = -0.099$, $p = 0.158$).

Table 3. Inferential statistics for ED symptoms by recent FI experiences.

	Recent FI				No Recent FI				Inferential Statistics			
	n	Mean (SD)	Median	Mean Rank	n	Mean (SD)	Median	Mean Rank	U	p	r	Power ($1-\beta$)
Eating Disorder Symptoms (EDDS)												
Fear of Weight Gain (n = 269)	125	5.11 (1.56)	6.00	131.87	144	5.16 (1.57)	6.00	137.72	8609	0.468	0.044	0.058
Weight/Shape Concern (n = 269)	125	5.30 (1.29)	6.00	139.00	144	5.10 (1.44)	6.00	131.52 [1]	8499.5	0.359	0.056	0.236
Frequency of Objective Binge Episodes (n = 269)	126	2.51 (3.95)	0.00	133.58	143	2.94 (4.45)	0.00	136.26	8829.5	0.748	0.020	0.140
Frequency of SIV (n = 264)	123	1.87 (4.05)	0.00	131.40	141	2.16 (4.35)	0.00	133.46	8536.5	0.790	0.016	0.089
Frequency of L/D use (n = 265)	124	1.84 (4.10)	0.00	136.13	141	1.82 (4.20)	0.00	130.24	8353.5	0.413	0.050	0.050
Frequency of Fasting (n = 265) *	124	6.67 (5.77)	6.00	145.38	141	4.95 (5.65)	2.00	122.12 [1]	7202.5	0.011	0.156	0.836
Frequency of ExE (n = 264) *	123	6.17 (5.78)	5.00	143.28	141	4.77 (5.48)	2.00	123.10 [1]	7346	0.027	0.136	0.681
Global ED Symptoms (n = 205)	95	42.11 (18.71)	-	-	110	38.73 (19.95)	-	-	1.154 [2]	0.250	0.162 [3]	0.534

SIV = self-induced vomiting, L/D = laxative or diuretic, ExE = excessive exercise. Please see the Supplementary Materials for full details of scale ranges. * Significant at p = 0.05; [1] Variables did not have similarly shaped distributions between both groups, and so, the mean rank should be used to interpret findings; [2] Variable met assumptions for parametric tests. Value represents results from t-test with degrees of freedom = 203; [3] Value represents Cohen's d for test.

Table 4. Inferential statistics for probable ED diagnosis by recent FI experiences.

	Recent FI		No Recent FI		Inferential Statistics
Probable ED Diagnosis (EDDS)	n	%	n	%	
Dichotomous (n = 205)					χ^2 (1) = 1.584, p = 0.208, OR = 0.620 (0.293, 1.311)
Any ED Diagnosis	82	86.32	86	79.63	
No Current Diagnosis	13	13.68	22	20.37	
Within ED Diagnosis (n = 168)					Fisher's exact = 4.548, p = 0.211, Cramer's V = 0.170
Anorexia Nervosa	59	71.95	58	67.44	
Bulimia Nervosa	19	23.17	17	19.77	
Binge Eating Disorder	0	0	4	4.65	
OSFED	4	4.88	7	8.14	

On average, participants espoused neither comfort nor discomfort with the notion of discussing FI with a healthcare professional during an appointment (M = 52.53, SD = 32.38, Range = 0–100). However, those with recent experiences of FI were significantly more likely to report discomfort discussing FI in this setting than those without recent FI experiences (see Table 4). Cost-of-living experiences, on average, were perceived to have a moderate impact on participants' day-to-day lives for all experiences, bar the reliance of zero-hour

https://doi.org/10.3390/nu18050852

or low-hour contracts, which was relatively unimpactful on participants (see Figure 2 for illustration). Significantly higher day-to-day impact was reported by participants with recent FI experiences on cost-of-living domains related to increases in the cost and affordability of energy, clothing, and transport, as well as the ability of participants to partake in non-food-related activities important for recovery, relative to participants without such experiences (Table 5). Small to moderate effect sizes were observed. All non-significant effects lacked adequate power.

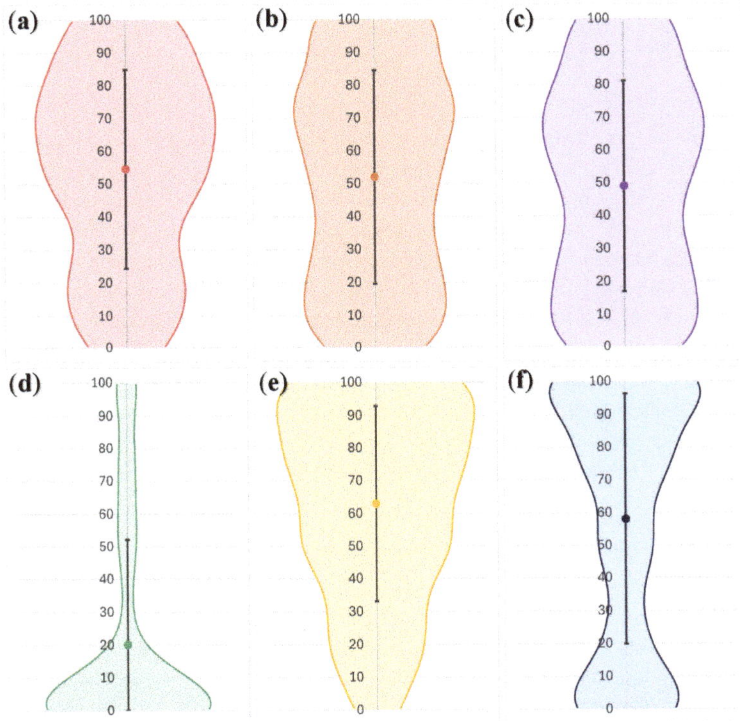

Figure 2. Participant ratings of the impact of several cost-of-living experiences on their day-to-day lives (0 = no impact, 100 = a great deal of impact). (**a**) Rising energy costs; (**b**) affordability of clothes; (**c**) rising transport costs; (**d**) reliance on zero-hour/low-hour contracts; (**e**) ability to do other, non-food-related things important for recovery/well-being; (**f**) taking time off work to focus on health and well-being/recovery.

Table 5. Inferential statistics for comfort discussing FI and cost-of-living experiences by recent FI experiences.

	Recent FI				No Recent FI				Inferential Statistics			
	n	Mean (SD)	Median	Mean Rank	*n*	Mean (SD)	Median	Mean Rank	*U*	*p*	*r*	Power (1 − β)
Comfort Discussing FI (*n* = 325) **	138	44.41 (31.61)	47.00	139.44	187	58.54 (31.69)	61.00	180.39 [1]	9651.5	<0.001	0.216	0.997
Cost-of-Living Experiences												
(a) Rising Energy Costs (*n* = 280) **	133	66.00 (29.54)	71.00	172.55	147	44.33 (29.26)	50.00	111.50 [1]	5512.5	<0.001	0.377	>0.999
(b) Affordability of Clothing (*n* = 286) **	130	59.89 (32.15)	66.50	163.83	156	45.51 (31.57)	46.00	126.56 [1]	7497	<0.001	0.225	0.995
(c) Rising Transport Costs (*n* = 284) **	130	55.92 (31.63)	59.00	160.21	154	43.27 (31.51)	46.50	127.55 [1]	7708	<0.001	0.198	0.981

https://doi.org/10.3390/nu18050852

Table 5. *Cont.*

	Recent FI				No Recent FI				Inferential Statistics			
	n	Mean (SD)	Median	Mean Rank	n	Mean (SD)	Median	Mean Rank	U	p	r	Power $(1-\beta)$
(d) Reliance on Zero/Low Hour Contracts (n = 248)	117	24.88 (36.24)	4.00	133.04	131	15.90 (27.55)	2.00	116.87 [1]	6664.5	0.068	0.116	0.631
(e) Partake in Activities for Recovery (n = 289) **	133	75.83 (25.31)	82.00	181.68	156	52.08 (29.22)	50.00	113.73 [1]	5495.5	<0.001	0.406	>0.999
(f) Time Off Work for Recovery (n = 277)	126	62.37 (38.75)	79.00	148.51	151	54.66 (37.66)	56.00	131.06	8314.5	0.069	0.109	0.525

** Significant at p <.001; [1] variables did not have similarly shaped distributions between both groups, and so the mean rank should be used to interpret findings.

3.2. *Qualitative Results*

Six themes emerged from the qualitative analysis: (1) FI sustains symptoms and hinders recovery; (2) FI impacts quality of life; (3) facilitators of help-seeking; (4) barriers to help-seeking; (5) community-level suggestions for guidance; and (6) systemic-level suggestions (Figure 3). Shame was a recurring topic that was common in responses to most questions and was related to each theme to a certain degree. Here, the following acronyms will be used for brevity: PD = previously diagnosed, ND = not previously diagnosed, UD = unknown diagnosis. Demographics are provided alongside illustrative quotes to describe the participant each quote comes from. Lastly, 231 participants provided useable responses to at least one of the qualitative questions included in the analysis. However, the number of responses to each question was variable, with some participants skipping over or providing responses that did not answer the question (e.g., if asked "How did X...", they answered "No".). Appendix A, Table A1 shows the total number of useable responses for each question.

3.2.1. Theme: FI Sustains Symptoms and Hinders Recovery

There were three subthemes under this theme: Relationship to Food and Eating, Access to/Engagement with Treatment, and, Relapse and Stability of Recovery.

Some participants described how childhood experiences of FI contributed to their ED development, while others reported that their ED preceded any experiences of FI. For example, P421 (29, F, White, PD) expressed that they felt "*like this [FI] contributed to, at times, an unhealthy attitude to food and having to finish eating even when I was full as a child. It warped the way I viewed food and eating and probably had an effect when I started to develop an eating disorder.*" Difficulties spending money on food was also described, particularly as participants felt undeserving of food: "*When I do spend money on food, it makes me feel really anxious. I'm constantly worrying about whether I 'deserve' to buy food.*" (P30, 18, F, Asian, PD). Eating behaviours, such as restricting food intake, binge eating, and hoarding food, were also described by participants as being impacted by FI. P156 (22, NB, White, PD), for instance, revealed that "*It [FI] has become an excuse for me not to eat, and to buy less food... it gives me a double sense of pride when I don't eat; I successfully fasted which means I neither gained weight, nor spent money*". P421 also described how the financial strain of binge eating episodes contributed to feelings of stress and in turn future binges: "*Bulimia is an expensive illness, when I've just been paid and can afford to I often spend a lot more on food, especially during binge episodes and it leaves me without the ability to buy nutritious foods later. The anxiety then leaves me more likely to binge again in future... so it's much harder to break the cycle.*"

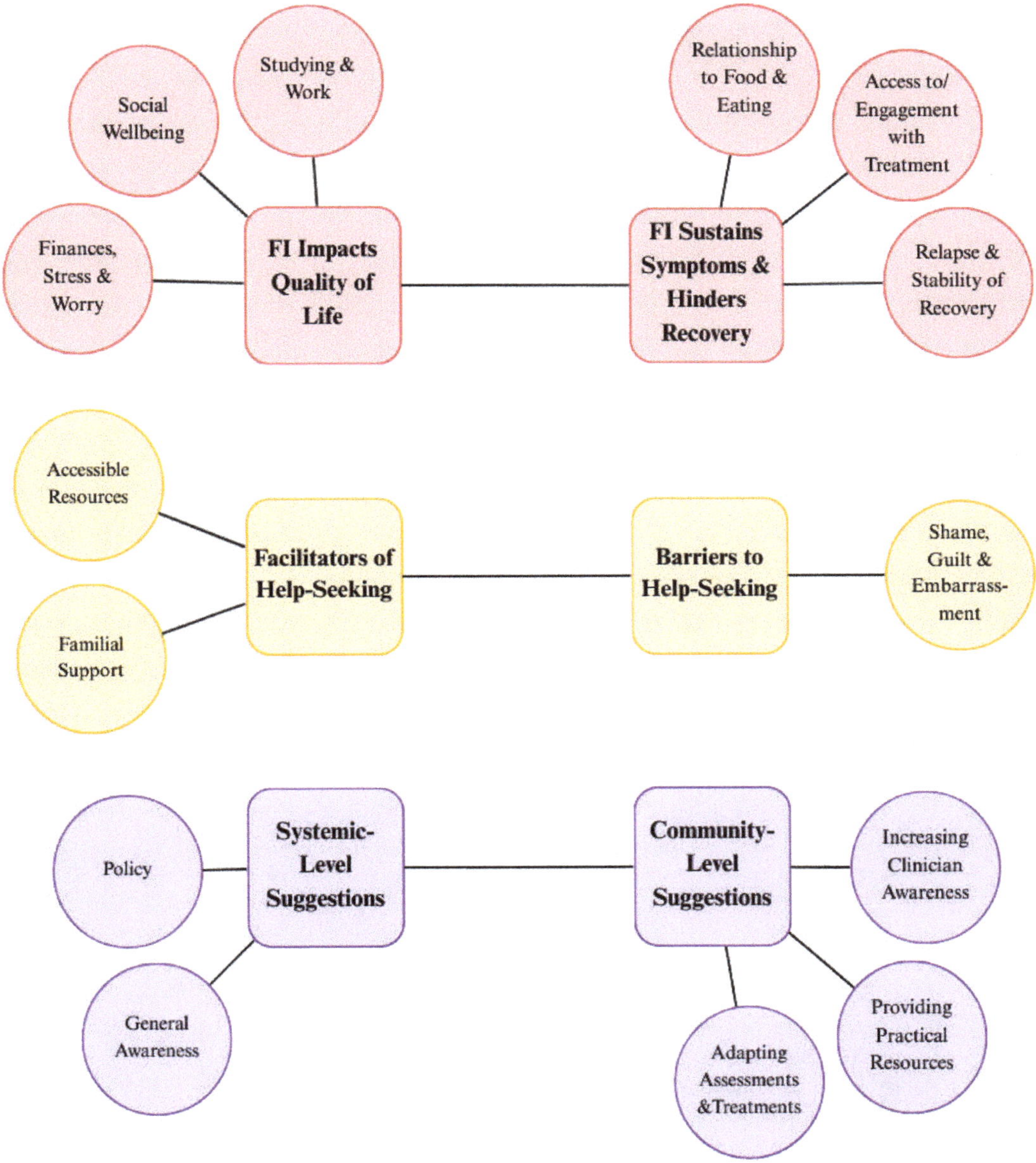

Figure 3. Thematic map. Themes are represented by squares, and the subthemes under them are represented by connected circles. Colours relate to the research question listed at the end of the introduction which are addressed by each theme. Circles in red relate to question 1 (interaction between FI and EDs), circles in yellow relate to question 2 (experiences of help-seeking), and circles in purple relate to question 3 (suggestions for guidance).

Participants also noted that FI and the cost of living had a negative impact on their ability to access treatments. Generally, undertaking recovery was noted to be a "*significant time commitment*" which "*financially… can be challenging.*" (P150, 34, M, White, PD). Physical challenges of accessing treatment were also described by P258 (16, F, White, PD) who stated "*Petrol costs make it incredibly difficult for travelling to my inpatient unit (170 miles away).*"

https://doi.org/10.3390/nu18050852

Once in treatment, participants perceived that FI could still be a barrier to engaging with treatment protocols. Specifically, P169 (22, F, Mixed, PD) reported ambivalence towards engaging in meal plans due to their financial cost: *"I know that I need to spend more money on food so that I am able to follow my meal plan, but I can't really afford to nor do I want to because it feels like a waste of money to spend what little I have on food"*. The inability to comply with these treatment demands was also attributed to a stagnation in recovery: *"It's [FI] stalling my treatment because I'm always so tired, cold and nauseous (through either hunger or eating food not really fit for consumption) and I can't justify buying things that, for example, my dietitian wants me to introduce."* (P174, 45, F, White, PD).

Lastly, for some participants, FI was perceived as increasing their risk of relapse. For example, P59 (40, F, White, PD) explained how *"Although I see myself as having recovered from my eating disorder* (i.e., *I rarely purge these days), the cost of food brings food back to the front of my mind or it's constantly there despite working hard for years to reduce my obsession with it."*. For others, the increase in food prices triggered the re-emergence of restrictive eating patterns, as P55 (26, F, Mixed, ND) noted, *"I feel the stress around affording enough nutritious food has highlighted my stress around eating cheap 'unhealthy' food and this has given me an excuse to start restricting my intake again"*. This increased risk of relapse was even present when participants had been in recovery for longer periods of time: *"[The] current cost-of-living crisis has caused me to relapse after 3 years in recovery as it's more economical to eat less, which in turn has triggered my guilt around food."* (P127, 26, NB, White, PD).

3.2.2. Theme: FI Impacts Quality of Life

Three subthemes emerged from this theme: Studying and Work, Social Well-being, and Finances, Stress, and Worry.

Experiences of FI had a wider impact on other aspects of participants' lives. Studying and working life were often cited as being negatively impacted by FI: *"Previously I have had to skip meals due to lack of money and would instead have a nap at meal times instead of [eating] food. I was at university at the time and struggling to get by on my student loan and rising cost-of-living. This definitely affected my ability to concentrate and focus on my work."* (P424, 23, F, White, ND). Disruption to participants' education/occupation was particularly difficult where it required physical exertion or concentration: *"[I'm] less able to do my job well as it is active and has some risk so needs high alertness and energy levels for long periods of time."* (P28, 30, F, Mixed, PD). Struggles with FI were also described as more acute when participants ability to work was disrupted by their ED, as P176 (43, F, White, PD) revealed, *"[I] need to eat more food in recovery and can't afford this because I am off sick from work"*.

Participants also perceived their social well-being as worsened by experiences of FI. For some, FI compounded anxiety around social eating. P269 (26, F, White, PD), for instance, stated, *"It [FI] has also limited my social interaction with people as I avoid social events where food is involved due to the costs, as well as the anxiety surrounding socialising and eating itself"*. Some participants also described a trade-off between affording food and socialising, such as P127 (26, NB, White, PD), who *"Started buying less food in order to still be able to enjoy life and have fun experiences* (i.e., *travelling to see friends, going to social events, keeping up hobbies)"*. Experiences of isolation were also perceived to be detrimental to participants' recovery efforts, as illustrated by P250's (29, F, White, PD) response, *"I use it [the cost-of-living crisis] as an excuse not to do certain things like go out for meals as it increases my anxiety- I worry about money so don't do things that will help challenge my eating disorder. As a result I do less and isolate myself more"*. Likewise, struggles with recovery compounded difficulties with socialising: *"It [FI] has slowed down my progress, I can feel really poorly some days and by not improving or trying new food, it means my relationship and friendships are impacted as it is not easy to socialise if any form of meal is involved"* (P238, 27, F, White, PD).

https://doi.org/10.3390/nu18050852

Lastly, experiences of FI contributed to feelings of stress and worry in participants' everyday lives. For example, participants experienced stress from increasing food prices, *"I am stressed, anxious, and depressed by the thought of eating nutritious meals as the shock of prices going up every time I go the shops is too much."* (P111, 40, F, Asian, ND). Participants also described other stressors related to FI, such as having to choose between accessing food over other household necessities *"I had to choose whether to pay my rent or eat and unfortunately often times rent would come before health"* (P374, 24, F, White, PD) or the need to prioritise food access for children in a household *"I will do anything for my kids even if that means starving myself"* (P216, 27, F, White, PD). Additionally, participants described increased stress as particularly detrimental to their ED. For P105 (24, F, White, ND), engaging in restrictive eating behaviours was used to manage the stress from both FI and their ED: *"it just makes me feel like spending more on food gives me stress and gaining weight makes me stressed so it's easier to control both by eating less"*.

3.2.3. Theme: Facilitators of Help-Seeking

Two subthemes were identified for this theme: Accessible Resources and Familial Support.

Positive experiences of help-seeking usually occurred where participants were provided with accessible resources. For P358 (20, F, White, PD), access to free food at school and validation from their GP was key to their help-seeking experience: *"My GP is amazing and made me feel less embarrassed. I got free food at school which was good. It was discreet and also packaged so I could take it home for my sister/mum and brother"*. Access to free, discrete food at work was also described by P79 (26, NB, White, ND) who said, *"at my induction with a major supermarket. I wasn't able to afford a meal deal for lunch as I had unplanned expenses, but their staff canteen had free pot noodles/pasta mug shots and other breakfast and lunch-type foods for staff to utilise in times of food insecurity"*.

Participants reported informal help-seeking via family members, for example, P355 (28, F, White, PD) stated, *"I asked my mum to help me financially to afford to get myself a variety of 'safe' snacks and meals"*. However, having to ask for help could also cause shame or guilt. P439 (47, F, White, ND), for instance, described guilt about burdening family, *"I've had to ask my mum for money at the end of lots of months for food for the last few days before payday. I feel ashamed and embarrassed. My mum helps me willingly but I'm a grown up and shouldn't be putting her in this position."* (P439, 47, F, White, ND). For others, like P26 (26, F, White, ND), shared experiences of struggling with FI and the cost-of-living crisis reduced shame and facilitated help-seeking, *"I wasn't scared of stigma or telling anyone, as I felt all of my friends and colleagues were going through the same and no one could really afford to heat their entire house/flat"*.

3.2.4. Theme: Barriers to Help-Seeking

Shame, Guilt and Embarrassment was the only subtheme to surface from this theme.

Feelings of guilt, shame, and embarrassment were widely noted barriers to help-seeking. P358 (20, F, White, PD), who described positive experiences with accessing food in school, also mentioned other attempts to ask directly for food left them feeling *"weak"* and *"disgusting"*. Another participant, P176 (43, F, White, PD), detailed how embarrassment around FI prevented them from seeking help from their treatment team: *"I wanted to ask my Eating Disorder team for a referral to a food bank but I was too embarrassed to do so. Also my eating disorder told me this was greedy"*. Resource use was also accompanied by marked guilt and shame, as said by P20 (22, F, White, PD): *"I am care experienced, I spoke to my leaving care workers, who were able to give me an emergency voucher for my local supermarket. I felt guilty for asking for help and felt guilty spending the voucher on food that I liked"*. Participants also worried about depriving others of resources, *"[I received an] Emergency food bank referral. Feel guilty for using it when other people need it"* (P28, 30, F, Mixed, PD), and were concerned about not fitting the intended service demographic, *"when I go to the foodbank, I feel a sense of shame because I think to myself "what the fuck am I doing here? I usually have money to eat! the foodbank is only for people who are dirt poor and I'm on maximum disability benefit!!""*.

3.2.5. Theme: Community-Level Suggestions for Guidance

There were three subthemes that surfaced under this theme: Adapting Assessments and Treatments, Providing Practical Solutions, and Increasing Clinician Awareness.

A majority of participants' suggestions for clinical guidance were related to creating adaptations to assessment and treatments. In terms of assessments, participants felt that discussions about FI should be standard for all patients, as illustrated by P382's (20, F, White, PD) response: *"There should be a discussion with each patient at start of the treatment to see if this is an issue or not"*. They additionally wanted clinicians to take initiative when starting these discussions: *"Clinicians could be given some prompt questions to approach the subject with kindness and to make the patient feel less anxious or shameful"* (P267, 39, F, White, PD). Preferences for assessment format varied among participants. P267 preferred questionnaires, *"perhaps a discreet questionnaire could be developed to be filled in"*, while other participants found these to be impersonal: "not via *a questionnaire that's then given to the GP as this can feel a bit impersonal and intrusive*" (P29, 16, F, White, PD). While many participants endorsed the idea of clinicians starting a conversation about FI, others disagreed: *"Prefer not to [discuss FI] as it's embarrassing"* (P93, 40, F, White, PD).

For treatment, participants noted that meal plans were sometimes untenable on a budget, and so they wanted clinicians to be able to provide plans that were more suited to participants' financial situations. For example, P26 (26, F, White, PD) suggested the clinicians could provide *"weekly varied meal plans with stretched budgets (so I can go food shopping once a week or so and thus have a better overview of my expenses)"*, as well as *"ideas for smaller, simple in-between meals to avoid going a day without eating"*. This sentiment was echoed by P50 (26, F, White, PD) who also recommended that guidance include information on *"low cost, nutritious recipe ideas for recovery e.g., using tinned foods, advice on how to mix up food brands—this is really hard in recovery and makes you rigid but some foods that are comfortable are more expensive now"*.

Outside of accommodations to assessment and treatment, participants wanted healthcare professionals to provide practical, useable advice for resources to receive food. For example, participants disliked the notion of clinicians offering them nothing but commiserations: *"[It's] helpful if they have something they offer. So not just say that it must be hard,* etc., *but actually provide practical solutions* (e.g., *food bank locations)."* (P52, 29, F, White, ND). Generic advice was also something participants wanted clinicians to avoid, as P19 (27, F, White, ND) shared, *"I would probably avoid recommending low cost foods* e.g., *pasta, rice, pulses* etc. *as this is information parroted back to people whenever issues of poverty/CoL [cost-of-living] crisis are raised and it can feel a bit condescending (like of course I'm trying to shop with a budget and aware of cheaper 'staple' items)"*. This generic advice was also sometimes described as being detrimental to ED symptoms: *"sometimes cooking from scratch, batch cooking and buying things in bulk are all not possible or advisable due … exacerbating eating disorder symptoms such as bingeing."* (P99, 40, F, White, PD). Additionally, participants wanted healthcare professionals to provide this information or for it to be freely available in clinical settings, rather than simply receiving encouragement to look for this information themselves, as P108 (31, F, White, PD) detailed, *"Real resources and the meaningful information to receive them—telling someone to google the resources in their area isn't actually helpful. Making this information, when possible, visibly accessible—much like signs to remind people to get their flu shots, encourage people to speak to their doctors if they are struggling with food insecurity or the cost-of-living because these are valid health questions/concerns"*.

https://doi.org/10.3390/nu18050852

Lastly, participants wanted healthcare professionals to be more knowledgeable and aware about FI and to work towards destigmatisation. P241 (17, F, White, PD), for instance, stated that "*…if this concept [financial struggles] was more respected and talked about, people may not feel as ashamed when admitting that they are having money problems*". Participants identified the need to raise awareness of how different diagnostic and social characteristics intersect with experiences of FI and recovery, such as those experiencing binge behaviours or ARFID. P197 (21, NB, Black, PD), for instance, suggested that "*clinicians should be aware of how food insecurity can affect several types of eating disorders, so not just restrictive but also binge eating*" (P197, 21, NB, Black, PD). Single parent households were also identified as being particularly vulnerable: "*Make the effort to understand that my recovery in a single parent, working class family is not the same as the recovery of somebody who lives in a middle-class family.*" (P30, 18, F, Asian, PD). Participants also identified the need for improved awareness for healthcare professionals, especially GPs, in understanding FI from lived experience perspectives: "*A guide on how to approach the subject [FI] and how to get across the seriousness of our concerns. I think GPs especially don't have much training in eating disorders so don't understand the underpinnings of the illness.*" (P221, 28, F, White, PD). Empathy and compassion from healthcare professionals was also consistently cited by participants: "*Clinician's [need] to be emphatic, maybe attend some training on how to approach the topic with someone with an ED*" (P70, 28, F, White, PD).

3.2.6. Theme: Systemic-Level Suggestions for Guidance

Two subthemes emerged under this theme: Policy and General Awareness.

Firstly, participants acknowledged that FI was a systemic issue that would require changes to policy to resolve. For example, it was suggested by P424 (23, F, White, ND) that guidance "*shouldn't only focus on the public and clinicians… it should… make them [the government] aware of the negative consequences of the rise in cost-of-living on food prices, people's lives and their health. Focusing just on clinicians and [the] public isn't going to tackle the heart of the problem*". P156 (22, NB, White, ND) linked "*the CoL crisis, food insecurity, and ED*" to systemic issues and "*real structures (government, capitalism, misogyny,* etc.*)*", noting they felt that "*any approach that forgets this is doomed to fail. Part of the way to address food insecurity is to ensure it is eliminated*". Involvement from clinicians in policy work was also suggested: "*I think mental health staff need to be more involved in policy solutions*" (P52, 29, F, White, ND).

Participants also wanted FI to be normalised by raising general awareness. For example, P272 (19, F, White, PD) stated they wanted "*Online platforms and more about the topic on the news to spread awareness and make people feel more comfortable around the topic rather than it being so secretive*". Other participants wanted to challenge stereotypes about FI, for instance, P368 (38, F, White, PF) responded, "*Food insecurity also needs to be seen as a problem faced by everyone, I have BED therefore my body shape is not 'typical' of someone with an eating disorder or someone facing food insecurity. I find both topics difficult to approach because of my size and the fear of being judged, this is also why I don't use food banks* etc." Table 6 summarises all participant suggestions.

https://doi.org/10.3390/nu18050852

Table 6. Participants' suggestions for community- and systemic-level guidance.

Level	Guidance Area	Explanation and Examples
Community		
	ED Assessment	FI should be screened for routinely at the ED assessment stage. Clinicians should initiate discussions about FI, rather than waiting for patients to elect to reveal this information, regardless of the patient's ethnicity, gender, diagnosis, disability status, or body size. FI should be assessed via questionnaires and/or discussions with patients. Care should be taken when broaching this subject, however, as many patients are likely to experience embarrassment about FI.
	ED Treatment	Once a clinician has identified that their patient experiences FI, adaptations to their treatment plans should be made. These may include providing budgeted meal plans, ideas for nutritious snacks, etc. Clinicians should be cognizant that many people experiencing FI are likely to be struggling financially in other areas, and that this may also impact their ability to implement treatment plans. Additionally, ED patients often experience difficulties with spending money and feelings of deservingness around food which are exacerbated by FI. Thus, these areas may be important targets for treatments.
	Practical Resources	Clinicians should not merely offer their commiserations; steps should be taken to provide practical resources to patients to help alleviate their FI. This may include information about how to access local foodbanks, voucher schemes, local charities, etc. Clinicians should avoid generic advice (i.e., batch cooking, buying in bulk, etc.) or just encouraging patients to look for this information themselves. This information can be made more widely available by placing it in common areas, like waiting rooms.
	Clinician Knowledge	Healthcare professionals (both primary and specialized) should receive training on FI. This should include, for example, how to identify FI, information on the ways that FI and different EDs may interact, and how FI may interfere with treatments, impede recovery, or facilitate relapse. Training should include perspectives of FI from those with lived experience of EDs.
	Reducing Stigma	FI can be more normalised in clinical settings by having posters around the hospital/practice which encourage patients to discuss their experiences of FI with their clinician. Placing psychoeducation materials about FI in common areas, such as waiting rooms, may also help. Empathy is necessary when discussing FI with patients as shame is a significant barrier to help-seeking.

https://doi.org/10.3390/nu18050852

Table 6. *Cont.*

Level	Guidance Area	Explanation and Examples
Systemic		
	General Awareness	Public awareness of FI should be raised. Awareness campaigns should focus on helping people to identify indicators of FI, the impact of FI on physical and mental health, and it should encourage people to seek help if they are experiencing FI. They should also seek to tackle stereotypes about who can experience FI, such as those with higher body weight. It may be helpful to look to other successful awareness campaigns in the UK, such as those for safe driving or smoking, and to work with established charities and organisations (e.g., the Trussell Trust or Food Foundation) to effectively design campaigns.
	Policy	The systemic nature of FI should be at the forefront of public discussions. FI is unlikely to be solved just through clinical intervention efforts, and solutions to FI will require policy changes. Awareness campaigns should also focus on illustrating the harm of FI and the cost-of-living crisis to government bodies, and they should acknowledge the interaction between FI and other forms of marginalisation (e.g., ethnicity, gender, etc.). Advocacy from clinicians may be a necessary adjunct to lived experience perspectives.

4. Discussion

This study examined the perspectives of PwEDs on the role of FI in the development, maintenance, and relapse of their illness, their experiences seeking help in clinical contexts, and their suggestions for clinical guidance. Quantitative analyses revealed that recent FI experiences in the current sample were related to self-reports of more frequent excessive exercise and fasting ED behaviours, less comfort discussing FI with a clinician, and being more adversely affected by multiple cost-of-living challenges, relative to participants without FI. Qualitative analysis illustrated that FI and the cost-of-living crisis were consistently reported to exacerbate restrictive and binge eating symptoms, and worsen quality of life. Those who experienced childhood FI believed it was linked to the onset of their ED. Recovery for participants with recent FI was also reportedly more difficult, with FI leading to a relapse of the ED in others. Help-seeking for FI was low in this sample, with shame, guilt, and embarrassment emerging as major barriers. Participants reported seeking help most frequently from family members; however, feelings of guilt and shame persisted in these cases. Participants also provided suggestions for clinical guidance which focused on community- and systemic-level changes.

In the current sample, 41.8% of participants reported experiencing at least one form of FI in the past month. This figure is elevated when compared to the national average (which ranges from 10 to 20% depending on the source [12,58,59]), as well as estimates from ED clinicians in the UK [47]. While this figure may be inflated by self-selection bias due to the wording of the study advertisement [60], previous research demonstrates that FI is two or even three times more prevalent in people with at least one mental health diagnosis or disability than those without [10,61]. Additionally, the specificity of the study advertisement has enabled the collection of a rich qualitative dataset in the current survey. Although untested in this sample, experiences of FI are likely to be acute in PwEDs from other vulnerable populations too (e.g., people from minoritized ethnic groups). These communities are known to also experience FI at higher rates [10], and are

https://doi.org/10.3390/nu18050852

typically underserved in ED research and practice [62]. However, little is known about how co-occurring minority status may impact the relationship between FI and EDs. Future epidemiological studies (e.g., [63]) are necessary to characterize the extent of FI in ED populations and to understand how troubling health inequalities may be worse in certain groups. Moreover, indicators of FI in the current study came from a single-item question based on the US Department of Agriculture Food Security Survey [53]. FI experiences in people with EDs may be better characterized in future by using multiple items from psychometrically tested surveys. Inclusion of some measure of past FI experiences may also provide a better understanding of the chronology of FI indicators and ED course.

Cost-of-living concerns were rated as having a moderate to high impact on participants' lives. This was especially true for participants with recent FI experiences. Nascent reports on this crisis suggest that, for instance, the inability to heat homes negatively impacts respiratory health in young children and the elderly [64], and financial uncertainty and stress related to increasing prices compromises mental well-being [16]. These outcomes are projected to worsen unless policy approaches are taken to mitigate the harm of the rising cost of living [65]. For PwEDs, the inability to afford heating their home is likely to be most detrimental to those with a low weight (e.g., those with AN or ARFID) who are particularly sensitive to feeling the cold [66]. Similar to what participants described in the sample, a 'heat or eat' dilemma—wherein individuals must choose between heating their homes or purchasing a sufficient amount of food—has been observed more widely as a consequence of the rising cost of living [67]. Vulnerable groups, such as single parents, also seem to bear the brunt of this, additionally feeling that they need to sacrifice their own food intake to ensure their children have nutritious diets [68]. Based on the descriptions from participants in the current sample, the added stress from the cost-of-living crisis is likely to worsen the symptoms of EDs.

Consistent with a social determinants framework [69], FI was described by participants as contributing to the development and maintenance of their ED. Participants who felt that FI contributed to their ED routinely reported that childhood experiences of FI created stressful scenarios around food which, in line with a life-course approach [70], later added to a poorer relationship with food. Participants also described a vicious cycle between FI, ED symptoms, and work and finances: (1) initial FI exacerbated ED symptoms, (2) the increased frequency and severity of ED symptoms hindered ones' ability to work, and (3) being out of work decreased personal finances which led to more FI, wherein the cycle started again. In this sample, FI impacted the frequency of restrictive behaviours (such as excessive exercise or fasting due to weight/shape concerns), and qualitative descriptions from participants also suggested that FI worsened binge behaviours. These findings are partially inconsistent with previous research which found that FI was most often related to reports of binge episodes, and a greater likelihood that participants would meet the diagnostic criteria for EDs like BN and BED [34–36]. The relationship between FI and binging is largely predicated on the concept of the "feast/famine" cycle where intermittent access to food is expected to lead to binging during times of food abundance [37]. Differences in the current study findings may be related to the sample being mostly comprised of participants with experiences of AN. A floor effect may have been observed for binge/purge symptoms (i.e., objective binge episodes, self-induced vomiting, etc.) as the median scores for these variables were zero for both groups (Table 3). Interpretability of these findings is also limited as the current study did not include any control participants. Future research with more balanced diagnostic groups and controls might therefore find differences in these binging and purging symptoms. Additionally, the current results suggest, at the very least, that the link between restrictive symptoms and FI (which has thus far been underexplored in the research literature [37]) is also worth further investigation, and that a cogent mechanistic model is needed.

Help-seeking for FI was very low in the current sample, at only 7.7%. Accessible resources and familial support aided help-seeking; however, participants still routinely cited feelings of shame, guilt, and embarrassment when receiving help. Shame was the largest barrier for participants to seek help for FI. These findings are consistent with previous literature which shows that FI users of food banks in the UK report large amounts of social stigma related to this use [71]. Additionally, individuals experiencing FI are known to encounter feelings of shame related to their financial situation and difficulties accessing food [72]. The relationship between shame, stigma and lack of help-seeking are also well understood. Negative attitudes towards seeking professional help for mental health concerns are higher in those that feel ashamed about having a mental health condition [73]. Furthermore, experiences of shame and self-stigma have been consistently associated with reduced help-seeking for EDs, especially BED [74]. There is likely to be an interaction between shame and stigma derived from FI and poverty, and of that seen in EDs, which should be explored further.

Alongside low rates of help-seeking, participants reported rarely discussing FI with healthcare professionals (11%). This aligns with accounts from ED clinicians in the UK. Despite clinicians noticing a marked rise in FI among patients, they felt they lacked sufficient knowledge of how to intervene [47]. In the current study, suggestions for clinical guidelines included: (a) for FI to be asked about routinely at the assessment stage and for clinicians to initiate this (either via questionnaires or conversations); (b) for accommodations to treatment plans for patients experiencing FI; (c) for shame and embarrassment to be combatted by having healthcare professionals be empathetic and knowledgeable about FI and its interaction with ED symptoms; and d) to be provided with practical advice to alleviate their FI (i.e., local foodbank referrals, food voucher schemes, etc.). Our earlier clinician survey study also found that many ED healthcare practitioners were positive about many of these suggestions, including routine screening and psychoeducation about the interaction between FI and EDs. Additionally, previous attempts to alleviate FI by implementing money advice alongside psychological interventions in the NHS have been shown to be feasible and acceptable [75]. Plans to co-produce interventions for FI also exist in other populations, such as in pregnancy [76]. PwEDs may benefit from a similar attempt to co-produce an FI intervention that includes advice on managing finances, with other necessary resources. Ultimately, there is a dire need for directions for clinicians as participants reported that FI not only exacerbated symptoms, but that it also jeopardized their recovery. Specifically, FI impeded recovery efforts in some participants, while for others it precipitated a relapse of ED cognitions and behaviours. To raise awareness of the issues in clinicians, health care commissioners, policy makers, and other relevant stakeholders and to start addressing participants' concerns, we have made a short animated film about FI and eating disorders (https://www.youtube.com/watch?v=lMhUHh4XpX8; accessed on 22 August 2025). We are also currently developing resources to aid ED clinicians in addressing FI in their practice, which we plan to disseminate nationally.

Participants also acknowledged that FI was a systemic problem that would require policy change to solve. A recent research briefing by the UK government acknowledged that the rise in the cost of living is affecting rates of FI and food bank use [58], while another report illustrates that household FI has increased since 2020, especially in low-income households and people with disabilities [77]. As discussed previously, current FI in the UK is likely related to austerity measures established and maintained by the UK government [15]. There have also been repeated calls for the government to implement critical policy changes to alleviate FI, with one article describing FI as a "public health issue left to fester" [14]. First steps towards policy solutions are being made. For example, the UK government is trialling the provision of free breakfasts before school in up to 750 schools, which may alleviate the burden of FI in some families. However, wider policy changes are still needed.

Strengths and Limitations

The current survey has elucidated that FI plays a role in the development, maintenance, and relapse risk of EDs and is the first of its kind in the UK. The use of an online survey has enabled rich data to be collected across the UK and for a wide array of perspectives to be considered. However, this mode of data collection is not without its challenges. For example, the current study was reliant on participants' self-report of previous and current ED diagnoses and symptoms, which could not be clinically validated due to the anonymous nature of the survey. Tools like the EDDS were implemented into the survey to provide information about probable diagnosis; however, as participants could end the survey early, this was not available for everyone. This limitation is likely to be present in future online survey studies of this nature, too. The cross-sectional design of the survey also limits the ability to draw any causal conclusions from the current research. Although the research literature suggests the relationship between FI and psychiatric conditions is likely bidirectional [27], longitudinal studies are necessary to properly parcellate these effects for PwEDs.

Additionally, participants in the current sample were largely white and female. As such, the generalisability of the current findings to minoritized ethnic and other PwEDs is questionable. As highlighted above, future research will need to delve into how minority status may impact the relationship between FI and EDs. Moreover, as efforts continue to make ED services more accessible to people from underserved communities, researchers will also need to consider the impact of this interaction on ED assessment and treatment. Lastly, as research develops in this field, it should consider weighting findings by the cost of living across UK regions. Inequities are usually concentrated in certain localities, so accounting for regional living costs may provide more nuanced information about which ED services are most likely to encounter referrals with co-occurring FI.

5. Conclusions

FI is a significant, yet understudied health issue for ED development and prognosis. Experiences of FI are quantitively and qualitatively associated with the maintenance of ED symptoms, and are antithetical to the stability of patients' recovery. Stress induced by FI and the cost of living is likely to cause PwEDs to engage in ED behaviours, slow recovery efforts, and lead some people to relapse. Despite the magnitude of FI and its consequences, many PwEDs do not feel comfortable discussing struggles with accessing food with healthcare professionals, nor is screening of this issue routinely included in clinical practice. Further work is needed to train ED clinicians and other healthcare professionals on identifying FI, adapting protocols for treatment, and providing necessary resources to patients. Additionally, stigma at both the clinical and cultural levels needs to be addressed to allow PwEDs to more confidently discuss FI experiences and seek support when needed. However, the problem of FI will not be solved by clinicians alone, as it is related more widely to systemic issues like poverty, austerity, and the cost of living. As such, policy change is critical to effectively resolve the issue of FI.

Supplementary Materials: The following supporting information can be downloaded at: https://www.mdpi.com/article/10.3390/nu18050852/s1, File S1: Survey of Food Insecurity and Eating Disorders.

https://doi.org/10.3390/nu18050852

Author Contributions: Conceptualization, C.B., B.İ., A.H., C.K., D.D., M.P., H.S. and U.S.; methodology, B.İ., A.H., C.K., M.P., H.S. and U.S.; formal analysis, C.B., J.W. and B.İ.; investigation and resources, C.B., J.W., B.İ., A.H., C.K., D.D., H.S. and U.S.; data curation, C.B.; writing—original draft preparation, C.B.; writing—review and editing, C.B., B.İ., J.W., A.H., C.K., H.S. and U.S.; visualization, C.B.; supervision, H.S. and U.S.; funding acquisition, H.S. and U.S. All authors have read and agreed to the published version of the manuscript.

Funding: This work is supported by the Medical Research Council/Arts and Humanities Research Council/Economic and Social Research Council Adolescence, Mental Health and the Developing Mind initiative as part of the EDIFY programme (grant number MR/W002418/1). This paper represents independent research funded by the National Institute of Health and Care Research (NIHR) Maudsley Biomedical Research Centre (BRC) at South London and Maudsley NHS Foundation Trust (SlaM) and King's College London (KCL). The views expressed are those of the authors and not necessarily those of the NIHR or the Department of Health and Social Care.

Institutional Review Board Statement: The study was conducted in accordance with the Declaration of Helsinki, and approved by the King's College London Research Ethics Committee (Review Reference: HR-22/23-34804, 28 April 2023).

Informed Consent Statement: Informed consent was obtained from all subjects involved in the study.

Data Availability Statement: The data presented in this study are available on request from the corresponding author due to ethical restrictions.

Acknowledgments: We would like to thank everyone who partook in the survey and provided their insights.

Conflicts of Interest: The authors declare no conflicts of interest. The funders had no role in the design of the study; in the collection, analyses, or interpretation of data; in the writing of the manuscript; or in the decision to publish the results.

Abbreviations

The following abbreviations are used in this manuscript and are presented in order of use:

FI	Food insecurity
UK	United Kingdom (of Great Britain and Northern Ireland)
US(A)	United States (of America)
PwEDs	People with current or past eating disorders
COVID-19	Coronavirus Disease 2019
UN	United Nations
EDs	Eating disorders
BED	Binge eating disorder
BN	Bulimia nervosa
AN	Anorexia nervosa
NHS	National Health Service
n	Number of participants
ARFID	Avoidant/Restrictive Food Intake Disorder
EDNOS	Eating Disorder Not Otherwise Specified
OSFED	Other Specified Feeding and Eating Disorder
EDDS	Eating Disorder Diagnostic Scale
SPSS	Statistical Package for the Social Sciences
SD	Standard deviation
SIV	Self-induced vomiting
L/D	Laxatives/diuretics
ExE	Excessive exercise
PD	Previously diagnosed
ND	Not previously diagnosed

https://doi.org/10.3390/nu18050852

UD	Unknown diagnosis
F	Female
NB	Non-binary
M	Male
GP	General practitioner
CoL	Cost of living
N/A	Not applicable

Appendix A

The number of responses to each question was variable. Table A1 shows the total number of useable responses to each question.

Table A1. Total number of responses to each qualitative question.

Question [1]	Useable [2]	No/Unsure [3]	Unusable [4]
Question 20 (n = 128)	128	-	-
Question 21 (n = 125)	90	33	2
Question 22 (n = 118)	102	-	16
Question 26 (n = 24)	11	-	13
Question 28 (n = 152)	137	9	6
Question 29 (n = 169)	145	20	4
Question 30 (n = 169)	139	26	4
Question 31 (n = 81)	55	14	12

[1] Shortened versions of the questions can be found below. For full questions, see Supplementary Materials, File S1. Question 20: How has your experience of FI impacted your daily life (e.g., practically/emotionally)? Question 21: Are there any ways FI has contributed to the development of your ED symptoms? Question 22: How has FI impacted your ED and ED treatment (if applicable)? Question 26: Please describe your experience [of help-seeking for FI] (e.g., who and where, what help received). Question 28: Is there anything you would like to share about how the CoL crisis has impacted you (e.g., your daily life, mood, mental state, etc.)? Question 29: Do you have any thoughts on what such [clinical] guidance should include? Question 30: When thinking about discussing FI or the CoL with a healthcare professional, is the anything that would help you to do so? Question 31: Thinking about FI and your ED treatment, is there anything your therapist could do to help your recovery journey? [2] Number of responses that were useable in the analysis. [3] Number of responses, where appropriate to answering the question, where participants responded something to the effect of "No", "Not sure", "I don't know" without elaborating. [4] Number of responses where it was either blank (e.g., responding "N/A" or "x") or where they responded with unusable data.

References

1. Sustainable Development Goals in the UK Follow Up: Hunger, Malnutrition and Food Insecurity in the UK. Available online: https://publications.parliament.uk/pa/cm201719/cmselect/cmenvaud/1491/149101.htm (accessed on 30 July 2025).
2. Definitions of Food Insecurity. Available online: https://www.ers.usda.gov/topics/food-nutrition-assistance/food-security-in-the-us/definitions-of-food-security (accessed on 17 August 2025).
3. COVID-19: Potential Impact on the World's Poorest People. Available online: https://www.wfp.org/publications/covid-19-potential-impact-worlds-poorest-people (accessed on 20 June 2025).
4. Vasconcelos-Neto, C.F.A.; Jacob, M.; Tregidgo, D.; Valle, D.; El Bizri, H.R.; Gomes, S.M.; Fa, J.E.; Morcatty, T.Q.; Monteiro, F.O.B.; Scofield, A.; et al. COVID-19 Pandemic Exacerbated Food Insecurity in South American Countries. *Food Secur.* **2025**, *17*, 1001–1022. [CrossRef]
5. Dasgupta, S.; Robinson, E.J.Z. Food Insecurity, Safety Nets, and Coping Strategies during the COVID-19 Pandemic: Multi-Country Evidence from Sub-Saharan Africa. *Int. J. Environ. Res. Public Health* **2021**, *18*, 9997. [CrossRef]
6. Kent, K.; Murray, S.; Penrose, B.; Auckland, S.; Visentin, D.; Godrich, S.; Lester, E. Prevalence and Socio-Demographic Predictors of Food Insecurity in Australia during the COVID-19 Pandemic. *Nutrients* **2020**, *12*, 2682. [CrossRef]
7. Niles, M.T.; Beavers, A.W.; Clay, L.A.; Dougan, M.M.; Pignotti, G.A.; Rogus, S.; Savoie-Roskos, M.R.; Schattman, R.E.; Zack, R.M.; Acciai, F.; et al. A Multi-Site Analysis of the Prevalence of Food Insecurity in the United States, before and during the COVID-19 Pandemic. *Curr. Dev. Nutr.* **2021**, *5*, nzab135. [CrossRef] [PubMed]
8. Louie, S.; Shi, Y.; Allman-Farinelli, M. The Effects of the COVID-19 Pandemic on Food Security in Australia: A Scoping Review. *Nutr. Diet.* **2022**, *79*, 28–47. [CrossRef] [PubMed]
9. Moseley, W.G.; Battersby, J. The Vulnerability and Resilience of African Food Systems, Food Security, and Nutrition in the Context of the COVID-19 Pandemic. *Afr. Stud. Rev.* **2020**, *63*, 449–461. [CrossRef]

https://doi.org/10.3390/nu18050852

10. Food Insecurity Tracking Round 15. Available online: https://foodfoundation.org.uk/initiatives/food-insecurity-tracking#tabs/Round-15 (accessed on 8 July 2025).
11. Food Insecurity Tracking Round 1. Available online: https://foodfoundation.org.uk/initiatives/food-insecurity-tracking#tabs/Round-1 (accessed on 8 July 2025).
12. Food Insecurity Tracking Round 16. Available online: https://foodfoundation.org.uk/initiatives/food-insecurity-tracking#tabs/Round-16 (accessed on 8 July 2025).
13. The State of Food Security and Nutrition in the World. Available online: https://openknowledge.fao.org/server/api/core/bitstreams/f5019ab4-0f6a-47e8-85b9-15473c012d6a/content (accessed on 30 July 2025).
14. The Lancet Gastroenterology & Hepatology. Food Insecurity in the UK: A Public Health Issue Left to Fester. *Lancet Gastroenterol. Hepatol.* **2022**, *7*, 585. [CrossRef]
15. Jenkins, R.H.; Aliabadi, S.; Vamos, E.P.; Taylor-Robinson, D.; Wickham, S.; Millett, C.; Laverty, A.A. The Relationship between Austerity and Food Insecurity in the UK: A Systematic Review. *EClinicalMedicine* **2021**, *33*, 100781. [CrossRef]
16. Jackson, S.E.; Cox, S.; Holmes, J.; Angus, C.; Robson, D.; Brose, L.; Brown, J. Paying the Price: Financial Hardship and Its Association with Psychological Distress among Different Population Groups in the Midst of Great Britain's Cost-of-Living Crisis. *Soc. Sci. Med.* **2025**, *364*, 117561. [CrossRef]
17. Moradi, S.; Arghavani, H.; Issah, A.; Mohammadi, H.; Mirzaei, K. Food Insecurity and Anaemia Risk: A Systematic Review and Meta-Analysis. *Public Health Nutr.* **2018**, *21*, 3067–3079. [CrossRef]
18. Seligman, H.K.; Jacobs, E.A.; Lopez, A.; Tschann, J.; Fernandez, A. Food Insecurity and Glycemic Control among Low-Income Patients with Type 2 Diabetes. *Diabetes Care* **2012**, *35*, 233–238. [CrossRef]
19. Ayasrah, A.I.I.; Shnaigat, S.F.; Obeidat, H.M.; Al-Najjar, K. Demographic, Health, and Socioeconomic Determinants of Food Insecurity and Its Association with Osteoporosis. *J. Tianjin Univ. Sci. Technol.* **2025**, *58*, 333–347.
20. Leung, C.W.; Kullgren, J.T.; Malani, P.N.; Singer, D.C.; Kirch, M.; Solway, E.; Wolfson, J.A. Food Insecurity Is Associated with Multiple Chronic Conditions and Physical Health Status among Older US Adults. *Prev. Med. Rep.* **2020**, *20*, 101211. [CrossRef] [PubMed]
21. Tamargo, J.A.; Strath, L.J.; Karanth, S.D.; Spector, A.L.; Sibille, K.T.; Anton, S.; Cruz-Almeida, Y. Food Insecurity Is Associated with Chronic Pain and High-Impact Chronic Pain in the USA. *Public Health Nutr.* **2024**, *27*, e7. [CrossRef]
22. Darling, K.E.; Fahrenkamp, A.J.; Wilson, S.M.; D'aUria, A.L.; Sato, A.F. Physical and Mental Health Outcomes Associated with Prior Food Insecurity among Young Adults. *J. Health Psychol.* **2017**, *22*, 572–581. [CrossRef]
23. Brian, T.; Cohen, M.J.; Meerman, J. World Food Insecurity and Malnutrition: Scope, Trends, Causes and Consequences. In *The Impact of Climate Change and Bioenergy on Nutrition*; Thompson, B., Cohen, M.J., Eds.; Springer: Dordrecht, The Netherlands, 2012; pp. 21–42. [CrossRef]
24. Dominick, S.R.; Widmar, N.J.O.; Ruple, A.; Weir, J.Z.G.; Acharya, L. The Intersection of Food Insecure Populations in the Midwest U.S. and Rates of Chronic Health Conditions. *Agric. Food Secur.* **2018**, *7*, 43. [CrossRef]
25. Poulos, N.S.; Pitman, S.A.; Velazquez, C.E.; Pasch, K.E. Food Insecurity Is Associated with Poor Mental Health Outcomes among a Diverse Sample of Young Adults. *Public Health Nutr.* **2025**, *28*, e108. [CrossRef]
26. Oh, H.; Smith, L.; Jacob, L.; Du, J.; Shin, J.I.; Zhou, S.; Koyanagi, A. Food Insecurity and Mental Health among Young Adult College Students in the United States. *J. Affect. Disord.* **2022**, *303*, 359–363. [CrossRef] [PubMed]
27. Abeldt, B. The Relationship between Food Insecurity and Mental Health. *Am. J. Psychiatry Resid. J.* **2024**, *20*, 15–17. [CrossRef]
28. American Psychiatric Association (Ed.) Feeding and Eating Disorders. In *Diagnostic and Statistical Manual of Mental Disorders*, 5th ed.; Text Revision (Dsm-5-Tr); American Psychiatric Publishing: Washington, DC, USA, 2022; pp. 372–399. [CrossRef]
29. Attia, E.; Guarda, A.S. Prevention and Early Identification of Eating Disorders. *JAMA* **2022**, *327*, 1029–1031. [CrossRef]
30. Bryant, E.; Spielman, K.; Le, A.; Marks, P.; National Eating Disorder Research Consortium; Touyz, S.; Maguire, S. Screening, Assessment and Diagnosis in the Eating Disorders: Findings from a Rapid Review. *J. Eat. Disord.* **2022**, *10*, 78. [CrossRef]
31. Treasure, J.; Duarte, T.A.; Schmidt, U. Eating Disorders. *Lancet Psychiatry* **2020**, *395*, 889–911. [CrossRef]
32. Royer, M.F.; Ojinnaka, C.O.; Bruening, M. Food Insecurity Is Related to Disordered Eating Behaviors among College Students. *J. Nutr. Educ. Behav.* **2021**, *53*, 951–956. [CrossRef]
33. Christensen, K.A.; Forbush, K.T.; Richson, B.N.; Thomeczek, M.L.; Perko, V.L.; Bjorlie, K.; Christian, K.; Ayres, J.; Wildes, J.E.; Chana, S.M. Food Insecurity Associated with Elevated Eating Disorder Symptoms, Impairment, and Eating Disorder Diagnoses in an American University Student Sample before and during the Beginning of the COVID-19 Pandemic. *Int. J. Eat. Disord.* **2021**, *54*, 1213–1223. [CrossRef]
34. Bruening, M.; MacLehose, R.; Loth, K.; Story, M.; Neumark-Sztainer, D. Feeding a Family in a Recession: Food Insecurity among Minnesota Parents. *Am. J. Public Health* **2012**, *102*, 520–526. [CrossRef]
35. Barry, M.R.; Sonneville, K.R.; Leung, C.W. Students with Food Insecurity Are More Likely to Screen Positive for an Eating Disorder at a Large, Public University in the Midwest. *J. Acad. Nutr. Diet.* **2021**, *121*, 1115–1124. [CrossRef]

36. Hazzard, V.M.; Barry, M.R.; Leung, C.W.; Sonneville, K.R.; Wonderlich, S.A.; Crosby, R.D. Food Insecurity and Its Associations with Bulimic-Spectrum Eating Disorders, Mood Disorders, and Anxiety Disorders in a Nationally Representative Sample of U.S. Adults. *Soc. Psychiatry Psychiatr. Epidemiol.* **2022**, *57*, 1483–1490. [CrossRef]
37. Hazzard, V.M.; Loth, K.A.; Hooper, L.; Becker, C.B. Food Insecurity and Eating Disorders: A Review of Emerging Evidence. *Curr. Psychiatry Rep.* **2020**, *22*, 74. [CrossRef] [PubMed]
38. Kosmas, J.A.; Wildes, J.E.; Graham, A.K.; O'connor, S.M. The Role of Stress in the Association among Food Insecurity, Eating Disorder Pathology, and Binge Eating-Related Appetitive Traits. *Eat. Behav.* **2023**, *49*, 101709. [CrossRef] [PubMed]
39. Campbell, I.C.; Mill, J.; Uher, R.; Schmidt, U. Eating Disorders, Gene–Environment Interactions and Epigenetics. *Neurosci. Biobehav. Rev.* **2011**, *35*, 784–793. [CrossRef]
40. Dinour, L.M.; Bergen, D.; Yeh, M.-C. The Food Insecurity–Obesity Paradox: A Review of the Literature and the Role Food Stamps May Play. *J. Am. Diet. Assoc.* **2007**, *107*, 1952–1961. [CrossRef] [PubMed]
41. Hazzard, V.M.; Loth, K.A.; Crosby, R.D.; Wonderlich, S.A.; Engel, S.G.; Larson, N.; Neumark-Sztainer, D. Relative Food Abundance Predicts Greater Binge-Eating Symptoms in Subsequent Hours among Young Adults Experiencing Food Insecurity: Support for the "Feast-or-Famine" Cycle Hypothesis from an Ecological Momentary Assessment Study. *Appetite* **2023**, *180*, 106316. [CrossRef]
42. Almeida, L.; Savoy, S.; Boxer, P. The Role of Weight Stigmatization in Cumulative Risk for Binge Eating. *J. Clin. Psychol.* **2011**, *67*, 278–292. [CrossRef]
43. Vizin, G.; Horváth, Z.; Vankó, T.; Urbán, R. Body-Related Shame or Guilt? Dominant Factors in Maladaptive Eating Behaviors among Hungarian and Norwegian University Students. *Heliyon* **2022**, *8*, e08817. [CrossRef]
44. Aceves-Martins, M.; Cruickshank, M.; Fraser, C.; Brazzelli, M. Child Food Insecurity in the UK: A Rapid Review. *Public Health Res.* **2018**, *6*. [CrossRef]
45. Sampson, K.; Memory, K.; Fazel, M.; Moran, P.; Bould, H. Does an Association Exist between Food Insecurity and Eating Disorder Symptoms among Young People Living in England? *BJPsych Open* **2024**, *10*, S78. [CrossRef]
46. Efstate, A.; Hazzard, V.M.; Burke, N.L.; Sonneville, K.R.; Hammond, D. Food Security and Eating Disorder Behaviors in the International Food Policy Study, 2018 to 2022. *Int. J. Epidemiol.* **2025**, *54*, dyaf060. [CrossRef]
47. Kuehne, C.; Hemmings, A.; Phillips, M.; İnce, B.; Chounkaria, M.; Ferraro, C.; Pimblett, C.; Sharpe, H.; Schmidt, U. A UK-Wide Survey of Healthcare Professionals' Awareness, Knowledge and Skills of the Impact of Food Insecurity on Eating Disorder Treatment. *Eat. Behav.* **2023**, *49*, 101740. [CrossRef]
48. Frayn, M.; Trainor, C.; Lin, M.; Pitts, A.; Drexler, S.A.; Patarinski, A.G.G.; Juarascio, A. Patient Perceptions of the Relationship between Food Insecurity and Eating Disorder Treatment: A Qualitative Exploration. *Int. J. Eat. Disord.* **2022**, *55*, 332–342. [CrossRef]
49. Sauerwein, J.; Austin, A.; Singh, M.; Pedram, P.; Allan, E.; Bruett, L.; Eckhardt, S.; Forsberg, S.; Keery, H.; Kimber, M.; et al. "Fbt Is for the Rich": A Qualitative Study Examining Clinicians' Experiences and Perceptions of Treatment Access and Engagement for Diverse Families in Family-Based Treatment. *Int. J. Eat. Disord.* **2025**, *58*, 554–563. [CrossRef]
50. Ali, K.; Radunz, M.; McLean, S.A.; O'Shea, A.; Mavrangelos, T.; Fassnacht, D.B.; Hart, L. The Unmet Treatment Need for Eating Disorders: What Has Changed in More Than 10 Years? An Updated Systematic Review and Meta-Analysis. *Int. J. Eat. Disord.* **2025**, *58*, 46–65. [CrossRef]
51. Nicula, M.; Pellegrini, D.; Grennan, L.; Bhatnagar, N.; McVey, G.; Couturier, J. Help-Seeking Attitudes and Behaviours among Youth with Eating Disorders: A Scoping Review. *J. Eat. Disord.* **2022**, *10*, 21. [CrossRef]
52. Food Insecurity Tracking Round 12. Available online: https://foodfoundation.org.uk/initiatives/food-insecurity-tracking#tabs/Round-12 (accessed on 8 July 2025).
53. Food Security in the U.S.—Survey Tools. Available online: https://www.ers.usda.gov/topics/food-nutrition-assistance/food-security-in-the-us/survey-tools (accessed on 12 September 2025).
54. Bohon, C.; Stice, E. Eating Disorder Diagnostic Scale. In *Encyclopedia of Feeding and Eating Disorders*; Wade, T., Ed.; Springer: Singapore, 2015; pp. 1–4. [CrossRef]
55. Stice, E.; Telch, C.F.; Rizvi, S.L. Development and Validation of the Eating Disorder Diagnostic Scale: A Brief Self-Report Measure of Anorexia, Bulimia, and Binge-Eating Disorder. *Psychol. Assess.* **2000**, *12*, 123. [CrossRef]
56. Krabbenborg, M.A.M.; Danner, U.N.; Larsen, J.K.; van der Veer, N.; van Elburg, A.A.; de Ridder, D.T.D.; Evers, C.; Stice, E.; Engels, R.C.M.E. The Eating Disorder Diagnostic Scale: Psychometric Features within a Clinical Population and a Cut-Off Point to Differentiate Clinical Patients from Healthy Controls. *Eur. Eat. Disord. Rev.* **2012**, *20*, 315–320. [CrossRef]
57. Braun, V.; Clarke, V. Using Thematic Analysis in Psychology. *Qual. Res. Psychol.* **2006**, *3*, 77–101. [CrossRef]
58. Food Poverty: Households, Food Banks and Free School Meals. Available online: https://commonslibrary.parliament.uk/research-briefings/cbp-9209/ (accessed on 30 August 2025).
59. Stanley, A.K.; Hadi, Y.; Newbold, D.; Heuvelman, H.; Krige, A. Identifying Predictors for Food Insecurity in England: A Cross-Sectional Database Analysis. *J. Health Popul. Nutr.* **2025**, *44*, 53. [CrossRef] [PubMed]

https://doi.org/10.3390/nu18050852

60. Kaźmierczak, I.; Zajenkowska, A.; Rogoza, R.; Jonason, P.K.; Ścigała, D. Self-Selection Biases in Psychological Studies: Personality and Affective Disorders Are Prevalent among Participants. *PLoS ONE* **2023**, *18*, e0281046. [CrossRef] [PubMed]
61. Teasdale, S.B.; Müller-Stierlin, A.S.; Ruusunen, A.; Eaton, M.; Marx, W.; Firth, J. Prevalence of Food Insecurity in People with Major Depression, Bipolar Disorder, and Schizophrenia and Related Psychoses: A Systematic Review and Meta-Analysis. *Crit. Rev. Food Sci. Nutr.* **2023**, *63*, 4485–4502. [CrossRef]
62. Asaria, A. Improving Eating Disorder Care for Underserved Groups: A Lived Experience and Quality Improvement Perspective. *J. Eat. Disord.* **2025**, *13*, 11. [CrossRef]
63. Investigating Food Insecurity and Eating Disorder Symptoms Among Adults in the UK: An Analysis of Epidemiological Data. Available online: https://proposals.epi.bristol.ac.uk/?q=node/131250 (accessed on 30 August 2025).
64. Meadows, J.; Montano, M.; Alfar, A.J.K.; Başkan, Ö.Y.; De Brún, C.; Hill, J.; McClatchey, R.; Kallfa, N.; Fernandes, G.S. The Impact of the Cost-of-Living Crisis on Population Health in the UK: Rapid Evidence Review. *BMC Public Health* **2024**, *24*, 561. [CrossRef]
65. Broadbent, P.; Thomson, R.; Kopasker, D.; McCartney, G.; Meier, P.; Richiardi, M.; McKee, M.; Katikireddi, S.V. The Public Health Implications of the Cost-of-Living Crisis: Outlining Mechanisms and Modelling Consequences. *Lancet Reg. Health-Eur.* **2023**, *27*, 100585. [CrossRef] [PubMed]
66. Swenne, I.; Engström, I. Medical Assessment of Adolescent Girls with Eating Disorders: An Evaluation of Symptoms and Signs of Starvation. *Acta Paediatr.* **2005**, *94*, 1363–1371. [CrossRef]
67. Barrett, C.; Lee, A.R.; Abrams, E.M.; Mayell, S.J.; Hawcutt, D.B.; Sinha, I.P. Eat or Heat: Fuel Poverty and Childhood Respiratory Health. *Lancet Respir. Med.* **2022**, *10*, 229. [CrossRef]
68. Younis, S.; Eberhardt, J. Heat or Eat: Exploring the Impact of the Cost-of-Living Crisis on Single Parents' Mental Wellbeing in the United Kingdom. *J. Poverty* **2025**, *29*, 176–200. [CrossRef]
69. Marmot, M.; Allen, J.; Bell, R.; Bloomer, E.; Goldblatt, P. Who European Review of Social Determinants of Health and the Health Divide. *Lancet* **2012**, *380*, 1011–1029. [CrossRef]
70. Allen, J.; Balfour, R.; Bell, R.; Marmot, M. Social Determinants of Mental Health. *Int. Rev. Psychiatry* **2014**, *26*, 392–407. [CrossRef]
71. Purdam, K.; Garratt, E.A.; Esmail, A. Hungry? Food Insecurity, Social Stigma and Embarrassment in the UK. *Sociology* **2016**, *50*, 1072–1088. [CrossRef]
72. Leung, C.W.; Stewart, A.L.; Portela-Parra, E.T.; Adler, N.E.; Laraia, B.A.; Epel, E.S. Understanding the Psychological Distress of Food Insecurity: A Qualitative Study of Children's Experiences and Related Coping Strategies. *J. Acad. Nutr. Diet.* **2020**, *120*, 395–403. [CrossRef]
73. Rüsch, N.; Müller, M.; Ajdacic-Gross, V.; Rodgers, S.; Corrigan, P.; Rössler, W. Shame, Perceived Knowledge and Satisfaction Associated with Mental Health as Predictors of Attitude Patterns Towards Help-Seeking. *Epidemiol. Psychiatr. Sci.* **2014**, *23*, 177–187. [CrossRef]
74. Ali, K.; Farrer, L.; Fassnacht, D.B.; Gulliver, A.; Bauer, S.; Griffiths, K.M. Perceived Barriers and Facilitators Towards Help-Seeking for Eating Disorders: A Systematic Review. *Int. J. Eat. Disord.* **2017**, *50*, 9–21. [CrossRef]
75. Belcher, H.L.; Parri, L.; Kilcoyne, I.; Evans, J.; Lewin, C.D.C.; Lau, R.; Bond, N.; D'aRcy, C.; Hatch, M.; Wykes, T. Feasibility and Potential Effects of a Combined Money Advice and Psychological Therapy Intervention within National Health Service Talking Therapies Services. *BJPsych Open* **2025**, *11*, e120. [CrossRef] [PubMed]
76. Hurley, K.L.; Jolly, K.; Brown, H.; Scott, S.; Akhter, Z.; Dyer, E.; Nguyen, G.; Lake, A.A.; Möller-Christensen, C.; Flint, N.; et al. Food, Pregnancy & Me: Exploring Food Insecurity in Pregnancy in the Uk to Inform Future Public Health Intervention Needs–a Mixed-Methods Study Protocol. *PLoS ONE* **2025**, *20*, e0321638. [CrossRef]
77. Department for Environmental, Food & Rural Affairs. *United Kingdom Food Security Report 2024: Introduction*; Department for Environmental, Food & Rural Affairs: London, UK, 2024.

https://doi.org/10.3390/nu18050852

nutrients

MDPI

Article

Relationships Between Consumption of High-Saturated-Fat Foods, Sleep Duration, BMI, Depression, Age and Sex, and Emotional Eating in Peruvian Adolescents: A Cross-Sectional Study

Yaquelin E. Calizaya-Milla [1,*], Ingrid Puente De La Vega-Fernández [1], David Javier-Aliaga [1], Mery Rodríguez-Vásquez [1], Christian Casas-Gálvez [2], Ana Valle-Chafloque [2] and Jacksaint Saintila [2,*]

1 School of Human Nutrition, Faculty of Health Sciences, Universidad Peruana Unión, Lima 15472, Peru; puentedelavegafernandezingridc@gmail.com (I.P.D.L.V.-F.); davidjavieraliaga@gmail.com (D.J.-A.); meryrv@upeu.edu.pe (M.R.-V.)

2 Research Group for Nutrition and Healthy Behaviors, Universidad Señor de Sipán, Chiclayo 14000, Peru; cgalvezchristic@uss.edu.pe (C.C.-G.); vchafloqueanali@uss.edu.pe (A.V.-C.)

* Correspondence: yaquelincalizaya@upeu.edu.pe (Y.E.C.-M.); jacksaintsaintila@gmail.com (J.S.)

Abstract

Background: Emotional eating, defined as the tendency to eat in response to emotions, has been associated with various biopsychosocial factors. However, in the Peruvian context, there is limited evidence regarding the specific predictors of this eating behavior in adolescents. **Objective:** To examine the associations between saturated fat intake, sleep duration, body mass index (BMI), depressive symptoms, age and sex, and emotional eating in Peruvian adolescents. **Methods:** This was a predictive cross-sectional study based on non-probabilistic sampling. A total of 722 adolescents from four schools located in East Lima were included. A multiple linear regression model was employed to examine the relationships between age, sex, saturated fat intake (SFI), sleep duration, BMI, and depressive symptoms and emotional eating. **Results:** The model was statistically significant (adjusted $R^2 = 0.301$; $F = 45.276$; $p < 0.001$), explaining 30.1% of the variance in emotional eating based on the explanatory variables. Being female ($\beta = 0.208$; $p = 0.011$), aged 15 to 18 versus 12 to 14 years ($\beta = 0.083$; $p < 0.001$), having a high SFI ($\beta = 0.186$; $p < 0.001$), sleeping ≥ 7 h ($\beta = -0.126$; $p < 0.001$), and a higher BMI ($\beta = -0.082$; $p = 0.011$) were significantly associated with emotional eating. Depressive symptoms ($\beta = 0.365$; $p < 0.001$) emerged as the strongest predictor in the model. **Conclusions:** Emotional eating among Peruvian adolescents is associated with psychological, behavioral, and sociodemographic factors. Depressive symptoms showed the strongest association, while longer sleep duration was linked to lower emotional eating scores. These findings highlight the need for integrated interventions targeting mental health, sleep hygiene, and healthy dietary behaviors in adolescents.

Keywords: emotional eating; adolescents; depression; saturated fat; body mass index; sleep duration; Peru

1. Introduction

Adolescence is a critical period for the development of eating habits and health-related behaviors [1]. According to recent estimates, mental health problems and disordered eating patterns affect approximately 15% and 22% of adolescents worldwide, respectively, representing a growing public health concern [2,3]. In the Peruvian context, 29.6% of adolescents aged 12 to 17 are at risk of experiencing a mental or emotional health problem [4]. Only 11.3% of the Peruvian population aged 15 and older meets the fruit and vegetable intake recommended by the World Health Organization (WHO) [5]. Studies conducted among Peruvian adolescents report a prevalence of eating disorder symptoms ranging from 7.3% to 13.9%, particularly among females and those with low family meal frequency, poor family communication, or sociocultural pressures related to thinness and body image [6,7]. Recent studies indicate that 62.1% of individuals engage in emotional eating [8]. In terms of body mass index (BMI), it is estimated that 62.7% of individuals aged 15 and older are overweight [9]. This situation is exacerbated by factors such as food insecurity, lack of nutritional education, and limited access to mental health services. For example, in Peru, eight out of ten individuals do not receive mental health care despite needing it [10]. Therefore, there is a clear need to investigate the contributing factors behind these behaviors to design more effective preventive and educational interventions.

Excessive consumption of foods high in saturated fat, along with factors such as BMI, sleep quality and duration, and depressive symptoms, significantly influences the development of emotional eating. However, the literature exploring these interactions in Peruvian adolescents remains limited, despite the fact that this population faces socioeconomic and cultural conditions that may heighten their vulnerability to such maladaptive eating behaviors [4,11].

Among the many psychosocial constructs related to disordered eating, body image dissatisfaction and poor body appreciation have emerged as critical mediators between internalized social ideals and maladaptive eating behaviors [12]. These constructs, particularly relevant during adolescence, interact with emotional regulation capacities and perceived stress to shape responses such as emotional eating [13–15]. Gross's Emotion Regulation Model posits that negative emotions elicit psychological distress, prompting individuals to adopt coping strategies to mitigate it—such as emotional eating [16]. From this perspective, emotional eating functions as a maladaptive regulatory mechanism that, while offering temporary relief, ultimately reinforces the cycle of emotional discomfort and dysfunctional behaviors [1]. Previous studies support this model; for instance, research conducted among Chinese adolescents found that higher levels of emotional suppression—and, in females, lower levels of cognitive reappraisal—were associated with greater consumption of energy-dense foods, with emotional eating serving as a key mediating factor [17]. Shriver et al. [1] demonstrated that poor emotional regulation in childhood predicts higher levels of emotional eating during adolescence, particularly among normal-weight adolescents and those with a negative body image. Therefore, emotional eating is a multifactorial phenomenon shaped by both emotional regulation strategies and body weight, underscoring the importance of implementing comprehensive interventions from early stages of development.

The consumption of foods high in saturated fat is a key dietary pattern linked to adverse physical and mental health outcomes [18]. This type of food, commonly found in ultra-processed products such as fried foods, cold cuts, industrial baked goods, and fast food, is characterized by high energy density and low nutritional value [19]. Saturated fats not only contribute to the development of metabolic diseases such as obesity and dyslipidemia, but have also been linked to the disruption of neurobiological mechanisms involved in mood regulation and eating behavior [19,20]. In adolescents, this developmental stage—characterized by hormonal, emotional, and social changes—can heighten vulnerability to these types of foods, particularly in situations of emotional stress or challenges in self-regulation [21].

Previous studies have shown associations between emotional eating and frequent consumption of foods high in saturated fat. For instance, a cross-sectional study conducted with women found that higher levels of emotional eating were positively associated with greater energy intake and more frequent consumption of items such as cakes, high-fat snacks, hydrogenated oils, and other calorie-dense foods [22]. Similarly, a study conducted with Taiwanese adolescents found that high levels of emotional eating were significantly associated with an increased likelihood of frequently consuming fast food, fatty snacks, processed meats, desserts, and sugar-sweetened beverages [23]. Furthermore, a study involving African American adolescents revealed that the relationship between emotional eating and dietary quality may be moderated by parental feeding practices, underscoring the critical role of the family environment in shaping emotional eating behaviors [24]. It should be noted that, although these studies provide valuable insights, most have focused on adult populations or culturally distinct settings, leaving a gap in our understanding of this relationship among Latin American adolescents. Therefore, it is essential to explore this link within local contexts, where emotional responses and eating behaviors may differ due to unique sociocultural influences.

Sleep is another factor increasingly associated with emotional eating [25]. Insufficient or poor-quality sleep can impair emotional regulation and heighten stress reactivity, thereby increasing the risk of maladaptive behaviors such as emotional eating [26]. Indeed, sleep disturbances have been associated with changes in the brain's reward and appetite regulation systems, which may promote the intake of high-calorie foods [27].

There is growing evidence of the correlation between sleep quality and emotional eating, as well as its importance in young people and adolescents. For example, short sleep duration and increased rates of insomnia have been found to correlate with increased emotional eating in adolescents, specifically with anxiety, anger, and sadness [28]. On the other hand, in Latino adults living in the United States, López-Cepero et al. found that poor sleep quality is associated with increased emotional eating and that the correlation occurs mainly through negative emotions such as depression, anxiety, and perceived stress. Similarly, Zhou et al. [29] reported that, in Chinese university students, poor sleep quality is an indicator of increased emotional eating. The studies mentioned provide evidence that lack of sleep or poor sleep quality can alter emotional regulation and lead people to eat as an emotional response. Most of these studies have been conducted in adults or young Asians, highlighting the importance of studying this correlation in young Latin Americans, among whom sleep and sociocultural patterns can vary significantly.

During adolescence, BMI is particularly important, as this stage involves rapid changes in body composition that can influence body image, self-esteem, and eating behavior [30]. Furthermore, in the context of this study, it is worth mentioning that a high BMI could be linked to a higher risk of developing disordered eating patterns, such as emotional eating [31–33].

Some investigations have analyzed the association between emotional eating and elevated BMI, but the findings were contradictory, mainly in adolescents. A systematic review carried out by Limbers and Summers [31], which gathered 13 studies, led to the conclusion that, on the whole, there is no significant association between emotional eating and excessive weight in adolescents. Of the six longitudinal analyses examined, only one evidenced a significant prospective association between emotional eating and weight status. In fact, one intervention trial included in the review signaled that emotional eating at the beginning of the intervention was not significantly associated with weight modifications two years after bariatric procedures in obese adolescents. These findings suggest the hypothesis that, in contrast to what has been observed in adults, emotional eating would not be an immediate weight-gain determinant in adolescents. Yet, other studies introduce nuances [32]. Thus, Wilson et al. [33] observed that the relationship between perceived stress and emotional eating in student college populations was moderated by the BMI:

emotional eating was more strongly associated with stress in those students with lower IMC, indicating that the effect of emotional stress on food consumption might vary according to whether or not another state of nutrition is considered. Taken together, these findings demonstrate that the association between emotional eating and BMI is intricate and may occur according to contextual elements such as stress level, access to coping resources, and the situation of development, which justifies continuing to explore this relationship in diverse adolescent populations.

Sociodemographic variables such as age and sex are also relevant. Age is a relevant factor in health, as it has an influence on the acquisition of healthy behaviors, including eating styles [34]. Thus, examining age as a variable associated with emotional eating enables us to understand how this behavior can be initiated or exacerbated during adolescent development.

Emotional eating changes as an individual ages, and emotions that trigger food consumption may change in the course of development, perhaps as a result of differences in emotional maturation [35]. In a study that compared children aged 9 to 10 years and young adults aged 19 years, it was observed that children had the desire to consume more snack foods when they were experiencing positive emotions, whereas young adults did so when they experienced negative emotions [36]. Likewise, Wu et al. [37] discovered that emotional eating is positively related to age among the female adolescents, while the relationship was not observed in the male adolescents. Also, in another study conducted with obese and overweight adolescents, it was found that greater instability in positive affect was linked with an increase in loss of control and overeating in the older individuals, whereas in the younger ones, this link was in the opposite direction [38]. These findings indicate that the impact of emotional instability on disordered eating behaviors may be higher as we progress in age.

While some studies point toward an increase in emotional eating with advancing age during adolescence, the empirical evidence is not conclusive, and the relationship between the two variables is not consistent. In one particular study, Heshmati et al. [39] found that age was not significantly correlated with emotional eating in a sample of American adolescents [39]. This result is consistent with earlier studies showing that age is not a valid predictor of emotional eating [40]. In fact, one study's findings showed that age acts as a protective factor against emotional eating in adolescence, as in both negative and positive emotional contexts, older adolescents have less opportunity to use eating as a response to these emotions [41]. Consequently, there is the necessity to carry out additional research using multivariate models with the aim of clarifying the precise role played by age in the expression and persistence of emotional eating at this vital phase of development.

On the other hand, gender is a social determinant of health that influences how individuals perceive, deal with, and react to a variety of emotional and environmental situations [42]. The hormonal and biological differences between women and men, along with the social and cultural constructions of gender, can influence food habits and emotional coping mechanisms from early life [43,44]. Evidence indicates that adolescent females have a higher incidence of emotional eating compared to males, which has been linked to higher emotional reactivity, greater internalization of stress, and a more pronounced tendency to use food as an emotional regulation mechanism, especially in response to feelings of sadness or anxiety [36,37]. Additionally, it is hypothesized that women have more intense hedonic reactions to rewarding foods under negative emotional situations [36,37]. Gender disparities can be ascribed to both hormonal factors and sociocultural standards that lead to greater concern for body image and body appearance among women, which further increases their susceptibility to experience negative emotions and food use as an emotional compensatory factor.

Depression is one of the most common mood disorders during adolescence, a stage of life in which emotional vulnerability increases due to hormonal, social, and cognitive changes [45]. Depressive symptoms, such as depressed mood, loss of interest, fatigue, and feelings of worthlessness, not only compromise overall psychological functioning but can also have a negative effect on eating behavior patterns [46]. From this perspective, emotional eating has been thought of as an adaptive coping strategy in response to aversive affective states, such as depressive symptomatology, potentially leading to the establishment of unhealthy or disorganized eating patterns within this population [29].

Recent studies have strengthened the association between depressive symptoms and emotional eating among adolescents, despite differences in context and design. A systematic review and meta-analysis conducted by Muha et al. [47], which included 37 studies with 26,000 participants, confirmed the association between depressive symptoms and emotional eating, finding a moderate positive correlation as identified by cross-sectional studies ($g = 0.48$) and longitudinal studies ($g = 0.37$). In an investigation of young Mexican university students, Lazarevich et al. [48] found that emotional eating acted as an overall mediator of the relationship between depressive symptoms and body mass index (BMI), thereby substantiating the hypothesis that emotional distress can lead to maladaptive eating patterns that negatively influence nutritional status. Similarly, in recent multicenter studies, Silva et al. [49] discovered that depressive symptoms, anxiety, and stress were independently related to higher scores of emotional eating during the pandemic, thereby substantiating adolescents' susceptibility to psycho-emotional risks during crisis conditions.

These findings consolidate the evidence on the relationship between depression and emotional eating, but also reveal the need for studies with culturally contextualized approaches to understand the underlying mechanisms in Latin American adolescent populations. In this context, it is necessary to examine this relationship considering other relevant variables, such as sleep, BMI, and consumption of high-fat foods, to generate a comprehensive view of the phenomenon.

Despite the growing interest in elucidating the factors that affect emotional eating in adolescence, the current evidence is fragmented and sometimes inconsistent [31]. Earlier investigations have sought to investigate the correlation between this behavior and other factors; however, a significant amount of this work has been conducted within specific cultural settings, essentially involving Western, adult, or clinical samples, thus limiting the generalizability of the findings. Furthermore, much of the literature has focused on the independent assessment of individual variables instead of integrating psychological, behavioral, and sociodemographic variables into a concerted predictive model.

In the context of Latin America, particularly in Peru, there is a pressing need for research that focuses on this issue among adolescent populations. This necessity arises from the high prevalence of overweight individuals, rapid changes in eating patterns, and mounting concerns regarding youth mental health. Moreover, there is a paucity of research addressing the potential moderating effects of variables such as gender or age on the relationship between individual factors and emotional eating. In light of the aforementioned limitations, the present study endeavors to make a meaningful contribution to the field by employing a predictive approach. This approach involves the examination of the joint association of six key variables: the consumption of foods high in saturated fat, sleep duration, BMI, symptoms of depression, age, and gender. The primary objective of this study is to elucidate the role of these variables in the phenomenon of emotional eating among Peruvian adolescents. The objective of this study is to identify the factors that exert the greatest influence on the predisposition to this behavior. The findings of this study will provide contextualized evidence that can serve as a basis for the development of future prevention and intervention strategies that are adapted to local realities.

Therefore, the present study examines the association between saturated fat intake, sleep duration, BMI, symptoms of depression, age, and sex and emotional eating in a sample of Peruvian adolescents.

2. Materials and Methods

2.1. Design and Participants

The methodology employed in this study was a cross-sectional design, according to the classification proposed by Ato et al. [50]. With regard to the participants, a sample of individuals who participated in the study was used. This study encompassed a series of predictor variables, including the consumption of foods rich in saturated fats, sleep duration, BMI, and symptoms of depression. The dependent variable of the study was defined as emotional eating. The field study was conducted in three public educational institutions located in the district of Lima Este, Peru. The study sample consisted of 722 school-going adolescents who were selected through non-probabilistic intentional sampling based on criteria of accessibility and institutional willingness. The study subjects met the following inclusion criteria: they were between 12 and 18 years of age, they were enrolled in the selected educational centers, and they provided informed consent (and assent in the case of minors).

The minimum sample size was estimated using the Soper A-priori Sample Size Calculator for Multiple Regression (http://www.danielsoper.com/statcalc, accessed on 7 July 2025) [51]. The following parameters were established: a significance level of $\alpha = 0.05$, a statistical power of $(1 - \beta) = 0.95$, an effect size $f^2 = 0.15$, and six predictors (consumption of foods rich in saturated fats, sleep duration, BMI, symptoms of depression, sex, and age). The calculation yielded a minimum required sample size of 146 participants. The final study sample, consisting of 722 adolescents, exceeded this value, ensuring adequate statistical power for the analysis.

Table 1 presents the sociodemographic characteristics of the 722 adolescents. The mean age of the participants was 15.59 years (SD = 1.88). With respect to gender, the distribution was relatively balanced, with 51.2% of subjects identified as male and 48.8% as female.

Table 1. Description of the sociodemographic characteristics of the study sample ($n = 722$).

Characteristic	*n*	%
Age	M = 15.59	SD = 1.88
Sex		
Female	352	48.8
Male	370	51.2

Note. M = mean; SD = standard deviation.

2.2. Variables and Instruments

Intake of foods rich in saturated fats: Saturated fat intake was assessed using a food frequency questionnaire (FFQ). This FFQ was previously designed [52] and used in studies conducted in the Peruvian population [53]. The instrument consisted of 16 items that collected the frequency of consumption of foods commonly recognized as sources of saturated fats. The participants were instructed to indicate how frequently they performed a specified action, and the responses were recorded on an ordinal scale with the following categories: "Once a month or less" (0 points), "2 to 3 times a month" (1 point), "1 to 2 times a week" (2 points), "3 to 4 times a week" (3 points), and "5 or more times a week" (4 points). The total score, ranging from 0 to 64, was treated as a continuous variable in the statistical analyses to preserve variability and enhance explanatory power. The FFQ included items such as hamburgers, ground beef, fried chicken, bacon, sausages, cold cuts, hard cheeses, butter or margarine used in cooking, and pizza, which are recognized as the primary dietary sources of saturated fat. The questionnaire demonstrated high levels of reliability in its prior validation, with an ordinal alpha of 0.94, an omega coefficient of 0.94, and an H coefficient of 0.95, supporting its use for consistently measuring saturated fat consumption in Peruvian adolescents [54].

2.3. Duration of Sleep

Sleep duration was assessed by asking participants a direct question: "How many hours of sleep does your average day consist of?" Responses were classified into three categories, following criteria previously established in the scientific literature. Sleep was considered short when participants reported sleeping less than 7 h per day, normal when between 7 and 9 h, and prolonged when the duration of sleep was greater than 9 h [13,55].

BMI: Anthropometric assessment was carried out by a nutrition professional early in the morning over the course of a week, following standardized protocols. Participants were asked to remove their shoes and clothing as much as possible to ensure accurate data collection. The BMI was then calculated using the following formula: weight (kg) divided by height squared (m^2). The adolescents were then classified according to the criteria established by the WHO, using BMI z-scores. According to this classification, underweight was defined as a BMI z-score less than −1, normal weight as a BMI z-score between −1 and +1, and overweight as a BMI z-score greater than +1 [56].

Symptoms of depression: Depressive symptoms were assessed using the Patient Health Questionnaire-2 (PHQ-2), which consists of the two core items from the PHQ-9 [57]: "Feeling down, depressed, or hopeless", and "Having little interest or pleasure in doing things." Participants were asked to indicate their experience over the past two weeks using a frequency scale ranging from 0 (no days) to 3 (almost every day). The total score ranges from 0 to 6, with a score of 3 or higher indicating clinically relevant depressive symptoms [58,59]. The scale has demonstrated acceptable internal consistency in the adult Peruvian population, with an alpha of 0.75 and an omega coefficient of 0.76 [60].

Emotional Eating: Emotional eating was assessed using the Spanish version of a specific questionnaire consisting of 10 items that probe the frequency with which participants eat in response to various emotions [61]. Each item was evaluated using a four-point Likert scale, with response options ranging from "never" (0) to "always" (3). The total score obtained allowed the adolescents to be classified into three levels of emotional eating: low or none (0–5 points), moderate (6–10 points), and high or very emotional (11–30 points) [62]. The instrument includes the following question: "Do you have particular dietary preferences or restrictions?" The questionnaire was originally developed in Spain and has been validated in the adolescent population in Chile [61,63]. Given that it has not yet been formally validated for Peruvian adolescents, the internal reliability of the scale was calculated in the total sample in the present study, obtaining a Cronbach's alpha coefficient of 0.74, which is considered acceptable. According to the findings of previous studies conducted on adolescent populations, the levels of internal consistency reported were similar, with coefficients close to 0.71 [64].

2.4. Statistical Analysis

First, descriptive analyses were performed, reporting means, standard deviations, and absolute and relative frequencies. To examine differences in the study variables according to sex and age, Student's *t*-tests for independent samples were applied, along with effect size calculation using Cohen's d statistic and 95% confidence intervals. Normality was assessed using the Kolmogorov–Smirnov test and visual inspection of histograms and

Q-Q plots. Homoscedasticity and linearity assumptions for the regression analysis were evaluated through residual plots. All assumptions were met. Subsequently, a multiple linear regression model was applied to identify significant predictors of emotional eating. The following were included as independent variables: consumption of foods rich in saturated fats, sleep duration (categories), z-BMI, symptoms of depression, age (categories), and sex. In addition, the assumptions of multicollinearity were verified using the TOL (Tolerance) and VIF (Variance Inflation Factor) indicators. Statistically significant values were determined as $p < 0.05$. The analysis was performed using IBM SPSS Statistics software version 26.

2.5. Ethical Considerations

The study was approved by the Research Ethics Committee of the Faculty of Health Sciences at the Universidad Peruana Unión (Ref. Code: 2025-CEB-FCS-UPeU-No.005. 7 January 2025), in accordance with the international ethical provisions established in the Declaration of Helsinki. Prior to data collection, formal authorization was requested from the participating educational institutions, as well as informed consent from the students' parents or legal guardians. Informed consent was also obtained from the adolescents, who were informed about the objectives of the study, the voluntary nature of their participation, the confidentiality of the data, and their right to withdraw from the study at any time without consequences.

3. Results

As shown in Table 2, there were notable differences in some variables based on sex and age. The results of the study indicated that women reported having less sleep and higher levels of depression and emotional eating in comparison to men ($p < 0.05$), with moderate effect sizes. No differences were observed between sexes in saturated fat consumption or BMI. In terms of age, older adolescents (15–18 years) had higher BMI and emotional eating than those aged 12–14 years ($p < 0.01$). There were no significant differences in the other variables.

Table 2. Analysis of variables related to consumption of foods rich in saturated fats, sleep, BMI, depression, and emotional eating according to sociodemographic variables.

Variables	SFI	Sleep	z-BMI	Depression	Emotional Eating
General M (SD)	14.10 (6.94)	1.99 (0.79)	23.91 (3.90)	2.48 (1.77)	9.42 (5.41)
Sex [1]					
p	0.095	0.028 *	0.379	<0.001 ***	<0.001 ***
95% CI	[−1.873, 0.153]	[−0.242, −0.014]	[−0.315, 0.826]	[0.791, 1.286]	[2.611, 4.116]
Cohen's d	−0.124	−0.164	0.066	0.613	0.654
Age [1]					
p	0.885	0.796	<0.001 ***	0.930	0.007 **
95% CI	[−1.092, 0.942]	[−0.130, 0.099]	[−2.412, −1.301]	[−0.248, 0.271]	[−1.877, −0.299]
Cohen's d	−0.011	−0.019	−0.489	0.007	−0.202

Note. M = mean; SD = standard deviation; Student's *t*-test [1]; z-BMI, body mass index z-score; CI = confidence interval at 95%; *p* = *p*-value; SFI = saturated fat intake, * $p < 0.05$, ** $p < 0.01$, *** $p < 0.001$.

Table 3 presents the bivariate correlations among SFI, sleep duration, z-BMI, depressive symptoms, and emotional eating. Emotional eating was positively and significantly associated with saturated fat intake (r = 0.190, $p < 0.001$), depressive symptoms (r = 0.465, $p < 0.001$), and z-BMI (r = 0.114, $p < 0.01$), while it was negatively associated with sleep duration (r = –0.180, $p < 0.001$). Additionally, depressive symptoms showed significant positive correlations with SFI (r = 0.078, $p < 0.05$) and z-BMI (r = 0.024), and a negative correlation with sleep duration (r = –0.191, $p < 0.001$). Notably, SFI and z-BMI were not significantly correlated (r = –0.031), and sleep duration showed no meaningful association with BMI (r = 0.008).

Table 3. Correlation analysis between consumption of foods rich in saturated fat, sleep, z-BMI, depression, and emotional eating.

Variables	1. SFI	2. Sleep Duration	3. z-BMI	4. Depression	5. Emotional Eating
1. SFI		0.068	−0.031	0.078 *	0.190 ***
2. Sleep Duration	-	-	0.008	−0.191 ***	−0.180 ***
3. z-BMI	-	-	-	0.024	0.114 **
4. Depression	-	-	-	-	0.465 ***
5. Emotional Eating	-	-	-	-	-

Note. SFI = saturated fat intake, z-BMI = body mass index z-score, * $p < 0.05$, ** $p < 0.01$, *** $p < 0.001$.

As shown in Table 4, the findings of the multiple regression model for predicting emotional eating in adolescents are noteworthy. The model was found to be statistically significant overall, with an adjusted R^2 value of 0.301 and a p-value less than 0.001. This indicates that the model explains 30.1% of the observed variance in emotional eating behaviors among adolescents. All predictors included in the analysis proved to be statistically significant. Higher saturated fat intake and higher levels of depressive symptoms were associated with higher emotional eating. Similarly, advanced age and female sex were shown to be associated with increased emotional eating tendencies. Conversely, sleeping seven hours or more exhibited a protective effect, significantly reducing this behavior. The model did not present multicolinearity problems (TOL > 0.69; VIF < 1.5), which supports its statistical validity.

Table 4. Factors associated with emotional eating in Peruvian adolescents.

Model		Standardized Coefficients		t	TOL	VIF	p
		β	CI				
	(Constant)			−1.24			0.214
1	SFI	0.186	[0.124, 0.248]	5.90	0.978	1.02	<0.001 ***
	Sleep (<7 h)			Reference			
	Sleep (7 h)	−0.094	[−0.167, −0.020]	−2.50	0.691	1.45	0.013 *
	Sleep (>7 h)	−0.126	[−0.199, −0.052]	−3.37	0.697	1.43	<0.001 ***
	z-BMI	0.082	[0.019, 0.146]	2.53	0.922	1.08	0.011 *
	Depression	0.365	[0.299, 0.431]	10.84	0.855	1.17	<0.001 ***
	15 to 18 years	0.083	[0.019, 0.146]	6.33	0.903	1.11	<0.001 ***
	Being female	0.208	[0.143, 0.272]	2.55	0.921	1.09	0.011 *

Note. Dependent variable: emotional eating; SFI = saturated fat intake; z-BMI = body mass index z-score; Model 1: Adjusted R^2 = 0.301, ANOVA F (F = 45.276, $p < 0.001$). * $p < 0.05$, *** $p < 0.001$.

4. Discussion

Adolescence is a critical stage in the formation of eating habits and the development of emotional regulation strategies. These aspects can be influenced by psychological, behavioral, and sociodemographic factors [1]. This study examined variables such as the consumption of foods rich in saturated fats, sleep duration, BMI, symptoms of depression, age, and sex to understand their relationship with emotional eating in Peruvian adolescents. The current study's findings indicate a significant association between higher saturated fat consumption and higher levels of depressive symptoms with greater emotional eating. In a similar vein, being female and older were associated with a higher propensity for this type of behavior. Conversely, sleeping seven hours or more was associated with a reduced likelihood of emotional eating. The model demonstrated an overall explanatory power of 30.1% for the variance in emotional eating among adolescents.

One of the study's primary findings was the identification of depression as the strongest predictor of emotional eating in adolescents. This result indicates that higher levels of depressive symptoms are associated with a greater tendency to use food as an emotional regulation strategy. These findings align with those reported in recent studies, which found a moderately strong positive association between depressive symptoms and emotional eating in adolescents, in both cross-sectional and longitudinal designs [47]. A similar study of university students demonstrated that symptoms of depression, anxiety, and stress are independently associated with an increase in emotional eating behaviors, underscoring the pivotal role of mental health in influencing eating patterns [49]. In the Peruvian context, a study we conducted among young adults yielded similar results [13]. However, while some studies have indicated a positive relationship, others have not reported significant associations [31]. These discrepancies can be attributed to methodological and contextual differences, as well as the influence of moderating factors such as social support, coping strategies, and the presence of other psychopathological symptoms.

Beyond the discrepancies, it has been suggested that depression can alter emotional regulation processes [65], increasing vulnerability to maladaptive eating behaviors [1,17]. Difficulty regulating emotions, a common characteristic in people with depressive symptoms, can encourage the use of food as an immediate strategy for emotional relief, as has been observed in contexts of induced hunger [66]. Furthermore, neurobiological alterations associated with depression, such as reward system dysfunction and hypothalamic-pituitary–adrenal axis dysregulation, have the potential to increase sensitivity to highly palatable foods [67]. This, in turn, could reinforce the vicious cycle between negative affect and overeating. These pathways underscore the necessity for interventions that integrate emotional management and the promotion of healthy eating habits as strategies to prevent eating disorders and mental health problems in adolescence.

Another salient finding was the positive association between the consumption of foods rich in saturated fats and emotional eating. This suggests that increased consumption of these foods is associated with a heightened tendency to overeat in response to negative emotions. These findings align with recent studies suggesting that highly palatable foods, particularly those high in saturated fat, function as hedonic reinforcers, providing temporary relief from unpleasant emotional states [22,68]. Furthermore, research conducted among adolescents indicates a correlation between emotional eating and increased consumption of ultra-processed foods [23], such as fatty snacks, pastries, and fast food items, which are high in saturated fat. However, the association between fat consumption and emotional eating may not be absolute, as food preferences can vary depending on cultural, economic, or food availability factors [69]. Therefore, while some cultures demonstrate a higher propensity for consuming fatty foods in response to emotions, others exhibit a stronger preference for sweet foods [70].

On the other hand, foods high in saturated fats have been shown to influence the brain's reward system, leading to increased dopamine release and a sensation of well-being [71]. This rapid reward effect could serve as an immediate strategy for managing negative emotions [21]. Furthermore, repeated exposure to these types of foods in emotional contexts has the potential to reinforce behaviors that seek short-term gratification, making it challenging to establish eating patterns regulated by physiological signals of hunger and satiety [72]. This neurobehavioral mechanism could explain why adolescents who regularly turn to fatty foods in response to stress or sadness tend to maintain or intensify these patterns over time [21].

The results of the present study indicated that adolescents who slept seven hours or more exhibited a lower tendency for emotional eating compared to those who slept less than seven hours. This finding suggests that adequate sleep may offer a protective effect against emotional eating behaviors in this population. A recent study found that adolescents who slept less tended to experience emotional eating more often, a tendency that was particularly strong among those who were dissatisfied with their bodies [28]. A recent study of university students also found that poor sleep quality is a predictor of emotional eating, with depression playing a partial mediating role [29]. This lends further support to the notion that insufficient sleep has a negative impact on emotional regulation, which in turn, can lead to changes in eating patterns. However, the association between the two variables is not entirely consistent. In fact, certain cross-sectional studies have not identified a significant association between sleep duration and emotional eating [73,74]. These differences could be explained by the way sleep is measured (self-reported hours vs. objective assessments), the age range of the samples, or the presence of other uncontrolled psychological factors in the analysis.

In any case, from a physiological and behavioral standpoint, there are various mechanisms that could explain the observed relationships. For instance, sleep deprivation has been shown to alter appetite regulation systems, increasing levels of ghrelin (a hormone that stimulates hunger) and reducing levels of leptin (a hormone that promotes satiety), which increases appetite, particularly for high-calorie and high-fat foods [75]. Additionally, insufficient sleep has been shown to impair executive functions, leading to diminished self-control and emotional regulation. This can result in impulsive reactions, such as overeating in response to stress or negative emotions [76]. Therefore, it is important to promote proper sleep hygiene as a strategy to prevent maladaptive eating behaviors in adolescents.

Regarding BMI, the results of this study indicated a positive association between higher BMI and higher levels of emotional eating in adolescents. Although the strength of this relationship was lower compared to other variables, the finding suggests that overweight adolescents may be more vulnerable to using eating as a strategy to cope with negative emotional states. This result is consistent with studies such as that of Lazarevich et al. [48], who reported that emotional eating mediated the relationship between depressive symptoms and higher BMI in young Mexican adults. Similarly, a systematic review concluded that, although longitudinal evidence is limited, several cross-sectional studies have found associations between emotional eating and higher body weight in adolescents, although not universally [31]. Indeed, research indicates that the association between emotional eating and weight gain can be influenced by external factors, including the level of social support or coping mechanisms available [33]. In some contexts, it has been observed that high BMI does not necessarily predict higher emotional eating independently. Rather, its impact may be modulated by psychological variables such as perfectionism [77].

Among the possible underlying mechanisms, it has been suggested that adolescents with higher BMI may experience greater social pressure and body stigmatization, which generates negative emotions that, in turn, encourage emotional eating as a coping mechanism [77]. In addition, being overweight may be associated with more dysfunctional dietary patterns—such as higher consumption of ultra-processed and high-fat foods—that perpetuate the cycle between emotional distress and overeating [32]. On the other hand, alterations in the brain's reward systems could also favor a more intense response to high-calorie foods in adolescents with greater adiposity, reinforcing the relationship between BMI and emotional eating [27,71].

Finally, the present study found that both gender and age were significant predictors of emotional eating. In particular, being female and older were associated with higher levels of this behavior. These findings are consistent with previous research that has documented a higher prevalence of emotional eating in women compared to men [36,37]. In fact, it has been suggested that adolescent girls tend to report greater use of maladaptive emotional strategies, including eating [8,78], possibly due to greater emotional sensitivity and higher levels of perceived stress during this stage of development.

Regarding age, the findings suggest that, as adolescents mature, they are more prone to using food as a means of emotional regulation. This pattern has also been reported by Wu et al. [37], who found that the relationship between age and emotional eating was positive in adolescent females but not in males. This suggests that emotional development and hormonal changes during puberty may intensify vulnerability in girls as they become older. Also, Moss et al. [36] observed discrepancies in the emotions that precipitated emotional eating in children and young adults, underscoring that the impact of age might also be contingent on the prevailing emotion. These findings suggest that, as adolescents transition into adulthood, heightened academic, social, and familial pressures may amplify their exposure to stressors, prompting them to utilize food as a coping mechanism for managing adverse emotions, despite the absence of more effective regulatory skills. However, not all studies concur entirely with this trend. In some cultural contexts or among specific populations, weak or non-significant associations between age, gender, and emotional eating have been reported [32,39,40]. These findings could reflect variations in sociocultural norms related to emotional expression, access to food, and learned coping models.

4.1. Limitations and Future Considerations

The findings of the current study should be interpreted considering several limitations. First, because we conducted a cross-sectional study, we cannot claim that the associations observed between the explanatory variables (sleep duration, BMI, depression, age, and sex) and the outcome variable (emotional eating) are causal. Therefore, longitudinal studies are suggested to better understand the direction and evolution of these relationships. Second, all variables were assessed using self-report, which can introduce social desirability bias or recall errors, particularly in measures such as sleep duration or food consumption. Furthermore, in the specific case of depression, we did not use clinical diagnoses of psychological symptoms made by a physician based on medical care data. This is especially important because the gold standard for establishing a psychiatric diagnosis requires a structured interview and functional neuroimaging [79–81]. Thirdly, although a questionnaire validated in other Spanish-speaking populations was used to measure emotional eating [61,63], we do not yet have a specific validation for Peruvian adolescents; therefore, this aspect must be taken into account when interpreting some items from a cultural perspective. Finally, the sample was limited to three public schools in eastern Lima; private schools and other educational institutions located in other geographical regions of Peru were not considered. Consequently, the results should be generalized to other geographical or socioeconomic contexts with caution. Future studies should broaden the geographic, cultural, and socioeconomic diversity of the samples, and incorporate clinical assessments of mental health along with objective measurements of variables such as sleep and dietary intake. This approach will help strengthen the empirical foundation and support the development of more specific and culturally relevant interventions to prevent emotional eating and promote comprehensive health among adolescents.

4.2. Implications for Public Health

Despite these limitations, we believe that this study provides valuable information that can serve as a basis for future research and interventions carried out in both school and community settings, aimed at promoting the mental and nutritional health of adolescents. Specifically, it is worth mentioning that the results of the current study support the design of strategies to prevent unhealthy eating behaviors and promote health among adolescents. In fact, since saturated fat consumption, inadequate sleep duration, high BMI, depressive symptoms, female gender, and older age are factors associated with emotional eating, policies and interventions should consider a multifactorial approach that integrates not only nutritional aspects but also emotional and behavioral aspects. Furthermore, since adolescents constitute a significant school population, it is essential that educational institutions promote not only healthy eating habits but also adaptive emotional regulation strategies, educating students about the importance of adequate sleep and encouraging psychosocial support activities aimed at adolescents. In addition, promoting the importance of mindful eating and depression prevention is suggested, as these could contribute to reducing the incidence of emotional eating and, consequently, reduce the risk of excess body weight and long-term metabolic disorders.

5. Conclusions

This study provides evidence on the factors associated with emotional eating in Peruvian adolescents, highlighting the fundamental role of depressive symptoms, consumption of foods rich in saturated fats, sleep duration, BMI, sex, and age. The findings underscore the multifactorial nature of emotional eating and the need to address both psychological and behavioral determinants in health promotion strategies targeting this population.

Author Contributions: Y.E.C.-M.: Conceptualization of the manuscript, literature review, writing—review and editing. M.R.-V. and Y.E.C.-M.: Project coordination, data collection, and institutional permissions; writing—review and editing. D.J.-A.: Statistical analysis, data interpretation, and critical review of the manuscript. C.C.-G. and A.V.-C.: Data entry and preparation of tables and figures; writing—review and editing. I.P.D.L.V.-F.: Contribution to writing—review and editing of the manuscript. J.S.: Principal investigator of the original research project, conceptual design, supervision of all research phases, writing, and final manuscript editing. All authors have read and agreed to the published version of the manuscript.

Funding: This research did not receive specific funding for data collection or analysis. However, Universidad Señor de Sipán and Universidad Peruana Unión have provided institutional support for the article processing charge (APC) related to the publication of this manuscript.

Institutional Review Board Statement: The study was approved by the Research Ethics Committee of the Faculty of Health Sciences at the Universidad Peruana Unión (Ref. Code: 2025-CEB-FCS-UPeU-No.005, 7 January 2025), in accordance with the international ethical provisions established in the Declaration of Helsinki.

Informed Consent Statement: Prior to data collection, formal authorization was requested from the participating educational institutions, as well as informed consent from the students' parents or legal guardians. Informed consent was also obtained from the adolescents, who were informed about the objectives of the study, the voluntary nature of their participation, the confidentiality of the data, and their right to withdraw from the study at any time without consequences.

Data Availability Statement: The data that support the findings of this study are available on request from the corresponding author. The data are not publicly available due to privacy or ethical restrictions.

Acknowledgments: The authors would like to thank the directors of the participating educational institutions in East Lima for facilitating access and support during data collection. We are also grateful to all the adolescents, parents, and guardians for their voluntary participation and commitment to this research. Special thanks to the Research Group for Nutrition and Healthy Behaviors at Universidad Señor de Sipán and to the academic team at Universidad Peruana Unión for their collaboration in the development and execution of this study.

Conflicts of Interest: The authors declare no conflict of interest.

Abbreviations

The following abbreviations are used in this manuscript:

SFI	Saturated fat intake
z-BMI	Body mass index z-score
SD	Sleep duration
EE	Emotional eating

References

1. Shriver, L.H.; Dollar, J.M.; Calkins, S.D.; Keane, S.P.; Shanahan, L.; Wideman, L. Emotional eating in adolescence: Effects of emotion regulation, weight status and negative body image. *Nutrients* **2021**, *13*, 79. [CrossRef] [PubMed]
2. WHO. Mental Health of Adolescents. Newsroom. 2024. Available online: https://www.who.int/news-room/fact-sheets/detail/adolescent-mental-health (accessed on 7 July 2025).
3. López-Gil, J.F.; García-Hermoso, A.; Smith, L.; Firth, J.; Trott, M.; Mesas, A.E.; Jimenez-Lopez, E.; Gutierrez-Espinoza, H.; Tarraga-Lopez, P.J.; Victoria-Montesinos, D. Global Proportion of Disordered Eating in Children and Adolescents. *JAMA Pediatr.* **2023**, *177*, 363. [CrossRef] [PubMed]
4. MINSA. Minsa: El 29.6% de Adolescentes Entre Los 12 y 17 Años Presenta Riesgo de Padecer Algún Problema de Salud Mental o Emocional—Noticias—Ministerio de Salud—Plataforma del Estado Peruano. 2024. Available online: https://www.gob.pe/institucion/minsa/noticias/536664-minsa-el-29-6-de-adolescentes-entre-los-12-y-17-anos-presenta-riesgo-de-padecer-algun-problema-de-salud-mental-o-emocional (accessed on 27 March 2025).
5. INEI; Gobierno del Perú. Solo el 11.3% de la Población Peruana Mayor de 15 Años Consume la Cantidad de Frutas y Verduras Que Recomienda la OMS. Lima, Perú, 2020. Available online: https://www.gob.pe/institucion/minsa/noticias/302155-solo-el-11-3-de-la-poblacion-peruana-mayor-de-15-anos-consume-la-cantidad-de-frutas-y-verduras-que-recomienda-la-oms (accessed on 5 January 2021).
6. Valero-Solis, S.; Granero-Perez, R.; Sanchez-Carracedo, D.; Valero-Solis, S.; Granero-Perez, R.; Sanchez-Carracedo, D. Frequency of family meals and risk of eating disorders in adolescents in Spain and Peru. *Rev. Latinoam. Psicol.* **2019**, *51*, 48–57. [CrossRef]
7. Risk Factors Associated with Eating Disorders in Adolescents from Metropolitan Lima. Available online: https://www.medigraphic.com/cgi-bin/new/resumenI.cgi?IDARTICULO=119436 (accessed on 29 June 2025).
8. Saintila, J.; Soriano-Moreno, A.N.; Basauri-Delgado, M.; Carranza-Cubas, S.P.; López-Gonzales, J.L.; Oblitas-Guerrero, S.M.; Calizaya-Milla, Y.E. Sex differences in social network addiction and emotional eating among adolescents in a Peruvian region: A cross-sectional analysis. *J. Eat. Disord.* **2024**, *12*, 168. [CrossRef] [PubMed]
9. MINSA. *En el Perú, el 62.7% de Personas de 15 Años de Edad a Más Padece de Exceso de Peso*; MINSA: Lima, Peru, 2022.
10. Defensoria del Pueblo Peru. Available online: https://www.defensoria.gob.pe/ocho-de-cada-10-personas-no-reciben-atencion-en-salud-mental-pese-a-requerirlo/ (accessed on 27 March 2025).
11. EsSalud. EsSalud advierte que 40% de Adolescentes Internados en Hospital Almenara Tienen Trastornos Alimenticios—Noticias—Seguro Social de Salud—Plataforma del Estado Peruano. 2024. Available online: https://www.gob.pe/institucion/essalud/noticias/901303-essalud-advierte-que-40-de-adolescentes-internados-en-hospital-almenara-tienen-trastornos-alimenticios (accessed on 27 March 2025).
12. Reichenberger, J.; Schnepper, R.; Arend, A.K.; Blechert, J. Emotional eating in healthy individuals and patients with an eating disorder: Evidence from psychometric, experimental and naturalistic studies. *Proc. Nutr. Soc.* **2020**, *79*, 290–299. [CrossRef] [PubMed]
13. Calderón-Asenjo, R.E.; Jalk-Muñoz, M.C.; Calizaya-Milla, Y.E.; Calizaya-Milla, S.E.; Ramos-Vera, C.; Saintila, J. Association Between Emotional Eating, Sociodemographic Characteristics, Physical Activity, Sleep Duration, and Mental and Physical Health in Young Adults. *J. Multidiscip. Healthc.* **2022**, *15*, 2845–2859. [CrossRef] [PubMed]
14. Liu, H.; Yang, Q.; Luo, J.; Ouyang, Y.; Sun, M.; Xi, Y.; Yong, C.; Xiang, C.; Lin, Q. Association between Emotional Eating, Depressive Symptoms and Laryngopharyngeal Reflux Symptoms in College Students: A Cross-Sectional Study in Hunan. *Nutrients* **2020**, *12*, 1595. [CrossRef] [PubMed]
15. van Strien, T.; Cebolla, A.; Etchemendy, E.; Gutiérrez-Maldonado, J.; Ferrer-García, M.; Botella, C.; Baños, R. Emotional eating and food intake after sadness and joy. *Appetite* **2013**, *66*, 20–25. [CrossRef] [PubMed]
16. Gross, J.J. The Emerging Field of Emotion Regulation: An Integrative Review. *Rev. Gen. Psychol.* **1998**, *2*, 271–299. [CrossRef]
17. Lu, Q.; Tao, F.; Hou, F.; Zhang, Z.; Ren, L.-L. Emotion regulation, emotional eating and the energy-rich dietary pattern. A population-based study in Chinese adolescents. *Appetite* **2016**, *99*, 149–156. [CrossRef] [PubMed]
18. Wilson, J.; McMullan, L.; Blackburn, N.; Klempel, N.; Yakkundi, A.; Amstrong, N.; Brolly, C.; Butler, L.; Barnett, Y.; Jacob, L.; et al. Changes in dietary fat intake and associations with mental health in a UK public sample during the COVID-19 pandemic. *J. Public Health* **2021**, *43*, 687–694. [CrossRef] [PubMed]

19. Brichacek, A.L.; Florkowski, M.; Abiona, E.; Frank, K.M. Ultra-Processed Foods: A Narrative Review of the Impact on the Human Gut Microbiome and Variations in Classification Methods. *Nutrients* **2024**, *16*, 1738. [CrossRef] [PubMed]
20. Abay, S.M.; Amelo, W. Assessment of self-medication practices among medical, pharmacy, and health science students in gondar university, ethiopia. *J. Young Pharm.* **2010**, *2*, 306–310. [CrossRef] [PubMed]
21. Sinai, T.; Axelrod, R.; Shimony, T.; Boaz, M.; Kaufman-Shriqui, V. Dietary Patterns among Adolescents Are Associated with Growth, Socioeconomic Features, and Health-Related Behaviors. *Foods* **2021**, *10*, 3054. [CrossRef] [PubMed]
22. Zare, H.; Rahimi, H.; Omidi, A.; Nematolahi, F.; Sharifi, N. Relationship between emotional eating and nutritional intake in adult women with overweight and obesity: A cross-sectional study. *Nutr. J.* **2024**, *23*, 129. [CrossRef] [PubMed]
23. Bui, C.; Lin, L.Y.; Wu, C.Y.; Chiu, Y.W.; Chiou, H.Y. Association between Emotional Eating and Frequency of Unhealthy Food Consumption among Taiwanese Adolescents. *Nutrients* **2021**, *13*, 2739. [CrossRef] [PubMed]
24. Quattlebaum, M.; Wilson, D.K.; Sweeney, A.M.; Zarrett, N. Moderating Effects of Parental Feeding Practices and Emotional Eating on Dietary Intake among Overweight African American Adolescents. *Nutrients* **2021**, *13*, 1920. [CrossRef] [PubMed]
25. De Longis, E.; Kassis, A.; Rémond-Derbez, N.; Thota, R.; Darimont, C.; Donato-Capel, L.; Hudry, J. Cognitive benefits of sleep: A narrative review to explore the relevance of glucose regulation. *Sleep Adv.* **2025**, *6*, zpae095. [CrossRef] [PubMed]
26. López Malque, J.J.; Chanducas Lozano, B.; Calizaya-Milla, Y.E.; Calizaya-Milla, S.E.; Morales-García, W.C.; Saintila, J. Relationship between sleep quality, eating habits, and anthropometric profile in adolescents: A cross-sectional survey. *Retos* **2023**, *48*, 341–348. [CrossRef]
27. Thellman, K.E.; Dmitrieva, J.; Miller, A.; Harsh, J.R.; LeBourgeois, M.K. Sleep timing is associated with self-reported dietary patterns in 9- to 15-year-olds. *Sleep Health* **2017**, *3*, 269–275. [CrossRef] [PubMed]
28. White, M.L.; Triplett, O.M.; Morales, N.; Van Dyk, T.R. Associations Among Sleep, Emotional Eating, and Body Dissatisfaction in Adolescents. *Child Psychiatry Hum. Dev.* 2024; *Online ahead of print*. [CrossRef]
29. Zhou, J.; Chen, Y.; Ji, S.; Qu, J.; Bu, Y.; Li, W.; Zhou, Z.; Wang, X.; Fu, X.; Liu, Y. Sleep quality and emotional eating in college students: A moderated mediation model of depression and physical activity levels. *J. Eat. Disord.* **2024**, *12*, 155. [CrossRef] [PubMed]
30. Reel, J.; Voelker, D.; Greenleaf, C. Weight status and body image perceptions in adolescents: Current perspectives. *Adolesc. Health Med. Ther.* **2015**, *6*, 149. [CrossRef] [PubMed]
31. Limbers, C.A.; Summers, E. Emotional Eating and Weight Status in Adolescents: A Systematic Review. *Int. J. Environ. Res. Public Health* **2021**, *18*, 991. [CrossRef] [PubMed]
32. Cuyan-Zumaeta, K.; Javier-Aliaga, D.; Rodríguez-Vásquez, M.; Saintila, J. Do mental wellbeing and emotional eating influence BMI similarly or differently? Evidence from a sample of Peruvian adolescents. *Front. Public Health* **2025**, *13*, 1564656. [CrossRef] [PubMed]
33. Wilson, S.M.; Darling, K.E.; Fahrenkamp, A.J.; D'Auria, A.L.; Sato, A.F. Predictors of Emotional Eating During Adolescents' Transition to College: Does Body Mass Index Moderate the Association Between Stress and Emotional Eating? *J. Am. Coll. Health* **2015**, *63*, 163–170. [CrossRef] [PubMed]
34. Perez, F.P.; Perez, C.A.; Chumbiauca, M.N. Insights into the Social Determinants of Health in Older Adults. *J. Biomed. Sci. Eng.* **2022**, *15*, 261–268. [CrossRef] [PubMed]
35. Fuente González, C.E.; Chávez-Servín, J.L.; de la Torre-Carbot, K.; Ronquillo González, D.; Aguilera Barreiro Mde los, Á.; Ojeda Navarro, L.R. Relationship between Emotional Eating, Consumption of Hyperpalatable Energy-Dense Foods, and Indicators of Nutritional Status: A Systematic Review. *J. Obes.* **2022**, *2022*, 4243868. [CrossRef] [PubMed]
36. Moss, R.H.; Conner, M.; O'Connor, D.B. Exploring the effects of positive and negative emotions on eating behaviours in children and young adults. *Psychol. Health Med.* **2021**, *26*, 457–466. [CrossRef] [PubMed]
37. Wu, J.; Willner, C.J.; Hill, C.; Fearon, P.; Mayes, L.C.; Crowley, M.J. Emotional eating and instructed food-cue processing in adolescents: An ERP study. *Biol. Psychol.* **2018**, *132*, 27–36. [CrossRef] [PubMed]
38. Egbert, A.H.; Smith, K.E.; Ranzenhofer, L.M.; Goldschmidt, A.B.; Hilbert, A. The Role of Affective Instability in Loss of Control Eating in Youth with Overweight/Obesity Across Development: Findings from Two EMA Studies. *Res. Child. Adolesc. Psychopathol.* **2022**, *50*, 945–957. [CrossRef] [PubMed]
39. Heshmati, S.; DavyRomano, E.; Chow, C.; Doan, S.N.; Reynolds, K.D. Negative emodiversity is associated with emotional eating in adolescents: An examination of emotion dynamics in daily life. *J. Adolesc.* **2023**, *95*, 115–130. [CrossRef] [PubMed]
40. Bell, B.M.; Spruijt-Metz, D.; Naya, C.H.; Lane, C.J.; Wen, C.K.F.; Davis, J.N.; Weigensberg, M.J. The mediating role of emotional eating in the relationship between perceived stress and dietary intake quality in Hispanic/Latino adolescents. *Eat. Behav.* **2021**, *42*, 101537. [CrossRef] [PubMed]
41. Schneider-Worthington, C.R.; Smith, K.E.; Roemmich, J.N.; Salvy, S.J. External food cue responsiveness and emotional eating in adolescents: A multimethod study. *Appetite* **2022**, *168*, 105789. [CrossRef] [PubMed]

42. Chaplin, T.M.; Hong, K.; Bergquist, K.; Sinha, R. Gender Differences in Response to Emotional Stress: An Assessment Across Subjective, Behavioral, and Physiological Domains and Relations to Alcohol Craving. *Alcohol. Clin. Exp. Res.* **2008**, *32*, 1242–1250. [CrossRef] [PubMed]
43. Feraco, A.; Armani, A.; Amoah, I.; Guseva, E.; Camajani, E.; Gorini, S.; Strollo, R.; Padua, E.; Caprio, M.; Lombardo, M. Assessing gender differences in food preferences and physical activity: A population-based survey. *Front. Nutr.* **2024**, *11*, 1348456. [CrossRef] [PubMed]
44. Colineaux, H.; Neufcourt, L.; Delpierre, C.; Kelly-Irving, M.; Lepage, B. Explaining biological differences between men and women by gendered mechanisms. *Emerg. Themes Epidemiol.* **2023**, *20*, 2. [CrossRef] [PubMed]
45. Bruggink, S.M.; Shomaker, L.B.; Kelly, N.R.; Drinkard, B.E.; Chen, K.Y.; Brychta, R.J.; Cassidy, O.; Demidowich, A.P.; Brady, S.M.; Tanofsky-Kraff, M.; et al. Insulin Sensitivity, Depression/Anxiety, and Physical Fitness in At-Risk Adolescents. *Sports Med. Int. Open* **2019**, *3*, E40–E47. [CrossRef] [PubMed]
46. Lu, W. Adolescent Depression: National Trends, Risk Factors, and Healthcare Disparities. *Am. J. Health Behav.* **2019**, *43*, 181–194. [CrossRef] [PubMed]
47. Muha, J.; Schumacher, A.; Campisi, S.C.; Korczak, D.J. Depression and emotional eating in children and adolescents: A systematic review and meta-analysis. *Appetite* **2024**, *200*, 107511. [CrossRef] [PubMed]
48. Lazarevich, I.; Irigoyen Camacho, M.E.; Velázquez-Alva Mdel, C.; Zepeda Zepeda, M. Relationship among obesity, depression, and emotional eating in young adults. *Appetite* **2016**, *107*, 639–644. [CrossRef] [PubMed]
49. Silva, I.; Meireles, A.L.; dos Santos Chagas, C.M.; Cardoso, C.S.; de Oliveira, H.N.; de Freitas, E.D.; de Carvalho Vidigal, F.; Nobre, L.N.; da Silva, L.S.; de Paula, W.; et al. Emotional Eating and Its Relationship with Symptoms of Anxiety, Depression, and Stress During the COVID-19 Pandemic: A Multicenter Study in College Students. *Int. J. Environ. Res. Public Health* **2025**, *22*, 354. [CrossRef] [PubMed]
50. Ato, M.; López, J.J.; Benavente, A. A classification system for research designs in psychology. *An. Psicol.* **2013**, *29*, 1038–1059.
51. Soper, D. A-Priori Sample Size Calculator for Multiple Regression. Software. 2022. Available online: https://www.danielsoper.com/statcalc/ (accessed on 4 January 2022).
52. Block, G.; Gillespie, C.; Rosenbaum, E.H.; Jenson, C. A rapid food screener to assess fat and fruit and vegetable intake. *Am. J. Prev. Med.* **2000**, *18*, 284–288. [CrossRef] [PubMed]
53. Lopez-Lopez, D.E.; Saavedra-Roman, I.K.; Calizaya-Milla, Y.E.; Saintila, J. Food Addiction, Saturated Fat Intake, and Body Mass Index in Peruvian Adults: A Cross-Sectional Survey. *J. Nutr. Metab.* **2021**, *2021*, 9964143. [CrossRef] [PubMed]
54. Saintila, J.; Morales García, W.C.; Calizaya-Milla, Y.E.; Ruiz Mamani, P.G.; Huancahuire-Vega, S.; Calizaya-Milla, S.E. Psychometric evaluation and invariance of the Spanish version of the Block Fat Screener (BFS-E) in university students. *Front. Psychol.* **2023**, *14*, 1042. [CrossRef] [PubMed]
55. Chen, X.; Wang, S.B.; Li, X.L.; Huang, Z.H.; Tan, W.Y.; Lin, H.C.; Hou, C.-L.; Jia, F.-J. Relationship between sleep duration and sociodemographic characteristics, mental health and chronic diseases in individuals aged from 18 to 85 years old in Guangdong province in China: A population-based cross-sectional study. *BMC Psychiatry* **2020**, *20*, 455. [CrossRef] [PubMed]
56. Hirschler, V.; Aranda, C.; De Luján, M.; Maccalini, G.; Jadzinsky, M. Can waist circumference identify children with the metabolic syndrome? *Arch. Pediatr. Adolesc. Med.* **2005**, *159*, 740–744. [CrossRef] [PubMed]
57. Staples, L.G.; Dear, B.F.; Gandy, M.; Fogliati, V.; Fogliati, R.; Karin, E.; Nielssen, O.; Titov, N. Psychometric properties and clinical utility of brief measures of depression, anxiety, and general distress: The PHQ-2, GAD-2, and K-6. *Gen. Hosp. Psychiatry* **2019**, *56*, 13–18. [CrossRef] [PubMed]
58. Duncan, D.; Goedel, W.; Mayer, K.; Safren, S.; Palamar, J.; Hagen y Gorardin, J. Poor sleep health and its association with mental health, substance use, and condomless anal intercourse among gay, bisexual, and other men who have sex with men. *Physiol. Behav.* **2016**, *2*, 316–321. [CrossRef] [PubMed]
59. Richardson, L.P.; Rockhill, C.; Russo, J.E.; Grossman, D.C.; Richards, J.; McCarty, C.; McCauley, E.; Katon, W. Evaluation of the PHQ-2 as a Brief Screen for Detecting Major Depression Among Adolescents. *Pediatrics* **2010**, *125*, e1097-103. [CrossRef] [PubMed]
60. Baños-Chaparro, J.; Ynquillay-Lima, P.; Lamas, F.; Fuster, F.G. Evidencias psicométricas del Patient Health Questionnarie-2 para la evaluación de síntomas depresivos en adultos peruanos. *Rev. Cienc. Médicas Pinar Del Río* **2021**, *25*, e5064.
61. Garaulet, M.; Canteras, M.; Morales, E.; López-Guimera, G.; Sánchez-Carracedo, D.; Corbalán-Tutau, M.D. Validation of a questionnaire on emotional eating for use in cases of obesity: The Emotional Eater Questionnaire (EEQ). *Nutr. Hosp.* **2012**, *27*, 645–651. [PubMed]
62. Betancourt-Núñez, A.; Torres-Castillo, N.; Martínez-López, E.; De Loera-Rodríguez, C.O.; Durán-Barajas, E.; Márquez-Sandoval, F.; Bernal-Orozco, M.F.; Garaulet, M.; Vizmanos, B. Emotional Eating and Dietary Patterns: Reflecting Food Choices in People with and without Abdominal Obesity. *Nutrients* **2022**, *14*, 1371. [CrossRef] [PubMed]
63. González, M. Validation of emotional eater questionnaire in Chile. *Gen* **2018**, *72*, 21–24.
64. Farhangi, M.A. Night Eating Syndrome and Its Relationship with Emotional Eating, Sleep Quality and Nutritional Status Among Adolescents' Boys. *Community Ment. Health J.* **2019**, *55*, 1411–1418. [CrossRef] [PubMed]

65. Wu, D.; Li, J.; Wang, J. Altered neural activities during emotion regulation in depression: A meta-analysis. *J. Psychiatry Neurosci.* **2024**, *49*, E334–E344. [CrossRef] [PubMed]
66. Ackermans, M.; Jonker, N.; de Jong, P. Adaptive and maladaptive emotion regulation skills are associated with food intake following a hunger-induced increase in negative emotions. *Appetite* **2024**, *193*, 107148. [CrossRef] [PubMed]
67. Chao, A.M.; Jastreboff, A.M.; White, M.A.; Grilo, C.M.; Sinha, R. Stress, cortisol, and other appetite-related hormones: Prospective prediction of 6-month changes in food cravings and weight. *Obesity* **2017**, *25*, 713–720. [CrossRef] [PubMed]
68. van Strien, T.; Gibson, E.L.; Baños, R.; Cebolla, A.; Winkens, L.H.H. Is comfort food actually comforting for emotional eaters? A (moderated) mediation analysis. *Physiol. Behav.* **2019**, *211*, 112671. [CrossRef] [PubMed]
69. Gherasim, A.; Arhire, L.I.; Niță, O.; Popa, A.D.; Graur, M.; Mihalache, L. The relationship between lifestyle components and dietary patterns. *Proc. Nutr. Soc.* **2020**, *79*, 311–323. [CrossRef] [PubMed]
70. Javadi Arjmand, E.; Bemanian, M.; Vold, J.H.; Skogen, J.C.; Sandal, G.M.; Arnesen, E.K.; Mæland, S.; Fadnes, L.T. Emotional Eating and Changes in High-Sugar Food and Drink Consumption Linked to Psychological Distress and Worries: A Cohort Study from Norway. *Nutrients* **2023**, *15*, 778. [CrossRef] [PubMed]
71. Wallace, C.W.; Fordahl, S.C. Obesity and dietary fat influence dopamine neurotransmission: Exploring the convergence of metabolic state, physiological stress, and inflammation on dopaminergic control of food intake. *Nutr. Res. Rev.* **2022**, *35*, 236–251. [CrossRef] [PubMed]
72. Ouwens, M.A.; van Strien, T.; van Leeuwe, J.F.J. Possible pathways between depression, emotional and external eating. A structural equation model. *Appetite* **2009**, *53*, 245–248. [CrossRef] [PubMed]
73. Papaconstantinou, E.; Quick, V.; Vogel, E.; Coffey, S.; Miller, A.; Zitzelsberger, H. Exploring Relationships of Sleep Duration with Eating and Physical Activity Behaviors among Canadian University Students. *Clocks Sleep* **2020**, *2*, 194–207. [CrossRef] [PubMed]
74. Richards, A.L.; Specker, B.L. Exploring Relationships of Eating and Physical Activity Behaviors with Sleep Behaviors Among Adult Weight Loss Participants. *Top. Clin. Nutr.* **2020**, *35*, 50–61. [CrossRef]
75. Liu, S.; Wang, X.; Zheng, Q.; Gao, L.; Sun, Q. Sleep Deprivation and Central Appetite Regulation. *Nutrients* **2022**, *14*, 5196. [CrossRef] [PubMed]
76. Tomaso, C.C.; Johnson, A.B.; Nelson, T.D. The effect of sleep deprivation and restriction on mood, emotion, and emotion regulation: Three meta-analyses in one. *Sleep* **2021**, *44*, zsaa289. [CrossRef] [PubMed]
77. Bernabéu-Brotóns, E.; Marchena-Giráldez, C. Emotional Eating and Perfectionism as Predictors of Symptoms of Binge Eating Disorder: The Role of Perfectionism as a Mediator between Emotional Eating and Body Mass Index. *Nutrients* **2022**, *14*, 3361. [CrossRef] [PubMed]
78. Jääskeläinen, A.; Nevanperä, N.; Remes, J.; Rahkonen, F.; Järvelin, M.R.; Laitinen, J. Stress-related eating, obesity and associated behavioural traits in adolescents: A prospective population-based cohort study. *BMC Public Health* **2014**, *14*, 321. [CrossRef] [PubMed]
79. Husain, S.F.; Ong, S.K.; Cuizhen, L.; Tran, B.; Ho, R.C.; Ho, C.S. Functional near-infrared spectroscopy during a decision-making task in patients with major depressive disorder. *Aust. N. Z. J. Psychiatry* **2021**, *55*, 485–493. [CrossRef] [PubMed]
80. Ho, C.S.H.; Lim, L.J.H.; Lim, A.Q.; Chan, N.H.C.; Tan, R.S.; Lee, S.H.; Ho, R.C.M. Diagnostic and Predictive Applications of Functional Near-Infrared Spectroscopy for Major Depressive Disorder: A Systematic Review. *Front. Psychiatry* **2020**, *11*, 378. [CrossRef] [PubMed]
81. Davila-Torres, D.M.; Vilcas-Solís, G.E.; Rodríguez-Vásquez, M.; Calizaya-Milla, Y.E.; Saintila, J. Eating habits and mental health among rugby players of the Peruvian pre-selection during the second quarantine due to the COVID-19 pandemic. *SAGE Open Med.* **2021**, *9*, 205031212110437. [CrossRef] [PubMed]

nutrients

MDPI

Article

Associations of Dietary Inflammatory and Antioxidant Indices with Mental Health Indicators Among University Students: A Cross-Sectional Study

Merve Esra Çıtar Dazıroğlu [1], Saniye Bilici [1] and Perim Fatma Türker [2,*]

[1] Department of Nutrition and Dietetics, Faculty of Health Sciences, Gazi University, 06560 Ankara, Türkiye; esracitar@gazi.edu.tr (M.E.Ç.D.); sgbilici@gazi.edu.tr (S.B.)

[2] Department of Nutrition and Dietetics, Faculty of Health Sciences, Acıbadem Mehmet Ali Aydınlar University, 34638 İstanbul, Türkiye

* Correspondence: perim.turker@acibadem.edu.tr

Abstract

Background/Objectives: Protecting students' mental health during university is essential for their future quality of life. Therefore, diet should be emphasized as a complementary and preventive strategy in supporting and maintaining mental health. This study aimed to examine the association between dietary inflammatory and antioxidant indices and mental health indicators (depression, anxiety, stress, and well-being) in university students. **Methods:** This cross-sectional study included 907 university students. We collected dietary data using a 24 h recall. Based on this data, we used 33 food parameters to calculate the Dietary Inflammatory Index (DII) and 6 antioxidant nutrients to calculate the Dietary Antioxidant Index (DAI). We evaluated mental health using the Depression, Anxiety, and Stress Scales-21 (DASS-21), and assessed well-being using the World Health Organization Five Well-Being Index (WHO-5). **Results:** Overall, 62.4% of participants reported symptoms of depression, 56.2% anxiety, and 40.7% stress. Anxiety and stress levels were significantly higher among females compared to males ($p < 0.001$ and $p = 0.005$, respectively). In fully adjusted models, depression scores were significantly higher in the highest DII tertile compared to the lowest (B = 1.74; 95% CI: 0.24–3.26), while well-being was lower (B = −0.82; 95% CI: −1.65 to −0.00). For DAI, participants in tertile 2 had significantly lower anxiety (B = −1.38; 95% CI: −2.63 to −0.14), depression (B = −1.69; 95% CI: −3.19 to −0.19), and stress (B = −1.70; 95% CI: −3.22 to −0.18) scores compared to tertile 1. No significant association was found between DAI and well-being. **Conclusions:** In this study, university students' pro-inflammatory diets were associated with poorer mental health profiles. Enhancing the diet's anti-inflammatory potential may be a promising strategy to support mental health in this population.

Keywords: mental health; university student; diet; inflammation; antioxidant

1. Introduction

Mental health refers to a state of well-being in which an individual realizes their abilities, copes with the everyday stresses of life, works productively, and contributes to the society in which they live [1]. Problems related to mental health, which have a very important place for everyone and everywhere, are unfortunately common [2]. Although mental disorders include a wide range of problems with different symptoms, they are often characterized by a combination of abnormal feelings, thoughts, behaviors, and relationships with others [1]. The latest data from the World Health Organization (WHO) has shown that 970 million people around the world continue to live with mental health problems. The majority of them are anxious, 31.0%, and depressed, 28.9% [2].

University students often struggle with numerous challenges, including increased academic pressures, social adjustments, and economic difficulties. They also become vulnerable to mental health concerns, including anxiety, depression, and stress, due to the stressors associated with navigating a new environment, balancing academic responsibilities, and adapting to greater independence, which can impact their academic performance, personal well-being, and overall quality of life [3]. Also, factors like food insecurity, housing instability, perfectionism, and lack of knowledge of how to shop and cook healthily can further impact their well-being [4].

Previous studies have indicated that biological pathways may affect the relationships between diet quality and mental health, such as the dysregulated hypothalamic–pituitary–adrenal (HPA) axis and inflammation [5].

For mental health, omega-3 fatty acids, phospholipids, cholesterol, niacin, folate, vitamin B_6, and vitamin B_{12} reflect nutrients that may be beneficial, while saturated fat and simple sugar are considered detrimental to cognitive function [6]. Also, inflammatory dietary patterns may be associated with mental well-being. The brain is particularly vulnerable to oxidative stress as it is rich in lipids in the neuronal membrane and is metabolically active [7,8].

In a systematic review and meta-analysis, it is mentioned that a one-unit increase in the dietary inflammatory index (DII) is associated with a 6% increased risk for symptoms of depression, and an increase in the inflammatory burden of diet was found to be significantly associated with various mental health outcomes [9]. Studies conducted among adolescents and adults suggest that a higher Dietary Antioxidant Index (DAI) may be related to better mental health outcomes. Antioxidants support mental health by reducing oxidative stress, a key contributor to depression, highlighting the potential role of an antioxidant- and anti-inflammatory-rich diet in improving psychological well-being [10]. During the transition to university, students may change their eating habits, such as increasing fast food consumption, relying more on take-out meals, and having a reduced intake of fresh food, which can lead to poor diet quality [11].

Studies investigating the associations between diet quality and mental health have previously focused on the general population, but studies involving the student population in Türkiye are scarce. Also, various studies conducted to date have revealed that the inflammatory load of the diet is associated with multiple mental health problems. However, well-being is less of an issue and addressing this in this study is very important. Moreover, the literature on the effects of DII and dietary antioxidant capacity on mental health and well-being is still limited. Therefore, this study aims to evaluate the impact of the DII and DAI on depression, anxiety, stress, and well-being among university students.

2. Materials and Methods

2.1. Study Design and Participants

This cross-sectional study was conducted with 907 volunteer university students (268 males, 639 females) in Ankara, the capital city of Türkiye, using convenience and snowball sampling methods. The university students agreed to participate in the study with written informed consent in accordance with the Declaration of Helsinki.

We used a demographic questionnaire, a 24 h dietary recall, the Depression, Anxiety, and Stress Scale (DASS-21), the WHO-5 Well-Being Index, and anthropometric measurements (body weight and height) as data collection tools. Body mass index (BMI) was calculated by dividing weight in kilograms by the square of height in meters (kg/m^2) [12]. The research data were collected by the students using the face-to-face interview technique.

We excluded individuals with chronic diseases, diagnosed psychological disorders, those using antidepressants, or those following a special diet or eating pattern from the study.

2.2. Depression, Anxiety, and Stress Scales

The Depression, Anxiety, and Stress Scales (DASS-21), developed by Lovibond and Lovibond to measure negative emotional states related to depression, anxiety, and stress [13,14], has been adapted into Turkish and validated by Sarıçam (2018) [15]. The scale in question consists of three subscales, namely depression, anxiety, and stress, and includes a total of 21 items, with 7 items in each category. The scale is a 4-point Likert-type scale from 0 to 3 for scoring the items, and it ranges from 0 to 21 for each subscale. Since the DASS-21 is the short version of the original 42-item DASS, the final score for each subscale is multiplied by two (*2). Based on these scores, depression, anxiety, and stress levels are categorized as normal, mild, moderate, severe, or extremely severe [13,14].

2.3. World Health Organization (WHO) (Five) Well-Being Index

Developed by the WHO, the WHO (Five) Well-Being Index is a short scale that evaluates emotional well-being in healthy and diseased individuals [16,17]. The Turkish validity and reliability study of the index was conducted by Eser et al. [18]. The scale includes 5 positive statements about the emotions of the participant in the last 2 weeks. Each item on the scale is between 0 and 5 points and is evaluated with a 6-point Likert type scale. A score of 0 on the scale indicates no positive emotions in the last two weeks, and a score of 5 indicates continuous positive emotions. On the scale, where the raw score ranges from 0 to 25 points, the raw score is multiplied by 4 to obtain a percentage score between 0 and 100. The higher the score from the index, the higher the well-being [16,17].

2.4. Assessment of Dietary Intake

We used the 24 h dietary recall method to evaluate the participants' food intake. For this, we asked the participants to record all the food and beverages they consumed the day before. To assess participants' energy and nutrient intake, we calculated the average daily values using the Nutrition Information System (BeBis) 8.2 program [19].

2.5. Assessment of Dietary Inflammatory Index (DII)

We used dietary data from the 24 h recall to calculate participants' DII scores. DII was first created by Cavicchia et al. in 2009 to measure the overall effect of diet on inflammatory potential [20], and was later developed by Shivappa et al. in 2014 [21]. In this study, we calculated the DII as described in the work of Shivappa et al. [21]. For the calculation, we subtracted the global average daily consumption amounts from the participants' average daily intake of foods and nutrients, and divided the result by the standard deviation. We converted these to percentiles to reduce the right skewness of the obtained z-scores. Then, we multiplied the percentile values by 2 and subtracted 1 from the result. We multiplied the centered percentile values obtained after this procedure by the customized Inflammatory Effect Score value of that food and nutrient. This way, we calculated the DII value of each food and nutrient. As a result of the sum of these values, the total DII scores from the foods in the diet of the individuals were calculated [21]. Since there are no data on some DII components (flavonoids and spices) these were not included in the calculation of DII in this study, and the calculation was based on a total of 33 nutrients and elements. A resulting negative DII score was associated with an anti-inflammatory effect, while a positive score was associated with a pro-inflammatory effect.

2.6. Assessment of Dietary Antioxidant Index (DAI)

We calculated the DAI using the method described by Wright et al. [22] to assess the overall antioxidant capacity of a diet. We determined the intake of six dietary antioxidants (vitamins A, C, and E, magnesium, selenium, and zinc) for all participants. We normalized each micronutrient intake by subtracting the mean intake and dividing by the standard deviation (SD). We summed the resulting standardized values for the six components to obtain the overall DAI score. The detailed calculation formula was as follows.

$$\mathrm{DAI} = \sum_{i=1}^{n=6} \frac{\text{Individual Intake} - \text{Mean}}{\text{SD}}$$

2.7. Data Analysis

The data collected via the questionnaire were analyzed and interpreted using a statistical software package. The Kolmogorov–Smirnov test was applied to assess the normality of the data distribution. We presented descriptive statistics as frequency (percentage) for categorical variables and mean ± standard deviation (SD) for continuous variables. We used Pearson's Chi-square test to examine the association between categorical variables. We performed Kruskal–Wallis/Mann–Whitney U analysis to determine the significance of the difference between the means of the groups. We conducted multivariable linear regression analyses to examine the independent effects of the DII and DAI on depression, anxiety, stress, and mental well-being. DII and DAI were included in each model as independent variables, with sex, age, and BMI added as covariates to control for potential confounding. Considering that the study sample predominantly consisted of female participants and individuals with a normal BMI, and that both variables are known potential confounders in the association between diet and mental health, adjusting for them contributed to improving the model accuracy. We examined the relationship between categorical variables using Chi-square analysis. We evaluated results at a 95% confidence interval and considered them statistically significant at a $p < 0.05$ level.

2.8. Ethical Considerations

The study protocol was approved by the Ethical Committee of Gazi University (Number: E-77082166-604.01.02-609239, Date: 10 March 2023).

3. Results

Table 1 compares sociodemographic characteristics, mental health scores, and dietary indices by gender. Females had significantly lower BMI, mental well-being, and dietary antioxidant index scores, but higher DII scores than males ($p < 0.05$). A substantial proportion of participants experienced depression (62.4%), anxiety (56.2%), and stress (40.7%), with moderate levels appearing to be the most prevalent for each condition. In addition, the prevalence of anxiety and stress was significantly higher among females compared to males ($p < 0.05$).

Figure 1 shows the mean scores of depression, anxiety, stress, and well-being according to the tertiles of the participants' DII scores. Accordingly, the mean well-being score in tertile 3 was significantly lower than in both tertiles 1 and 2.

The mean scores of depression, anxiety, stress, and well-being according to the tertiles of the participants' DAI scores are given in Figure 2. Accordingly, we observed no statistically significant difference between the tertiles' mean values for any mental health indicators.

Table 1. Some general features of participants according to gender.

	Overall (n = 907)	Male (n = 268)	Female (n = 639)	Z	χ^2	p-Value
Age (year), $\overline{X} \pm SS$	21.7 ± 1.63	22.0 ± 1.63	21.6 ± 1.61	−3.826		**0.000**
BMI (kg/m^2), $\overline{X} \pm SS$	22.6 ± 3.18	24.4 ± 2.98	21.9 ± 2.94	−11.857		**0.002**
BMI category, n (%)						
<18.5	61 (6.7%)	4 (1.5%)	57 (8.9%)			
18.5–24.9	651 (71.8%)	152 (56.7%)	499 (78.1%)		100.360	**0.000**
≥25.0	195 (21.5%)	112 (41.8%)	83 (13.0%)			
DASS scores						
Depression, $\overline{X} \pm SS$	13.2 ± 9.42	12.4 ± 8.71	13.6 ± 9.69	−1.169		0.242
Depression status, n (%)	566 (62.4%)	167 (62.3%)	399 (62.4%)		28.665	0.122
Normal	341 (37.6%)	101 (37.7%)	240 (37.6%)			
Mild	152 (16.8%)	42 (15.7%)	110 (17.2%)			
Moderate	242 (26.7%)	87 (32.5%)	155 (24.3%)			
Severe	96 (10.6%)	25 (9.3%)	71 (11.1%)			
Extremely severe	76 (8.4%)	13 (4.9%)	63 (9.9%)			
Anxiety, $\overline{X} \pm SS$	9.8 ± 7.99	7.3 ± 6.93	10.9 ± 8.16	−6.571		**0.000**
Anxiety status, n (%)	510 (56.2%)	113 (42.2%)	397 (62.1%)		59.916	**0.000**
Normal	397 (43.8%)	155 (57.8%)	242 (37.9%)			
Mild	96 (10.6%)	31 (11.6%)	65 (10.2%)			
Moderate	201 (22.2%)	46 (17.2%)	155 (24.3%)			
Severe	93 (10.3%)	15 (5.6%)	78 (12.2%)			
Extremely severe	120 (13.2%)	21 (7.8%)	99 (15.5%)			
Stress ($\overline{X} \pm SS$)	14.2 ± 9.64	12.4 ± 9.28	14.9 ± 9.70	−3.464		**0.001**
Stress status, n (%)	369 (40.7%)	90 (33.6%)	279 (43.7%)		7.950	**0.005**
Normal	538 (59.3%)	178 (66.4%)	360 (56.3%)			
Mild	112 (12.3%)	26 (9.7%)	86 (13.5%)			
Moderate	137 (15.1%)	36 (13.4%)	101 (15.8%)			
Severe	71 (7.8%)	18 (6.7%)	53 (8.3%)			
Extremely severe	49 (5.4%)	10 (3.7%)	39 (6.1%)			
Mental well-being score, $\overline{X} \pm SS$	12.1 ± 5.18	12.9 ± 5.00	11.7 ± 5.22	−3.072		**0.002**
Dietary inflammatory index, $\overline{X} \pm SS$	2.1 ± 1.76	1.8 ± 1.81	2.2 ± 1.72	−3.415		**0.001**
Dietary antioxidant index, $\overline{X} \pm SS$	0.0 ± 3.45	0.7 ± 3.32	−0.3 ± 3.47	−4.268		**0.000**

Statistically significant p-values are shown in bold.

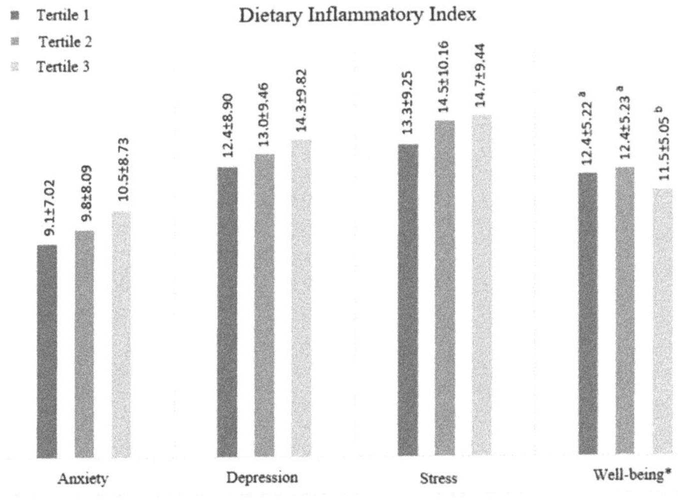

Figure 1. Mean scores of participants' mental health and well-being traits according to DII. Significant differences (p < 0.05) are indicated with an asterisk (*) on the figure. [a,b] represent the statistically significant differences among the groups.

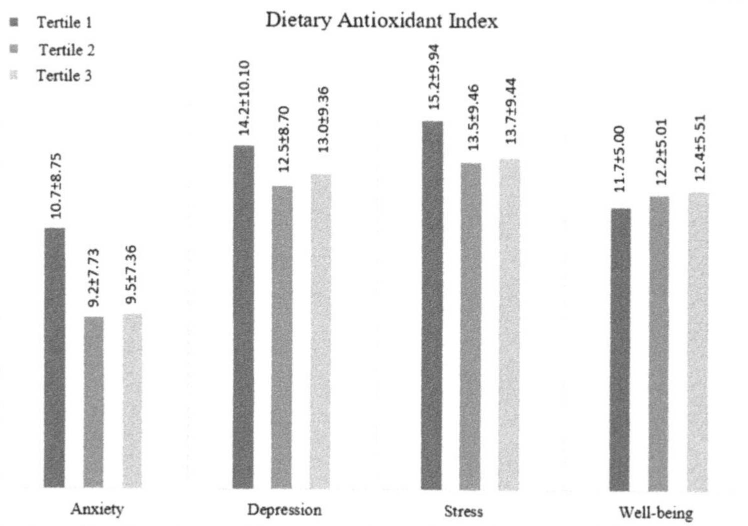

Figure 2. Mean scores of participants' mental health and well-being traits according to DAI.

We conducted multivariable regression analyses based on DII tertiles to examine the associations between DII and depression, anxiety, stress, and well-being (Table 2). According to the initial unadjusted analysis (Model 1), the group with the most pro-inflammatory diet (tertile 3) had significantly higher anxiety (B = 1.33; 95% CI: 0.06–2.61) and depression (B = 1.90; 95% CI: 0.40–3.40) scores compared to the reference group (tertile 1). In addition, well-being scores were significantly lower in this group (B = −0.98; 95% CI: −1.81 to −0.16). After adjusting for sex (Model 2), depression scores remained significantly higher in the tertile 3 group (B = 1.78; 95% CI: 0.27–3.29), and well-being scores remained significantly lower (B = −0.84; 95% CI: −1.67 to −0.01). In Model 3, which was adjusted for both sex and BMI, depression (B = 1.74; 95% CI: 0.24–3.26) and well-being (B= −0.82; 95% CI: −1.65–0.00) scores in the tertile 3 group remained significantly higher.

Table 2. Associations of DII with depression, anxiety, stress, and well-being.

Mental Health Profile	Dietary Inflammatory Index		
	Tertile 1 (*n* = 302)	**Tertile 2 (*n* = 303) B (95% CI)**	**Tertile 3 (*n* = 302) B (95% CI)**
Anxiety			
Model 1	Ref	0.73 (−0.54 to 2.00) $p = 0.261$	1.33 (0.06 to 2.61) $\mathbf{p = 0.041}$
Model 2	Ref	0.48 (−0.77 to 1.73) $p = 0.449$	0.89 (−0.37 to 2.15) $p = 0.164$
Model 3	Ref	0.42 (−0.83 to 1.67) $p = 0.507$	0.88 (−0.38 to 2.13) $p = 0.170$
Depression			
Model 1	Ref	0.59 (−0.91 to 2.09) $p = 0.443$	1.90 (0.40 to 3.40) $\mathbf{p = 0.013}$
Model 2	Ref	0.52 (−0.99 to 2.02) $p = 0.500$	1.78 (0.27 to 3.29) $\mathbf{p = 0.021}$
Model 3	Ref	0.48 (−1.02 to 1.98) $p = 0.533$	1.74 (0.24 to 3.26) $\mathbf{p = 0.023}$

Table 2. *Cont.*

Mental Health Profile	Dietary Inflammatory Index		
	Tertile 1 (*n* = 302)	**Tertile 2 (*n* = 303) B (95% CI)**	**Tertile 3 (*n* = 302) B (95% CI)**
Stress			
Model 1	Ref	1.21 (−0.32 to 2.75) $p = 0.122$	1.43 (−0.11 to 2.97) $p = 0.068$
Model 2	Ref	1.05 (−0.49 to 2.58) $p = 0.180$	1.14 (−0.40 to 2.68) $p = 0.147$
Model 3	Ref	0.96 (−0.56 to 2.45) $p = 0.216$	1.11 (−0.41 to 2.65) $p = 0.152$
Well-being			
Model 1	Ref	−0.06 (−0.89 to 0.76) $p = 0.885$	−0.98 (−1.81 to −0.16) **$p = 0.020$**
Model 2	Ref	0.02 (−0.81 to 0.84) $p = 0.967$	−0.84 (−1.67 to −0.01) **$p = 0.047$**
Model 3	Ref	0.06 (−0.76 to 0.88) $p = 0.891$	−0.82 (−1.65 to 0.00) **$p = 0.050$**

Model 1: crude, Model 2: adjusted for sex, Model 3: Additionally adjusted for age and BMI. Statistically significant *p*-values are shown in bold.

According to Table 3, which examines the associations between DAI tertiles and depression, anxiety, stress, and well-being, in Model 2 adjusted for sex, anxiety (B: −1.34; 95% CI: −2.59 to −0.09), depression (B: −1.70; 95% CI: −3.21 to −1.00), and stress (B: −1.63; 95% CI: −3.16 to −0.10) scores were significantly lower in the tertile 2 group compared to the tertile 1 group. In Model 3, additionally adjusted for age and BMI, these associations remained significant, and the tertile 2 group had significantly lower anxiety (B: −1.38; 95% CI: −2.63 to −0.14), depression (B: −1.69; 95% CI: −3.19 to −0.19), and stress (B: −1.70; 95% CI: −3.22 to −0.18) scores compared to the tertile 1 group.

Table 3. Associations of DAI with depression, anxiety, stress, and well-being. (95% CI).

Mental Health Profile	Dietary Antioxidant Index		
	Tertile 1 (*n* = 303)	**Tertile 2 (*n* = 301) B (95% CI)**	**Tertile 3 (*n* = 303) B (95% CI)**
Anxiety			
Model 1	Ref	−1.45 (−2.72 to −0.18) **$p = 0.026$**	−1.22 (−2.49 to 0.06) $p = 0.061$
Model 2	Ref	−1.34 (−2.59 to −0.09) **$p = 0.035$**	−0.75 (−2.00 to 0.51) $p = 0.242$
Model 3	Ref	−1.38 (−2.63 to −0.14) **$p = 0.030$**	−0.69 (−1.95 to 0.56) $p = 0.277$
Depression			
Model 1	Ref	−1.73 (−3.24 to −0.23) **$p = 0.024$**	−1.19 (−2.69 to 0.31) $p = 0.120$
Model 2	Ref	−1.70 (−3.21 to −1.00) **$p = 0.027$**	−1.04 (−2.55 to 0.47) $p = 0.175$
Model 3	Ref	−1.69 (−3.19 to −0.19) **$p = 0.028$**	−0.93 (−2.44 to 0.58) $p = 0.228$

Table 3. *Cont.*

Mental Health Profile	Dietary Antioxidant Index		
	Tertile 1 (n = 303)	**Tertile 2 (n = 301) B (95% CI)**	**Tertile 3 (n = 303) B (95% CI)**
Stress			
Model 1	Ref	−1.71 (−3.24 to −0.17) **p = 0.030**	−1.53 (−3.06 to 0.01) p = 0.051
Model 2	Ref	−1.63 (−3.16 to −0.10) **p = 0.036**	−1.21 (−2.75 to 0.32) p = 0.121
Model 3	Ref	−1.70 (−3.22 to −0.18) **p = 0.029**	−1.15 (−2.68 to 0.38) p = 0.141
Well-being			
Model 1	Ref	0.46 (−0.37 to 1.28) p = 0.279	0.64 (−0.19 to 1.46) p = 0.131
Model 2	Ref	0.42 (−0.40 to 1.25) p = 0.317	0.49 (−0.34 to 1.31) p = 0.250
Model 3	Ref	0.43 (−0.39 to 1.26) p = 0.301	0.43 (−0.40 to 1.25) p = 0.314

Model 1: crude, Model 2: adjusted for sex, Model 3: Additionally adjusted for age and BMI. Statistically significant *p*-values are shown in bold.

4. Discussion

In addition to coping with academic pressure, university can be stressful for some students for various reasons, including separation from family and the addition of individualization or job responsibilities. In this context, many university students experience the first onset of mental health problems or the exacerbation of their symptoms during this period [23].

Anxiety and depression are the most common mental health issues among university students, but also problems such as eating disorders, attention deficit/hyperactivity disorder, or schizophrenia can be encountered [23]. A study has shown that 11.94% of university students have anxiety and 7.04% have major depressive disorder [24]. In a study conducted by another group of researchers, it was reported that the prevalence of depression was 17.3% and anxiety was 9.8% [25]. In another study conducted among university students, approximately half of the participants were found to experience depression (48.2%), anxiety (59.8%), and stress (48.2%). Anxiety and stress levels were significantly higher in the female group. When examining severity levels, a greater number of individuals were found in the mild category; however, it is also noteworthy that there were individuals with the highest severity levels, particularly in anxiety, but also in depression and stress [26]. Early detection of these mental health problems, which are common among university students, can reduce attrition and improve educational and psychosocial functionality with effective treatments [27]. In our study, we observed high rates of depression (62.4%), anxiety (56.2%), and stress (40.7%) among participants. Across all three domains, moderate severity levels were the most commonly reported. However, we also observed severe and extremely severe levels in both genders across all three subscales, particularly in the anxiety dimension, indicating that psychological distress was not limited to moderate severity. Furthermore, female participants exhibited significantly higher levels of anxiety and stress than their male counterparts ($p < 0.05$) (Table 1).

DII was developed to determine the inflammatory potential of the diet [21], and this index has been associated with some inflammatory markers such as CRP and IL-6 in various studies [28–31]. In our study, we found that the majority of participants (approximately 72%) had a BMI within the normal range, suggesting that the influence of obesity-related inflammation may have been limited. Moreover, by including BMI as a covariate in the adjusted regression models, we aimed to ensure that the associations observed between dietary indices (e.g., DII) and mental health outcomes more accurately reflected diet-related effects independent of body weight status. This approach strengthens the interpretability of the findings by minimizing the potential confounding effect of obesity. Low-grade, chronic systemic inflammation is now recognized to be associated with most noncommunicable diseases (NCDs), including obesity, diabetes, cardiovascular diseases, respiratory and musculoskeletal disorders, and cancers, as well as impaired neurodevelopment and adverse mental health outcomes [32]. Relatedly, the focus has been on whether the quality of diet contributes to the psychopathology of widespread mental problems such as depression and anxiety [33]. On the contrary, antioxidants come to the forefront in preventing this and support brain health [34].

In our study, the significant associations between both DII and DAI and depression remained in the fully adjusted models. For DII, depression scores were significantly higher in tertile 3 compared to tertile 1 across all models. In contrast, for DAI, all adjusted models showed that participants in tertile 2 had significantly lower depression scores compared to those in tertile 1 (Tables 2 and 3). Other investigators have supported similar findings to those in our study, and these studies reported an increased risk of depression among those on the most pro-inflammatory diets [35,36]. For example, women on the most anti-inflammatory diets were found to have an approximately 20% lower risk of developing depression than women on the most pro-inflammatory diet [36]. Salari-Moghaddam et al. [37] found that adherence to a pro-inflammatory diet was positively associated with psychological disorders. Individuals in the highest quintile of the DII score had higher depression compared to those in the lowest quartile (6.56 ± 0.16 vs. 5.48 ± 0.16; $p < 0.001$), anxiety (3.85 ± 0.17 vs. 3.09 ± 0.17; $p = 0.006$), and had psychological distress (2.42 ± 0.13 vs. 1.77 ± 0.13; $p = 0.001$) [37]. Similarly, a pro-inflammatory diet has been associated with a higher risk of various mental health problems in several other studies in different populations [38,39]. Contrastingly, Bergmans et al. [40] found that higher DII scores were also associated with more than twice the likelihood of depression in adults in the US (OR (95% CI) = 1.81 (1.20, 2.71) for the highest vs. lowest quintile, Type III p- value = 0.0167), but found no significant results for anxiety [40]. In a study conducted among middle-aged and older American adults, the composite dietary antioxidant index (CDAI) was found to be linearly and inversely associated with depression, and nonlinearly and inversely related to all-cause mortality [41]. Similar findings have been supported in different study populations, highlighting the inverse relationship between depression and CDAI [42,43].

For anxiety, according to the initial unadjusted analysis (Model 1) participants in tertile 3 had significantly higher anxiety scores compared to tertile 1. However, this association lost its statistical significance after adjustments for confounding variables. Regarding DAI, we found that tertile 2 was associated with significantly lower levels of anxiety compared to tertile 1 in all adjusted models (Tables 2 and 3). Focusing specifically on anxiety, Torabynasab et al. [44] calculated the dietary inflammatory index (EDII) scores of 85 patients with anxiety and healthy individuals ($n = 85$) by taking the frequency of food consumption. As a result, they observed that individuals in the highest category of EDII score were 2.09 times more likely to have an anxiety disorder compared to those in the lower category (OR: 2.09, %95 GA: 1.01, 4.33) [44].

In our study, for DAI all of the adjusted models showed that participants in tertile 2 had significantly lower stress levels than those in tertile 1 (Tables 2 and 3). In a study conducted with university students living in dormitories in the United Arab Emirates, the association of stress, in addition to anxiety, with EDII scores was highlighted. Logistic regression analysis results showed each point increased anxiety (OR = 1.35; 95% CI: 1.07–

1.69; $p = 0.01$) and stress symptoms (OR = 1.41; 95% CI: 1.12–1.77; $p = 0.003$) [45]. Adolescent girls with the highest level of pro-inflammatory diet in Iran were found to have higher stress scores calculated by DASS-21 [46]. Chronic stress contributes to the development of oxidative stress in the brain, while antioxidants play an active role in its prevention and management [47]. However, it is important to emphasize that the relationship is bidirectional. While dietary changes can trigger stress by directly affecting mood, the development of stress can also lead to negative eating behaviors [48]. Stress has been reported to be associated with unhealthy diets in university students [49].

Mental well-being is essential to overall quality of life. When the level of well-being is high, the probability of experiencing mental illness decreases [50]. According to the initial unadjusted analysis (Model 1), participants in the most pro-inflammatory diet group (tertile 3) had significantly lower well-being scores compared to the reference group (tertile 1). This association remained significant after adjustment for sex, with well-being scores still significantly lower in tertile 3 (Table 2). The results of a cross-sectional study showed that while the risk of depression and anxiety is higher in the tertile with the highest EDII score, well-being is lower. Also, this only applies to women [51].

The different results between studies on the relationship of DII and DAI with mental health outcomes may be related to the gender, race, or many other general characteristics of the studied groups. In addition, reasons such as the difference in the scales used to evaluate mental health problems or the non-standardity of the components used for calculating DII or DAI may explain the difference between studies.

This study has some limitations. First, the gender distribution of the sample was unbalanced, with a higher proportion of female participants. Although we adjusted for gender in the regression models to mitigate this effect, caution is warranted when generalizing the findings to a more gender-balanced population. In addition, depression, anxiety, stress, and well-being are closely interconnected, and their impact on each other is undeniable. Therefore, the relationship between these mental health indicators and the nutritional indices examined may reflect a general mental health pattern rather than a domain-specific effect. This possibility should be taken into account when interpreting the results. And finally, we did not assess factors such as smoking status, socioeconomic level, academic performance, physical activity levels, or sleep quality, as these variables were not included in the survey. These unmeasured variables may act as potential confounders and limit the interpretation of the observed associations. Future studies that include these variables and use more representative sampling methods are needed to strengthen the evidence.

5. Conclusions

The findings of this study provide additional evidence supporting the relationship between dietary patterns and mental health outcomes among young adults. In this study, higher dietary inflammatory potential, as reflected by increased DII scores, was significantly associated with higher depression levels and lower well-being, even after adjusting for confounding variables. Conversely, moderate dietary antioxidant intake (tertile 2 of DAI) was linked to lower depression, anxiety, and stress scores compared to lower antioxidant intake. These findings suggest that pro-inflammatory and antioxidant dietary patterns may influence young adults' mental health. University years are essential for mental health, with long-term effects on overall life outcomes. Therefore, supporting students' nutrition through public catering services in the university environment and designing menus suitable for the Mediterranean diet profile may be beneficial for promoting students' well-being. Further studies with larger samples are recommended to determine nutritional strategies specific to university students.

Author Contributions: Conceptualization, S.B. and M.E.Ç.D.; methodology, S.B., M.E.Ç.D. and P.F.T.; software, M.E.Ç.D.; formal analysis, M.E.Ç.D.; investigation, S.B., M.E.Ç.D. and P.F.T.; resources, M.E.Ç.D.; data curation, S.B. and M.E.Ç.D.; writing—original draft preparation, M.E.Ç.D.; writing—review and editing, S.B. and P.F.T.; visualization, M.E.Ç.D.; supervision, S.B. All authors have read and agreed to the published version of the manuscript.

Funding: This research received no external funding.

Institutional Review Board Statement: The study protocol was approved by the Ethical Committee of Gazi University (Number: E-77082166-604.01.02-609239, 10 March 2023).

Informed Consent Statement: The university students agreed to participate in the study with written informed consent in accordance with the Declaration of Helsinki.

Data Availability Statement: Due to privacy restrictions, the data are available from the corresponding author upon request.

Conflicts of Interest: The authors declare no conflicts of interest.

References

1. World Health Organization. *Mental Health Action Plan 2013–2020*; World Health Organization: Geneva, Switzerland, 2013.
2. World Health Organization. *World Mental Health Report: Transforming Mental Health for All*; World Health Organization: Geneva, Switzerland, 2022.
3. Ghatpande, A.C.; Anand, S.K. Mental Health and Stress Management Among College Students: A Critical Analysis. *Int. J. Sci. Res. Eng. Manag.* **2025**, *9*, 1–3. [CrossRef]
4. Shi, Y.; Grech, A.; Allman-Farinelli, M. Diet quality among students attending an Australian university is compromised by food insecurity and less frequent intake of home cooked meals. A cross-sectional survey using the validated healthy eating index for Australian adults (HEIFA-2013). *Nutrients* **2022**, *14*, 4522. [CrossRef]
5. Marx, W.; Lane, M.; Hockey, M.; Aslam, H.; Berk, M.; Walder, K.; Borsini, A.; Firth, J.; Pariante, C.M.; Berding, K.; et al. Diet and depression: Exploring the biological mechanisms of action. *Mol. Psychiatry* **2021**, *26*, 134–150. [CrossRef]
6. Lim, S.Y.; Kim, E.J.; Kim, A.; Lee, H.J.; Choi, H.J.; Yang, S.J. Nutritional factors affecting mental health. *Clin. Nutr. Res.* **2016**, *5*, 143–152. [CrossRef]
7. Conner, T.S.; Brookie, K.L.; Carr, A.C.; Mainvil, L.A.; Vissers, M.C.M. Let them eat fruit! The effect of fruit and vegetable consumption on psychological well-being in young adults: A randomized controlled trial. *PLoS ONE* **2017**, *12*, e0171206. [CrossRef]
8. Lycett, K.M.; Wijayawickrama, D.J.; Liu, M.; Grobler, A.; Burgner, D.P.; Baur, L.A.; Liu, R.; Lange, K.; Wake, M.; Kerr, J.A. Does an inflammatory diet affect mental well-being in late childhood and mid-life? A cross-sectional study. *Br. J. Nutr.* **2022**, *127*, 939–947. [CrossRef]
9. Chen, G.-Q.; Peng, C.-L.; Lian, Y.; Wang, B.-W.; Chen, P.-Y.; Wang, G.-P. Association between dietary inflammatory index and mental health: A systematic review and dose–response meta-analysis. *Front. Nutr.* **2021**, *8*, 662357. [CrossRef]
10. Pourmontaseri, H.; Bazmi, S.; Sepehrinia, M.; Mostafavi, A.; Arefnezhad, R.; Homayounfar, R.; Vahid, F. Exploring the application of dietary antioxidant index for disease risk assessment: A comprehensive review. *Front. Nutr.* **2025**, *11*, 1497364. [CrossRef]
11. Solomou, S.; Robinson, H.; Perez-Algorta, G. The association of diet quality with the mental health of students during their transition to university. *PLoS ONE* **2024**, *19*, e0312123. [CrossRef]
12. World Health Organization. *Obesity: Preventing and Managing the Global Epidemic: Report of a WHO Consultation*; World Health Organization: Geneva, Switzerland, 2000; p. 894.
13. Lovibond, P.F.; Lovibond, S.H. The structure of negative emotional states: Comparison of the Depression Anxiety Stress Scales (DASS) with the Beck Depression and Anxiety Inventories. *Behav. Res. Ther.* **1995**, *33*, 335–343. [CrossRef]
14. Lovibond, S.H.; Lovibond, P.F. *Manual for the Depression Anxiety Stress Scales*, 2nd ed.; Psychology Foundation: Sydney, Australia, 1995.
15. Sarıçam, H. The psychometric properties of Turkish version of Depression Anxiety Stress Scale-21 (DASS-21) in health control and clinical samples. *J. Cogn.-Behav. Psychother. Res.* **2018**, *7*, 19–30.
16. Bech, P.; Gudex, C.; Johansen, K.S. The WHO (Ten) well-being index: Validation in diabetes. *Psychiatry Psychol.* **1996**, *65*, 183–190.
17. Topp, C.W.; Østergaard, S.D.; Søndergaard, S.; Bech, P. The WHO-5 Well-Being Index: A systematic review of the literature. *Psychiatry Psychol.* **2015**, *84*, 167–176. [CrossRef]

18. Eser, E.; Çevik, C.; Baydur, H.; Güneş, S.; Esgin, T.A.; Öztekin, Ç.S.; Eker, E.; Gümüşsoy, U.; Eser, G.B.; Özyurt, B. Reliability and validity of the Turkish version of the WHO-5, in adults and older adults for its use in primary care settings. *Prim. Health Care Res. Dev.* **2019**, *20*, e100. [CrossRef]
19. *BeBis*, version 8.2. Nutrition Data Base Software: The German Food Code and Nutrient Data Base (BLS II.3, 1999) with Additions from USDA-SR and Other Sources [Computer Program]. Beslenme Bilgi Sistemleri Ltd.: Istanbul, Turkey, 2004.
20. Cavicchia, P.P.; Steck, S.E.; Hurley, T.G.; Hussey, J.R.; Ma, Y.; Ockene, I.S.; Hébert, J.R. A new dietary inflammatory index predicts interval changes in serum high-sensitivity C-reactive protein. *J. Nutr.* **2009**, *139*, 2365–2372. [CrossRef]
21. Shivappa, N.; Steck, S.E.; Hurley, T.G.; Hussey, J.R.; Hébert, J.R. Designing and developing a literature-derived, population-based dietary inflammatory index. *Public Health Nutr.* **2014**, *17*, 1689–1696. [CrossRef]
22. Wright, M.E.; Mayne, S.T.; Stolzenberg-Solomon, R.Z.; Li, Z.; Pietinen, P.; Taylor, P.R.; Virtamo, J.; Albanes, D. Development of a comprehensive dietary antioxidant index and application to lung cancer risk in a cohort of male smokers. *Am. J. Epidemiol.* **2004**, *160*, 68–76. [CrossRef]
23. Pedrelli, P.; Nyer, M.; Yeung, A.; Zulauf, C.; Wilens, T. College students: Mental health problems and treatment considerations. *Acad. Psychiatry* **2015**, *39*, 503–511. [CrossRef]
24. Blanco, C.; Okuda, M.; Wright, C.; Hasin, D.S.; Grant, B.F.; Liu, S.-M.; Olfson, M. Mental health of college students and their non-college-attending peers: Results from the national epidemiologic study on alcohol and related conditions. *Arch. Gen. Psychiatry* **2008**, *65*, 1429–1437. [CrossRef]
25. Eisenberg, D.; Hunt, J.; Speer, N. Mental health in American colleges and universities: Variation across student subgroups and across campuses. *J. Nerv. Mental Dis.* **2013**, *201*, 60–67. [CrossRef]
26. Bayram, N.; Bilgel, N. The prevalence and socio-demographic correlations of depression, anxiety and stress among a group of university students. *Soc. Psychiatry Psychiatr. Epidemiol.* **2008**, *43*, 667–672. [CrossRef]
27. Auerbach, R.P.; Alonso, J.; Axinn, W.G.; Cuijpers, P.; Ebert, D.D.; Green, J.G.; Hwang, I.; Kessler, R.C.; Liu, H.; Mortier, P.; et al. Mental disorders among college students in the World Health Organization world mental health surveys. *Psychol. Med.* **2016**, *46*, 2955–2970. [CrossRef]
28. Wirth, M.D.; Burch, J.; Shivappa, N.; Violanti, J.M.; Burchfiel, C.M.; Fekedulegn, D.; Andrew, M.E.; Hartley, T.A.; Miller, D.B.; Mnatsakanova, A.; et al. Association of a dietary inflammatory index with inflammatory indices and the metabolic syndrome among police officers. *J. Occup. Environ. Med.* **2014**, *56*, 986–989. [CrossRef]
29. Shivappa, N.; Hébert, J.R.; Rietzschel, E.R.; De Buyzere, M.L.; Langlois, M.; Debruyne, E.; Marcos, A.; Huybrechts, I. Associations between dietary inflammatory index and inflammatory markers in the Asklepios Study. *Br. J. Nutr.* **2015**, *113*, 665–671. [CrossRef]
30. Vahid, F.; Shivappa, N.; Hekmatdoost, A.; Hebert, J.R.; Davoodi, S.H.; Sadeghi, M. Association between Maternal Dietary Inflammatory Index (DII) and abortion in Iranian women and validation of DII with serum concentration of inflammatory factors: Case-control study. *Appl. Physiol. Nutr. Metab.* **2017**, *42*, 511–516. [CrossRef]
31. Shivappa, N.; Wirth, M.D.; Hurley, T.G.; Hébert, J.R. Association between the dietary inflammatory index (DII) and telomere length and C-reactive protein from the National Health and Nutrition Examination Survey-1999–2002. *Mol. Nutr. Food Res.* **2017**, *61*, 1600630. [CrossRef]
32. Phillips, C.M.; Chen, L.-W.; Heude, B.; Bernard, J.Y.; Harvey, N.C.; Duijts, L.; Mensink-Bout, S.M.; Polanska, K.; Mancano, G.; Suderman, M.; et al. Dietary inflammatory index and non-communicable disease risk: A narrative review. *Nutrients* **2019**, *11*, 1873. [CrossRef]
33. Berk, M.; Williams, L.J.; Jacka, F.N.; O'Neil, A.; Pasco, J.A.; Moylan, S.; Allen, N.B.; Stuart, A.L.; Harley, A.C.; Byrne, M.L.; et al. So depression is an inflammatory disease, but where does the inflammation come from? *BMC Med.* **2013**, *11*, 200. [CrossRef]
34. Oyovwi, M.O.; Chijiokwu, E.A.; Ben-Azu, B.; Atere, A.D.; Joseph, U.G.; Ogbutor, U.G.; Udi, O.A. Potential Roles of Natural Antioxidants in Modulating Neurodegenerative Disease Pathways. *Mol. Neurobiol.* **2025**, *62*, 10367–10397. [CrossRef]
35. Akbaraly, T.N.; Kerlau, C.; Wyart, M.; Chevallier, N.; Ndiaye, L.; Shivappa, N.; Hebert, J.R.; Kivimäki, M. Dietary inflammatory index and recurrence of depressive symptoms: Results from the Whitehall II Study. *Clin. Psychol. Sci.* **2016**, *4*, 1125–1134. [CrossRef]
36. Shivappa, N.; Schoenaker, D.A.J.M.; Hebert, J.R.; Mishra, G.D. Association between inflammatory potential of diet and risk of depression in middle-aged women: The Australian Longitudinal Study on Women's Health. *Br. J. Nutr.* **2016**, *116*, 1077–1086. [CrossRef]
37. Salari-Moghaddam, A.; Keshteli, A.H.; Afshar, H.; Esmaillzadeh, A.; Adibi, P. Association between dietary inflammatory index and psychological profile in adults. *Clin. Nutr.* **2019**, *38*, 2360–2368. [CrossRef]
38. Ghazizadeh, H.; Yaghooti-Khorasani, M.; Asadi, Z.; Zare-Feyzabadi, R.; Saeidi, F.; Shabani, N.; Safari-Ghalezou, M.; Yadegari, M.; Nosrati-Tirkani, A.; Shivappa, N.; et al. Association between dietary inflammatory index (DII®) and depression and anxiety in the Mashhad stroke and heart atherosclerotic disorder (MASHAD) study population. *BMC Psychiatry* **2020**, *20*, 282. [CrossRef]
39. Haghighatdoost, F.; Feizi, A.; Esmaillzadeh, A.; Feinle-Bisset, C.; Keshteli, A.H.; Afshar, H.; Adibi, P. Association between the dietary inflammatory index and common mental health disorders profile scores. *Clin. Nutr.* **2019**, *38*, 1643–1650. [CrossRef]

40. Bergmans, R.S.; Malecki, K.M. The association of dietary inflammatory potential with depression and mental well-being among U.S. adults. *Prev. Med.* **2017**, *99*, 313–319. [CrossRef]
41. Luo, J.; Xu, X.; Sun, Y.; Lu, X.; Zhao, L. Association of composite dietary antioxidant index with depression and all-cause mortality in middle-aged and elderly population. *Sci. Rep.* **2024**, *14*, 9809. [CrossRef]
42. Zhang, T.; Zhang, R.; Song, T.; Chen, F.; Wei, Y. The impact of Composite Dietary Antioxidant Index on the relationship between eczema and depression symptoms in US adults. *Front. Nutr.* **2024**, *11*, 1470833. [CrossRef]
43. Zhao, L.; Zhang, X.; Guo, S.; Han, K.; Sun, Y.; Li, X.; Yan, Z.; Peng, W. Relationship between composite dietary antioxidant index and depression among overweight and obese adults. *J. Affect. Disord.* **2023**, *341*, 358–365. [CrossRef]
44. Torabynasab, K.; Shahinfar, H.; Effatpanah, M.; Jazayeri, S.; Azadbakht, L.; Abolghasemi, J.; Jamali, S. Association between empirical dietary inflammatory index, odds, and severity of anxiety disorders: A case–control study. *Food Sci. Nutr.* **2023**, *11*, 6349–6359. [CrossRef]
45. Attlee, A.; Saravanan, C.; Shivappa, N.; Wirth, M.D.; Aljaberi, M.; Alkaabi, R.; Bataineh, M.F.; Hebert, J.R. Higher dietary inflammatory index scores are associated with stress and anxiety in dormitory-residing female university students in the United Arab Emirates. *Front. Nutr.* **2022**, *9*, 814409. [CrossRef]
46. Shivappa, N.; Hebert, J.R.; Rashidkhani, B. Association between inflammatory potential of diet and stress levels in adolescent women in Iran. *Arch. Iran. Med.* **2017**, *20*, 108–112.
47. Juszczyk, G.; Mikulska, J.; Kasperek, K.; Pietrzak, D.; Mrozek, W.; Herbet, M. Chronic stress and oxidative stress as common factors of the pathogenesis of depression and Alzheimer's disease: The role of antioxidants in prevention and treatment. *Antioxidants* **2021**, *10*, 1439. [CrossRef]
48. Bremmer, J.D.; Moazzami, K.; Wittbrodt, M.T.; Nye, J.A.; Lima, B.B.; Gillespie, C.F.; Rapaport, M.H.; Pearce, B.D.; Shah, A.J.; Vaccarino, V. Diet, Stress and Mental Health. *Nutrients* **2020**, *12*, 2428. [CrossRef]
49. Solomou, S.; Logue, J.; Reilly, S.; Perez-Algorta, G. A systematic review of the association of diet quality with the mental health of university students: Implications in health education practice. *Health Educ. Res.* **2023**, *38*, 28–68. [CrossRef]
50. Gautam, S.; Jain, A.; Chaudhary, J.; Gautam, M.; Gaur, M.; Grover, S. Concept of mental health and mental well-being, it's determinants and coping strategies. *Indian. J. Psychiatry* **2024**, *66*, S231–S244. [CrossRef]
51. Phillips, C.M.; Shivappa, N.; Hébert, J.R.; Perry, I.J. Dietary inflammatory index and mental health: A cross-sectional analysis of the relationship with depressive symptoms, anxiety and well-being in adults. *Clin. Nutr.* **2018**, *37*, 1485–1491. [CrossRef]

nutrients

MDPI

Article

Dyslipidemia in Anorexia Nervosa Is Associated with Decreased Plasma Tauroursodeoxycholic Acid and a Specific Fatty Acid Pattern

Aleš Žák [1], Marek Vecka [1,2,*], Peter Szitanyi [3], Marcela Floriánková [1], Barbora Staňková [1,2], Petra Uhlíková [3], Veronika Dostálová [4] and Michal Burda [5]

[1] 4th Department of Medicine, 1st Faculty of Medicine, Charles University in Prague and the General University Hospital in Prague, 128 08 Prague, Czech Republic; azak@vfn.cz (A.Ž.); marcela.floriankova@vfn.cz (M.F.); barsta@atlas.cz (B.S.)
[2] Institute of Clinical Chemistry and Laboratory Diagnostics, 1st Faculty of Medicine, Charles University in Prague and the General University Hospital in Prague, 128 08 Prague, Czech Republic
[3] Department of Pediatrics and Inherited Metabolic Disorders, 1st Faculty of Medicine, Charles University in Prague and the General University Hospital in Prague, 128 08 Prague, Czech Republic; szitanyi@yahoo.com (P.S.); petra.uhlikova@vfn.cz (P.U.)
[4] Department of Psychiatry, 1st Faculty of Medicine, Charles University in Prague and the General University Hospital in Prague, 128 08 Prague, Czech Republic; veronika.dostalova2@vfn.cz
[5] Institute for Research and Applications of Fuzzy Modeling, CE IT4Innovations, University of Ostrava, 701 03 Ostrava, Czech Republic; michal.burda@osu.cz
* Correspondence: marek.vecka@lf1.cuni.cz

Abstract

Background: Dyslipidemia and distorted fatty acid (FA) metabolism are frequent biochemical abnormalities associated with anorexia nervosa (AN). Gut microbiota is supposed to play an important role in the etiopathogenesis of AN. Apart from the digestive function of bile acids (BAs), these compounds have multiple metabolic functions due to the activation of specific receptors. Objective/aims: The aims of the study were to investigate biochemical measures, including plasma lipids (lipoproteins, respectively), fatty acid (FA) patterns, and the profile of plasma Bas, in AN patients and healthy controls (CON). Methods: Plasma phospholipid FA and BAs profiles were analyzed in 39 women with a restrictive type of AN (AN-R; median age 17 years) and in 35 CON women (median age 20 years). Results: Compared to CON, AN had an increased concentration of HDL-C, increased content of palmitic acid, and decreased proportion of linoleic acid. Moreover, AN had a drop in the level of the sum of PUFA*n*-6 and increased delta 9 desaturase activity for stearic acid. In AN, we found decreased levels of plasma tauroursodeoxycholic acid (TUDCA). In AN, concentrations of 22:5*n*-6, 16:0, 20:3*n*-6 and fat mass index were predic-tors of HDL-C levels (R^2 = 0.43). Conclusions: Patients with AN-R had an increased concentration of HDL-C, decreased levels of total PUFA *n*-6, and increased activity of D9D for stearic acid. Furthermore, AN exerted decreased levels of TUDCA. Therefore, a decreased level of TUDCA could potentially serve as a marker of AN.

Keywords: anorexia nervosa; lipids and lipoproteins; fatty acid pattern; plasma bile acid composition; multiple linear regression analysis; long-chain polyunsaturated fatty acids of *n*-6 family

1. Introduction

Anorexia nervosa (AN) is a serious psychiatric disorder with a peak onset in both men and women between 15 and 19 years, which has the highest mortality and relapse rate of all psychiatric illnesses. AN is characterized by persistent, pathological weight and shape concerns, leading to a restricted oral intake and, consequently, low body weight, with a reduction in fat mass and fat-free mass at the expense of adipose tissue [1–3].

The etiology of AN remains unclear and is supposed to be complex and multifactorial, with substantial environmental and genetic influences. The main risk factors predisposing individuals to the development of AN include environmental and social aspects, biological influences, psychological traits, and genetic factors, with the heritability of AN ranging from 20 to 58% [4–6].

Energy deprivation and malnutrition have a major impact on several organs and systems in patients with AN. Patients with AN present multiple psychiatric and somatic comorbidities/complications related to prolonged starvation and altered eating behaviors. The most common psychiatric comorbidities include mood and anxiety disorders, obsessive-compulsive disorder, personality traits (anxiety, depression, perfectionism, and low self-esteem), substance use disorders, and neurodevelopmental disorders (autism spectrum and attention deficit hyperactivity disorder) [7]. Furthermore, AN is associated with several somatic comorbidities.

The phenotype of AN depends on many factors, such as the age at AN onset, duration, and severity of illness [3,7,8]. AN is associated with several somatic comorbidities, the most serious of which are cardiac complications (Supplementary Table S1).

Dyslipidemia and impaired fatty acid (FA) metabolism are the common biochemical abnormalities found in AN. Lipid (lipoprotein, respectively) alterations in AN have been known since the 1960s [9,10]. The results of studies analyzing lipid (lipoprotein, respectively) concentrations in AN seem to be inconsistent. Several studies have described hypercholesterolemia in 20 to 50% of patients with AN [11–13], whilst other studies found normal or reduced plasma lipid concentrations. On the other hand, Crisp et al. [10] found nearly normal levels of plasma total cholesterol (TC), with only two persons out of twelve who were hypercholesterolemic. Other authors [14] have described only elevated levels of HDL-C in AN. However, in normolipidemic patients with AN, changes in the lipoprotein spectrum toward more atherogenic subclasses have been described [15]. A large-scale meta-analysis described the effect of AN on plasmatic TC, LDL-cholesterol (LDL-C), HDL-cholesterol (HDL-C), and triacylglycerols (TAG). Patients with acute AN had, compared to healthy controls, on average, increased levels of TC by 0.60 mmol/L, LDL-C by 0.32, HDL-C by 0.09, and TAG by 0.09 mmol/L [16].

The pathophysiological mechanisms underlying hypercholesterolemia in anorexia nervosa are not yet fully understood; increased cholesterol synthesis seems unlikely [17]. Other studies have suggested increased absorption of exogenous cholesterol [18,19]. Several studies have described a disturbed hormonal milieu that could lead to secondary dyslipidemia (reviewed in Refs. [16,17,20]).

Dysregulated plasma fatty acid (FA) patterns have been found in patients with eating disorders (EDs) such as obesity and AN in several studies [21–24]. Apart from inconsistent changes in concentrations of saturated (SFAs) and monounsaturated FAs of the n-9 family (MFA n-9), the most consistent changes in the FA profiles in AN patients include alterations in polyunsaturated FAs (PUFAs) [25].

Among the biological factors involved in the etiopathogenesis of AN, the gut microbiota plays a significant role. In recent years, the importance of the gut microbiota in the pathogenesis of eating disorders (ED) such as AN and bulimia nervosa has been intensively studied [7,26–28]. The composition of the gut microbiota is highly variable between individuals and depends on many endogenous and exogenous factors. The most important factor that influences the size and composition of gut microbiota is the diet [29,30].

It is generally accepted that the gut microbiota plays a crucial role in the gut microbiota–brain axis. Gut dysbiosis (disturbed size and composition of the gut microbiota) influences communication between the gut/pancreas, brain, and adipose tissue. The gut microbiota affects the synthesis of many compounds/substances, such as hormones and short-chain fatty acids (SCFAs), with an impact on intestinal and blood–brain barrier permeability, subclinical inflammation of the intestine and central nervous system (CNS), the expression of hormones and neurotransmitters affecting appetite and satiety [28].

Furthermore, the gut microbiota significantly affects the size and composition of the bile acid (BA) pool. BAs have been recognized as signaling molecules with many pleiotropic physiological functions. BAs act as metabolic integrators of lipid, glucose, and energy metabolism. BAs also control gastrointestinal motility, inflammation, size, and configuration/growth of the gut microbiome.

The BA pool in the human body is maintained by efficient enterohepatic circulation, preserving up to 95% of conjugated BA. Absorbed BA enter the portal bloodstream and are rapidly taken up by hepatocytes and resecreted into bile. A small fraction of BA escapes enterohepatic recirculation and spills into the systemic circulation, which allows BA signaling to occur in other organs and tissues. Only a small amount (~5%) of BA enters the colon, where the gut microbiota can convert primary BA into more hydrophobic secondary BAs—deoxycholic acid (DCA) and lithocholic acid (LCA). These secondary BAs can be passively reabsorbed from the colon. Primary BAs are further metabolized in the intestine by the gut microbiota in processes that involve the action of three groups of bacterial enzymes: bile salt hydrolases, hydroxysteroid dehydrogenases that oxidize and epimerize hydroxy groups of the BA molecule, yielding the secondary/tertiary BAs—ursodeoxycholic acid (UDCA), iso-DCA, and iso-LCA. The third reaction is the 7α-dehydroxylation of unconjugated BA in the colon. In the intestine, conjugated primary BA [cholic acid (CA), chenodeoxycholic acid (CDCA), respectively] can be deconjugated and 7α-dehydroxylated by the gut microbiota to form secondary (DCA, LCA, UDCA, respectively). The gut microbiota controls BA diversity and vice versa; the size of the BA pool and its composition mediate gut microbiome patterns [31–33]. However, until now, changes in the size and composition of plasma BA have not been systematically studied in AN.

TUDCA exerts many beneficial functions in human metabolism: (a) TUDCA stabilizes the endoplasmic reticulum thus inhibiting endoplasmic reticulum stress [34] that induces leptin resistance [35] and activates several inflammatory pathways [36]; (b) stabilizes mitochondrial membranes, probably acting as molecular chaperone by blocking the activation of unfolded protein response and consequent apoptosis [37]; (c) activates TGR5 receptors which results in the attenuation of the production of proinflammatory cytokines, also during activation of microglia and astrocytes [38]. Neuroinflammatory processes are known to be present in the hypothalamus in AN [39]. In obesity models, TUDCA restored hypothalamic sensitivity to leptin. In AN, hypothalamic leptin signalization also changes [40].

In our previous study, changes in plasma lipids, fatty acid pattern, and non-cholesterol sterols (lathosterol, β-sitosterol, campesterol) were found in AN [18]. The aims of the study were to investigate clinical features, biochemical measures that include plasma lipids (lipoproteins, respectively), FA patterns, and the profile of plasma BA in AN patients and healthy controls (CON). Furthermore, using multiple linear regression analysis, concentrations of plasma lipids/lipoproteins (as dependent variables) and levels of individual FAs (as independent variables) were studied in both groups (i.e., AN and CON).

2. Materials and Methods

2.1. Study Design and Participants

This case-control study was carried out at the Department of Pediatrics and Inherited Metabolic Disorders and the 4th Department of Medicine. Thirty-nine women with a restrictive type of anorexia nervosa (AN-R), recruited from the consecutive outpatients of the Department of Pediatrics and Inherited Metabolic Disorders from September 2018 to August 2022, and thirty-five sex and age-matched healthy controls (CON) were enrolled in the study. All women studied were of Caucasian descent. All patients with AN-R met the Diagnostic and Statistical Manual-V [1] criteria of this illness, and diagnosis was confirmed by two independent pediatric and adolescent psychiatrists/psychologists.

The study protocol was approved by the Ethics Committee of the General University Hospital in Prague (decision no. 611/18 S; 2018) and performed in accordance with the principles of the Declaration of Helsinki. Written informed consent was obtained from all participants. The medical examination was performed during the acute stage of the disease. The patients did not suffer from any somatic disorder. A bulimic type of anorexia was excluded. Other exclusion criteria were chronic somatic diseases or other mental/neurodevelopmental disorders (a primary disease related to eating disorders), hereditary disorders (first-degree, such as familial hypercholesterolemia), pharmacotherapy, hormonal therapy, pregnancy, contraception, dietary supplements, and smoking. The patients and controls did not use drugs known to affect lipid and lipoprotein metabolism, vitamins, antioxidants, and supplements enriched with *n*-3 and/or *n*-6 PUFA. The control group consisted of eumenorrheic and generally healthy girls who agreed to participate in the study. Patients attending urgent or non-routine treatment were excluded from the control group. No control subject reported eating disorders in the past. Other exclusion criteria in the CON group related to general health were chronic somatic diseases, mental or neurodevelopmental disorders, hereditary disorders, such as familial dyslipidemia (in first-degree relatives), pregnancy or breastfeeding, pharmacotherapy, dietary supplements, or contraception. Neither a family history of premature coronary heart disease nor familial dyslipidemia was detected.

2.2. Blood Sampling, Diet Evaluation, and Anthropometry

Blood samples were taken after 12 h of fasting. Routine biochemical and hematological analyses were performed immediately, and samples for special analyses were stored at −80 °C until use. Basic clinical, nutritional, and anthropometric data, including assessment of body fat, were examined using standard methods, as described previously [18,41].

2.3. Indirect Calorimetry

Resting energy expenditure (REE) and respiratory quotient were analyzed with a computerized, open-circuit indirect calorimetry system that measured resting oxygen uptake and resting carbon dioxide production using a ventilated canopy (Omnia 1.5—Quark RMR, Cosmed, Srl, Italy, Rome).

2.4. Laboratory Measurements

Total cholesterol (TC) was analyzed in serum using a commercially purchased enzymatic-colorimetric test (CHOD-PAP) (Biola-test cholesterol 2500 kit; Pliva-Lachema, Czech Republic). Serum TAGs were measured using a standard enzymatic-colorimetric kit (GPO-PAP) (Pliva-Lachema, Czech Republic). HDL-C concentration was measured in the supernatant of serum samples after selective precipitation of LDL-C using a BIO-LA-TEST HDL-Cholesterol kit (Pliva-Lachema, Czech Republic) on a Cobas Mira analyzer (Roche, Switzerland). The levels of non-esterified fatty acids (NEFAs) were determined using an enzymatic-colorimetric method (Randox Laboratories Ltd., Crumlin, UK). Apolipoprotein B concentration was analyzed nephelometrically using a standard kit (Beckman Coulter Inc., Brea, CA, USA) on an Image analyzer. Insulin concentrations were measured using diagnostic sets and a modular analyzer (Roche Diagnostic, Indianapolis, IN, USA) by electrochemiluminescence.

The fatty acid profiles in the main plasma lipid classes (phospholipids, triacylglycerols, and cholesteryl-esters) were examined by analytical procedures described previously [32]. The homeostasis model assessment method, HOMA-IR, was used as an index of insulin resistance [33]. Desaturase activities were estimated using FA product/precursor ratios [42,43]. The ratio of palmitoleic to linoleic acid (16:1*n*-7/18:2*n*-6) greater than 0.086 was used as a surrogate marker of *n*-6 essential fatty acid deficiency (EFAD) [44]. The plasma BA spectrum was measured by the LC-MS/MS method [45].

2.5. Statistical Analyses

All statistical analyses were performed using the R statistical software version 4.1.3. or with STATISTICA® software version 12 for Windows [46]. Categorical data were summarized by absolute and relative frequencies. Continuous data are expressed as median and interquartile range (IQR, 25th–75th percentile). The normality of the distribution was tested using the Shapiro–Wilk test. Comparisons between groups were carried out using the two-sample Mann–Whitney test. The p-values for continuous and categorical data were adjusted for multiple comparisons using Holm's correction.

Stepwise multivariate linear regression was used to assess the relationship between plasma lipids (lipoproteins, respectively), such as dependent variables, and plasma phospholipid FA, body mass index (BMI), fat mass index (FMI), glucose, and insulin, such as independent variables. To avoid collinearity, these relationships were observed using two models. In the first model, the concentrations of FA and the values of BMI and FMI were included as independent variables; in the second model, concentrations of FA, insulin, and glucose were used as independent variables. A stepwise multivariate linear regression analysis was performed to determine the coefficients of determination (R^2) using FA concentrations, anthropometric measures (BMI and FMI), and biochemical parameters (glucose and insulin).

We performed post hoc power analyses to better quantify the sensitivity of the statistical tests. For comparisons based on the largest available subsample ($n = 39 + 35$), the analyses indicate a power of 0.89 to detect large effect sizes (Cohen's d ≈ 0.8, $\alpha = 0.05$, two-tailed). However, for smaller subsamples (e.g., $n = 21 + 13$), the power to detect large effects drops to 0.56. This illustrates that while some parts of the study were sufficiently powered to detect large effects, other parts were underpowered, particularly to detect moderate or small effects. We have clarified in the text that due to these limitations, the findings should be interpreted with caution and viewed as exploratory. The results may serve as a basis for generating hypotheses to be tested in future studies with larger and more balanced samples.

3. Results

3.1. Basic Clinical, Anthropometric, and Biochemical Characteristics

The basic clinical, anthropometric, and biochemical characteristics of the study groups (i.e., AN, CON) are shown in Table 1. The anthropometric parameters of patients with AN are coherent with the marantic type of malnutrition (simple starvation, respectively). As expected, the patients with AN had, in comparison with the healthy CON group, decreased BMI (by 21%), fat mass (by 51%), lean body mass (by 13%), and fat mass index (by 45%). These data show that weight loss is linked with adipose tissue reduction. The AN group had decreased REE (by 36%), levels of triiodothyronine as well as thyroxine (by 45%, and by 21%, respectively). Biochemical characteristics are completed by a reduced insulin concentration (by 55%) and a decrease in the HOMA-IR index (by 62%). In the AN group, we found only an increase in the concentration of HDL-C fraction (by 22%). Although the number of patients with high concentrations of HDL-C (>2.07 mmol/L), considered as dysfunctional, was higher in the AN group (4 of them met the criteria), we did not prove a significant difference in the distribution (chi-square test with Yates' correction; $p = 0.422$). Dysfunctional HDL is not believed to have protective effects in relation to cardiovascular disease [47,48].

Table 1. Basic clinical and biochemical characteristics of the studied groups.

Parameter	AN ($n = 39$)	CON ($n = 35$)
Age (years)	17 (14–21) [1]	20 (16–22)
BMI (kg·m^{-2})	16.4 (13.6–18.2) ***	20.8 (19.8–22.4)
Fat mass (kg)	7.6 (4.2–10.6) ***	15.5 (12.4–18.5)
Fat mass index (kg·m^{-2})	3.1 (1.5–4.0) ***	5.6 (4.8–6.5)
Lean body mass (kg)	36.3 (30.2–41.1) *	41.8 (39.1–43.6)
LBMI (kg·m^{-2})	13.3 (11.7–15.0) **	15.4 (14.4–16.3)
REE (kcal)	998 (866–1309) **	1569 (1503–1645)
NEFA (mmol/L)	0.410 (0.155–0.780)	0.420 (0.322–0.532)
T3I (nmol/L)	3.350 (2.775–3.855) ***	6.100 (5.900–6.500)
T4I (nmol/L)	12.300 (11.750–13.225) **	15.500 (14.200–16.100)
TSH (mIU/L)	1.928 (1.375–2.280)	2.670 (1.943–3.821)
TC (mmol/L)	4.76 (4.23–5.59)	4.18 (3.95–4.88)
TAG (mmol/L)	0.92 (0.80–1.24)	0.73 (0.61–1.03)
Apo B (g/L)	0.74 (0.60–0.85)	0.72 (0.64–0.77)
HDL-C (mmol/L)	1.56 (1.40–1.85) ***	1.28 (1.07–1.42)
LDL-C (mmol/L)	2.62 (2.18–3.31)	2.61 (2.24–3.20)
Non-HDL-C	3.16 (2.390– 3.96)	3.07 (2.69–3.54)
LDL/HDL (ratio)	1.74 (1.24–2.25)	2.14 (1.72–2.84)
Glucose (mmol/L)	4.6 (4.1–5.0)	4.7 (4.5–4.9)
Insulin (mU/L)	5.12 (3.57–6.36) **	11.36 (7.84–16.30)
HOMA-IR (ratio)	0.98 (0.59–1.56) *	2.57 (1.57–3.26)
CRP (mg/L)	2.10 (0.54–4.38)	2.30 (0.50–4.38)

[1] Data are given as median (25th–75th percentile); statistical analysis: Mann-Whitney test: * $p < 0.05$, ** $p < 0.01$, *** $p < 0.001$; after adjustment for multiple comparisons using Holm's corrections. Abbreviations: AN—anorexia nervosa; BMI—body mass index; CON—control group; CRP—C-reactive protein; TC—total cholesterol; TAG—triacylglycerols; LDL—low density lipoproteins; HDL—high density lipoproteins; Apo—apolipoprotein; HOMA-IR—homeostasis model assessment for insulin resistance (f-insulin (μU/mL) × f-glucose (mmol/L)/22.5); REE—resting energy expenditure; T3I—triiodothyronine; T4I—thyroxine; TSH—thyroid stimulating hormone; NEFA—non-esterified fatty acids; LBMI—lean body mass index; FMI—fat mass index.

The analyses of CRP concentrations did not reveal differences between the studied groups. However, the molar ratio of TUDCA exhibited a negative correlation with the CRP values in the AN group ($r = -0.58$; $p = 0.05$, Pearson correlation coefficient).

The composition of the diets of both studied groups is presented in Supplementary Table S5. The AN group had lower energy and fat intake, as documented by lower cholesterol and saturated fat content in the diet.

3.2. Fatty Acid Profiles

The plasma phospholipid FA profile is shown in Table 2. In the group with AN, we found, in comparison with healthy controls, a statistically significant increased concentration of palmitic acid (PA, 16:0) by 10%, and a decreased level of linoleic acid (LA;

18:2*n*-6). Anorectic patients had decreased concentrations of the sum of all polyunsaturated fatty acids (ΣPUFA *n*-6) and an increased index of D9D 18 (delta 9 desaturase for stearic acid) (Table 3). Neither patients in the AN group nor subjects in the CON group showed biochemical signs of essential fatty acid deficiency using surrogate markers (Table 3).

Table 2. Plasma phospholipid fatty acid composition of the studied groups.

Parameter	AN (n = 39)	CON (n = 35)
14:0 [1]	0.24 (0.20–0.40) [2]	0.26 (0.24–0.37)
16:0	29.53 (27.31–30.92) [3*]	26.81 (25.55–29.05)
16:1*n*-9	0.16 (0.13–0.18)	0.17 (0.15–0.21)
16:1*n*-7	0.72 (0.52–0.95)	0.63 (0.57–0.70)
18:0	12.95 (11.52–13.68)	13.49 (12.42–14.46)
18:1tra*ns*	0.11 (0.08–0.14)	NA
18:1*n*-9	11.31 (10.70–12.63)	10.81 (10.28–11.75)
18:1*n*-7	1.87 (1.63–2.14)	1.96 (1.71–2.35)
18:2*n*-6	23.65 (21.02–25.28) *	25.53 (24.38–26.46)
18:3*n*-6	0.08 (0.05–0.11)	0.08 (0.06–0.10)
18:3*n*-3	0.21 (0.08–0.38)	0.30 (0.08–0.34)
20:0	0.06 (0.05–0.15)	0.07 (0.06–0.16)
20:1*n*-9	0.15 (0.13–0.18)	0.17 (0.14–0.19)
20:2*n*-6	0.44 (0.34–0.76)	0.40 (0.33–0.46)
20:3*n*-6	3.11 (2.35–3.61)	3.11 (2.74–3.29)
20:4*n*-6	10.46 (9.00–11.33)	10.23 (9.38–11.59)
20:5*n*-3	0.60 (0.51–0.80)	0.66 (0.54–0.81)
22:4*n*-6	0.37 (0.32–0.42)	0.37 (0.35–0.40)
22:5*n*-6	0.28 (0.20–0.35)	0.24 (0.21–0.28)
22:5*n*-3	0.92 (0.69–1.14)	0.90 (0.82–1.06)
22:6*n*-3	2.61 (1.95–3.43)	2.91 (2.17–3.80)

[1] shorthand notation of fatty acids: number of carbon atoms; number of double bonds; *n*—number of carbon atoms from the methyl end to the nearest double bond; NA—not available; [2] numbers are given as median (25th–75th percentile; mol%); [3] statistical analysis: Mann–Whitney test: * $p < 0.05$, after adjustment for multiple comparisons using Holm's corrections.

Table 3. Plasma phospholipid fatty acids of the studied groups (calculated parameters).

Parameter	AN (n = 39)	CON (n = 35)
Σ SFA	42.07 (41.18–43.57) [2]	40.73 (39.86–43.35)
Σ MFA	14.38 (13.42–15.74)	13.82 (12.99–14.85)
Σ PUFA *n*-6	38.36 (36.97–39.77) [3**]	39.82 (38.77–41.47)
Σ PUFA *n*-3	4.88 (3.61–5.66)	5.12 (3.65–5.82)
D5D*n*-6 (20:4*n*-6/20:3*n*-6) [1]	3.216 (2.642–4.817)	3.338 (3.027–4.127)
D6D*n*-6 (18:3*n*-6/18:2*n*-6)	0.003 (0.002–0.005)	0.003 (0.002–0.004)
D9D16 (16:1*n*-7/16:0)	0.025 (0.019–0.032)	0.023 (0.020–0.026)
D9D18 (18:1*n*-9/18:0)	0.908 (0.829–1.031) *	0.811 (0.736–0.888)
ADA *n*-6 [4]	0.615 (0.536–0.540)	0.572 (0.511–0.614)
22:4*n*-6/22:5*n*-6	1.369 (1.211–1.637) [5]	1.522 (1.414–1.644)
n-6 EFAD index	0.030 (0.021–0.075)	0.025 (0.019–0.028)
n-6 EFAD index (≥0.086/<0.086)	none/39	none/35

[1] shorthand notation of fatty acids: number of carbon atoms; number of double bonds; *n*—number of carbon atoms from the methyl end to the nearest double bond; [2] numbers are given as median (25th–75th percentile; mol%); [3] statistical analysis: Mann–Whitney test: * $p < 0.05$, ** $p < 0.01$, after adjustment for multiple comparisons using Holm's corrections; [4] ADA *n*-6 (aggregated desaturase activity for PUFA *n*-6)—ratio of all PUFA *n*-6 except LA (18:2*n*-6) to LA (18:2*n*-6); [5] ratio 22:4*n*-6/22/5*n*-6 (adrenic to Osbond acid)—biochemical marker of functional DHA status; Abbreviations: Σsatur—sum of saturated fatty acids; ΣMFA—sum of monounsaturated fatty acids; Σ*n*-6—sum of *n*-6 polyunsaturated fatty acids; Σ*n*-3—sum of *n*-3 polyunsaturated fatty acids; *n*-6 EFAD—*n*-6 essential fatty acid deficiency; EFAD index = 16:1*n*-7/18:2*n*-6.

3.3. Bile Acid Composition

When comparing the profile of plasma bile acids, we found reduced concentrations of tauroursodeoxycholic acid (TUDCA) in the AN group, both when evaluating absolute concentrations [0.003 (0.002–0.006) vs. 0.010 (0.006–0.021); μmol/L; median (25th–75th percentile), $p < 0.05$)], and when comparing their proportion [0.140 (0.068–0.251) vs. 0.397 (0.295–0.493); mol%; median (25th–75th percentile) $p < 0.05$] (Supplementary Tables S2 and S3). Although the data were available only for a subset of the studied groups (21 participants in the AN group and 13 individuals in the CON group), we did not observe a selection bias between those with analyzed BA concentrations and those without the BA measurements.

3.4. Regression Analysis

The results of multivariate linear regression analysis between plasma lipids (lipoproteins, respectively, that is, TC, LDL-C, HDL-C, TAG, apo B, and LDL-C/HDL-C) as dependent variables and plasma phospholipid FA, BMI, FMI, glucose, and insulin as independent variables in the AN patients and CON group are given in Table 4/Supplementary Table S4. In the AN group, a moderate correlation ($R^2 = 0.43$) was found between FA (22:5*n*-6, 16:0, 20:3*n*-6), FMI, and HDL-C, as well as between FA (20:0, 16:1*n*-9), insulin, and TAG ($R^2 = 0.45$). The coefficients of determination between TC and LDL-C, and plasma FAs were mild ($R^2 = 0.28$–0.33), while the independent variables were 22:4*n*-6 and 18:1*n*-9 for TC and LDL-C.

Table 4. Independent predictors of plasma HDL-cholesterol concentrations in the studied groups.

HDL-C									
AN					CON				
Model 1: FAs + BMI + FMI					Model 1: FAs + BMI + FMI				
variable	**estimate**	SE	*p*	Adjusted R^2	variable	estimate	SE	*p*	Adjusted R^2
22:5*n*-6	−0.4932	0.1321	0.0007	0.43	20:0	0.3894	0.1603	0.0208	0.15
FMI	−0.4044	0.1319	0.0042						
16:0	0.3646	0.1347	0.0106						
20:3*n*-6	−0.2568	0.1309	NS						
Model 2: FAs + Glu + Ins					Model 2: FAs + Glu + Ins				
variable	estimate	SE	*p*	Adjusted R^2	variable	estimate	SE	*p*	Adjusted R^2
22:5*n*-6	−0.3896	0.1514	0.0142	0.15	20:0	0.3894	0.1603	0.0208	0.15

FAs—fatty acids (see Table 3); BMI—body mass index; FMI—fat mass index; AN—anorexia nervosa; CON—control group; R^2—coefficient of determination (in%); SE—standard error. Model 1 suggests an independent association between individual FA, BMI, FMI, and HDL-C. Model 2 suggests an independent association between individual FA, glucose, insulin, and HDL-C.

In the CON group, a weak correlation was found between HDL-C and the 20:0 level ($R^2 = 0.15$). The moderate correlation between the TAG level and plasma phospholipid FA was found in both models. TAG levels were dependent on levels of 22:5*n*-6 and 20:5*n*-3 ($R^2 = 0.37$). Similarly, a moderate (strong resp.) correlation between TC and LDL-C ($R^2 = 0.46$, 0.64, resp.) and 16:0, and the sum of PUFA n-6 was found. Apo B levels were dependent on four FAs (16:0, 18:2*n*-6, 20:4*n*-6, and 20:0) and BMI, with a strong coefficient of determination ($R^2 = 0.61$).

As it follows from the regression analysis, an increase in HDL-C concentration is associated with a decrease in DPA-6 (22:5*n*-6; 4,7,10,13,16-docosapentaenoic acid) and DHGLA (dihomo-γ-linolenic acid, 20:3*n*-6). In contrast, an increase in TC (LDL-C, respectively) is associated with an increase in adrenic acid (22:4*n*-6; 7,10,13,16-docosatetraenoic acid) and a decrease in oleic acid (18:1*n*-9).

4. Discussion

The main results of our study are the association of HDL-C concentrations with changes in the concentrations of specific FA and the finding of reduced TUDCA concentrations in AN. The clinical and biochemical data of our study are consistent with the published results of other authors [3,16,49,50]. In agreement with the literature [14,16], we demonstrated only a significant increase in HDL-C concentration in AN. In our previous study, we demonstrated an increase in TC, TAG, and HDL-C, as well as an elevation in NEFA levels in AN [18]. This difference may be due to a general change in the dietary habits of the Czech population in recent years [51].

In the group with AN, we found, compared to healthy controls, a statistically increased content of palmitic acid (PA, 16:0) by 10%, and a decreased level of linoleic acid (LA; 18:2*n*-6). Anorectic patients had decreased concentrations of the sum of all polyunsaturated fatty acids (ΣPUFA *n*-6) as well as increased index of D9D 18 (delta 9 desaturase for stearic acid. These results are consistent with the results of our previous study, i.e., an increase in 16:0, 18:1*n*-9, SFA, and MFA, and a decrease in *n*-6 PUFA and 18:2*n*-6 [18].

Changes in FA metabolism in ED (especially in AN) have been studied by several authors. Nguyen et al. [52] found an increased concentration of lauric acid (12:0), eicosapentaenoic acid (EPA, 20:5*n*-3), DPA-3 (22:5*n*-3), and ALA (α-linolenic acid, 18:3*n*-3) in AN compared to healthy controls, while food intake shifted the pattern of FA toward a less pathological FA profile. French authors studied the composition of FA in plasma phospholipids and erythrocyte membranes. They did not find EFAD, a decrease in LA, or ALA, respectively, and no increase in 20:3*n*-9. However, they observed decreased levels of LC-PUFA, mainly those in the *n*-3 family [53]. A meta-analysis investigating the composition of PUFAs in ED (mainly in AN, 6 of 7 studies) found, compared to controls, higher plasma levels of ALA, EPA, stearidonic acid (18:4*n*-3), Osbond acid (DPA*n*-6; 22:5*n*-6), palmitoleic acid (POA, 16:1*n*-7), oleic acid (18:1*n*-9), and total PUFA *n*-3 fatty acids, together with lower levels of total n-6 fatty acids and a ratio of PUFA*n*-6/PUFA*n*-3. Eating disorders were associated with significantly higher levels of palmitoleic acid and oleic acid in the red blood cell membrane and lower levels of adrenic acid (22:4*n*-6), arachidonic acid (20:4*n*-6), and total n-6 fatty acids [24]. Japanese authors in a case-control study found in AN-R, compared to controls, increased levels of 18:3*n*-3, 20:0, 20:1*n*-9, 20:5*n*-3, 22:0, and 22:1*n*-9 [23].

Differences in the composition of FAs when comparing our work with that of other authors may be partly due to methodological aspects. In our study, we express the individual FA in mol%, just like some other authors [24]; other authors express the concentrations of FAs in absolute units (μmol/L) [23,25,52]. We did not find indirect signs of EFAD [LA/POA ratio] or Mead's acid content in the AN group.

The relationship between the amount of fat in the diet and its qualitative composition and human health, especially the occurrence of cardiovascular diseases, has been known since the late 1950s [54]. In subsequent years, research focused on the effects of individual saturated FAs, trans MFA, cis MFA, *n*-6 and *n*-3 PUFA on plasma lipids, and lipoprotein (including lipoprotein [a]), and enzymes of lipoprotein metabolism (reviewed in Refs. [55,56]). HDL-C concentrations in AN were positively associated with PA and negatively associated with DPA-6 and DHGLA. This means that a decrease in DPA-6 and DHGLA was reflected in AN by an increase in HDL-C concentration, and an increase in PA similarly leads to an increase in HDL-C. The lack of LC PUFA n-6 is probably causally related to the increase in HDL-C in AN. DPA-6 is an indicator of DHA (docosahexaenoic acid, 22:6*n*-3) deficiency and is related to several other disease states [24,57–59].

In the study by Muralidharan et al., a relationship was demonstrated between the composition of LC-PUFA n-6 in cell membranes, the size and function of HDL, and peripheral inflammation (levels of interleukin-6 and -8, respectively) [60]. Furthermore, patients with phenylketonuria revealed changes in plasma *n*-6 PUFA [higher LA, adrenic acid (AdA), and DPA-6] [61]. Women with gestational diabetes had lower concentrations of DHGLA, DHA, arachidonic acid (AA), AdA, DPA-6, and the AdA/DPA-6 ratio, which is a biochemical marker of DHA insufficiency [62]. On the other hand, a study by Dutch authors did not demonstrate a relationship between AA, AdA, DPA-6, EPA, and DHA acids and cognitive performance in non-pregnant women [63].

In a large meta-analysis of 379 patients with ED, higher plasma concentrations of ALA, EPA, 18:4*n*-3, DPA-6, POA, 18:1*n*-9 (oleic acid), and ΣPUFA*n*-6 and a higher ratio of *n*-6 PUFA to *n*-3 PUFA were found, as well as lower concentrations of AdA, AA, and the total *n*-6 PUFA [24].

Changes in liver and plasma phospholipids were demonstrated in obese patients. Obese patients showed lower levels of AA, DPA-3, DHA, total LC-PUFA, and total *n*-3 LC-PUFA and higher levels of DPA*n*-6, and higher ratios of *n*-6/*n*-3 LC-PUFA. Obese patients with nonalcoholic fatty liver disease showed marked alterations in the PUFA patterns in the liver. These changes are significantly correlated with those found in erythrocytes [64]. Zec et al. (2019) described the association of LC-PUFA *n*-6 with blood pressure and hypertension in black South African adults [58]. These authors found a negative association of DPA-6 with diastolic blood pressure [58]. The levels of DPA-6 (AdA/DPA-6 ratio) are considered a biochemical marker of the functional DHA status [59].

A surprising finding was the positive association of arachidic acid (20:0) with HDL-C levels in the CON group and the negative association of 20:0 with TAG in the AN group, and its positive association of 20:0 with apo B concentration in the CON group. These associations reached only low-to-moderate strength. Arachidic acid is a very-long-chain saturated fatty acid (VLCSFA). The concentrations of VLCSFA show negative associations with the risk of CV disease and are also a negative indicator of de novo lipogenesis. Increased VLCSFA concentrations are a biochemical marker of reduced lipogenesis. They appeared to be directly involved in reduced lipogenesis [65,66].

Changes in the gut microbiota, the synonym "dysbiosis", are characterized by low microbial diversity, the presence of pathobionts, and the lack of beneficial bacteria. Dysbiosis has been described in a growing number of diseases, such as in patients with inflammatory bowel disease, irritable bowel syndrome, asthma, obesity, and various neuropsychiatric disorders, including AN [67,68]. The decreased plasma TUDCA concentration, found in our study, is likely a surrogate marker of intestinal dysbiosis. Furthermore, decreased plasma TUDCA concentrations may be involved in the etiopathogenesis of AN through at least two other mechanisms. As we did not analyze SCFA concentrations or gut microbiota composition, these phenomena cannot be supported by our data. The gut microbiota, in addition to the gastrointestinal tract and CNS, are involved in the synthesis of several compounds with orexigenic (appetite-stimulating) and anorexigenic (appetite-suppressing) effects. Balance and interactions between the anorexigenic α–melanocyte-stimulating hormone, cholecystokinin, peptide YY, and orexigenic peptides (ghrelins) originating from the gastrointestinal tract appear to play an important role in the regulation of food intake by affecting hypothalamic energetic homeostasis (satiety, resp.) regulating centers. The imbalance influences feeding behavior with subsequent weight loss or weight regain in AN patients [69].

Experimental studies have shown that plasma concentrations of BA correlate with their levels in the brain [70]. Therefore, we can assume that TUDCA concentrations in the central nervous system might be reduced in patients with AN. In recent years, TUDCA has shown important anti-apoptotic and neuroprotective activities, with numerous experimental and clinical evidence suggesting its possible therapeutic use as a disease-modifier in neurodegenerative diseases. Experimental evidence on the mechanisms underlying TUDCA's neuroprotective action derives from animal models of Alzheimer's disease, Parkinson's disease, Huntington's disease, amyotrophic lateral sclerosis, and cerebral ischemia. Preclinical studies indicate that TUDCA exerts its effects not only by regulating and inhibiting the apoptotic cascade but also by reducing oxidative stress, protecting mitochondria, producing an anti-neuroinflammatory action, and acting as a chemical chaperone to maintain the stability and correct folding of proteins [71]. Therefore, the lack of TUDCA in the CNS could potentiate and/or exacerbate low-grade inflammation and neurodegenerative changes in AN.

Another mechanism by which changes in the spectrum of BA can be applied in AN is the anorexigenic effects of BA, which are mediated by receptor TGR5 [72,73]. However, individual BAs and free, tauro-, and glycoconjugates show different activity towards TGR5 and TUDCA, as the most hydrophilic BA has the lowest affinity for TGR5 [74,75]. Therefore, it is unlikely that a decrease in TUDCA contributes to the anorexigenic effect in AN.

Strengths and Limitations of the Study

This study had several strengths. To our knowledge, this study is the first to report decreased plasma concentrations of TUDCA in AN. Second, the experimental group consists exclusively of subjects with a restrictive type of AN, without psychiatric treatment and any nutritional support. Third, we present an innovative statistical approach evaluating the dependence of plasma lipid (lipoprotein, respectively) concentrations on FA levels in plasma phospholipids.

This study has some limitations. First, this is a retrospective cross-sectional study with a relatively small number of individuals in both groups. Second, not all subjects in both groups had analyses of BA concentrations, and third, there was a lack of intestinal microbiota and SCFA analyses.

5. Conclusions

Patients with AN-R had an increased concentration of HDL-C, decreased levels of the total PUFA *n*-6, and increased activity of D9D for stearic acid. Furthermore, AN exerts decreased levels of TUDCA. The HDL-C level was determined by levels of 22:5*n*-6, 20:3*n*-6, 16:0, and FMI. TC, LDL-C, and the LDL-C/HDL-C ratios were influenced by 22:4*n*-6 and 18:1*n*-9. In conclusion, dyslipidemia (increased HDL-C) is associated with a specific FA pattern.

The unexpected finding of decreased TUDCA levels, probably due to changes in the gut microbiota, could potentially serve as a marker of AN. The considerations regarding the possibility of correcting the decrease in TUDCA by its substitution are still speculative and will be the subject of further research.

Supplementary Materials: The following supporting information can be downloaded at https://www.mdpi.com/article/10.3390/nu17142347/s1, Table S1: Somatic complications of anorexia nervosa; Table S2: Plasma bile acid composition of the studied groups; Table S3: Plasma bile acid relative concentrations of the studied groups; Table S4: Independent predictors of plasma lipids (lipoproteins, respectively) in the studied groups; Table S5: Dietary and additional clinical parameters of the studied groups.

Author Contributions: Conceptualization, A.Ž., M.F. and M.V.; methodology, M.F.; software, M.B.; validation, M.V., B.S. and M.B.; formal analysis, B.S.; investigation, M.F., P.U. and V.D.; resources, P.S., M.F. and V.D.; data curation, M.B.; writing—original draft preparation, A.Ž., M.V., M.F. and M.B.; writing—review and editing, A.Ž., M.V., M.B. and M.F.; supervision, M.F. and A.Ž.; project administration, M.F.; funding acquisition, A.Ž. and M.V. All authors have read and agreed to the published version of the manuscript.

Funding: This research was funded by the Czech Ministry of Health grant MH CZ-DRO-VFN64165, the Ministry of Education, Youth and Sports of the Czech Republic—the Cooperatio Program at Charles University, University Research program/Cooperatio—Gastroenterology, and the project "Research of Excellence on Digital Technologies and Wellbeing CZ.02.01.01/00/22_008/0004583" which is co-financed by the European Union; the APC was funded by the Czech Ministry of Health grant MH CZ-DRO-VFN64165.

Institutional Review Board Statement: The study was conducted in accordance with the Declaration of Helsinki and approved by the Ethics Committee of the General University Hospital in Prague (decision no. 611/18 S; 19 July 2018).

Informed Consent Statement: Informed consent was obtained from all subjects involved in the study.

Data Availability Statement: The raw data supporting the conclusions of this article will be made available by the authors on request.

Conflicts of Interest: The authors declare no conflicts of interest. The funders had no role in the design of the study; in the collection, analyses, or interpretation of data; in the writing of the manuscript; or in the decision to publish the results.

Abbreviations

The following abbreviations are used in this manuscript:

AN-R	Anorexia nervosa (restrictive type)
FA	Fatty acid
TC	Total cholesterol
LDL-C	Low-density lipoprotein-cholesterol
HDL-C	High-density lipoprotein-cholesterol
TAG	Triacylglycerols
EDs	Eating disorders
SFA	Saturated fatty acids
MFA	Monounsaturated fatty acids
PUFA	Polyunsaturated fatty acids
SCFA	Short-chain fatty acids
CNS	Central nervous system
BA	Bile acid
DCA	Deoxycholic acid
LCA	Lithocholic acid
UDCA	Ursodeoxycholic acid
CA	Cholic acid
CDCA	Chenodeoxycholic acid
CON	Control group
REE	Resting energy expenditure
NEFA	Non-esterified fatty acids
HOMA-IR	Homeostasis model assessment method of insulin resistance
EFAD	Essential fatty acid deficiency
BMI	Body mass index
FMI	Fat mass index
D9D	Delta-9 desaturase
TUDCA	Tauroursodeoxycholic acid
apo B	Apolipoprotein B-100
DPA-6	Docosapentaenoic acid (*n*-6 family), Osbond acid
DHGLA	Dihomo-γ-linolenic acid
PA	Palmitic acid

LA	Linoleic acid
ALA	α-linolenic acid
EPA	Eisocapentaenoic acid
POA	Palmitoleic acid
LC-PUFA	Long-chain polyusaturated fatty acids
DHA	Docosahexaenoic acid
AdA	Adrenic acid
AA	Arachidonic acid
GLA	γ-linolenic acid
VLCSFA	Very-long-chain saturated fatty acids

References

1. DSM-5. *Diagnostic and Statistical Manual of Mental Disorders*, 5th ed.; American Psychiatric Association: Arlington, VA, USA, 2013. [CrossRef]
2. Katzman, D.K. Medical complications in adolescents with anorexia nervosa: A review of the literature. *Int. J. Eat. Disord.* **2005**, *37*, S52–S59. discussion S87–S89. [CrossRef] [PubMed]
3. Katzman, D.K.; Kearney, S.A.; Becker, A.E. Feeding and Eating Disorders. In *Slesinger and Fordtran's Gastrointestinal and Liver Disease*, 10th ed.; Feldman, M., Friedman, L.S., Brandt, L.J., Eds.; Saunders Elsevier: Philadelphia, PA, USA, 2016; Volume 1, pp. 130–147.
4. Watson, H.J.; Yilmaz, Z.; Thornton, L.M.; Hübel, C.; Coleman, J.R.I.; Gaspar, H.A.; Bryois, J.; Hinney, A.; Leppä, V.M.; Mattheisen, M.; et al. Genome-Wide Association Study Identifies Eight Risk Loci and Implicates Metabo-Psychiatric Origins for Anorexia Nervosa. *Nat. Genet.* **2019**, *51*, 1207–1214. [CrossRef]
5. Mayo-Martínez, L.; Rupérez, F.J.; Martos-Moreno, G.Á.; Graell, M.; Barbas, C.; Argente, J.; García, A. Unveiling Metabolic Phenotype Alterations in Anorexia Nervosa through Metabolomics. *Nutrients* **2021**, *13*, 4249. [CrossRef]
6. Mack, T.; Sanchez-Roige, S.; Davis, L.K. Genetic investigation of the contribution of body composition to anorexia nervosa in an electronic health record setting. *Transl. Psychiatry* **2022**, *12*, 486. [CrossRef]
7. Frostad, S. Are the Effects of Malnutrition on the Gut Microbiota-Brain Axis the Core Pathologies of Anorexia Nervosa? *Microorganisms* **2022**, *10*, 1486. [CrossRef] [PubMed]
8. Winston, A.P. The clinical biochemistry of anorexia nervosa. *Ann. Clin. Biochem.* **2012**, *49*, 132–143. [CrossRef] [PubMed]
9. Klinefelter, H.F. Hypercholesterolemia in anorexia nervosa. *J. Clin. Endocrinol. Metab.* **1965**, *25*, 1520–1521. [CrossRef]
10. Crisp, A.H.; Blendis, L.M.; Pawan, G.L. Aspects of fat metabolism in anorexia nervosa. *Metabolism* **1968**, *17*, 1109–1118. [CrossRef]
11. Mordasini, R.; Klose, G.; Greten, H. Secondary type II hyperlipoproteinemia in patients with anorexia nervosa. *Metabolism* **1978**, *27*, 71–79. [CrossRef]
12. Mira, M.; Stewart, P.M.; Vizzard, J.; Abraham, S. Biochemical abnormalities in anorexia nervosa and bulimia. *Ann. Clin. Biochem.* **1987**, *24*, 29–35. [CrossRef]
13. Gotto, A.M., Jr.; Pownall, H.J. *Manual of Lipid Disorders*; Williams & Wilkins: Baltimore, MD, USA, 1999.
14. Arden, M.R.; Weiselberg, E.C.; Nussbaum, M.P.; Shenker, I.R.; Jacobson, M.S. Effect of weight restoration on the dyslipoproteinemia of anorexia nervosa. *J. Adolesc. Health Care* **1990**, *11*, 199–202. [CrossRef]
15. Stadler, J.T.; Lackner, S.; Mörkl, S.; Meier-Allard, N.; Scharnagl, H.; Rani, A.; Mangge, H.; Zelzer, S.; Holasek, S.J.; Marsche, G. Anorexia Nervosa Is Associated with a Shift to Pro-Atherogenic Low-Density Lipoprotein Subclasses. *Biomedicines* **2022**, *10*, 895. [CrossRef]
16. Hussain, A.A.; Hübel, C.; Hindborg, M.; Lindkvist, E.; Kastrup, A.M.; Yilmaz, Z.; Støving, R.K.; Bulik, C.M.; Sjögren, J.M. Increased lipid and lipoprotein concentrations in anorexia nervosa: A systematic review and meta-analysis. *Int. J. Eat. Disord.* **2019**, *52*, 611–629. [CrossRef]
17. Feillet, F.; Feillet-Coudray, C.; Bard, J.M.; Parra, H.J.; Favre, E.; Kabuth, B.; Fruchart, J.C.; Vidailhet, M. Plasma cholesterol and endogenous cholesterol synthesis during refeeding in anorexia nervosa. *Clin. Chim. Acta* **2000**, *294*, 45–56. [CrossRef] [PubMed]
18. Zák, A.; Vecka, M.; Tvrzická, E.; Hrubý, M.; Novák, F.; Papezová, H.; Lubanda, H.; Veselá, L.; Stanková, B. Composition of plasma fatty acids and non-cholesterol sterols in anorexia nervosa. *Physiol. Res.* **2005**, *54*, 443–451. [CrossRef] [PubMed]
19. Nestel, P.J. Cholesterol metabolism in anorexia nervosa and hypercholesterolemia. *J. Clin. Endocrinol. Metab.* **1974**, *38*, 325–328. [CrossRef]
20. Föcker, M.; Cecil, A.; Prehn, C.; Adamski, J.; Albrecht, M.; Adams, F.; Hinney, A.; Libuda, L.; Bühlmeier, J.; Hebebrand, J.; et al. Evaluation of Metabolic Profiles of Patients with Anorexia Nervosa at Inpatient Admission, Short- and Long-Term Weight Regain-Descriptive and Pattern Analysis. *Metabolites* **2020**, *11*, 7. [CrossRef]

21. Yehuda, S.; Rabinovitz, S. The Role of Essential Fatty Acids in Anorexia Nervosa and Obesity. *Crit. Rev. Food Sci. Nutr.* **2016**, *56*, 2021–2035. [CrossRef] [PubMed]
22. Kunesová, M.; Hainer, V.; Tvrzicka, E.; Phinney, S.D.; Stich, V.; Parízková, J.; Zák, A.; Stunkard, A.J. Assessment of dietary and genetic factors influencing serum and adipose fatty acid composition in obese female identical twins. *Lipids* **2002**, *37*, 27–32. [CrossRef]
23. Shimizu, M.; Kawai, K.; Yamashita, M.; Shoji, M.; Takakura, S.; Hata, T.; Nakashima, M.; Tatsushima, K.; Tanaka, K.; Sudo, N. Very long chain fatty acids are an important marker of nutritional status in patients with anorexia nervosa: A case control study. *Biopsychosoc. Med.* **2020**, *14*, 14, Erratum in *Biopsychosoc. Med.* **2020**, *14*, 18. https://doi.org/10.1186/s13030-020-00192-w. [CrossRef]
24. Satogami, K.; Tseng, P.T.; Su, K.P.; Takahashi, S.; Ukai, S.; Li, D.J.; Chen, T.Y.; Lin, P.Y.; Chen, Y.W.; Matsuoka, Y.J. Relationship between polyunsaturated fatty acid and eating disorders: Systematic review and meta-analysis. *Prostaglandins Leukot. Essent. Fatty Acids* **2019**, *142*, 11–19. [CrossRef]
25. Shih, P.B.; Morisseau, C.; Le, T.; Woodside, B.; German, J.B. Personalized polyunsaturated fatty acids as a potential adjunctive treatment for anorexia nervosa. *Prostaglandins Other Lipid Mediat.* **2017**, *133*, 11–19. [CrossRef]
26. Fetissov, S.O.; Hökfelt, T. On the origin of eating disorders: Altered signaling between gut microbiota, adaptive immunity and the brain melanocortin system regulating feeding behavior. *Curr. Opin. Pharmacol.* **2019**, *48*, 82–91. [CrossRef]
27. Smitka, K.; Prochazkova, P.; Roubalova, R.; Dvorak, J.; Papezova, H.; Hill, M.; Pokorny, J.; Kittnar, O.; Bilej, M.; Tlaskalova-Hogenova, H. Current Aspects of the Role of Autoantibodies Directed Against Appetite-Regulating Hormones and the Gut Microbiome in Eating Disorders. *Front. Endocrinol.* **2021**, *12*, 613983. [CrossRef] [PubMed]
28. Butler, M.J.; Perrini, A.A.; Eckel, L.A. The Role of the Gut Microbiome, Immunity, and Neuroinflammation in the Pathophysiology of Eating Disorders. *Nutrients* **2021**, *13*, 500. [CrossRef]
29. Iannone, L.F.; Preda, A.; Blottière, H.M.; Clarke, G.; Albani, D.; Belcastro, V.; Carotenuto, M.; Cattaneo, A.; Citraro, R.; Ferraris, C.; et al. Microbiota-gut brain axis involvement in neuropsychiatric disorders. *Expert Rev. Neurother.* **2019**, *19*, 1037–1050. [CrossRef] [PubMed]
30. Monteleone, A.M.; Troisi, J.; Serena, G.; Fasano, A.; Dalle Grave, R.; Cascino, G.; Marciello, F.; Calugi, S.; Scala, G.; Corrivetti, G.; et al. The Gut Microbiome and Metabolomics Profiles of Restricting and Binge-Purging Type Anorexia Nervosa. *Nutrients* **2021**, *13*, 507. [CrossRef]
31. Winston, J.A.; Theriot, C.M. Diversification of host bile acids by members of the gut microbiota. *Gut Microbes* **2020**, *11*, 158–171. [CrossRef] [PubMed]
32. Vecka, M.; Dušejovská, M.; Staňková, B.; Rychlík, I.; Žák, A. A Matched Case-Control Study of Noncholesterol Sterols and Fatty Acids in Chronic Hemodialysis Patients. *Metabolites* **2021**, *11*, 774. [CrossRef]
33. Matthews, D.R.; Hosker, J.P.; Rudenski, A.S.; Naylor, B.A.; Treacher, D.F.; Turner, R.C. Homeostasis model assessment: Insulin resistance and beta-cell function from fasting plasma glucose and insulin concentrations in man. *Diabetologia* **1985**, *28*, 412–419. [CrossRef]
34. Sarvani, C.; Sireesh, D.; Ramkumar, K.M. Unraveling the role of ER stress inhibitors in the context of metabolic diseases. *Pharmacol. Res.* **2017**, *119*, 412–421. [CrossRef]
35. Hosoi, T.; Sasaki, M.; Miyahara, T.; Hashimoto, C.; Matsuo, S.; Yoshii, M.; Ozawa, K. Endoplasmic reticulum stress induces leptin resistance. *Mol. Pharmacol.* **2008**, *74*, 1610–1619. [CrossRef]
36. Yin, Y.; Guo, Q.; Zhou, X.; Duan, Y.; Yang, Y.; Gong, S.; Han, M.; Liu, Y.; Yang, Z.; Chen, Q.; et al. Role of brain-gut-muscle axis in human health and energy homeostasis. *Front. Nutr.* **2022**, *9*, 947033. [CrossRef]
37. Alotaibi, G.; Alkhammash, A. Pharmacological landscape of endoplasmic reticulum stress: Uncovering therapeutic avenues for metabolic diseases. *Eur. J. Pharmacol.* **2025**, *998*, 177509. [CrossRef] [PubMed]
38. Romero-Ramírez, L.; Mey, J. Emerging Roles of Bile Acids and TGR5 in the Central Nervous System: Molecular Functions and Therapeutic Implications. *Int. J. Mol. Sci.* **2024**, *25*, 9279. [CrossRef] [PubMed]
39. Amerio, A.; Escelsior, A.; Martino, E.; Strangio, A.; Giacomini, C.; Montagna, E.; Aguglia, A.; Bellomo, M.; Sukkar, S.G.; Saverino, D. Dysfunction of Inflammatory Pathways and Their Relationship with Anti-Hypothalamic Autoantibodies in Patients with Anorexia Nervosa. *Nutrients* **2023**, *15*, 2199. [CrossRef] [PubMed]
40. Hebebrand, J.; Hildebrandt, T.; Schlögl, H.; Seitz, J.; Denecke, S.; Vieira, D.; Gradl-Dietsch, G.; Peters, T.; Antel, J.; Lau, D.; et al. The role of hypoleptinemia in the psychological and behavioral adaptation to starvation: Implications for anorexia nervosa. *Neurosci. Biobehav. Rev.* **2022**, *141*, 104807. [CrossRef]
41. Floriánková, M.; Uhlíková, P.; Dostálová, V.; Vecka, M.; Szitányi, P.; Žák, A. Nutritional and Clinical Status of Czech Adolescents with Anorexia Nervosa before and during the SARS-CoV-2 Pandemic. *Bratisl. Med. J.* **2025**, *126*, 609–618. [CrossRef]
42. Tosi, F.; Sartori, F.; Guarini, P.; Olivieri, O.; Martinelli, N. Delta-5 and delta-6 desaturases: Crucial enzymes in polyunsaturated fatty acid-related pathways with pleiotropic influences in health and disease. *Adv. Exp. Med. Biol.* **2014**, *824*, 61–81. [CrossRef]

43. Zák, A.; Tvrzická, E.; Vecka, M.; Jáchymová, M.; Duffková, L.; Stanková, B.; Vávrová, L.; Kodydková, J.; Zeman, M. Severity of metabolic syndrome unfavorably influences oxidative stress and fatty acid metabolism in men. *Tohoku J. Exp. Med.* **2007**, *212*, 359–371. [CrossRef]
44. Siguel, E.N.; Lerman, R.H. Prevalence of essential fatty acid deficiency in patients with chronic gastrointestinal disorders. *Metabolism* **1996**, *45*, 12–23. [CrossRef]
45. Žížalová, K.; Vecka, M.; Vítek, L.; Leníček, M. Enzymatic methods may underestimate the total serum bile acid concentration. *PLoS ONE* **2020**, *15*, e0236372. [CrossRef] [PubMed]
46. The R Development Core Team: R. *A Language and Environment for Statistical Computing;* R Foundation for Statistical Computing: Vienna, Austria, 2015; Available online: https://www.r-project.org/ (accessed on 28 April 2025).
47. Huang, Y.Q.; Liu, X.C.; Lo, K.; Liu, L.; Yu, Y.L.; Chen, C.L.; Huang, J.Y.; Feng, Y.Q.; Zhang, B. The U Shaped Relationship Between High-Density Lipoprotein Cholesterol and All-Cause or Cause-Specific Mortality in Adult Population. *Clin. Interv. Aging.* **2020**, *15*, 1883–1896. [CrossRef] [PubMed]
48. Chen, L.; Zhao, Y.; Wang, Z.; Wang, Y.; Bo, X.; Jiang, X.; Hao, C.; Ju, C.; Qu, Y.; Dong, H. Very high HDL-C (high-density lipoprotein cholesterol) is associated with increased cardiovascular risk in patients with NSTEMI (non-ST-segment elevation myocardial infarction) undergoing PCI (percutaneous coronary intervention). *BMC Cardiovasc. Disord.* **2023**, *23*, 357. [CrossRef] [PubMed]
49. Schorr, M.; Miller, K.K. The endocrine manifestations of anorexia nervosa: Mechanisms and management. *Nat. Rev. Endocrinol.* **2017**, *13*, 174–186. [CrossRef]
50. Jafar, W.; Morgan, J. Anorexia nervosa and the gastrointestinal tract. *Frontline Gastroenterol.* **2021**, *13*, 316–324. [CrossRef]
51. Králová Lesná, I.; Suchánek, P.; Kovář, J.; Poledne, R. Life style change and reverse cholesterol transport in obese women. *Physiol. Res.* **2009**, *58*, S33–S38. [CrossRef]
52. Nguyen, N.; Dow, M.; Woodside, B.; German, J.B.; Quehenberger, O.; Shih, P.B. Food-Intake Normalization of Dysregulated Fatty Acids in Women with Anorexia Nervosa. *Nutrients* **2019**, *11*, 2208. [CrossRef]
53. Caspar-Bauguil, S.; Montastier, E.; Galinon, F.; Frisch-Benarous, D.; Salvayre, R.; Ritz, P. Anorexia nervosa patients display a deficit in membrane long chain polyunsaturated fatty acids. *Clin. Nutr.* **2012**, *31*, 386–390. [CrossRef]
54. Keys, A. Diet and the epidemiology of coronary heart disease. *J. Am. Med. Assoc.* **1957**, *164*, 1912–1919. [CrossRef]
55. Kremmyda, L.S.; Tvrzicka, E.; Stankova, B.; Zak, A. Fatty acids as biocompounds: Their role in human metabolism, health and disease: A review. Part 2: Fatty acid physiological roles and applications in human health and disease. *Biomed. Pap. Med. Fac. Univ. Palacky Olomouc Czech Repub.* **2011**, *155*, 195–218. [CrossRef]
56. Zeman, M. Fatty acids and cardiovascular disease. In *Fatty Acids and Fats in Health and Disease*, 1st ed.; Zeman, M., Macášek, J., Vecka, M., Eds.; Grada Publishing: Prague, Czech Republic, 2024; pp. 109–126. (In Czech)
57. van der Wurff, I.S.M.; von Schacky, C.; Bergeland, T.; Leontjevas, R.; Zeegers, M.P.; Kirschner, P.A.; de Groot, R.H.M. Exploring the association between whole blood Omega-3 Index, DHA, EPA, DHA, AA and n-6 DPA, and depression and self-esteem in adolescents of lower general secondary education. *Eur. J. Nutr.* **2019**, *58*, 1429–1439, Erratum in *Eur. J. Nutr.* **2020**, *59*, 843.. [CrossRef]
58. Zec, M.M.; Schutte, A.E.; Ricci, C.; Baumgartner, J.; Kruger, I.M.; Smuts, C.M. Long-Chain Polyunsaturated Fatty Acids Are Associated with Blood Pressure and Hypertension over 10-Years in Black South African Adults Undergoing Nutritional Transition. *Foods* **2019**, *8*, 394. [CrossRef]
59. de Groot, R.H.; van Boxtel, M.P.; Schiepers, O.J.; Hornstra, G.; Jolles, J. Age dependence of plasma phospholipid fatty acid levels: Potential role of linoleic acid in the age-associated increase in docosahexaenoic acid and eicosapentaenoic acid concentrations. *Br. J. Nutr.* **2009**, *102*, 1058–1064. [CrossRef] [PubMed]
60. Muralidharan, J.; Papandreou, C.; Soria-Florido, M.T.; Sala-Vila, A.; Blanchart, G.; Estruch, R.; Martínez-González, M.A.; Corella, D.; Ros, E.; Ruiz-Canela, M.; et al. Cross-Sectional Associations between HDL Structure or Function, Cell Membrane Fatty Acid Composition, and Inflammation in Elderly Adults. *J. Nutr.* **2022**, *152*, 789–795. [CrossRef] [PubMed]
61. van Gool, C.J.; van Houwelingen, A.C.; Hornstra, G. The essential fatty acid status in phenylketonuria patients under treatment. *J. Nutr. Biochem.* **2000**, *11*, 543–547. [CrossRef] [PubMed]
62. Thomas, B.A.; Ghebremeskel, K.; Lowy, C.; Offley-Shore, B.; Crawford, M.A. Plasma fatty acids of neonates born to mothers with and without gestational diabetes. *Prostaglandins Leukot. Essent. Fatty Acids* **2005**, *72*, 335–341. [CrossRef]
63. de Groot, R.H.; Hornstra, G.; Jolles, J. Exploratory study into the relation between plasma phospholipid fatty acid status and cognitive performance. *Prostaglandins Leukot. Essent. Fatty Acids* **2007**, *76*, 165–172. [CrossRef]
64. Elizondo, A.; Araya, J.; Rodrigo, R.; Poniachik, J.; Csendes, A.; Maluenda, F.; Díaz, J.C.; Signorini, C.; Sgherri, C.; Comporti, M.; et al. Polyunsaturated fatty acid pattern in liver and erythrocyte phospholipids from obese patients. *Obesity* **2007**, *15*, 24–31. [CrossRef]
65. Lemaitre, R.N.; King, I.B. Very long-chain saturated fatty acids and diabetes and cardiovascular disease. *Curr. Opin. Lipidol.* **2022**, *33*, 76–82. [CrossRef]

66. Lai, K.Z.H.; Yehia, N.A.; Semnani-Azad, Z.; Mejia, S.B.; Boucher, B.A.; Malik, V.; Bazinet, R.P.; Hanley, A.J. Lifestyle Factors Associated with Circulating Very Long-Chain Saturated Fatty Acids in Humans: A Systematic Review of Observational Studies. *Adv. Nutr.* **2023**, *14*, 99–114. [CrossRef]
67. Roubalová, R.; Procházková, P.; Papežová, H.; Smitka, K.; Bilej, M.; Tlaskalová-Hogenová, H. Anorexia nervosa: Gut microbiota-immune-brain interactions. *Clin. Nutr.* **2020**, *39*, 676–684. [CrossRef]
68. Shapiro, H.; Kolodziejczyk, A.A.; Halstuch, D.; Elinav, E. Bile acids in glucose metabolism in health and disease. *J. Exp. Med.* **2018**, *215*, 383–396. [CrossRef]
69. Galmiche, M.; Achamrah, N.; Déchelotte, P.; Ribet, D.; Breton, J. Role of microbiota-gut-brain axis dysfunctions induced by infections in the onset of anorexia nervosa. *Nutr. Rev.* **2022**, *80*, 381–391. [CrossRef]
70. Higashi, T.; Watanabe, S.; Tomaru, K.; Yamazaki, W.; Yoshizawa, K.; Ogawa, S.; Nagao, H.; Minato, K.; Maekawa, M.; Mano, N. Unconjugated bile acids in rat brain: Analytical method based on LC/ESI-MS/MS with chemical derivatization and estimation of their origin by comparison to serum levels. *Steroids* **2017**, *125*, 107–113. [CrossRef] [PubMed]
71. Khalaf, K.; Tornese, P.; Cocco, A.; Albanese, A. Tauroursodeoxycholic acid: A potential therapeutic tool in neurodegenerative diseases. *Transl. Neurodegener.* **2022**, *11*, 33. [CrossRef] [PubMed]
72. Wu, X.; Li, J.Y.; Lee, A.; Lu, Y.X.; Zhou, S.Y.; Owyang, C. Satiety induced by bile acids is mediated via vagal afferent pathways. *JCI Insight* **2020**, *5*, e132400. [CrossRef] [PubMed]
73. Perino, A.; Velázquez-Villegas, L.A.; Bresciani, N.; Sun, Y.; Huang, Q.; Fénelon, V.S.; Castellanos-Jankiewicz, A.; Zizzari, P.; Bruschetta, G.; Jin, S.; et al. Central anorexigenic actions of bile acids are mediated by TGR5. *Nat. Metab.* **2021**, *3*, 595–603. [CrossRef]
74. Sato, H.; Macchiarulo, A.; Thomas, C.; Gioiello, A.; Une, M.; Hofmann, A.F.; Saladin, R.; Schoonjans, K.; Pellicciari, R.; Auwerx, J. Novel potent and selective bile acid derivatives as TGR5 agonists: Biological screening, structure-activity relationships, and molecular modeling studies. *J. Med. Chem.* **2008**, *51*, 1831–1841. [CrossRef]
75. Li, R.; Andreu-Sánchez, S.; Kuipers, F.; Fu, J. Gut microbiome and bile acids in obesity-related diseases. *Best Pract. Res. Clin. Endocrinol. Metab.* **2021**, *35*, 101493. [CrossRef]

nutrients

Article

The Association Between Identity Functioning and Personality Pathology in Female Patients with Eating Disorders

Laurence Claes [1,2,*], Annabel Bogaerts [3], Tim Bastiaens [4], Glenn Kiekens [1,5,6], Eva Dierckx [7,8], Katrien Schoevaerts [7] and Koen Luyckx [1,9]

[1] Faculty of Psychology and Educational Sciences, KU Leuven, 3000 Leuven, Belgium; glenn.kiekens@kuleuven.be or g.kiekens@tilburguniversity.edu (G.K.); koen.luyckx@kuleuven.be (K.L.)
[2] Faculty of Medicine and Health Sciences, University Antwerp, 2000 Antwerp, Belgium
[3] Department of Psychology, Clinical Developmental Psychology Program, University of Amsterdam, 1001 Amsterdam, The Netherlands; a.bogaerts@uva.nl
[4] Campus Kortenberg, University Psychiatric Centre, KU Leuven, 3070 Kortenberg, Belgium; tim.bastiaens@upckuleuven.be
[5] Department of Neurosciences, Center for Contextual Psychiatry, KU Leuven, 3000 Leuven, Belgium
[6] Department of Medical and Clinical Psychology, Tilburg University, 5037 Tilburg, The Netherlands
[7] Psychiatric Hospital Alexianen Zorggroep Tienen, 3300 Tienen, Belgium; eva.dierckx@azt.broedersvanliefde.be or eva.dierckx@vub.be (E.D.); katrien.schoevaerts@azt.broedersvanliefde.be (K.S.)
[8] Department of Clinical Psychology, Vrije Universiteit Brussel, 1050 Brussels, Belgium
[9] Educational Unit for Professional Training and Service in the Behavioural Sciences (UNIBS), University of the Free State, Bloemfontein 9301, South Africa
* Correspondence: laurence.claes@kuleuven.be or laurence.claes@uantwerpen.be; Tel.: +32-16326133

Abstract

Aims. In the present study, we investigated the associations between the three identity dimensions of Kaufman (Consolidated Identity, Disturbed Identity, Lack of Identity) and symptoms of personality disorders (PDs) in 176 female inpatients with an eating disorder (ED). We examined five aspects: the prevalence of categorical PD diagnoses in patients with EDs; the relationship between dimensional PD scores and identity dimensions as well as their relationships with age and ED subtype; and the unique variance in dimensional PD scores explained by identity dimensions, while controlling for age and ED subtype. Methods. To assess identity functioning, we made use of the Self-Concept and Identity Measure, and to assess PDs, we used the categorical and dimensional scores of the Assessment of DSM-IV Personality Disorders. Results. The findings showed that the avoidant, obsessive–compulsive, and borderline categorical PDs were the most frequently reported PDs. Age was negatively related to all Cluster B PDs and Disturbed Identity, and binge-eating/purging ED patients reported significantly more Cluster B PD features compared to restrictive ED patients. ED subtype and identity dimensions were unrelated. Correlational analysis showed that all dimensional PD scores were positively related to Disturbed Identity and Lack of Identity and negatively related to Consolidated Identity. The results of the hierarchical regression analyses showed that Cluster A PDs were significantly predicted by Lack of Identity, controlled for age and ED subtype. Additionally, Cluster B PDs were significantly predicted by Disturbed Identity. Finally, two of the three cluster C PDs were predicted by Lack of Identity (avoidant and obsessive–compulsive PD), whereas the dependent PD was explained by Disturbed Identity. Conclusions. The co-occurrence of identity issues in both PDs and EDs underscores the role of identity as a transdiagnostic feature. Accordingly, using identity-based interventions in treatment may have broad therapeutic benefits across these disorders.

Keywords: identity; personality disorders; eating disorders

 https://doi.org/10.3390/nu17142329

1. Introduction

Understanding the associations between identity functioning and personality disorders (PDs) in eating disorders (EDs) offers critical insights into the co-occurrence of these complex conditions. Identity disturbance not only underpins many of the core features of EDs but also serves as a bridge linking EDs to co-occurring personality pathology. In the present study, we will investigate the prevalence of categorical PDs in patients with EDs, examine the associations between identity functioning and dimensional PD scores as well as their relationships with age and ED subtype, and research the unique variance that identity dimensions can explain in dimensional PD scores (while controlling for age and ED subtype).

1.1. Identity

In Erikson's [1] influential lifespan theory, identity formation is conceptualized as a dynamic tension between identity synthesis and identity confusion. Successful development requires individuals to achieve a balance that favors synthesis over confusion. Identity synthesis reflects the extent to which different aspects of the self are integrated, contributing to a subjective sense of continuity and coherence across time and situations. In contrast, identity confusion is characterized by difficulties in making and sustaining long-term commitments, as well as a lack of clear purpose and direction in life [1–3].

To advance the study of identity in both community and clinical populations, Kaufman et al. [4] proposed a multidimensional model of identity, grounded in both developmental and clinical theoretical frameworks [1,5]. This model delineates three core dimensions of identity functioning. (1) Consolidated Identity reflects a stable and coherent sense of self, characterized by a clear understanding of who one is, commitment to personal values and beliefs, consistency across time and situations, and a sense of positive self-worth [4]. (2) Disturbed Identity captures disruptions in this coherence, including internal inconsistencies in values, beliefs, and opinions, as well as an overreliance on external sources—such as others' expectations or approval—to define the self [4]. (3) Lack of Identity, a dimension that has received comparatively less empirical attention, refers to a profound sense of inner emptiness and disconnection of the self. Individuals scoring high on this dimension often report feeling lost, broken, or devoid of a coherent self-concept, with little or no sense of who they are [4]. This tripartite framework offers a nuanced understanding of identity functioning and its impairments, with relevance for both normative development and psychopathology. To assess the three identity dimensions, Kaufman et al. [4] developed the Self-Concept and Identity Measure (SCIM), a reliable and valid questionnaire that has demonstrated convergent validity with measures of borderline PD, emotion dysregulation, and various other indicators of psychopathology [4,6].

1.2. Identity and Eating Disorders

Bruch [7,8] proposed that EDs, particularly anorexia nervosa, arise from fundamental disturbances in identity development and autonomy, rather than purely sociocultural ideals. Contemporary perspectives support this view, highlighting maladaptive identity functioning as central across restrictive and binge/purge EDs [3,9]. In restrictive EDs, individuals often exhibit a poorly differentiated self, linking identity to control over food and body [10–12]. The pursuit of thinness serves as a compensatory strategy for fragmented identity and perceived ineffectiveness [7,8,10,11]. In binge/purge EDs, individuals experience chronic emptiness, using bingeing to fill emotional voids and purging to regain control, reflecting an unstable self-concept and impaired emotion regulation [3,13–15].

Numerous empirical studies have shown that individuals with eating disorders (EDs) exhibit greater identity confusion, and that maladaptive identity functioning is positively correlated with ED symptom severity [14,16–19]. Verschueren et al. [20] found that ED patients scored lower on adaptive and higher on maladaptive identity processes compared to controls, identifying an "identity disorder" status exclusively among ED patients. Although many studies have examined the link between identity and EDs, the directionality of this relationship has been less explored. In a two-year longitudinal study, Verschueren et al. [21] demonstrated that identity confusion increased vulnerability to body dissatisfaction and bulimia symptoms, while identity synthesis was protective. Moreover, bulimia symptoms predicted increased identity confusion and decreased identity synthesis, highlighting a bidirectional relationship. Recent findings further show that reductions in identity confusion and increases in identity synthesis during treatment are associated with decreases in drive for thinness and body dissatisfaction [22]. These results suggest that recovery involves relinquishing an ED-centered identity and developing a more integrated self [23–25]. Finally, Rohde et al. [18] found that patients with bulimia nervosa exhibited greater identity impairment than those with restrictive-type anorexia nervosa.

1.3. Identity and Personality Disorders in Patients with Eating Disorders

Given the high prevalence of identity disturbances among individuals with eating disorders (EDs) and their established association with personality disorders (PDs) [26], it is unsurprising that many ED patients also exhibit PD features. Most studies examining PDs in ED populations have employed the categorical approach outlined in DSM-5 Section II [27], which defines ten PDs grouped into three clusters: Cluster A (odd/eccentric: paranoid, schizoid, and schizotypal PDs), Cluster B (dramatic/emotional: narcissistic, antisocial, borderline, and histrionic PDs), and Cluster C (anxious/fearful: avoidant, dependent, and obsessive–compulsive PDs). Approximately 50–70% of individuals with an ED meet criteria for at least one PD [28–30], with Cluster C PDs being most prevalent, followed by Cluster B and Cluster A PDs [31].

By subtype, individuals with ED binge/purge type (ED-BP) show higher rates of Cluster B PDs, especially the borderline PD, compared to restrictive-type ED (ED-R) patients [30,32]. No consistent differences have been observed for Cluster C PDs between subtypes [28,29,33]. Additionally, PD prevalence tends to decrease with age in ED populations [31].

While identity disturbance is a diagnostic criterion for the borderline PD, the Alternative Model for Personality Disorders (AMPD) in DSM-5 Section III [27] considers identity impairment a core feature of all PDs. The AMPD conceptualizes PDs dimensionally, defined by impairments in self-functioning (identity, self-direction) and interpersonal functioning (empathy, intimacy) (Criterion A), along with maladaptive personality traits (Criterion B).

To date, only two studies have examined identity impairments—as conceptualized by Kaufman [4]—and their relationship with dimensional scores of PDs in clinical populations. First, Bogaerts et al. [34] investigated this association in a sample of 153 psychiatric inpatients, using the Self-Concept and Identity Measure (SCIM) [4]. Their findings indicated that Lack of Identity was not significantly associated with age, Disturbed Identity was negatively correlated with age, and Consolidated Identity was positively associated with age. Correlation analyses revealed that Consolidated Identity was negatively associated with all PDs, except the narcissistic and obsessive–compulsive PDs. Disturbed Identity was positively associated with all PDs except the schizoid PD, while Lack of Identity was positively related to all PDs except the narcissistic PD. Regression analyses further demonstrated that Consolidated Identity did not significantly predict variance in any PDs other than the narcissistic PD. In contrast, Disturbed Identity was a significant positive predictor of all PDs except the schizoid and avoidant PDs. Lastly, Lack of Identity significantly predicted variance in all Cluster A PDs, as well as the borderline, avoidant, and dependent PDs.

Second, Tressova et al. [35] examined the bivariate correlations between the SCIM subscales and personality pathology as defined in Section III of the DSM-5, in a sample of 92 male forensic patients and 139 healthy controls. Disturbed Identity and Lack of Identity were positively associated with all six assessed personality disorders—antisocial, avoidant, borderline, narcissistic, obsessive–compulsive, and schizotypal PD. In contrast, Consolidated Identity was not significantly associated with any of the PDs.

1.4. The Present Study

The present study aimed to examine the prevalence of categorical PDs in patients with EDs and was the first to investigate the associations between identity functioning, as conceptualized by Kaufman et al. [4], and dimensional PD symptom scores in individuals with EDs. Specifically, this study pursued five main objectives. First, we assessed the prevalence of categorical PD diagnoses among individuals with EDs. Drawing on prior research [29], we hypothesized the highest prevalence rates for obsessive–compulsive, avoidant, borderline, dependent, and paranoid PDs. Furthermore, we anticipated that Cluster C PDs would be the most frequent, followed by Cluster B, with Cluster A PDs being the least prevalent [31].

Second, we investigated whether age and ED subtype—restrictive (ED-R) versus binge/purge (ED-BP)—were associated with dimensional symptom scores of PDs. Prior research in ED populations has demonstrated significantly negative associations between age and PD symptoms, with younger individuals typically exhibiting more pronounced PD traits [31]. Within Cluster B, we expected ED-BP patients to exhibit higher levels of borderline PD symptoms compared to those with ED-R. In contrast, we anticipated either no significant differences within Cluster C or a slightly higher prevalence of obsessive–compulsive PD among ED-R patients [30,32].

Third, we explored associations between age, ED subtype, and Kaufman's et al. [4] three dimensions of identity functioning: Lack of Identity, Disturbed Identity, and Consolidated Identity. Based on previous findings [34], we hypothesized that age would be positively associated with Consolidated Identity and negatively associated with Disturbed Identity, while no significant association was expected with Lack of Identity. Guided by the findings of Rohde et al. [18], we further anticipated that patients engaging in binge-eating/purging behaviors would demonstrate higher levels of identity-related deficits, compared to those with restrictive behaviors.

Fourth, we examined associations between the three identity dimensions and the dimensional symptom scores of PDs, by controlling for age and ED subtype. Consistent with the existing literature [34,35], we expected that both Disturbed Identity and Lack of Identity would show positive associations with most PDs, except the narcissistic PD [34]. In contrast, we hypothesized that Consolidated Identity would be negatively associated with all PDs (except the narcissistic and obsessive–compulsive PD) [34] or would be unrelated to all PDs [35].

Fifth, we investigated the unique contribution of each identity dimension to the variance in dimensional symptoms scores of PDs while controlling for age and ED subtype. Specifically, we expected that Cluster A PDs would be primarily predicted by Lack of Identity, whereas Cluster B PDs would be significantly associated with Disturbed Identity [34]. Given that the borderline PD is characterized by Disturbed Identity and chronic feelings of emptiness (as described in DSM-5, Section II), we also expected that Lack of Identity, related to feelings of emptiness, would further predict variance in the borderline PD [34]. Moreover, considering the DSM-5 criteria for narcissistic PD—marked by grandiosity and an inflated sense of self—we hypothesized that Consolidated Identity would predict additional variance in the narcissistic PD, and potentially in the antisocial

PD as well [34]. Finally, we hypothesized that the dependent and obsessive–compulsive PDs (Cluster C) would be uniquely predicted by Disturbed Identity, while the avoidant PD would be uniquely predicted by Lack of Identity. This expectation was based on findings by previous research [34,36] and the well-documented high comorbidity between the avoidant and Cluster A PDs [37].

2. Materials and Methods

2.1. Participants and Procedure

Data were collected from the clinical records of female inpatients treated at a specialized unit for EDs in Flanders (Belgium). The current sample included 176 female inpatients (age $\geq$ 18 years), of whom 46 (26.1%) were diagnosed as AN-R, 16 as AN-BP (9.1%), 23 as BN (13.1%), 8 (4.5%) as BED, and 83 (47.2%) as EDNOS by means of the EDI-3 Symptom Checklist (EDI-3 SC) [38]. The mean age of the patients was 25.23 (SD = 6.91; range: 18–48 years). Regarding the highest level of education, 5 (2.8%) patients had completed primary education, 50 (28.4%) secondary education, and 121 (68.8%) higher education. Given that personality functioning is often related to ED subtype, we divided our ED sample into a restrictive (ED-R; N = 96, 54.5%) and a binge-eating/purging (ED-BP; N = 80, 45.5%) subgroup. The mean BMI of both groups was significantly different [$F(1, 173) = 24.58$, $p < 0.001$, partial $\eta 2 = 0.13$], with restrictive patients (M_{BMI} = 16.31, SD_{BMI} = 2.53) reporting a significantly lower BMI than patients with ED-BP (M_{BMI} = 19.17, SD_{BMI} = 4.91). The mean age difference between both groups was borderline-significant [$F(1, 174) = 3.94$, $p = 0.049$, partial $\eta 2 = 0.02$], with restrictive patients being slightly younger (M_{Age} = 24.29, SD_{Age} = 6.78) than patients with ED-BP (M_{Age} = 26.35, SD_{Age} = 6.94). Importantly, since the sample consisted exclusively of female patients with EDs, no conclusions can be drawn regarding male patients.

Patients gave written informed consent and permission to the pseudonymized use of their data for research purposes by signing an informed consent form at admission and before filling out the questionnaires on the PC. This procedure was approved by the medical–ethical committee of the clinic and the Social and Societal Ethics Committee of KU Leuven. Patients were not compensated for their participation in this study.

2.2. Instruments

All ED patients completed the Self-Concept and Identity Measure (SCIM [4]; Dutch version: [34,39]) and the Assessment of DSM-IV Personality Disorders (APD-IV [40,41]) to assess identity functioning and PD symptomatology.

The Self-Concept and Identity Measure (SCIM [4]; Dutch translation: [34,39]) comprises 27 items, each rated on a 7-point Likert scale ranging from 1 ("completely disagree") to 7 ("completely agree"). The SCIM yields three subscales: Consolidated Identity (10 items, e.g., "I know who I am"), Disturbed Identity (11 items, e.g., "I change a lot depending on the situation"), and Lack of Identity (6 items, e.g., "I feel empty inside, like a person without a soul"). Subscale scores are calculated as the mean score of the corresponding item scores. The Dutch version of the SCIM has been validated in both the general population and clinical samples [34,39]. In the clinical sample, confirmatory factor analysis supported the three-factor model of the SCIM, with a good model fit achieved after the exclusion of items 3, 11, and 14 from the Consolidated Identity Scale and item 23 from the Disturbed Identity scale [34]. In the present study, the internal consistency (Cronbach's alpha) for the revised subscales was as follows: $\alpha = 0.68$ for Consolidated Identity (7 items), $\alpha = 0.81$ for Disturbed Identity (10 items), and $\alpha = 0.86$ for Lack of Identity (6 items). According to George and Mallery [42], alpha values above 0.70, 0.80, and 0.90 indicate acceptable, good, and excellent reliability, respectively. The Disturbed Identity and Lack of Identity Scales demonstrated good reliability coefficients, while the Consolidated Identity Scale exhibited marginally acceptable reliability. These results align with previous studies employing the Dutch version of the SCIM [34,39]. Excluding the item "I am basically the same person that I've always been" from the Consolidated Identity Scale would have increased the alpha coefficient to $\alpha = 0.72$, indicating acceptable reliability. However, to ensure comparability with prior findings [34,39], this item was retained.

The Assessment of DSM-IV Personality Disorders (ADP-IV [40,41]) was used to assess personality disorder symptomatology. The ADP-IV is a Dutch self-report questionnaire consisting of 94 items, covering the diagnostic criteria for the 12 personality disorders (PDs) defined in the DSM-IV [43]. The structure of the ADP-IV allows for both dimensional trait scoring and categorical PD diagnosis. Each item (e.g., a borderline PD item: "I absolutely cannot bear the idea that someone would leave or abandon me; therefore, I will do anything to prevent this") is rated on a 7-point Likert scale, ranging from 1 ("totally disagree") to 7 ("totally agree"), yielding a trait score. If a trait score is 5 ("rather agree") or higher, respondents are further asked to indicate the degree of distress the feature causes themselves or others, using a 3-point scale (1 = "not at all"; 3 = "most certainly"). Mean dimensional trait scores are calculated by summing the trait scores and dividing by the number of items corresponding to each specific PD. Categorical diagnoses are derived according to the DSM-IV criteria, using combined trait and distress scores within validated scoring algorithms (e.g., a criterion is considered present if Trait > 4 and Distress > 1) [40,41]. In the present study, both categorical diagnoses and dimensional trait scores were used. Internal consistency (Cronbach's alpha) for the ADP-IV dimensional scales ranged from 0.68 (marginally acceptable reliability; the antisocial PD) to 0.81 (good reliability; the schizotypal PD). Excluding the item "I experience little or no feelings of guilt or remorse when I have done something wrong" from the Antisocial PD Scale would have increased the alpha coefficient to $\alpha = 0.71$, indicating acceptable reliability. Nevertheless, this item was preserved to allow for direct comparison with earlier studies [34,39].

2.3. Analyses

All analyses were performed by means of the program SPSS, version 29. First, to determine the prevalence of the categorical PDs in our ED sample, we calculated the number (percentages) of the patients who met the diagnostic criteria of the 10 categorical PDs. Second, we calculated the descriptive statistics of the dimensional symptom scores of PDs. To investigate the association between the dimensional symptom scores of PDs and age, we calculated the Pearson correlation coefficients. To investigate whether the dimensional symptoms scores of PDs differed between ED subtype (ED-R vs. ED-BP), we performed a MANOVA with the dimensional symptom scores of PDs as dependent variables and ED subtype as independent variable. Third, to investigate the descriptive statistics of the three SCIM identity scales, we calculated the means and standard deviations of the three scales. Associations between the SCIM scales and age were calculated by means of the Pearson correlation coefficients. To investigate differences in the three SCIM scales between ED subtype, we performed a MANOVA with the SCIM scales as dependent variables and ED subtype as independent variable. Fourth, to determine the associations between the three SCIM identity scales and the dimensional symptom scores of PDs (controlled for age and ED subtype depending on the outcomes of the prior analyses), we calculated partial correlations. Hemphill [44] suggests that correlation coefficients below 0.20, between 0.20 and 0.30, and above 0.30 indicate small, medium, and large effects, respectively. Finally, to investigate which SCIM scales predicted the most variance in each of the 10 dimensional symptom scores of PDs, while controlling for age and ED subtype, we performed 10 hierarchical regression analyses with each of the dimensional symptom scores of PDs as dependent variables, and in step 1 (age) and step 2 (ED subtype) the control variables, and in step 3 (the three SCIM scales) the predictors.

3. Results

3.1. Prevalence of Categorical PDs in Patients with EDs

The prevalence rates of the categorical PDs in our ED sample are displayed in Table 1. The obsessive–compulsive PD (66.5%), the avoidant PD (58.8%), and the borderline PD (46%) were the most frequently reported PDs, followed by the dependent PD (23.3%) and the Cluster A PDs.

Table 1. Numbers (percentages) of categorical PDs, means (standard deviations) of the dimensional PD and identity scores, correlations with age, and differences in means (standard deviations) in dimensional PD and identity scores between restrictive and binge-eating/purging patients with an ED.

	Categorical PDs (N = 176)		Dimensional PDs (N = 176)							
						Restrictive (N = 96)		Binge/Purge (N = 80)		
ADP-IV	N	(%)	M	(SD)	r(age)	M	(SD)	M	(SD)	F
Paranoid	33	(18.8)	3.31	(1.12)	−0.05	3.30	(1.18)	3.33	(1.05)	0.045
Schizoid	31	(17.6)	3.26	(1.09)	0.03	3.24	(1.04)	3.30	(1.16)	0.138
Schizotypal	29	(16.5)	3.09	(1.08)	−0.14	3.12	(1.09)	3.05	(1.08)	0.168
Antisocial	0	(0.0)	1.75	(0.67)	−0.16 *	1.60	(0.61)	1.93	(0.69)	10.749 ***
Borderline	81	(46.0)	3.86	(1.01)	−0.23 **	3.76	(0.96)	3.99	(1.07)	2.303
Histrionic	7	(4.0)	2.95	(0.88)	−0.27 **	2.82	(0.83)	3.11	(0.91)	5.077 *
Narcissistic	2	(1.1)	2.21	(0.81)	−0.21 **	2.22	(0.81)	2.20	(0.81)	0.031
Avoidant	103	(58.8)	4.50	(1.13)	−0.06	4.50	(1.14)	4.50	(1.13)	0.001
Dependent	41	(23.3)	3.75	(0.96)	−0.24 **	3.79	(0.95)	3.70	(0.96)	0.371
Obsessive–Compulsive	117	(66.5)	4.52	(0.94)	−0.07	4.64	(0.90)	4.37	(0.97)	3.713
SCIM			M	(SD)	r(age)	M	(SD)	M	(SD)	F
Disturbed identity			3.21	(0.98)	−0.26 ***	3.12	(0.96)	3.31	(1.00)	1.59
Lack of Identity			4.52	(1.29)	−0.06	4.57	(1.31)	4.46	(1.26)	0.33
Consolidated identity			4.19	(0.88)	0.08	4.21	(0.86)	4.17	(0.82)	0.07

* $p < 0.05$; ** $p < 0.01$; *** $p < 0.001$; ADP-IV = Assessment of DSM-IV Personality Disorders; SCIM: Self-Concept and Identity Measure; ED = eating disorder.

3.2. Associations Between Dimensional Symptom Scores of PDs and Age and ED Subtype

The means (standard deviations) of the dimensional symptom scores of PDs are shown in Table 1. Age showed a significantly negative association with the dimensional scores of all Cluster B PDs and the dimensional score of the dependent PD, with a medium effect size. Regarding ED subtype, ED-BP patients reported significantly higher dimensional scores for the antisocial and the histrionic PD (Cluster B) compared to restrictive patients.

3.3. Associations Between Dimensional SCIM Identity Scale Scores and Age and ED Subtype

The mean scores on the three SCIM identity scale scores are displayed in Table 1, and the highest mean score is indicated for Lack of Identity ($M = 4.52$; 4 = neither agree nor disagree, 5 = somewhat agree), followed by Consolidated Identity ($M = 4.19$; 4 = neither agree nor disagree) and Disturbed Identity ($M = 3.21$; 3 = somewhat disagree). Age showed a significant negative association with Disturbed Identity (medium effect size), while no associations were found with Lack of Identity and Consolidated Identity. Finally, no significant differences emerged between the two ED subtypes (ED-R vs. ED-BP) on the three SCIM scales.

3.4. Correlations Between SCIM Identity Scale Scores and Dimensional Symptom Scores of PDs Controlled for Age and ED Subtype

The partial correlations between the three SCIM identity scales and the dimensional PD scales (controlled for age and ED subtype (ED-R vs. ED-BP); Table 2) showed that all PDs were significantly positively related to Disturbed Identity and Lack of Identity (except the narcissistic and histrionic PDs), and significantly negatively related to Consolidated Identity (except the narcissistic, histrionic, and obsessive–compulsive PDs). The strongest positive correlations (large effect sizes) were observed between Disturbed Identity and the Cluster A and Cluster B PDs, as well as between Lack of Identity and the Cluster A PDs, avoidant PD, and borderline PD. Finally, the strongest negative correlations were found between Consolidated Identity and the Cluster A PDs and avoidant PD.

Table 2. Partial correlations between APD-IV and SCIM dimensional scores controlled for age and ED subtype (ED-R vs. ED-BP).

	SCIM Identity Disturbance	**SCIM Lack of Identity**	**SCIM Consolidated Identity**
ADP-IV	Partial *r*	Partial *r*	Partial *r*
Paranoid	0.35 ***	0.50 ***	−0.35 ***
Schizoid	0.16 *	0.39 ***	−0.23 **
Schizotypal	0.33 ***	0.46 ***	−0.31 ***
Antisocial	0.29 ***	0.18 *	−0.16 *
Borderline	0.33 ***	0.44 ***	−0.29 ***
Histrionic	0.52 ***	0.15	−0.15
Narcissistic	0.31 ***	0.10	0.03
Avoidant	0.22 **	0.40 ***	−0.35 ***
Dependent	0.37 ***	0.22 **	−0.26 ***
Obsessive–Compulsive	0.20 **	0.27 ***	−0.15
SCIM			
Disturbed Identity	-	0.46 ***	−0.40 ***
Lack of Identity		-	−0.62 ***
Consolidated Identity			-

* $p < 0.05$; ** $p < 0.01$; *** $p < 0.001$; ADP-IV = Assessment of DSM-IV Personality Disorders; SCIM: Self-Concept and Identity Measure; ED = eating disorder; ED-R = ED-restrictive type; ED-BP = ED-binge/purge type.

3.5. Prediction of Dimensional Symptom Scores of PDs by Means of SCIM Identity Scale Scores Controlled for Age and ED Subtype

The results of the hierarchical regression analyses with the dimensional PD scales as dependent variables are displayed in Table 3. Overall, the findings indicate that adding the three identity scales explained a significant amount of additional variance in all dimensional PD scores, above and beyond the effects of age and ED subtype. The largest increases in explained variance were observed for the Cluster A paranoid PD ($\Delta R^2 = 0.263$), schizotypal PD ($\Delta R^2 = 0.226$), and histrionic PD ($\Delta R^2 = 0.245$). When examining the total variance explained across all PDs by age, ED subtype, and identity dimensions, the proportion of explained variance ranged from $R^2 = 0.100$ (obsessive–compulsive PD) to $R^2 = 0.360$ (histrionic PD). These results suggest that there remains substantial room for improving the prediction of dimensional PDs beyond age, ED subtype, and identity dimensions.

Table 3. Hierarchical regression analyses with dimensional PD scores as dependent variables (ADP-IV), age and ED subtype as control variables, and identity dimensions (SCIM) as predictors.

	ADP-IV									
	PAR	**SZ**	**ST**	**AS**	**BPD**	**HIS**	**NAR**	**AV**	**DEP**	**OC**
	β	β	β	β	β	β	β	β	β	β
Age	−0.05	0.03	−0.14	−0.16 *	−0.23 **	−0.27 ***	−0.21 **	−0.06	−0.24 ***	−0.07
R^2	0.003	0.001	0.019	0.024 *	0.055 **	0.073 ***	0.044 **	0.004	0.056 ***	0.004
Age	−0.06	0.02	−0.14	−0.20 **	−0.26 ***	−0.30 ***	−0.21 **	−0.07	−0.24 **	−0.05
R/BP	0.02	0.03	−0.01	0.27 ***	0.15 *	0.21 **	0.02	0.01	−0.01	−0.14
R^2	0.003	0.001	0.019	0.096	0.078	0.117	0.044	0.004	0.057	0.023
ΔR^2	0.001	0.001	0.000	0.072 ***	0.023 *	0.044 **	0.000	0.000	0.000	0.019
Age	0.01	0.04	−0.07	−0.12	−0.19 **	−0.15 *	−0.12	−0.03	−0.13	−0.01
R/BP	0.02	0.04	−0.02	0.24 ***	0.14 *	0.13 *	−0.02	0.01	−0.06	−0.14
Disturbed Identity	0.15	−0.03	0.16	0.25 ***	0.17 *	0.56 ***	0.37 ***	0.02	0.33 ***	0.11
Lack of Identity	0.40 ***	0.41 ***	0.37 ***	0.05	0.34 ***	−0.11	0.06	0.29 **	−0.02	0.24 **
Consolidated Identity	−0.05	0.01	−0.02	−0.03	−0.00	0.01	0.22 *	−0.17	−0.14	0.04
R^2	0.267	0.151	0.245	0.174	0.272	0.362	0.165	0.181	0.199	0.100
ΔR^2	0.263 ***	0.150 ***	0.226 ***	0.078 **	0.195 ***	0.245 ***	0.121 ***	0.177 ***	0.143 ***	0.077 ***

* $p < 0.05$; ** $p < 0.01$; *** $p < 0.001$; ADP-IV = Assessment of DSM-IV Personality Disorders; SCIM: Self-Concept and Identity Measure; ED = eating disorder; R/BP = restrictive/binge-eating/purging ED subtype. PAR = paranoid; SZ = schizoid; ST = schizotypal; AS = antisocial; BPD = borderline; NAR = narcissistic; AV = avoidant; DEP = dependent; OC = obsessive–compulsive dimensional personality disorder scores.

Concerning Cluster A PDs, Lack of Identity positively predicted the dimensional scores of all three Cluster A PDs (paranoid, schizoid, and schizotypal), while controlling for age, ED subtype, and the other SCIM scales. Regarding Cluster B PDs, age was significantly negatively related to the dimensional scores of all Cluster B PDs (step 1), indicating that Cluster B PDs are more frequently reported by younger female patients with an ED. After controlling for age, ED subtype also significantly predicted the dimensional scores of three out of four Cluster B PDs (excluding the narcissistic PD), suggesting that Cluster B PDs are more prevalent in patients with binge-eating/purging-type EDs compared to restrictive-type EDs. Furthermore, Disturbed Identity positively predicted unique variance in all dimensional Cluster B PDs, after controlling for age and ED subtype. Additionally, the dimensional borderline PD was also positively predicted by Lack of Identity, and the narcissistic PD by Consolidated Identity. Finally, for Cluster C PDs, the dependent PD was significantly positively predicted by Disturbed Identity, whereas the avoidant and obsessive–compulsive PDs were significantly predicted by Lack of Identity, in line with the findings for Cluster A PDs.

4. Discussion

Given the high comorbidity between eating disorders (EDs) and personality disorders (PDs) [28–30], it may be crucial to consider identity dysfunction as a potential transdiagnostic mechanism underlying this co-occurrence. This perspective aligns with contemporary dimensional models of psychopathology, such as the Research Domain Criteria (RDoC) framework proposed by the National Institute of Mental Health [45]. This model emphasizes the importance of shared underlying psychological processes—such as impairments in self and identity functioning—that surpass traditional diagnostic boundaries. Identity dysfunction, characterized by difficulties in establishing a coherent and stable sense of self, has been increasingly recognized as a core feature in both EDs and PDs [4,34]. As such, conceptualizing identity dysfunction as a transdiagnostic vulnerability factor may offer a more integrative understanding of the high comorbidity between these disorders and inform more targeted interventions.

4.1. Prevalence of Categorical PDs in Patients with EDs

In line with prior research [29], we found that the obsessive–compulsive, avoidant, and borderline categorical PDs were the most prevalent categorical PDs among individuals with EDs. Overall, Cluster C PDs were most prevalent, followed by Cluster B and Cluster A PDs, respectively [31]. This pattern suggests that anxiety-related traits (Cluster C) and emotional dysregulation (Cluster B) are particularly common among ED patients [28,29].

4.2. Associations Between Dimensional Symptom Scores of PDs and Age and ED Subtype

In line with previous research, we observed significant negative associations between age and dimensional scores of all Cluster B PDs, as well as the dependent PD [31,37,46]. The decline in dependent traits with age may reflect increased autonomy and social maturity over time [47]. Similarly, reduction in Cluster B traits is consistent with findings indicating that impulsivity and affective instability typically decrease with age [48]. Furthermore, patients with binge-eating/purging behaviors showed higher Cluster B PD scores compared to those with restrictive eating behaviors. This supports evidence that impulsivity—a core feature of Cluster B PDs—is more pronounced in ED subtypes involving bingeing and purging, emphasizing the link between behavioral dysregulation and identity disturbances in these groups [28,49].

4.3. Associations Between Dimensional SCIM Identity Scale Scores and Age and ED Subtype

As hypothesized and in line with prior findings [34], Disturbed Identity was negatively associated with age, indicating some normative improvement in identity integration over time. However, Lack of Identity was unrelated to age, and contrary to our expectations, Consolidated Identity was not significantly related to age. While identity consolidation typically increases in community samples [20], this trend may be disrupted in clinical ED samples, where chronic psychopathology can hinder the development of a coherent and synthesized identity. Unlike Rohde et al. [18], we did not observe significant differences in SCIM dimensions between ED subtypes (ED-R vs. ED-BP). This divergence may be due to differences in subgroup definitions: our ED-BP group included both BN and AN-BP patients, possibly diluting subtype-specific effects.

4.4. Correlations Between SCIM Identity Scale Scores and Dimensional Symptom Scores of PDs Controlled for Age and ED Subtype

In line with earlier research, Disturbed Identity and Lack of Identity were significantly positively associated with nearly all dimensional scores of PDs, except the narcissistic and histrionic PDs, which were not significantly correlated with Lack of Identity. Conversely, Consolidated Identity was negatively associated with most dimensional scores of PDs, supporting its role as a protective factor [4,34]. These findings support the importance of identity dysfunction as a core diagnostic criterion of most PDs, as recognized in the Alternative Model for Personality Disorders of the DSM-5 [50,51].

4.5. Prediction of Dimensional Symptom Scores of PDs by Means of SCIM Identity Scale Scores Controlled for Age and ED Subtype

Finally, when predicting PD symptoms controlled for age and ED subtype, Lack of Identity significantly predicted all Cluster A PDs (paranoid, schizoid, and schizotypal) and two Cluster C PDs (avoidant and obsessive–compulsive). These PDs are characterized by impaired identity integration. In Cluster A PDs, identity is often fragmented or unintegrated, resulting in bizarre thoughts, social withdrawal, and suspiciousness. As individuals with Cluster A PDs often present with a psychotic personality structure [5,52], their reality testing and sense of identity may be compromised, leading to blurred self-other boundaries and a fragmented self [34]. In Cluster C PDs, patients tend to be overly contingent, either on others' approval (avoidant PD) or rigid performance standards (obsessive–compulsive PD).

All dimensional Cluster B PDs scores were predicted by Disturbed Identity, typically expressed through a fluctuating self-image, externalized self-worth, and fragmented internal cohesion [53,54]. Notably, the borderline PD was predicted by both Disturbed Identity and Lack of Identity. This aligns with the literature highlighting chronic feelings of emptiness and dissociative states marked by feelings of nothingness, numbness, and disconnection from self and others as central to borderline pathology [34,53,55]. The narcissistic PD also involves both disturbed and partially integrated identity structures. In grandiose narcissism, individuals often maintain a highly idealized and inflated self-image; however, this self-concept is fragile, defensive, and dependent on external validation, achievement, and dominance, making it vulnerable to destabilization by criticism or failure [34,56].

Finally, the dependent PD was also predicted by Disturbed Identity alone, suggesting a failure in the individuation processes, resulting in an identity excessively reliant on close relationships and vulnerable to interpersonal disruptions [47].

When considering age, ED subtype, and identity dimensions, the proportion of explained variance in PD scores ranged from R^2 = 0.100 (obsessive–compulsive PD) to R^2 = 0.360 (histrionic PD). This indicates that substantial variance remains unexplained, highlighting the need to include additional factors. According to the Alternative Model for Personality Disorders (AMPD) in DSM-5 Section III [50,51], personality disorders arise from impairments in self and interpersonal functioning (Criterion A) and specific maladaptive personality traits (Criterion B). While our study focused on self-functioning through identity dimensions, incorporating measures of interpersonal dysfunction and personality traits could further improve the prediction and understanding of PD symptoms in ED patients.

4.6. Clinical Implications

The co-occurrence of identity disturbance in both PDs and EDs underscores its role as a transdiagnostic feature. Given its central role, identity disturbance can be considered a valuable treatment target in both PDs and EDs. Schema therapy (ST), for example, addresses maladaptive schemas underlying identity disturbance, helping patients develop a more integrated and stable sense of self; it has shown efficacy for both PDs and chronic EDs [57,58]. Mentalization-based treatment (MBT), originally developed for BPD, focuses on improving reflective functioning and self-understanding, and has been adapted successfully for EDs to enhance self-structure and emotional regulation [59]. Dialectical behavior therapy (DBT) targets identity disturbance indirectly through skills modules focused on emotion regulation, mindfulness, and interpersonal effectiveness, and has demonstrated effectiveness in patients with comorbid EDs and BPD [60,61]. By explicitly addressing identity disturbance, these approaches provide promising avenues for targeting the shared vulnerabilities underlying both PDs and EDs.

4.7. Limitations and Suggestions for Future Research

The present cross-sectional study examining the association between identity dimensions and dimensional scores of PDs in female patients with an ED via self-report measures presents several limitations that warrant consideration. These limitations pertain to the sample and the methodological constraints inherent in self-report designs and the cross-sectional nature of the study, which collectively impact the interpretability and generalizability of the findings. The exclusive focus on a female inpatient sample limits the generalizability of the findings to male patients and individuals receiving outpatient treatment. Additionally, EDNOS represents a heterogeneous category, and collapsing it into restrictive versus binge/purge groups may mask important clinical differences. Furthermore, we did not have access to patients' medical files and therefore lacked information on detailed sociodemographic variables as well as physical and psychological comorbidities, which should be addressed in future studies. Finally, as most participants were White and from Western backgrounds (i.e., Flemish), the findings may not be generalizable to individuals from other ethnic, cultural, or regional groups. The reliance on self-report measures introduces susceptibility to social desirability bias and may be particularly problematic in individuals with EDs and comorbid personality disorders, who may have impaired introspective capacity [62]. The use of self-report for all study variables also raises concerns about shared method variance, potentially inflating observed associations [63]. Additionally, the reliability of the Consolidated Identity Scale and the Antisocial PD Scale was marginally adequate; however, these scales were retained in their original form to allow for direct comparison with earlier studies [34,39]. Moreover, the cross-sectional design precludes causal inference and limits insight into the temporal dynamics between identity issues and personality pathology. Future research should address these limitations by incorporating clinician-administered assessments and informant reports to reduce bias and enhance construct validity. Longitudinal designs are also recommended to elucidate the directionality of relationships. Finally, future research could also make use of assessment instruments specifically designed to measure the PD criteria outlined in the Alternative Model for Personality Disorders [64]. Such methodological improvements would strengthen the validity and clinical utility of findings in this population.

5. Conclusions

In sum, the co-occurrence of identity issues in both PDs and EDs underscores its role as a transdiagnostic feature. Addressing identity issues in treatment may therefore have broad therapeutic benefits across these disorders.

Author Contributions: Conceptualization, L.C., A.B., T.B., G.K. and K.L.; methodology, L.C., G.K. and K.L.; software, L.C. and K.L.; validation, L.C., A.B., T.B., G.K., E.D., K.S. and K.L.; formal analysis, L.C.; investigation, L.C., A.B., T.B., G.K. and K.L.; resources, K.L. and L.C.; data curation, L.C., E.D., K.S. and K.L.; writing—original draft preparation, L.C.; writing—review and editing, L.C., A.B., T.B., G.K., E.D., K.S. and K.L.; visualization, L.C. and K.L.; supervision, L.C. and K.L.; project administration, L.C. and K.L.; funding acquisition, K.L. and L.C. All authors have read and agreed to the published version of the manuscript.

Funding: This research was funded by INTERNE FONDSEN KU LEUVEN (IF), grant number C14/21/052.

Institutional Review Board Statement: The study was conducted in accordance with the Declaration of Helsinki and approved by the Social and Societal Ethics Committee of KU LEUVEN (protocol code: G-2025-10006-R2(AMD); date of approval: 10 June 2025).

Informed Consent Statement: Informed consent was obtained from all subjects involved in the study.

Data Availability Statement: Data are available upon request at laurence.claes@kuleuven.be.

Conflicts of Interest: The authors declare no conflicts of interest.

References

1. Erikson, E.H. *Identity: Youth and Crisis*; W.W. Norton: New York, NY, USA, 1968.
2. Schwartz, S.J.; Zamboanga, B.L.; Wang, W.; Olthuis, J.V. Measuring identity from an Eriksonian perspective: Two sides of the same coin? *J. Personal. Assess.* **2009**, *91*, 143–154. [CrossRef] [PubMed]
3. Verschueren, M.; Claes, L.; Gandhi, A.; Luyckx, K. Identity and psychopathology: Bridging developmental and clinical research. *Emerg. Adulthood* **2020**, *8*, 319–332. [CrossRef]
4. Kaufman, E.A.; Cundiff, J.M.; Crowell, S.E. The development, factor structure, and validation of the Self-Concept and Identity Measure (SCIM): A self-report assessment of clinical identity disturbance. *J. Psychopathol. Behav. Assess.* **2015**, *37*, 122–133. [CrossRef]
5. Kernberg, O.F. Identity: Recent findings and clinical implications. *Psychoanal. Q.* **2006**, *75*, 969–1004. [CrossRef] [PubMed]
6. Kaufman, E.A.; Puzia, M.E.; Crowell, S.E.; Price, C.J. Replication of the Self-Concept and Identity Measure (SCIM) among a treatment-seeking sample. *Identity* **2019**, *19*, 18–28. [CrossRef] [PubMed]
7. Bruch, H. Developmental considerations of anorexia nervosa and obesity. *Can. J. Psychiatry* **1981**, *26*, 212–217. [CrossRef] [PubMed]
8. Bruch, H. Anorexia nervosa: Therapy and theory. *Am. J. Psychiatry* **1982**, *139*, 1531–1538. [CrossRef] [PubMed]
9. Vartanian, L.R.; Hayward, L.E.; Smyth, J.M.; Paxton, S.J.; Touyz, S.W. Risk and resiliency factors related to body dissatisfaction and disordered eating: The identity disruption model. *Int. J. Eat. Disord.* **2018**, *51*, 322–330. [CrossRef] [PubMed]
10. Corning, A.F.; Heibel, H.D. Re-thinking eating disorder prevention: The case for prioritizing the promotion of healthy identity development. *Eat. Disord.* **2016**, *24*, 106–113. [CrossRef] [PubMed]
11. Polivy, J.; Herman, P. Is the body the self? Women and body image. *Coll. Antropol.* **2007**, *31*, 63–67. [PubMed]
12. Casper, R.C. Some provisional ideas concerning psychological structure in anorexia nervosa and bulimia. In *Anorexia Nervosa: Recent Developments in Research*; Darby, P.L., Garfinkel, P.E., Garner, D.M., Coscina, D.V., Eds.; Alan R. Liss: New York, NY, USA, 1983; pp. 378–392.
13. Heatherton, T.F.; Baumeister, R.F. Binge eating as escape from self-awareness. *Psychol. Bull.* **1991**, *110*, 86–108. [CrossRef] [PubMed]
14. Schupak-Neuberg, E.; Nemeroff, C.J. Disturbances in identity and self-regulation in bulimia nervosa: Implications for a metaphorical perspective of "body as self". *Int. J. Eat. Disord.* **1993**, *13*, 335–347. [CrossRef] [PubMed]
15. Wheeler, H.A.; Adams, G.R.; Keating, L. Binge eating as a means for evading identity issues: The association between an avoidance identity style and bulimic behavior. *Identity* **2001**, *1*, 161–178. [CrossRef]
16. Biberdzic, M.; Tang, J.; Tan, J. Beyond difficulties in self-regulation: The role of identity integration and personality functioning in young women with disordered eating behaviours. *J. Eat. Disord.* **2021**, *9*, 93. [CrossRef] [PubMed]
17. Klein, E.M.; Benecke, C.; Kasinger, C.; Brahler, E.; Ehrenthal, J.C.; Straus, B.; Ernst, M. Eating disorder psychopathology: The role of attachment anxiety, attachment avoidance, and personality functioning. *J. Psychosom. Res.* **2022**, *160*, 110975. [CrossRef] [PubMed]
18. Rohde, J.; Obbarius, A.; Voigt, B.; Sarrar, L.; Biesenthal-Matthes, S.; Kind, C.-S.; Rose, M.; Hofmann, T. Differences and similarities in personality functioning across different types of eating disorders. *Front. Psychiatry* **2023**, *14*, 1155725. [CrossRef] [PubMed]
19. Schumacher, A.M.; Tschitsaz, A.; Lerch, S.; Wyssen, A.; Schlensog-Schuster, F.; Mürner-Lavanchy, I.; Koenig, J.; Cavelti, M.; Kaess, M. Impairments in personality functioning in adolescents with anorexia nervosa. *Eur. Eat Disord. Rev.* **2025**, *33*, 360–373. [CrossRef] [PubMed]
20. Verschueren, M.; Luyckx, L.; Kaufman, E.A.; Vansteenkiste, M.; Moons, P.; Sleuwaegen, E.; Berens, A.; Schoevaerts, K.; Claes, L. Identity processes and statuses in patients with and without eating disorders. *Eur. Eat. Disord. Rev.* **2017**, *25*, 26–35. [CrossRef] [PubMed]
21. Verschueren, M.; Claes, L.; Bogaerts, A.; Palmeroni, N.; Gandhi, A.; Moons, P.; Luyckx, K. Eating disorder symptomatology and identity formation in adolescence: A cross-lagged longitudinal approach. *Front. Psychol.* **2018**, *9*, 816. [CrossRef] [PubMed]
22. Verschueren, M.; Claes, L.; Palmeroni, N.; Raemen, L.; Moons, P.; Bruckers, L.; Molenberghs, G.; Dierckx, E.; Schoevaerts, K.; Luyckx, K. Identity functioning in patients with and eating disorder: Developmental trajectories throughout treatment. *Nutrients* **2024**, *16*, 591. [CrossRef] [PubMed]
23. Conti, J.E.; Joyce, C.; Hay, P.; Meade, T. Finding my own identity: A qualitative meta-synthesis of adult anorexia nervosa treatment experiences. *BMC Psychol.* **2020**, *8*, 110. [CrossRef] [PubMed]
24. Croce, S.R.; Malcolm, A.C.; Ralph-Nearman, C.; Phillipou, A. The role of identity in anorexia nervosa. *New Ideas Psychol.* **2024**, *72*, 101060. [CrossRef]
25. Lamoureux, M.M.H.; Bottorff, J.L. Becoming the real me: Recovering from anorexia nervosa. *Health Care Women Int.* **2005**, *26*, 170–188. [CrossRef] [PubMed]

26. Links, P.S.; Aslam, H.; O'Donnell, M. Personality disorders and clinical disorders: The challenge of comorbid autism spectrum disorder (ASD), eating disorders (EDs), posttraumatic stress disorder (PTSD), or somatic symptom disorder (SSD). *Curr. Psychiatry Rep.* **2025**, *27*, 1–9. [CrossRef] [PubMed]
27. American Psychiatric Association. *Diagnostic and Statistical Manual of Mental Disorders*, 5th ed.; American Psychiatric Association: Washington, DC, USA, 2013.
28. Cassin, S.E.; von Ranson, K.M. Personality and eating disorders: A decade in review. *Clin. Psychol. Rev.* **2005**, *25*, 895–916. [CrossRef] [PubMed]
29. Farstad, S.M.; McGeown, L.M.; von Ranson, K.M. Eating disorders and personality, 2004–2016: A systematic review and meta-analysis. *Clin. Psychol. Rev.* **2016**, *46*, 91–105. [CrossRef]
30. Grilo, C.M. Recent research of relationships among eating disorders and personality disorders. *Curr. Psychiatry Rep.* **2002**, *4*, 18–24. [CrossRef] [PubMed]
31. Martinussen, M.; Friborg, O.; Schmierer, P.; Kaiser, S.; Øvergård, K.T.; Neunhoeffer, A.L.; Martinsen, E.W.; Rosenvinge, J.H. The comorbidity of personality disorders in eating disorders: A meta-analysis. *Eat. Weight Disord.* **2017**, *22*, 201–209. [CrossRef] [PubMed]
32. Rosenvinge, J.H.; Martinussen, M.; Ostensen, E. The comorbidity of eating disorders and personality disorders: A meta-analytic review of studies published between 1983 and 1998. *Eat. Weight Disord.* **2000**, *5*, 52–61. [CrossRef] [PubMed]
33. Eielsen, H.P.; Vrabel, K.; Hoffart, A.; Rø, Ø.; Rosenvinge, J.H. Reciprocal relationships between personality disorders and eating disorders in a prospective 17-year follow-up study. *Int. J. Eat. Disord.* **2022**, *55*, 1753–1764. [CrossRef] [PubMed]
34. Bogaerts, A.; Luyckx, K.; Bastiaens, T.; Sleuwaegen, E.; Berens, A.; Claes, L. The Self-Concept and Identity Measure in patients with personality disorders: A psychometric evaluation and associations with identity processes, core domains of self-functioning, and personality disorder symptoms. *Assessment* **2023**, *30*, 2184–2197. [CrossRef] [PubMed]
35. Tressová, D.; De Caluwé, E.; Bogaerts, S. Identity and personality pathology in adult forensic psychiatric patients and healthy controls. *Int. J. Offender Ther. Comp. Criminol.* **2024**, *68*, 1558–1578. [CrossRef] [PubMed]
36. D'Agostino, A.; Pepi, R.; Monti, M.R.; Starcevic, V.; Price, A. Measuring emptiness: Validation of the Italian version of the Subjective Emptiness Scale in clinical and non-clinical populations. *J. Affect. Disord.* **2021**, *6*, 100226. [CrossRef]
37. Lenzenweger, M.F. Epidemiology of personality disorders. *Psychiatr. Clin. N. Am.* **2008**, *31*, 395–403. [CrossRef] [PubMed]
38. Garner, D.M. *Eating Disorders Inventory-3 (EDI-3). Professional Manual*; Psychological Assessment Resources: Odessa, FL, USA, 2004.
39. Bogaerts, A.; Claes, L.; Verschueren, M.; Bastiaens, T.; Kaufman, E.A.; Smits, D.; Luyckx, K. The Dutch Self-Concept and Identity Measure (SCIM): Factor structure and associations with identity dimensions and psychopathology. *Personal. Individ. Differ.* **2018**, *123*, 56–64. [CrossRef]
40. De Doncker, D.; Schotte, C.K.W.; Cosyns, P. ADP-IV questionnaire: Aspects of reliability and validity. *Eur. Psychiatry* **2000**, *15*, 73.
41. Schotte, C.K.W.; De Doncker, D.; Vankerckhoven, C.; Vertommen, H.; Cosyns, P. Self-report assessment of the DSM-IV personality disorders, measurement of trait and distress characteristics: The ADP-IV. *Psychol. Med.* **1998**, *28*, 1179–1188. [CrossRef] [PubMed]
42. George, D.; Mallery, P. *SPSS for Windows Step by Step: A Simple Guide and Reference*, 4th ed.; Allyn & Bacon: Boston, MA, USA, 2003.
43. American Psychiatric Association. *Diagnostic and Statistical Manual of Mental Disorders*, 4th ed.; American Psychiatric Association: Washington, DC, USA, 1994.
44. Hemphill, J.F. Interpreting the magnitudes of correlation coefficients. *Am. Psychol.* **2003**, *58*, 78–79. [CrossRef] [PubMed]
45. Insel, T.; Cuthbert, B.; Garvey, M.; Heinssen, R.; Pine, D.S.; Quinn, K.; Sanislow, C.; Wang, P. Research domain criteria (RDoC): Toward a new classification framework for research on mental disorders. *Am. J. Psychiatry* **2010**, *167*, 748–751. [CrossRef] [PubMed]
46. Paris, J. Personality disorders over time: Precursors, course and outcome. *J. Personal. Disord.* **2003**, *17*, 479–488. [CrossRef] [PubMed]
47. Chasidy, F. Dependent personality disorder: A review of etiology and treatment. *Grad. J. Couns. Psychol.* **2009**, *1*, 7.
48. Steinberg, L.; Albert, D.; Cauffman, E.; Banich, M.; Graham, S.; Woolard, J. Age differences in sensation seeking and impulsivity as indexed by behavior and self-report: Evidence for a dual systems model. *Dev. Psychol.* **2008**, *44*, 1764–1778. [CrossRef] [PubMed]
49. Wonderlich, S.A.; Crosby, R.D.; Mitchell, J.E.; Thompson, K.M.; Redlin, J.; Demuth, G.; Smyth, J.; Haseltine, B. Eating disturbance and sexual trauma in childhood and adulthood. *Int. J. Eat. Disord.* **2001**, *30*, 401–412. [CrossRef] [PubMed]
50. Sharp, C.; Wall, K. DSM-5 level of personality functioning: Refocusing personality disorder on what it means to be human. *Annu. Rev. Clin. Psychol.* **2021**, *17*, 313–337. [CrossRef] [PubMed]
51. Widiger, T.A.; Bach, B.; Chmielewski, M.; Clark, L.A.; DeYoung, C.; Hopwood, C.J.; Kotov, R.; Krueger, R.F.; Miller, J.D.; Morey, L.C.; et al. Criterion A of the AMPD in HiTOP. *J. Personal. Assess.* **2019**, *101*, 345–355. [CrossRef] [PubMed]
52. Kernberg, O.F.; Caligor, E. A psychoanalytic theory of personality disorders. In *Major Theories of Personality Disorder*, 2nd ed.; Lenzenweger, M.F., Clarkin, J.F., Eds.; Guilford Press: New York, NY, USA, 2005; pp. 114–156.

53. Jorgensen, C.R.; Boye, R. How does it feel to have a disturbed identity? The phenomenology of identity diffusion in patients with borderline personality disorder: A qualitative study. *J. Personal. Disord.* **2021**, *35*, 526. [CrossRef] [PubMed]
54. Morey, L.C.; Skodol, A.E.; Oldham, J.M. Clinician judgments of clinical utility: A comparison of the DSM-IV-TR personality disorders and the alternative model for DSM-5 personality disorders. *J. Abnorm. Psychol.* **2014**, *123*, 398–405. [CrossRef] [PubMed]
55. Price, A.L.; Mahler, H.I.M.; Hopwood, C.J. Construction and validation of a self-report subjective emptiness scale. *Assessment* **2022**, *29*, 397–409. [CrossRef] [PubMed]
56. Pincus, A.L.; Lukowitsky, M.R. Pathological narcissism and narcissistic personality disorder. *Annu./Rev. Clin. Psychol.* **2010**, *6*, 421–446. [CrossRef] [PubMed]
57. Joshua, P.R.; Lewis, V.; Kelty, S.F.; Boer, D.P. Is schema therapy effective for adults with eating disorders? A systematic review into the evidence. *Cogn. Behav. Ther.* **2023**, *52*, 213–231. [CrossRef] [PubMed]
58. Farrell, J.M.; Shaw, I.A.; Webber, M.A. A schema-focused approach to group psychotherapy for outpatients with borderline personality disorder: A randomized controlled trial. *J. Behav. Ther. Exp. Psychiatry.* **2009**, *40*, 317–328. [CrossRef] [PubMed]
59. Skårderud, F. Eating one's words: Part 3. Mentalisation-based psychotherapy for anorexia nervosa: An outline for a treatment and training manual. *Eur. Eat Disord. Rev.* **2007**, *15*, 323–339. [CrossRef] [PubMed]
60. Bankoff, S.M.; Karpel, M.G.; Forbes, H.E.; Pantalone, D.W. A systematic review of dialectical behavior therapy for the treatment of eating disorders. *Eat. Disord.* **2012**, *20*, 196–215. [CrossRef] [PubMed]
61. Ben-Porath, D.; Duthu, F.; Luo, T.; Gonidakis, F.; Compte, E.J.; Wisniewski, L. Dialectical behavioral therapy: An update and review of the existing treatment models adapted for adults with eating disorders. *Eat. Disord.* **2020**, *28*, 101–121. [CrossRef] [PubMed]
62. Zimmerman, M. Diagnosing personality disorders. A review of issues and research methods. *Arch. Gen. Psychiatry* **1994**, *51*, 225–245. [CrossRef] [PubMed]
63. Podsakoff, P.M.; MacKenzie, S.B.; Lee, J.-Y.; Podsakoff, N.P. Common method biases in behavioral research: A critical review of the literature and recommended remedies. *J. Appl. Psychol.* **2003**, *88*, 879–903. [CrossRef] [PubMed]
64. Zimmermann, J.; Kerber, A.; Rek, K.; Hopwood, C.J.; Krueger, R.F. A Brief but Comprehensive Review of Research on the Alternative DSM-5 Model for Personality Disorders. *Curr. Psychiatry Rep.* **2019**, *21*, 92. [CrossRef] [PubMed]

nutrients

MDPI

Article

Overweight, Obesity, and Depression in Multimorbid Older Adults: Prevalence, Diagnostic Agreement, and Associated Factors in Primary Care—Results from a Multicenter Observational Study

Daniel Christopher Bludau [1], Alexander Pabst [1], Franziska Bleck [1], Siegfried Weyerer [2], Wolfgang Maier [3], Jochen Gensichen [4], Karola Mergenthal [5], Horst Bickel [6], Angela Fuchs [7], Ingmar Schäfer [8], Hans-Helmut König [9], Birgitt Wiese [10], Gerhard Schön [11], Karl Wegscheider [11], Martin Scherer [8], Steffi G. Riedel-Heller [1] and Margrit Löbner [1,*]

1 Institute for Social Medicine, Occupational Health and Public Health, University of Leipzig, 04103 Leipzig, Germany
2 Central Institute of Mental Health, Medical Faculty Mannheim, Heidelberg University, 68159 Mannheim, Germany
3 Department of Neurodegenerative Diseases and Geriatric Psychiatry, University Hospital Bonn, 53127 Bonn, Germany
4 Institute of General Practice and Family Medicine, University Hospital of LMU Munich, 80336 Munich, Germany
5 Institute of General Practice, Goethe-University Frankfurt, 60590 Frankfurt am Main, Germany
6 Department of Psychiatry, Technical University of Munich, 81675 Munich, Germany
7 Institute of General Practice, Medical Faculty of the Heinrich Heine University Düsseldorf, 40225 Düsseldorf, Germany
8 Department of Primary Medical Care, Center of Psychosocial Medicine, University Medical Center Hamburg-Eppendorf, 20246 Hamburg, Germany
9 Department of Health Economics and Health Services Research, Hamburg Center for Health Economics, University Medical Center Hamburg-Eppendorf, 20246 Hamburg, Germany
10 MHH Information Technology, Hannover Medical School, 30625 Hannover, Germany
11 Department of Medical Biometry and Epidemiology, Center for Experimental Medicine, University Medical Center Hamburg-Eppendorf, 20251 Hamburg, Germany
* Correspondence: margrit.loebner@medizin.uni-leipzig.de; Tel.: +49-(0)341-97-24591; Fax: +49-(0)341-97-24569

Abstract: Background/Objectives: Obesity and depression, in conjunction with multimorbidity, are interconnected conditions increasingly managed in general practitioner (GP) settings, yet these associations remain insufficiently studied in older patients. This study investigates the prevalence of depression across different body mass index (BMI) classes and includes age and gender differences in multimorbid older patients, offering a novel perspective on subgroup-specific patterns. Further the agreement between GP depression diagnoses and the Geriatric Depression Scale (GDS) is studied and patient-specific factors that may affect the agreement are explored, aiming to improve future diagnostics for vulnerable subgroups. **Methods**: Data were provided by the baseline assessment of the MultiCare Study, a prospective multicenter observational cohort of multimorbid patients aged 65+ years recruited from 158 GP practices across eight study centers in Germany. Data from 2568 study participants were analyzed based on GP-coded International Classification of Diseases (ICD) diagnoses, structured GP questionnaires, and patient questionnaires. Assessments included data on the BMI and depression (15 item version of the GDS). Agreement between GP diagnoses of depression and GDS assessment was measured using Cohen's kappa. Four logistic regression models were used to examine the effects of patient-specific factors on the agreement of depression diagnosis (match or mismatch). **Results**: GPs diagnosed depression in 17.3% of cases, compared to the detection of depressive symptoms in 12.4% of the patients by GDS (cut-off $\geq$ 6 points). The highest prevalence rates were observed in patients with obesity class III (25.0% by GP; 21.7% by GDS). Women were significantly more likely to receive a depression diagnosis by a GP across most BMI classes (except obesity classes II and III). The detection of depressive symptoms by GDS was significantly more prevalent in older multimorbid obese patients (≥75 years), except for patients with obesity class III. The overall agreement between GP diagnosis and GDS assessment was weak ($\kappa = 0.156$, $p < 0.001$). The highest agreement was found for people with obesity class III ($\kappa = 0.256$, $p < 0.05$). Factors associated with a True Positive depression diagnosis (match by both GDS and GP) were female gender (odds ratio (OR) = 1.83, $p < 0.05$), widowhood (OR = 2.43, $p < 0.01$), limited daily living skills (OR = 3.14, $p < 0.001$), and a higher level of education (OR = 2.48, $p < 0.01$). A significantly lower likelihood of a False Negative depression diagnosis was found for patients with obesity class III. **Conclusions**: This study highlights the significant prevalence of depression among multimorbid older adults across different BMI classes, particularly in those with obesity class III. The weak diagnostic agreement between GP diagnosis and GDS assessment suggests a need for improved diagnostic practices in primary care. Implementing standardized screening tools and fostering collaboration with mental health specialists could enhance the identification and management of depression in this vulnerable population.

Keywords: body mass index; depression; Geriatric Depression Scale; late life; multimorbidity; obesity; primary care

1. Introduction

Recognizing their growing global impact, the World Health Organization (WHO) has increasingly been monitoring both obesity and depression, spurring research to investigate effective strategies for prevention, diagnosis, and integrated care and underscoring the need to address these pressing global health issues [1–3]. Obesity is a common non-communicable disease with far-reaching health consequences. It has shown a rapid increase in global prevalence over the last decades, with adult obesity rates more than doubling since 1990 [4,5]. The problem of obesity cuts across generations; among older adults, the rate of overweight and obese individuals has been rising, with particularly large increases in the last 40 years [6,7]. Overweight and obesity, which are quantifiable by body mass index (BMI), increase with age in both sexes and cause a range of adverse health outcomes [8]. Examples include the development of a metabolic syndrome consisting of type 2 diabetes or cardiovascular manifestations, as well as other conditions like steatohepatitis, osteoarthritis, the increased likelihood of cancer, and the development of depressive disorders [9]. Often, more than one of these chronic diseases coexist, creating multimorbidity. Obesity and multimorbidity are closely associated [10]. As overweight and obesity levels increase, so does the prevalence of multimorbidity [11]. This association has become more evident over the past 25 years, with increasing BMI leading to a greater prevalence of multimorbidity [12]. This association between obesity and multimorbidity is particularly strong in older patients [12].

In old age, in particular, lifestyle factors appear to play a significant role in modifying BMI, with physical activity playing the most critical role [13]. Genetic; biological (age and gender); and social determinants of health (such as education, income, and having a partner) interact with these factors in a complex way, in part, because they influence eating and activity behavior [9].

Depression is a common, growing, and increasingly relevant condition, recently seeing a rise in public awareness and media coverage [14]. Worldwide, it is among the leading contributors to disability-adjusted life years (DALYs) across a broad range of age groups. The trend over the last 30 years has been upward, with a more than 60% increase in DALYs due to depressive disorders [15]. For younger and middle-aged adults, depression ranks between first and third as the most common cause of years lived with disability (YLDs); for older adults (aged 65 or older), depression is still one of the top five causes for years spent with a disability. The trend of depression increasingly becoming a cause of disability has been particularly pronounced in recent decades, especially among older patients and compared to other diseases [16].

For older patients, depression is influenced by the number of additional medical conditions, and multimorbidity is related to both the presence and the severity of depression [17,18]. Depressive symptoms are significantly more frequent in multimorbid patients, and furthermore, multimorbid patients also show higher depression severity levels than non-multimorbid persons [18]. A cumulative effect of the number of conditions on the prevalence of depression is assumed [19].

As with the multimorbidity that often accompanies it, there is strong evidence that obesity has a major impact on mental health and vice versa [20]. Especially for younger patient groups, it has been shown that there is a positive association between childhood or adolescent obesity and depression. Similarly, more severe depressive symptoms were found in obese adolescents [21]. The question of an association in old age has been studied less frequently, but associations between depression and obesity in older populations have also been pointed out. For instance, studies indicate a bidirectional relationship between obesity and depression [22], with the likelihood of depression appearing to increase with increasing the BMI [23].

The relationship between differentiated BMI classes and depression in a multimorbid age cohort has so far been little researched. Furthermore, it has not yet been investigated whether biological and social determinants of health are adequately taken into consideration when diagnosing depression in general practitioner (GP) practices, where, in addition to multimorbidity management, more than half of the ongoing psychiatric care (estimated 60%) and the majority of antidepressant prescriptions are carried out [24]. Finally, previous studies point out inconsistencies in the diagnosis of depression between GPs and screening instruments such as the Geriatric Depression Scale (GDS) [25], as well as gender differences in this regard [26].

This study aims to investigate possible gaps in the outpatient primary care treatment of depression in obese, multimorbid patients in old age and to identify determinants of health influencing the diagnosis. It is the first study to explore age- and gender-specific depression prevalence across BMI classes and examine diagnostic agreement between GP diagnoses and GDS assessments while accounting for the BMI in a large sample of multimorbid older adults in primary care.

The following research questions will be addressed:

1. What are the age- and gender-specific prevalence rates of depression, and how do they differ between individuals with under- and normal weight, overweight, and with varying degrees of obesity?
2. What is the rate of agreement comparing depression diagnoses made by GPs and detected by a validated instrument (GDS) with regards to different BMI classes?
3. Which factors are associated with a match (True Positive or True Negative), and which factors are associated with a mismatch (False Positive or False Negative) between the GP's clinical judgment and the GDS-based screening outcome? What role does the BMI class play in this context?

2. Materials and Methods

2.1. Sample

Data were obtained from the baseline assessment of the MultiCare study, a prospective multicenter observational cohort in Germany. The study includes randomly selected GP patients aged 65 years or older with multimorbidity and comprises a baseline survey and three follow-up surveys. The baseline survey took place between July 2008 and October 2009. The mean age of the patient collective at baseline was 74 years. A total of N = 3189 patients were enrolled, in accordance with the study protocol, which targeted a minimum enrollment of 3050 patients [27]. The proportion of women was 59%, and 56% of the study population were married [28]. This sample can be considered representative of the population distribution of Germany in terms of gender and marital status for the age group of 65 years and older [29].

From 158 GP practices in the eight participating German study centers in Bonn, Düsseldorf, Frankfurt/Main, Hamburg, Jena, Leipzig, Mannheim, and Munich, study participants in the relevant age group with a date of birth between July 1923 and June 1943 who had consulted their GP during the last quarter were identified. Using a random number table, 50 patients per GP were selected from all eligible patients, contacted by the GP, and invited to participate in the study. Interested patients were then given information about the study and asked for written informed consent.

The study excluded individuals who were residing in nursing homes (short life expectancy) or who had a severe illness expected to be fatal within three months according to the GP. Further exclusion criteria included insufficient proficiency in speaking and reading German, inadequate capacity to provide consent (e.g., dementia), inability to participate in interviews (e.g., blindness and deafness), being unfamiliar to the GP (e.g., accidental consultation), or current participation in other studies.

Only patients who simultaneously had at least three chronic diseases from a defined (International Classification of Diseases [ICD]-10 codes) catalogue of 29 diseases were eligible for inclusion in the study. Following this selection process, a total of 3317 patients agreed to participate in the study. As part of the data analyses, 128 patients had to be excluded retrospectively due to situational circumstances (e.g., premature death) and 621 patients due to incomplete or missing data on the factors investigated. The final analytical sample comprised 2568 patients, as illustrated in Figure 1.

2.2. Data Collection and Assessment Procedure

The multimorbid disease burden of the patients was recorded using three approaches: Firstly, a chart review was used to record all ICD-10 diagnoses for each patient as recorded in the GP's database in the last quarter. Secondly, structured GP interviews were conducted. Thirdly, each patient was interviewed by the same interviewer over the entire duration of the study using standardized clinical questionnaires.

Patient age, gender, and current diagnoses were obtained through a chart review of the respective GP's database. Medical checkup data such as the patient's BMI were transmitted by the GP. Sociodemographic data (education level determined by CASMIN classification, marital status, and income) were collected from the direct patient interview. Furthermore, information on the mental state of the patients was obtained in direct dialogue with the patients using the GDS. The ability to carry out daily activities independently was assessed using the Instrumental Activities of Daily Living (IADL) Scale and pain perception was quantified using the Graded Chronic Pain Scale (GCPS). In the interviews, patients also provided information on physical activity (International Physical Activities Questionnaire IPAQ-S7S) and social integration (F-SozU K14).

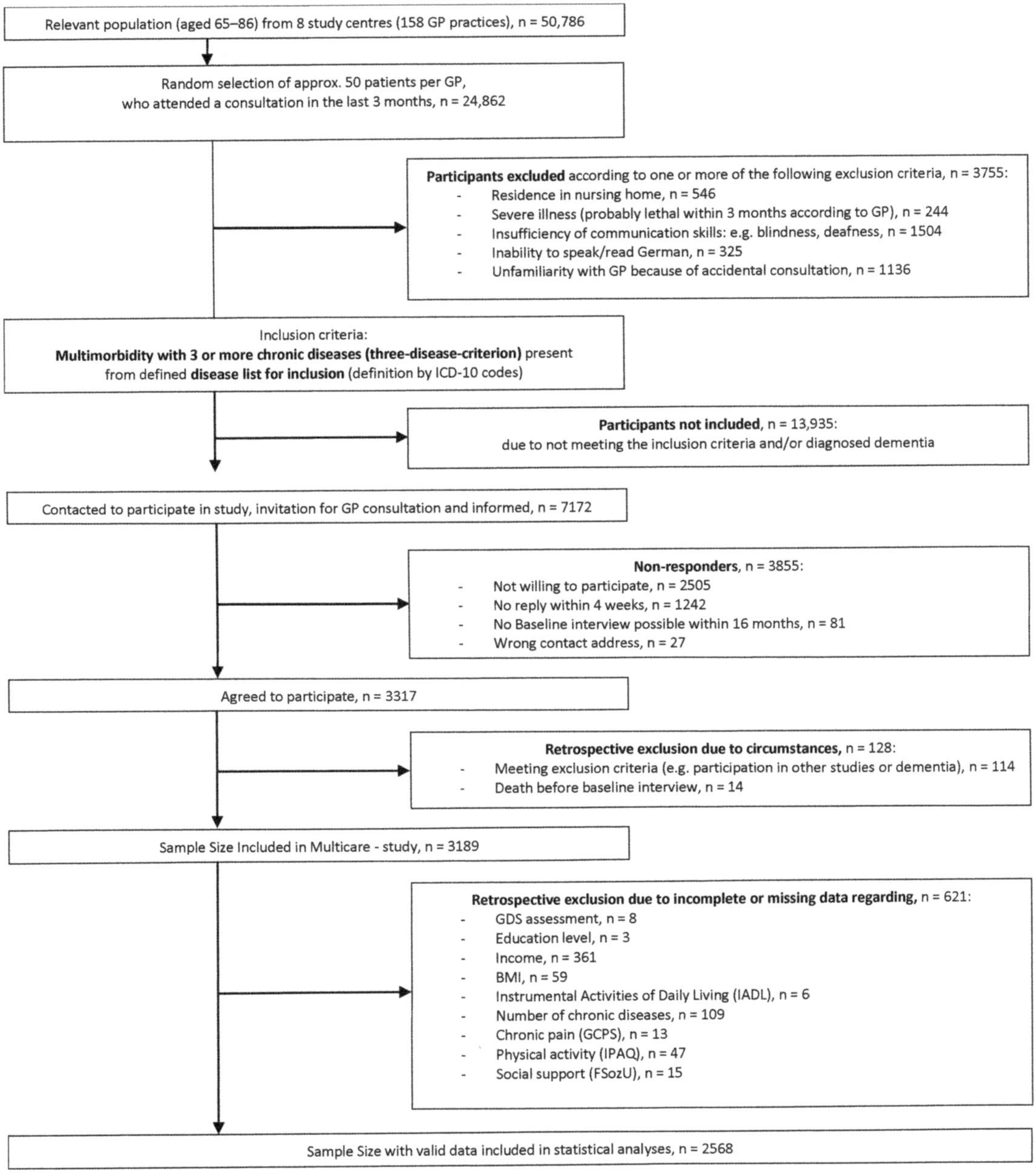

Figure 1. Sample flowchart; total sample of the MultiCare baseline survey.

2.3. Sociodemographic Data

The sociodemographic variables collected were age, gender, education level, marital status, and income. Two age groups were distinguished (young old people: 65–74 years and older old people: over 75 years) [30]; the education level was determined using the CASMIN classification (low, medium, and high); and marital status was categorized into married, single, divorced, and widowed. The monthly household net income was recorded and assigned to 1 of 23 graduated income levels, ranging from 1 (below 150 EUR) to 23

(10,000–18,000 EUR). These income levels were converted into continuous values (e.g., 150–300 EUR corresponds to 225 EUR) to calculate the equivalized disposable income. For international comparability, the equivalized disposable income according to the modified OECD equivalence scale was used, whereby the head of household was weighted with a factor of 1 and each additional household member with a factor of 0.5 ($\geq$15 years) or 0.3 (<15 years), according to age [31]. This equivalized disposable income was then scaled for a better overview and divided by a factor of 1000.

2.4. Resources and Risk Factors

Body weight and height were measured, and the BMI was calculated (body weight in kilograms divided by squared height in meters). According to the guidelines, the classification was made into BMI classes (under- and normal weight $\leq$ 24.9 kg/m^2, overweight 25–29.9 kg/m^2, and obesity $\geq$ 30 kg/m^2) [32], whereby obesity was additionally subdivided into its obesity classes I (30–34.9 kg/m^2), II (35–39.9 kg/m^2), and III ($\geq$40 kg/m^2).

The IADL score was used to assess whether participants could still manage an independent daily life. The skills assessed include aspects of household management, personal health care, telecommunication skills, financial and schedule management, and mobility [33]. The summary score usually varies from 0 to 8 for women and, to prevent gender bias, from 0 to 5 for men. Lower scores signify reduced function and dependence on assistance, while higher scores indicate enhanced function and independence [34]. For better comparability of the obtained score between men and women in this cohort, the three items "food preparation", "housekeeping", and "laundry" were not included in the analysis, so that each participant could now obtain a maximum score of 5. For better interpretation of the score, dichotomization into not limited (5 points) versus limited (0–4 points) was performed.

To determine the severity of chronic pain, the Graded Chronic Pain Scale (GCPS) was used [35]. Based on the first three questions concerning pain intensity (involving the items "Pain Right Now", "Worst Pain" during the last 4 weeks, and "Average Pain" during the last 4 weeks) the "Characteristic Pain Intensity" was calculated, providing information on the presence of pain (yes versus no) and the subjective intensity of perceived pain on a scale from 0 to 100.

Through a separate questionnaire listing the chronic diseases included in the study, multimorbidity was quantified by adding up the chronic diseases as reported by the patients [27].

Physical activity was assessed using the International Physical Activities Questionnaire (IPAQ-S7S). The self-reported physical activity of the last 7 days was assessed by a series of 7 items. The activity level was then classified as a low, moderate, or high activity level. The evaluation of the data is based on the "Guidelines for Data Processing and Analysis of the IPAQ" [36].

The questionnaire F-SozU in its short form (K-14) was used to survey social integration by measuring perceived and anticipated social support with 14 items using a five-point Likert scale. The participants were presented with 14 positively formulated statements about their social environment, and the extent of their agreement was assessed on a scale ranging from 1 (strongly disagree) to 5 (strongly agree). The individual item values were summed and divided by the number of items to yield an average, with a score of 5 corresponding to the maximum and a score of 1 corresponding to the minimum perceived social support. To interpret the obtained value, one can refer to normalization against a representative German sample, where an average scale value of 3.97 with a standard deviation of 0.68 serves as a reference [37,38].

2.5. Dependent Variables

GDS assessment. The GDS was used in its abbreviated form (GDS-15) in the patient questionnaire as an established assessment instrument for the detection of depression in older age [39]. In the questionnaire, patients can respond affirmatively or negatively to 15 questions regarding mental well-being (e.g., "Have you dropped many of your activities and interests?"). A total score is then calculated based on the responses. A total of 0–5 points was considered normal, while a cut-off of ≥6 points defined the assumption of a depressive disorder [40,41].

GP-diagnosis. In order to determine whether a diagnosis of depression had been detected by a doctor, the responsible GP was asked in a standardized questionnaire whether the patient had a depression diagnosis according to ICD groups F32-F33 of the ICD-10 medical classification list [27,28,42].

The abovementioned assessments of depression were used to describe either a concordance or discordance between the GP's clinical judgment and the GDS-based screening outcome, hereafter referred to as "diagnostic agreement" in this study. For clarity, the following categories were defined:

True Positive (Indication of depression by both the GDS and the GP);

True Negative (No indication of depression by either the GDS or the GP);

False Positive (No indication of depression by the GDS but clinical diagnosis of depression by the GP);

False Negative (Indication of depression by the GDS but no clinical diagnosis of depression by the GP).

2.6. Statistical Analyses

All statistical analyses were performed using STATA SE, version 18 (StataCorp., College Station, TX, USA) for Windows. The significance level for the analyses was set at alpha $\leq$ 0.05. Sociodemographic and clinical characteristics of the study sample were presented descriptively, and gender differences were analyzed statistically (a chi-squared test was used for categorical variables, a t-test for normally distributed continuous variables, and a Wilcoxon rank-sum (Mann–Whitney) test for non-normally distributed continuous variables).

A descriptive presentation of the prevalence of depression (GDS assessment and GP diagnosis respectively) was made for the entire population, as well as categorized into BMI classes (under- and normal weight, overweight, obese, and stratified into obesity classes I–III). In the same course, the prevalence of depression was additionally presented categorized according to gender and according to age group (younger old people 65–74 years; older old people $\geq$ 75 years) and each tested for significant group differences with a chi-squared test or a Fisher's exact test (in case of small sample sizes with observations of less than 5).

The depression assessments according to the GDS and GP questionnaire were then compared for agreement in a second analysis, using Cohen's kappa as a statistical measure for interrater reliability. Bias-corrected Cohen's kappa with a 95% confidence interval was calculated for the total population, as well as separately for the categories of the respective BMI classes.

In order to examine the patient-specific factors gender, age, marital status, education level, income, BMI, independence in daily life, perceived pain, number of chronic diseases, physical activity, and social support with regards to their influence on the indication of depression according to the GP's clinical judgment and the GDS-based screening outcome, four logistic regression models were calculated to estimate the probability of a concordance (True Positive or True Negative) or a discordance (False Positive or False Negative) in indicating depression, respectively, depending on the presence of patient-specific risk and protective factors. The calculated odds ratios (ORs) were tested for significance and described the association between the patient-specific factor and the corresponding scenarios of either a depression diagnosis or no depression diagnosis made by the GP and their (mis)match in this regard with the assessment by the GDS.

3. Results

3.1. Sample Characteristics

The study population of 2568 participants consisted of people aged 65–86 years, 1498 (58.3%) of whom were female (see Table 1). The majority of both genders were married, while noticeably the majority of the widowed were female.

Table 1. Sociodemographic and clinical characteristics.

	Overall (n, (%))		Women (n, (%))		Men (n, (%))		p-Value
n (%)	2568	(100)	1498	(58.3)	1070	(41.7)	
Age							0.169 [a]
<75 years old	1505	(58.6)	861	(57.5)	644	(60.2)	
≥75 years old	1063	(41.4)	637	(42.5)	426	(39.8)	
Education							**<0.001** [a]
Low	1579	(61.5)	966	(64.5)	613	(57.3)	
Middle	694	(27.0)	443	(29.6)	251	(23.5)	
High	295	(11.5)	89	(5.9)	206	(19.3)	
Marital status							**<0.001** [a]
Married	1506	(58.6)	664	(44.3)	842	(78.7)	
Single	156	(6.1)	110	(7.3)	46	(4.3)	
Divorced	209	(8.1)	154	(10.3)	55	(5.1)	
Widowed	697	(27.1)	570	(38.1)	127	(11.9)	
Income							**<0.001** [b]
Mean (s.d.)	1.4	(0.7)	1.3	(0.6)	1.5	(0.8)	
BMI							**<0.001** [a,d]
Under- and normal weight	627	(24.4)	393	(26.2)	234	(21.9)	
Overweight	1120	(43.6)	579	(38.7)	541	(50.6)	
Obesity in total (I–III)	821	(32.0)	526	(35.1)	295	(27.6)	
Obesity I	609	(23.7)	379	(25.3)	230	(21.5)	
Obesity II	152	(5.9)	101	(6.7)	51	(4.8)	
Obesity III	60	(2.3)	46	(3.1)	14	(1.3)	
IADL							0.901 [a]
Limited	628	(24.5)	365	(24.4)	263	(24.6)	
Not limited	1940	(75.6)	1133	(75.6)	807	(75.4)	
GCPS pain presence							**<0.001** [a]
Yes	2019	(78.6)	1258	(84.0)	761	(71.1)	
No	549	(21.4)	240	(16.0)	309	(28.9)	
GCPS pain intensity (0–100)							**<0.001** [b]
Mean (s.d.)	34.0	(25.1)	38.2	(24.8)	28.2	(24.2)	
Number of chronic diseases							**<0.001** [b]
Mean (s.d.)	7.4	(3.1)	7.7	(3.1)	7.1	(3.2)	
IPAQ							**<0.001** [a]
Low	805	(31.4)	524	(35.0)	281	(26.3)	
Moderate	1121	(43.7)	647	(43.2)	474	(44.3)	
High	642	(25.0)	327	(21.8)	315	(29.4)	

Table 1. *Cont.*

	Overall (n, (%))		Women (n, (%))		Men (n, (%))		p-Value
Social support							0.507 [b]
Mean (s.d.)	4.1	(0.7)	4.1	(0.7)	4.1	(0.7)	
GDS							**<0.001** [c]
Mean (s.d.)	2.5	(2.6)	2.7	(2.7)	2.3	(2.5)	

NOTE: n (%) represents the sample size (n) and the percentage (%) of participants/observations in each category. Variables are shown in bold, while their categories are presented in regular font. [a] Comparison between women and men based on the chi-squared test, [b] comparison between women and men based on the t-test, [c] comparison between women and men based on the Wilcoxon rank-sum (Mann–Whitney) test, [d] comparison between the groups: under- and normal weight, overweight, obesity I, obesity II, and obesity III. Bold formatting of p-values is used to indicate statistical significance.

While only one-fifth (21.9%) of the men were of under- and normal weight, this was the case for around one-fourth (26.2%) of the women. The largest group in both sexes was overweight (50.6% of men and 38.7% of women). Obese patients made up the second largest group in terms of BMI class (27.6% of men and 35.1% of women), with class I obesity being the most common form in both genders.

3.2. Prevalence of Depressive Symptoms According to Body Mass Index, Gender, and Age

Using the GDS, a total of 319 patients (12.4%) were classified as depressed, while GPs diagnosed 444 patients (17.3%) with depression (see Table 2). In general, across almost all BMI classes (with the exception of obesity class II), GPs more frequently issued a diagnosis of depression compared to the GDS (under- and normal weight: 18.5% by GP versus 12.3% by GDS, overweight: 16.4% by GP versus 10.4% by GDS, and obesity in total: 17.5% by GP versus 15.4% by GDS).

Table 2. Gender- and age-specific depression prevalence according to GP and the GDS questionnaire, distributed by BMI class.

	Overall		Under- and Normal Weight		Overweight		Obesity in Total (Classes I–III)		Obesity Class I		Obesity Class II		Obesity Class III	
	n (%)	p	n (%)	p	n (%)	p	n (%)	p	n (%)	p	n (%)	p	n (%)	p
Depression prevalence according to GP														
Total	444 (17.3)		116 (18.5)		184 (16.4)		144 (17.5)		104 (17.1)		25 (16.5)		15 (25.0)	
Gender														
Female	331 (22.1)	**<0.001**	85 (21.6)	**0.009**	126 (21.8)	**<0.001**	120 (22.8)	**<0.001**	86 (22.7)	**<0.001**	21 (20.8)	0.062 [a]	13 (28.3)	0.483 [a]
Male	113 (10.6)		31 (13.3)		58 (10.7)		24 (8.1)		18 (7.8)		4 (7.8)		2 (14.3)	
Age														
<75 years old	274 (18.2)	0.144	78 (21.9)	**0.012**	108 (17.1)	0.498	88 (17.0)	0.611	63 (16.6)	0.674	13 (13.4)	0.182	12 (30.0)	0.343 [a]
≥75 years old	170 (16.0)		38 (14.0)		76 (15.6)		56 (18.4)		41 (17.9)		12 (21.8)		3 (15.0)	
Depression prevalence according to GDS questionnaire														
Total	319 (12.4)		77 (12.3)		116 (10.4)		126 (15.4)		85 (14.0)		28 (18.4)		13 (21.7)	
Gender														
Female	216 (14.4)	**<0.001**	56 (14.3)	0.052	74 (12.8)	**0.006**	86 (16.4)	0.288	59 (15.6)	0.142	18 (17.8)	0.790	9 (19.6)	0.478 [a]
Male	103 (9.6)		21 (9.0)		42 (7.8)		40 (13.6)		26 (11.3)		10 (19.6)		4 (28.6)	
Age														
<75 years old	170 (11.3)	**0.040**	44 (12.4)	0.945	57 (9.0)	0.095	69 (13.4)	**0.039**	44 (11.6)	**0.030**	13 (13.4)	**0.036**	12 (30.0)	**0.043** [a]
≥75 years old	149 (14.0)		33 (12.2)		59 (12.1)		57 (18.8)		41 (17.9)		15 (27.3)		1 (5.0)	

NOTE: n represents number of cases. (%) Percentage share is related to the corresponding intersection in each case. Variables are shown in bold, while their categories are presented in regular font. All p-values were calculated using the chi-squared test, except for the values labelld with [a] calculated using Fisher's exact test. Bold formatting of p-values is used to indicate statistical significance.

In both diagnostic approaches, with the slight exception of obesity II in GP-diagnosed depression, more severe degrees of obesity also showed increased depression prevalence in their respective BMI class (obesity I: 17.1% by GP and 14.0% by GDS and obesity II: 16.5%

by GP and 18.4% by GDS, with the maximum observed for obesity III: 25.0% by GP and 21.7% by GDS).

A gender-specific analysis showed that GPs diagnosed depression significantly more often in women. This phenomenon was found for the overall study sample ($p \leq 0.001$) and for women with under- and normal weight ($p = 0.009$), overweight ($p \leq 0.001$), and obesity in total ($p \leq 0.001$), as well as for obesity class I ($p \leq 0.001$). In contrast, when assessed by GDS, only women as a group across all BMI classes of the overall study sample ($p \leq 0.001$) and overweight women especially ($p = 0.006$) showed a significantly higher rate of depression. All other BMI classes did not show any significant differences in terms of gender distribution when assessed by GDS.

When looking at age-specific differences, only amongst the under- and normal weight did the GP-made depression diagnoses show a significant shift ($p = 0.012$) towards patients aged below 75 years. Meanwhile, the GDS revealed a contrary shift, with significantly increased depression rates on the part of older patients aged 75 years or above for the overall study sample ($p = 0.040$) and for obesity in total ($p = 0.039$), as well as obesity I ($p = 0.030$) and obesity II ($p = 0.036$) in particular. Only for obesity III did the GDS show a significant depression prevalence shift towards the younger patients aged below 75 years ($p = 0.043$).

3.3. *Diagnostic Agreement of Depression Analyzed by BMI Classes*

When comparing the agreement (Figure 2) between GDS assessment and GP diagnosis, a weak agreement was found for the overall study sample with a kappa coefficient [95% confidence interval, p-value] of $\kappa = 0.156$ [95% CI: 0.133–0.174, $p < 0.001$] (illustrated in Figure 3). Likewise, weak agreements were found when broken down by BMI class, with $\kappa = 0.179$ [95% CI: 0.120–0.231, $p < 0.001$] for under- and normal weight, $\kappa = 0.114$ [95% CI: 0.093–0.162, $p < 0.001$] for overweight, and $\kappa = 0.185$ [95% CI: 0.157–0.241, $p < 0.001$] for obese patients in total. A further distinction into obesity classes showed similarly weak agreements with $\kappa = 0.194$ [95% CI: 0.148–0.270, $p < 0.001$] for obesity I and a non-significant $\kappa = 0.109$ [95% CI: −0.016–0.184, $p = 0.088$] for obesity II but a slight improvement of $\kappa = 0.256$ [95% CI: 0.090–0.510, $p < 0.05$] for obesity III. Similarly, Receiver Operating Characteristic (ROC) analyses indicate that the GDS does not adequately fit with the GP diagnosis in distinguishing between individuals with and without depression symptoms (area under the curve = 0.640 [95% CI: 0.623–0.656]; standard error = 0.0134; sensitivity at cut-off score 6 = 0.43; specificity at cut-off score 6 = 0.78) (see Figure S1).

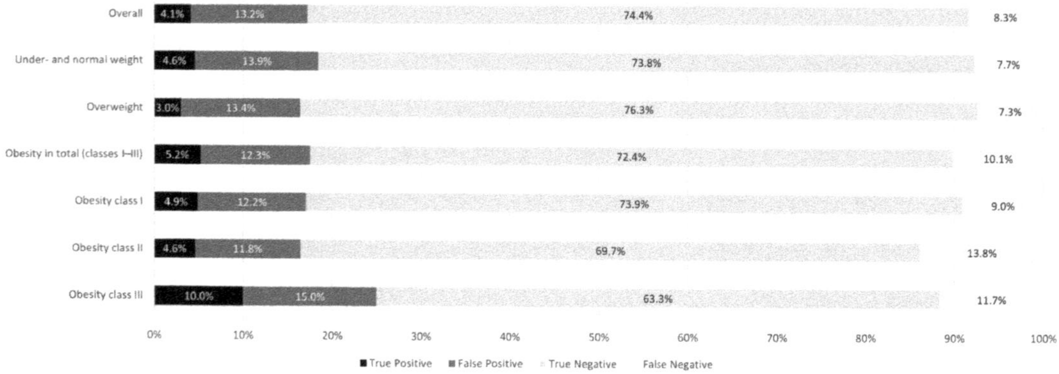

Figure 2. Agreement between GP diagnosis and GDS assessment: percentage distribution of True/False Positives and Negatives.

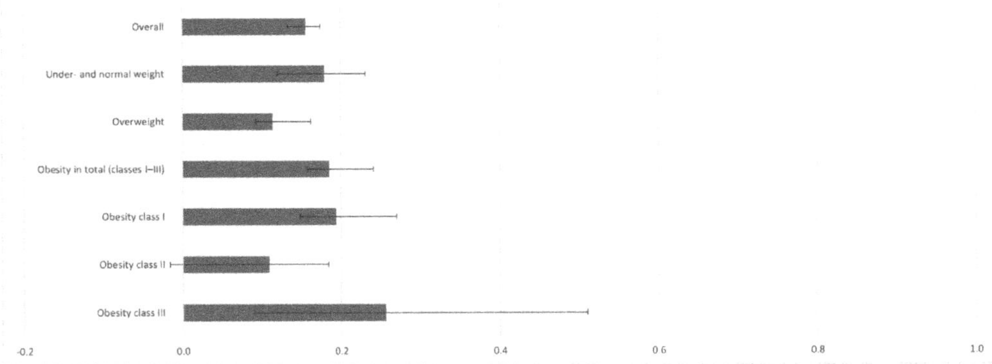

Figure 3. Agreement between GP diagnosis and GDS assessment: Cohen's kappa with 95% CI as error bars.

3.4. Patient-Specific Factors and Their Influence on the Outcome of GP Diagnosis Versus GDS-Based Depression Assessment

Four logistic regression models were used to examine the influence of patient-specific factors on the diagnostic agreement of indicating depression (see Table 3). True Positive describes the indication of depression by both the GDS and the GP, while True Negative shows no indication of depression by either the GDS or the GP. False Positive describes no indication of depression by the GDS but clinical diagnosis of depression by the GP, and False Negative describes the indication of depression by the GDS but no clinical diagnosis of depression by the GP.

Table 3. Results of cross-sectional analyses for the association of depression.

	True Positive Pseudo-R^2: 0.198			**True Negative Pseudo-R^2: 0.110**			**False Positive Pseudo-R^2: 0.035**			**False Negative Pseudo-R^2: 0.186**		
	OR	**(95% CI)**	***p*-Value**	**OR**	**(95% CI)**	***p*-Value**	**OR**	**(95% CI)**	***p*-Value**	**OR**	**(95% CI)**	***p*-Value**
Gender (Ref.: men)												
Women	1.83	(1.05–3.18)	**0.033**	0.58	(0.47–0.73)	**<0.001**	2.01	(1.51–2.68)	**<0.001**	0.96	(0.68–1.36)	0.824
Age (Ref.: <75 years old)												
≥75 years old	0.66	(0.43–1.01)	0.057	1.34	(1.09–1.65)	**0.005**	0.79	(0.61–1.02)	0.070	0.99	(0.71–1.38)	0.952
Marital status (Ref.: married)		Wald/F: 13.75	**0.003**		Wald/F: 8.68	**0.034**		Wald/F: 2.30	0.513		Wald/F: 0.47	0.925
Single	0.91	(0.35–2.41)	0.855	0.85	(0.57–1.28)	0.437	1.15	(0.70–1.89)	0.587	1.20	(0.66–2.18)	0.553
Divorced	1.57	(0.76–3.27)	0.227	0.67	(0.47–0.95)	**0.024**	1.37	(0.91–2.07)	0.135	1.14	(0.64–2.01)	0.656
Widowed	2.43	(1.47–4.01)	**0.001**	0.75	(0.59–0.94)	**0.015**	1.07	(0.79–1.44)	0.665	1.03	(0.70–1.51)	0.880
Education (Ref.: low)		Wald/F: 7.96	**0.019**		Wald/F: 0.72	0.698		Wald/F: 5.77	0.056		Wald/F: 2.98	0.226
Middle	1.05	(0.64–1.72)	0.860	1.06	(0.85–1.32)	0.630	0.78	(0.59–1.03)	0.077	1.31	(0.93–1.86)	0.127
High	2.48	(1.30–4.72)	**0.006**	0.91	(0.65–1.27)	0.571	0.63	(0.40–1.00)	0.050	1.38	(0.79–2.41)	0.253
Income	0.90	(0.66–1.22)	0.483	1.38	(1.16–1.64)	**<0.001**	0.96	(0.80–1.16)	0.678	0.47	(0.33–0.66)	**<0.001**
BMI (Ref.: ≤ 24.9 kg/m^2)		Wald/F: 3.11	0.539		Wald/F: 6.24	0.182		Wald/F: 3.25	0.517		Wald/F: 6.83	0.145
Overweight	0.63	(0.36–1.08)	0.092	1.14	(0.89–1.45)	0.312	1.04	(0.78–1.40)	0.769	0.84	(0.56–1.27)	0.413
Obesity I	0.76	(0.42–1.37)	0.366	1.35	(1.02–1.78)	**0.036**	0.82	(0.58–1.15)	0.252	0.75	(0.47–1.19)	0.217
Obesity II	0.63	(0.25–1.56)	0.314	1.21	(0.79–1.84)	0.377	0.77	(0.45–1.33)	0.353	1.08	(0.57–2.04)	0.822
Obesity III	0.65	(0.20–2.07)	0.461	1.79	(0.94–3.41)	0.076	0.93	(0.44–1.99)	0.859	0.33	(0.13–0.84)	**0.020**
IADL (Ref.: not limited)												
Limited	3.14	(1.98–5.00)	**<0.001**	0.61	(0.49–0.76)	**<0.001**	0.82	(0.61–1.11)	0.203	2.14	(1.54–2.99)	**<0.001**
GCPS pain presence (Ref.: no)												
Yes	1.07	(0.44–2.57)	0.884	0.97	(0.68–1.37)	0.842	1.41	(0.93–2.13)	0.106	0.73	(0.40–1.33)	0.301
GCPS pain intensity	1.01	(0.99–1.02)	0.281	0.99	(0.98–1.00)	**<0.001**	1.00	(1.00–1.01)	0.449	1.02	(1.01–1.02)	**<0.001**
Number of chronic diseases	1.05	(0.98–1.12)	0.161	0.95	(0.91–0.98)	**0.001**	0.99	(0.95–1.03)	0.509	1.13	(1.07–1.18)	**<0.001**
IPAQ (Ref.: low)		Wald/F: 1.63	0.442		Wald/F: 13.18	**0.001**		Wald/F: 1.10	0.576		Wald/F: 13.31	**0.001**
Moderate	0.89	(0.54–1.46)	0.644	1.24	(1.00–1.55)	0.055	1.01	(0.76–1.34)	0.969	0.71	(0.50–1.01)	0.059
High	0.62	(0.30–1.29)	0.202	1.68	(1.27–2.22)	**<0.001**	0.86	(0.61–1.21)	0.395	0.37	(0.22–0.64)	**<0.001**
Social support	0.36	(0.28–0.46)	**<0.001**	1.74	(1.51–2.00)	**<0.001**	1.16	(0.97–1.38)	0.102	0.49	(0.40–0.60)	**<0.001**

Notes: Variables are shown in bold, while their categories are presented in regular font. OR = odds ratio; CI = confidence interval; Ref. = reference category. Bold formatting of *p*-values is used to indicate statistical significance.

3.5. Concordance in Indicating and Not Indicating Depression

Patients who were significantly more likely to suffer from depression (identified through a match by both GDS and GP) in the True Positive model were women (OR = 1.83 [95% CI: 1.05–3.18]), widowed (OR = 2.43 [95% CI: 1.47–4.01]), those with limited IADL (OR = 3.14 [95% CI: 1.98–5.00]), and people with a high level of education (OR = 2.48 [95% CI: 1.30–4.72]). Along with divorced individuals, those also showed a lower probability of receiving a matching non-indication of depression in the True Negative model (women: OR = 0.58 [95% CI: 0.47–0.73], widowed: OR = 0.75 [95% CI: 0.59–0.94], limited IADL: OR = 0.61 [95% CI: 0.49–0.76], and divorced: OR = 0.67 [95% CI: 0.47–0.95]).

In contrast, the factors associated with a significantly increased probability of concordant non-indication of depression were age of ≥75 years (OR = 1.34 [95% CI: 1.09–1.65]), higher income (OR = 1.38 [95% CI: 1.16–1.64]), high physical activity (OR = 1.68 [95% CI: 1.27–2.22]), and social support (OR = 1.74 [95% CI: 1.51–2.00]), the latter being simultaneously associated with a lower probability of a True Positive indication of depression (social support: OR = 0.36 [95% CI: 0.28–0.46]).

Regarding BMI classes, there was only one significant effect with a slightly increased probability of receiving a matching non-indication of depression belonging to the obesity I class (OR = 1.35 [95% CI: 1.02–1.78]). The other BMI classes did not show any significant effects regarding matching depression diagnoses.

3.6. Discordance in Indicating and Not Indicating Depression

Women were significantly more likely than men to receive False Positive depression diagnosis from their GP (OR = 2.01 [95% CI: 1.51–2.68]). There were no significant associations between any BMI class and a False Positive depression diagnosis.

While limited daily activities (OR = 2.14 [95% CI: 1.54–2.99]) and, to a lesser extent, pain intensity (OR = 1.02 [95% CI: 1.01–1.02]) and the number of chronic diseases (OR = 1.13 [95% CI: 1.07–1.18]) were associated with a significantly increased likelihood of a False Negative depression diagnosis, the factors income (OR = 0.47 [95% CI: 0.33–0.66]), high physical activity (OR = 0.37 [95% CI: 0.22–0.64]), and social support (OR = 0.49 [95% CI: 0.40–0.60]) were significantly less likely to be associated with False Negative depression diagnoses. Looking at the BMI classes, there was a significantly lower likelihood of a False Negative depression diagnosis exclusively for the obesity III class (OR = 0.33 [95% CI: 0.13–0.84]).

4. Discussion

The aim of this study was to investigate the prevalence of depression in different BMI classes among multimorbid older patients (aged 65+ years) and to explore differences amongst obesity grades I to III, as well as possible gender and age differences. We also examined potential differences in the identification of depression between the GP's clinical judgment and the outcomes of the GDS, a scientifically well-established screening instrument. In addition to analyzing for agreement, physical and biopsychosocial factors were examined for their influence on depression diagnosis with the aim of identifying possible weaknesses in depression screening and sensitizing GPs, who are important providers of basic psychiatric care for this patient group.

It is interesting to note that the percentage of overweight people (according to BMI) reported in European and German studies of older age cohorts is very similar to our data, while the percentage of under- and normal weight patients in our multimorbid study sample is about 10–18% lower with a roughly equal increase in the percentage of obese people instead [43,44].

Like a previous study comparing depression diagnoses by GPs and GDS assessments, this study confirms that GPs diagnosed depression overall more frequently than the GDS [25]. The data from the present study show that this phenomenon remained constant across almost all BMI classes (except for obesity II). The lowest prevalence of depression was measured by GPs and GDS in the overweight class and differed by more than 10 percentage points from the highest prevalence of depression, which was found in the obese III class. Significant gender differences appeared to exist particularly when diagnosed by GPs, as women were significantly more likely to receive a depression diagnosis across almost all BMI classes. When the obese subgroups were broken down, this phenomenon was particularly significant in the early stage (obesity I). In contrast, significant age group differences dominated in the GDS. Except for the obesity III class, older patients (≥75 years) in the other obesity classes tended to suffer from depression more frequently than the younger comparison group (65–74 years).

The overall weak agreement between GP diagnosis and GDS assessment in direct comparison with a kappa of 0.16 was to be expected based on similar previous studies of this multimorbid cohort, which reported a $\kappa = 0.18$ [25] and a moderate $\kappa = 0.28$ in a different age cohort aged 75+ years [26]. These studies suggested this could be due to the two approaches taking different variables into account when diagnosing depression, with screening tools like the GDS being more sensitive to subliminal depression that does not qualify (yet) for a clinical diagnosis [26]. Even when controlling with other depression screening tools apart from the GDS, the kappa values remain within this range [26], so that the weak to moderate agreement appears to be a GDS-independent effect. When looking at BMI classes, the analysis did not show any better or worse agreement in individual subgroups. This goes against the expectation that weight or obesity stigma might affect GP diagnoses of mental disorders like depression, as suggested in a previous study [45]. In fact, the statistically highest agreement was observed for people with obesity III. Although the analysis of the kappa values indicates a poor agreement, it should be noted that these low kappa values still bring an agreement of around 75%, which means that, despite recognizable discrepancies, the GPs and the GDS came to the same conclusion in three quarters of the cases. For international comparison, this result can be juxtaposed with an Indian study with 306 participants (60+ years) in which there was, in principle, a good agreement between GDS and ICD-10 diagnosis with a kappa of 0.85, although the comparison was not based on the documented GP diagnosis of depression but on the ICD-10 criteria findings surveyed during the study, which could explain the higher agreement rate [46].

In our cohort, the diagnosis of depression was influenced by gender. GPs appear to be more sensitive to female patients and more likely to correctly diagnose existing depression as such. At the same time, women are also often mistakenly diagnosed with depression, whereas men are less likely to be suspected of having depression, and thus, more depression is correctly ruled out. The postulation of this effect is supported by research that attributed an increased probability of a GP diagnosis of depression to women [26].

GPs often correctly ruled out depression in patients over the age of 75. Widowhood, which incidentally mostly affects women, was usually correctly recognized as a risk factor and an indication of an accompanying depression. However, widowed and divorced people were probably also more often overdiagnosed by "cautious" doctors who less frequently correctly ruled out depression in them. The relationship between widowhood and depression was recently analyzed in a meta-analysis and found that the prevalence of depression, although decreasing over time from around 38% to 11%, remains above average, particularly in the first five years after the loss of a partner [47].

Higher education was associated with an increased likelihood of correct depression recognition. Similarly, people with higher incomes were more likely to correctly be excluded from depression, and the risk of overlooked depression was lower. These effects could possibly be due to better access to the healthcare system and preventative measures for these groups, as well as a better ability to articulate their own symptoms. Other studies confirm the protective effect of education and income on the prevalence of depression [48] and suggest that cytokines like IL-1β, TNFα, or the NF-κB pathway, which play a role in both obesity and depression, could explain the link [49]. Education as protective against obesity, which is more strongly correlated in women than in men, could therefore also have an influence on depression [50].

While physically active patients according to the IPAQ were more likely to be correctly ruled out for depression, people with limited daily activities according to the IADL showed diagnostic uncertainties with more correct depression diagnoses, fewer correct depression exclusions, and an increased probability of overlooked depression. Meanwhile, both pain and the number of chronic diseases showed only a weak influence on the diagnosis of depression.

In contrast, social support seemed to act as a protective factor against depression, leading more likely to correct depression exclusions. It was also associated with fewer overlooked depression diagnoses, potentially due to diagnosis-promoting hints from the patients' social environment. Social support has been described in the literature elsewhere as a possible protective factor against depression, particularly in lonely older people [51,52]. On the other hand, socially supported patients in our study were also less likely to receive correct positive depression diagnoses, which could indicate that depression may be less obvious and therefore more difficult to recognize in socially well-integrated patients.

Contrary to expectations, the BMI class did not play a pronounced role in the process of diagnosing and the diagnosis quality of depression. Significance was only found in minimum and maximum levels of obesity. Mild obesity was associated with an increased probability of correctly ruling out depression. This may be due to doctors being sufficiently sensitized to recognize physical manifestations related to obesity that can mimic depressive symptoms and therefore not immediately assuming a diagnosis of depression. On the other hand, extreme obesity seemed to reduce the likelihood of existing depression being overlooked by the GP. It is possible that most GPs are aware of the interplay between (extreme) obesity and depression. The literature also provides the explanation that, in particular, multimorbid obese people, in view of low self-esteem and learned helplessness, are more likely to utilize health services and seek help [53]. Overall, we found only a few significant correlations, which were not systematic and tended to relate to marginal categories. This leads to the conclusion that, in the German outpatient GP setting, contrary to original concerns, depression is probably diagnosed largely independently of body weight; thus weight-associated stigma appears to play less of a role than previously assumed [54,55]. At the same time, a detailed analysis of the differentiated degrees of obesity revealed a possible increased awareness of GPs for mental health in patients with extreme obesity (obesity III). Nevertheless, the results could also indicate that weight-associated mental consequences are not (yet) sufficiently reflected, as there was no systematic positive influence on correct diagnoses (matches). Either way, there does not appear to be a systematically increased rate of overlooked depression in overweight or obese patients.

Strengths and Limitations

The strengths of this study were its multicenter design and a large sample size of a so far insufficiently investigated patient collective of multimorbid older patients, a group that has growing relevance in the future due to demographic changes.

Limitations of the present study include the fact that only cross-sectional data from the baseline survey between July 2008 and October 2009 were analyzed, which means that correlations could be identified but no causal link could be proven. This study design cannot determine the causal direction of the bidirectional relationship between obesity and depression [22,23]. Future studies should examine these associations using more recent data and longitudinal study designs.

The GDS with 15 items was used as a well-established screening standard in our patient group (using a cut-off of ≥6 points for a likely depressive disorder), although more sensitive or restrictive cut-off values of ≥5 to ≥8 points are also discussed in the literature, which may, however, be associated with the risk of over- or underestimating the prevalence of depression [56]. It can be assumed that using a different cut-off value in our study would have influenced the estimated prevalence rates and the level of agreement between GDS assessments and GP diagnoses. A recent meta-analysis identified a cut-off of ≥8 as providing the best agreement with the Structured Clinical Interview for Diagnostic and Statistical Manual of Mental Disorders (SCID), the diagnostic gold standard. However, due to substantial heterogeneity across studies, this threshold was not considered suitable for routine clinical use [56].

It should be noted that the GDS remains a screening tool and can only provide indications of depression but cannot be considered the gold standard for its diagnosis. Like other screening tools, the GDS has inherent limitations due to its respective sensitivity and specificity, which influence its positive predictive value and utility in accurately identifying true cases of depression [57]. The diagnosis by the GP was assumed in our study exclusively on the basis of coded ICD diagnoses, although there are indications that this approach underestimates the "awareness" of GPs and therefore rather represents a "lack of registration" instead, which could be ameliorated by considering further indications from the medical record such as free text notes or antidepressant medication prescriptions [58]. The experience of GPs in the treatment of depressive disorders is another factor that seems to influence the diagnosis [26] and was not considered further in the present study.

In addition, other factors that we did not investigate may have influenced our findings. Previous studies highlight lifestyle-related variables such as diet, alcohol use, and smoking as relevant variables that can affect the relationship between obesity and depression. [59]. While the GDS is designed to minimize the impact of somatic health on depression screening in older adults, prior research suggests that the clinical diagnosis of depression, as made by GPs, may be confounded by residual symptoms, such as fatigue or weight loss in the context of cancer diseases [60]. Although these factors were not considered in our study, they might have contributed to differences in diagnostic agreement. These factors should be taken into account in future research.

The four logistic regressions in our study were able to reveal some clear correlations between the factors examined and the diagnostic outcome; however, the pseudo-R^2 values of our models with the factors examined only explain up to a maximum of just about 20% of the variance and varied within the same dataset in our four different models from 0.035 to 0.198. More research is needed in the future to identify possible other factors that could play a role in this complex interaction.

5. Conclusions

The present study is the first to examine age- and gender-specific prevalence rates of depression across different BMI classes in a large sample of multimorbid older adults in primary care. It is also the first to provide information on diagnostic agreement between GP diagnoses and GDS assessments while taking the BMI into account. The study highlights important factors associated with a poorer concordance between GP's clinical judgment and the GDS-based screening outcome among older adults with multiple health conditions in primary care. The results provide important insights into potential target groups that could benefit from intervention programs designed to improve depression diagnostics and treatment. A substantial proportion of multimorbid patients suffer from depression across all BMI classes, with GP patients in obesity class III identified as having the highest risk of depressive symptoms. Overall, agreement between depression diagnoses by GPs and the GDS assessments was weak, regardless of the BMI. These findings suggest that diagnostic agreement could be improved. The standardized evaluation of depression diagnoses in primary care could provide a basis upon which the current clinical diagnostic routine could be enhanced. For instance, improving diagnostic precision for depression in multimorbid older patients in primary care might be achieved through a combination of standardized screening tools (such as the GDS), targeted training, and structured screening of high-risk groups. Trained medical assistants or nurses could, in a first step, identify high-risk patients using a checklist with risk factors and administer a depression screening tool (like the GDS) prior to GP consultation. GPs could then, in a second step, leverage this information to detect (sub)clinical depression, guiding decisions on observation or further diagnostic evaluation. In a third step, identified depression cases could be managed through integrated care pathways involving case managers and mental health specialists. These could, for example, support home-based therapies or interventions to improve problem-solving skills or social and physical activity [61]. A rise in False Positive misidentifications and overtreatment of the respective groups (at the cost of under-provision for other patient groups) could be counteracted through re-evaluation of depression cases over an extended time rather than one-time depression assessments [62]. Before implementation, such approaches would need to be evaluated through feasibility and intervention studies. Collaborative care models, involving mental health specialists, also support the earlier and more effective identification of depression [63]. Finally, allowing more consultation time and building stronger patient–doctor relationships are essential for recognizing depressive symptoms more reliably.

Supplementary Materials: The following supporting information can be downloaded at: https://www.mdpi.com/article/10.3390/nu17081394/s1, Figure S1: Receiver Operating Characteristic (ROC) analyses.

Author Contributions: Conceptualization, study design, and project administration: S.W., W.M., J.G., K.M., H.B., A.F., I.S., H.-H.K., B.W., G.S., K.W., M.S., M.L. and S.G.R.-H. Data curation: B.W., G.S. and K.W. Investigation: S.W., W.M., J.G., K.M., H.B., A.F., I.S., H.-H.K., B.W., G.S., K.W., M.S., M.L. and S.G.R.-H. Analyses and interpretation of the results: D.C.B., A.P., F.B. and M.L. Writing—original draft preparation: D.C.B., A.P., S.G.R.-H. and M.L. Writing—review and editing and critical revision of the manuscript: all authors. All authors have read and agreed to the published version of the manuscript.

Funding: The study was funded by the German Federal Ministry of Education and Research (MultiCare Study, grant numbers 01ET0725-31 and 01ET1006A-K). The funding bodies had no impact on the design of the study, data collection, analysis, interpretation of data, or on writing the manuscript. M.L. was funded by the @ktivPLUS study (German Federal Ministry of Education and Research, grant number 01GY2108).

Institutional Review Board Statement: The study was approved by the Ethics Committee of the Medical Association of Hamburg (approval no. 2881; date of approval: 14 February 2008). The ethics committees of the other participating centers also approved the study. All procedures contributing to this work were specifically approved by the Ethics committee and comply with the Helsinki Declaration of 1975, as revised in 2008, and the ethical standards of the relevant national and institutional committees on human experimentation.

Informed Consent Statement: All participants gave written informed consent for their participation. Participants acknowledged that they cannot be identified via the paper and were fully anonymized.

Data Availability Statement: The data that support the findings of this study are not publicly available due to privacy and ethical restrictions. The data are, however, available from the authors upon reasonable request and with permission of Martin Scherer (principal investigator).

Acknowledgments: This article was written on behalf of the MultiCare Cohort Study Group, which consists of Attila Altiner, Horst Bickel, Wolfgang Blank, Monika Bullinger, Hendrik van den Bussche†, Anne Dahlhaus, Lena Ehreke, Michael Freitag, Angela Fuchs, Jochen Gensichen, Ferdinand Gerlach, Heike Hansen, Sven Heinrich, Susanne Höfels, Olaf von dem Knesebeck, Hans-Helmut König, Norbert Krause, Hanna Leicht, Margrit Löbner, Melanie Luppa, Wolfgang Maier, Manfred Mayer, Christine Mellert, Anna Nützel, Thomas Paschke, Juliana Petersen, Jana Prokein, Steffi Riedel-Heller, Heinz-Peter Romberg, Ingmar Schäfer, Martin Scherer, Gerhard Schön, Susanne Steinmann, Sven Schulz, Karl Wegscheider, Klaus Weckbecker, Jochen Werle, Siegfried Weyerer, and Birgitt Wiese. We thank Lisa Wittenburg for proofreading the article. We are grateful to the general practitioners in Bonn, Düsseldorf, Frankfurt/Main, Hamburg, Jena, Leipzig, Mannheim, and Munich who supplied clinical information on their patients. We would like to thank all study participants for taking part in the study.

Conflicts of Interest: The authors declare no conflicts of interest. The funders had no role in the design of the study; in the collection, analyses, or interpretation of data; in the writing of the manuscript; or in the decision to publish the results.

Abbreviations

The following abbreviations are used in this manuscript:

BMI	Body Mass Index
CASMIN	Comparative Analysis of Social Mobility in Industrial Nations
CI	Confidence interval
GCPS	Graded Chronic Pain Scale
GDS	Geriatric Depression Scale
GP	General practitioner
IADL	Instrumental Activities of Daily Living (scale)
ICD	International Classification of Diseases
IPAQ	International Physical Activities Questionnaire
OR	Odds ratio
ROC	Receiver Operating Characteristic
SCID	Structured Clinical Interview for Diagnostic and Statistical Manual of Mental Disorders
WHO	World Health Organization

References

1. World Health Organization. *MhGAP: Mental Health Gap Action Programme: Scaling up Care for Mental, Neurological, and Substance Use Disorders*; World Health Organization: Geneva, Switzerland, 2008; ISBN 978-92-4-159620-6.
2. World Health Organization (Ed.) *Mental Health Atlas 2017*; World Health Organization: Geneva, Switzerland, 2018; ISBN 978-92-4-151401-9.
3. World Health Organization (Ed.) *Global Strategy on Diet, Physical Activity and Health*; World Health Organization: Geneva, Switzerland, 2004; ISBN 92-4-159222-2.
4. Bentham, J.; Di Cesare, M.; Bilano, V. Worldwide Trends in Body-Mass Index, Underweight, Overweight, and Obesity from 1975 to 2016: A Pooled Analysis of 2416 Population-Based Measurement Studies in 128·9 Million Children, Adolescents, and Adults. *Lancet* **2017**, *390*, 2627. [CrossRef]
5. World Health Organization. Obesity and Overweight. Available online: https://www.who.int/news-room/fact-sheets/detail/obesity-and-overweight (accessed on 21 February 2025).
6. Batsis, J.A.; Zagaria, A.B. Addressing Obesity in Aging Patients. *Med. Clin. N. Am.* **2018**, *102*, 65–85. [CrossRef]

7. Flegal, K.M.; Kruszon-Moran, D.; Carroll, M.D.; Fryar, C.D.; Ogden, C.L. Trends in Obesity Among Adults in the United State 2005 to 2014. *JAMA* **2016**, *315*, 2284. [CrossRef] [PubMed]
8. Max Rubner-Institut. Ergebnisbericht, Teil 1 Nationale Verzehrsstudie II; 2008. Available online: https://www.mri.bund.de fileadmin/MRI/Institute/EV/NVS_II_Abschlussbericht_Teil_1_mit_Ergaenzungsbericht.pdf (accessed on 25 February 2025).
9. Haslam, D.W.; James, W.P.T. Obesity. *Lancet* **2005**, *366*, 1197–1209. [CrossRef]
10. Delpino, F.M.; dos Santos Rodrigues, A.P.; Petarli, G.B.; Machado, K.P.; Flores, T.R.; Batista, S.R.; Nunes, B.P. Overweight, Obesi and Risk of Multimorbidity: A Systematic Review and Meta-Analysis of Longitudinal Studies. *Obes. Rev.* **2023**, *24*, e1356 [CrossRef] [PubMed]
11. Kivimäki, M.; Strandberg, T.; Pentti, J.; Nyberg, S.T.; Frank, P.; Jokela, M.; Ervasti, J.; Suominen, S.B.; Vahtera, J.; Sipilä, P.N.; et a Body-Mass Index and Risk of Obesity-Related Complex Multimorbidity: An Observational Multicohort Study. *Lancet Diabet Endocrinol.* **2022**, *10*, 253–263. [CrossRef]
12. Lebenbaum, M.; Zaric, G.S.; Thind, A.; Sarma, S. Trends in Obesity and Multimorbidity in Canada. *Prev. Med.* **2018**, *116*, 173–17 [CrossRef]
13. Sikorski, C.; Luppa, M.; Weyerer, S.; König, H.-H.; Maier, W.; Schön, G.; Petersen, J.J.; Gensichen, J.; Fuchs, A.; Bickel, H.; et a Obesity and Associated Lifestyle in a Large Sample of Multi-Morbid German Primary Care Attendees. *PLoS ONE* **2014**, *9*, e10258 [CrossRef]
14. Speerforck, S.; Schomerus, G. "Mental Health Awareness"—Eine Entwicklung ohne Nebenwirkungen? *Psychiatr. Prax.* **202** *51*, 293–295. [CrossRef]
15. Vos, T.; Lim, S.S.; Abbafati, C.; Abbas, K.M.; Abbasi, M.; Abbasifard, M.; Abbasi-Kangevari, M.; Abbastabar, H.; Abd-Alla F.; Abdelalim, A.; et al. Global Burden of 369 Diseases and Injuries in 204 Countries and Territories, 1990–2019: A Systemati Analysis for the Global Burden of Disease Study 2019. *Lancet* **2020**, *396*, 1204–1222. [CrossRef]
16. GBD 2015 Disease and Injury Incidence and Prevalence Collaborators. Global, Regional, and National Incidence, Prevalence, an Years Lived with Disability for 310 Diseases and Injuries, 1990–2015: A Systematic Analysis for the Global Burden of Diseas Study 2015. *Lancet* **2016**, *388*, 1545–1602. [CrossRef] [PubMed]
17. Ye, B.; Xie, R.; Mishra, S.R.; Dai, X.; Chen, H.; Chen, X.; Li, D.; Yuan, C.; Xu, X. Bidirectional Association between Physic Multimorbidity and Subclinical Depression in Chinese Older Adults: Findings from a Prospective Cohort Study. *J. Affect. Disor* **2022**, *296*, 169–174. [CrossRef]
18. Spangenberg, L.; Forkmann, T.; Brähler, E.; Glaesmer, H. The Association of Depression and Multimorbidity in the Elderl Implications for the Assessment of Depression. *Psychogeriatrics* **2011**, *11*, 227–234. [CrossRef]
19. Agustini, B.; Lotfaliany, M.; Woods, R.L.; McNeil, J.J.; Nelson, M.R.; Shah, R.C.; Murray, A.M.; Ernst, M.E.; Reid, C.M.; Tonkin, A et al. Patterns of Association between Depressive Symptoms and Chronic Medical Morbidities in Older Adults. *J. Am. Geriat Soc.* **2020**, *68*, 1834–1841. [CrossRef]
20. Moetteli, S.; Mueller-Stierlin, A.S. Ernährungsinterventionen in der Psychiatrie—Ein vernachlässigter Baustein für einen gesü deren Lebensstil. *Psychiatr. Prax.* **2024**, *51*, 235–237. [CrossRef] [PubMed]
21. Quek, Y.-H.; Tam, W.W.S.; Zhang, M.W.B.; Ho, R.C.M. Exploring the Association between Childhood and Adolescent Obesity an Depression: A Meta-Analysis. *Obes. Rev.* **2017**, *18*, 742–754. [CrossRef] [PubMed]
22. Mannan, M.; Mamun, A.; Doi, S.; Clavarino, A. Is There a Bi-Directional Relationship between Depression and Obesity amon Adult Men and Women? Systematic Review and Bias-Adjusted Meta Analysis. *Asian J. Psychiatry* **2016**, *21*, 51–66. [CrossRef]
23. Pan, A.; Sun, Q.; Czernichow, S.; Kivimaki, M.; Okereke, O.I.; Lucas, M.; Manson, J.E.; Ascherio, A.; Hu, F.B. Bidirection Association between Depression and Obesity in Middle-Aged and Older Women. *Int. J. Obes.* **2012**, *36*, 595–602. [CrossRef]
24. Park, L.T.; Zarate, C.A. Depression in the Primary Care Setting. *N. Engl. J. Med.* **2019**, *380*, 559–568. [CrossRef]
25. Schwarzbach, M.; Luppa, M.; Hansen, H.; König, H.-H.; Gensichen, J.; Petersen, J.J.; Schön, G.; Wiese, B.; Weyerer, S.; Bickel, H et al. A Comparison of GP and GDS Diagnosis of Depression in Late Life among Multimorbid Patients—Results of the MultiCar Study. *J. Affect. Disord.* **2014**, *168*, 276–283. [CrossRef]
26. Dorow, M.; Stein, J.; Pabst, A.; Weyerer, S.; Werle, J.; Maier, W.; Miebach, L.; Scherer, M.; Stark, A.; Wiese, B.; et al. Categoric and Dimensional Perspectives on Depression in Elderly Primary Care Patients—Results of the AgeMooDe Study. *Int. J. Metho Psychiatr. Res.* **2018**, *27*, e1577. [CrossRef] [PubMed]
27. Schäfer, I.; Hansen, H.; Schön, G.; Maier, W.; Höfels, S.; Altiner, A.; Fuchs, A.; Gerlach, F.M.; Petersen, J.J.; Gensichen, J.; et al. Th German MultiCare-Study: Patterns of Multimorbidity in Primary Health Care—Protocol of a Prospective Cohort Study. *BM Health Serv. Res.* **2009**, *9*, 145. [CrossRef]
28. Van Den Bussche, H.; Scherer, M. Das Verbundvorhaben "Komorbidität und Multimorbidität in der hausärztlichen Versorgung (MultiCare). *Z. Gerontol. Geriatrie* **2011**, *44*, 73–100. [CrossRef]
29. Die Generation 65+ in Deutschland 2015. Statistisches Bundesamt, Wiesbaden. Available online: https://www statistischebibliothek.de/mir/servlets/MCRFileNodeServlet/DEMonografie_derivate_00001454/Generation65.pdf (accesse on 25 February 2025).

30. Lachman, M.E. Psychology of Adult Development. In *International Encyclopedia of the Social & Behavioral Sciences*; Elsevier: Amsterdam, The Netherlands, 2001. [CrossRef]
31. Glossary: Equivalised Disposable Income. Available online: https://ec.europa.eu/eurostat/statistics-explained/index.php?title=Glossary:Equivalised_disposable_income (accessed on 21 February 2025).
32. Hauner, H.; Moss, A.; Berg, A.; Bischoff, S.C.; Colombo-Benkmann, M.; Ellrott, T.; Heintze, C.; Kanthak, U.; Kunze, D.; Stefan, N.; et al. Interdisziplinäre Leitlinie der Qualität S3 zur "Prävention und Therapie der Adipositas": Der Deutschen Adipositas-Gesellschaft e.V.; der Deutschen Diabetes Gesellschaft; der Deutschen Gesellschaft für Ernährung e.V.; der Deutschen Gesellschaft für Ernährungsmedizin e.V. Version 2.0 (April 2014); AWMF-Register Nr. 050-001. *Adipositas Ursachen Folgeerkrankungen Ther.* **2014**, *8*, 179–221. [CrossRef]
33. Lawton, M.P.; Brody, E.M. Assessment of Older People: Self-Maintaining and Instrumental Activities of Daily Living. *Gerontologist* **1969**, *9*, 179–186. [CrossRef] [PubMed]
34. Graf, C. Lawton—Brody Instrumental Activities of Daily Living Scale (IADL). *AJN Am. J. Nurs.* **2008**, *108*, 59.
35. Klasen, B.W.; Hallner, D.; Schaub, C.; Willburger, R.; Hasenbring, M. Validation and Reliability of the German Version of the Chronic Pain Grade Questionnaire in Primary Care Back Pain Patients. *Psychosoc. Med.* **2004**, *1*, Doc07.
36. The IPAQ Group. Guidelines for Data Processing and Analysis of the International Physical Activity Questionnaire (IPAQ)—Short and Long Forms; 2005. Available online: https://biobank.ndph.ox.ac.uk/showcase/ukb/docs/ipaq_analysis.pdf (accessed on 25 February 2025).
37. Fydrich, T.; Geyer, M.; Hessel, A.; Sommer, G.; Brähler, E. Fragebogen Zur Sozialen Unterstützung (F-SozU): Normierung an Einer Repräsentativen Stichprobe. *Diagnostica* **1999**, *45*, 212–216. [CrossRef]
38. Fydrich, T.; Sommer, G.; Tydecks, S.; Brähler, E. Fragebogen zur sozialen Unterstützung (F-SozU): Normierung der Kurzform (K-14). *Z. Med. Psychol.* **2009**, *18*, 43–48.
39. Stone-Bury, L.; Granier, K.; Segal, D. Geriatric Depression Scale. In *Encyclopedia of Gerontology and Population Aging*; Springer: Cham, Switzerland, 2019; ISBN 978-3-319-69892-2. [CrossRef]
40. Gauggel, S.; Birkner, B. Validität und Reliabilität einer deutschen Version der Geriatrischen Depressionsskala (GDS). *Z. Klin. Psychol. Psychotherapie* **1999**, *28*, 18–27. [CrossRef]
41. Deppermann, K.-M.; Friedrich, C.; Herth, F.; Huber, R.M. Geriatrische Assessments Und Diagnostik Beim Älteren Patienten. *Onkologie* **2008**, *31*, 6–14. [CrossRef]
42. BfArM—ICD-10-GM Version 2024. Available online: https://klassifikationen.bfarm.de/icd-10-gm/kode-suche/htmlgm2024/block-f30-f39.htm (accessed on 21 February 2025).
43. Schienkiewitz, A.; Kuhnert, R.; Blume, M.; Mensink, G.B.M. Overweight and Obesity among Adults in Germany—Results from GEDA 2019/2020-EHIS. *J. Health Monit.* **2022**, *7*, 21–28. [CrossRef] [PubMed]
44. Peralta, M.; Ramos, M.; Lipert, A.; Martins, J.; Marques, A. Prevalence and Trends of Overweight and Obesity in Older Adults from 10 European Countries from 2005 to 2013. *Scand. J. Public Health* **2018**, *46*, 522–529. [CrossRef] [PubMed]
45. Pearl, R.L.; Hernandez, M.; Bach, C.; Groshon, L.; Wadden, T.A. Prevalence of Diagnosed Psychiatric Disorders among Adults Who Have Experienced and Internalized Weight Stigma. *Obes. Sci. Pract.* **2023**, *9*, 681–687. [CrossRef]
46. Nagar, S.; Patel, H.B.; Nagar, N.; Mahyavanshi, D.; Nagar, S.S.; Godara, N. Study on Factors Associated with Depression among Elderly and Comparison of Two Scales Used for Screening. *Indian J. Community Med.* **2021**, *46*, 446–449. [CrossRef] [PubMed]
47. Kristiansen, C.B.; Kjær, J.N.; Hjorth, P.; Andersen, K.; Prina, A.M. The Association of Time since Spousal Loss and Depression in Widowhood: A Systematic Review and Meta-Analysis. *Soc. Psychiatry Psychiatr. Epidemiol.* **2019**, *54*, 781–792. [CrossRef]
48. Li, L.; Sun, W.; Luo, J.; Huang, H. Associations between Education Levels and Prevalence of Depressive Symptoms: NHANES (2005–2018). *J. Affect. Disord.* **2022**, *301*, 360–367. [CrossRef]
49. Hryhorczuk, C.; Sharma, S.; Fulton, S.E. Metabolic Disturbances Connecting Obesity and Depression. *Front. Neurosci.* **2013**, *7*, 177. [CrossRef]
50. Hsieh, T.-H.; Lee, J.J.; Yu, E.W.-R.; Hu, H.-Y.; Lin, S.-Y.; Ho, C.-Y. Association between Obesity and Education Level among the Elderly in Taipei, Taiwan between 2013 and 2015: A Cross-Sectional Study. *Sci. Rep.* **2020**, *10*, 20285. [CrossRef]
51. Shin, J.; Kang, H.; Choi, S.; Choi, J. Exploring Social Activity Patterns among Community-Dwelling Older Adults in South Korea: A Latent Class Analysis. *BMC Geriatr.* **2024**, *24*, 697. [CrossRef]
52. Song, C.; Yao, L.; Chen, H.; Song, Y.; Liu, L. Prevalence and Factors Influencing Depression among Empty Nesters in China: A Meta-Analysis. *BMC Geriatr.* **2023**, *23*, 333. [CrossRef] [PubMed]
53. Hilbert, A.; Braehler, E.; Haeuser, W.; Zenger, M. Weight Bias Internalization, Core Self-Evaluation, and Health in Overweight and Obese Persons. *Obesity* **2014**, *22*, 79–85. [CrossRef]
54. Puhl, R.M.; Heuer, C.A. The Stigma of Obesity: A Review and Update. *Obesity* **2009**, *17*, 941–964. [CrossRef] [PubMed]
55. Emmer, C.; Bosnjak, M.; Mata, J. The Association between Weight Stigma and Mental Health: A Meta-Analysis. *Obes. Rev.* **2020**, *21*, e12935. [CrossRef] [PubMed]

56. Parsons, M.; Qiu, L.; Levis, B.; Fan, S.; Sun, Y.; Amiri, L.S.N.; Harel, D.; Markham, S.; Vigod, S.N.; Ziegelstein, R.C.; et a Depression Prevalence of the Geriatric Depression Scale-15 Was Compared to Structured Clinical Interview for DSM Usin Individual Participant Data Meta-Analysis. *Sci. Rep.* **2024**, *14*, 17430. [CrossRef]
57. Krishnamoorthy, Y.; Rajaa, S.; Rehman, T. Diagnostic Accuracy of Various Forms of Geriatric Depression Scale for Screening c Depression among Older Adults: Systematic Review and Meta-Analysis. *Arch. Gerontol. Geriatr.* **2020**, *87*, 104002. [CrossRef]
58. Joling, K.J.; Van Marwijk, H.W.J.; Piek, E.; Der Horst, H.E.V.; Penninx, B.W.; Verhaak, P.; Van Hout, H.P.J. Do GPs' Medical Record Demonstrate a Good Recognition of Depression? A New Perspective on Case Extraction. *J. Affect. Disord.* **2011**, *133*, 522–52 [CrossRef]
59. Hung, C.-F.; Rivera, M.; Craddock, N.; Owen, M.J.; Gill, M.; Korszun, A.; Maier, W.; Mors, O.; Preisig, M.; Rice, J.P.; et a Relationship between Obesity and the Risk of Clinically Significant Depression: Mendelian Randomisation Study. *Br. J. Psychiatr* **2014**, *205*, 24–28. [CrossRef]
60. Nelson, C.J.; Cho, C.; Berk, A.R.; Holland, J.; Roth, A.J. Are Gold Standard Depression Measures Appropriate for Use in Geriatri Cancer Patients? A Systematic Evaluation of Self-Report Depression Instruments Used With Geriatric, Cancer, and Geriatri Cancer Samples. *J. Clin. Oncol.* **2010**, *28*, 348–356. [CrossRef]
61. Ciechanowski, P.; Wagner, E.; Schmaling, K.; Schwartz, S.; Williams, B.; Diehr, P.; Kulzer, J.; Gray, S.; Collier, C.; LoGerfc J. Community-Integrated Home-Based Depression Treatment in Older Adults: A Randomized Controlled Trial. *JAMA* **200** *291*, 1569. [CrossRef]
62. Mitchell, A.J.; Vaze, A.; Rao, S. Clinical Diagnosis of Depression in Primary Care: A Meta-Analysis. *Lancet* **2009**, *374*, 609–61 [CrossRef] [PubMed]
63. Habtamu, K.; Birhane, R.; Demissie, M.; Fekadu, A. Interventions to Improve the Detection of Depression in Primary Healthcar Systematic Review. *Syst. Rev.* **2023**, *12*, 25. [CrossRef] [PubMed]

nutrients

MDPI

Article

#BodyPositivity: The Role of Body Appreciation and Body Mass Index for Muscle Dysmorphia, Body Attitudes and Exercise Motives Among Men

Kamila Czepczor-Bernat [1,*], Adriana Modrzejewska [2] and Justyna Modrzejewska [3]

1 Department of Pediatrics, Pediatric Obesity and Metabolic Bone Diseases, Faculty of Medical Sciences in Katowice, Medical University of Silesia, 40-055 Katowice, Poland
2 Department of Medical Anthropology, Faculty of Medical Sciences in Katowice, Medical University of Silesia, 40-055 Katowice, Poland; adriana.modrzejewska@sum.edu.pl
3 Institute of Pedagogy, University of Bielsko-Biała, 43-300 Bielsko-Biala, Poland; jmodrzejewska@ubb.edu.pl
* Correspondence: k.czepczor.bernat@gmail.com

Abstract: Objectives: The main aim of this study was to investigate the hypothesis that men with high body appreciation and healthy (normal) weight would have significantly lower levels of muscle dysmorphia and the non-adaptive (negative) multiple dimensions of body attitudes, as well as higher levels of the selected pro-health and adaptive exercise motives, than those men with low body appreciation and excess body weight. **Methods**: A total of 374 Polish men ($M_{age} = 28.96 \pm 8.52$) completed the following questionnaires: (a) the Body Appreciation Scale-2, (b) the Muscle Dysmorphic Disorder Inventory, (c) the Male Body Attitude Scale, and (d) the Exercise Motivations Inventory-2. **Results**: By analyzing the most important findings, it was discovered, as hypothesized, that significant differences (in terms of most of the assessed scale/subscales) were found between men who had high body appreciation and healthy weight (Cluster 4), and men with low body appreciation and excess body weight (Cluster 3). Cluster 4 (vs. Cluster 3) was characterized as follows: (a) considering muscle dysmorphia, these participants had lower levels in terms of the total score and subscale of appearance intolerance; (b) they had fewer non-adaptive (negative) body attitudes, with lower total scores and lower scores on two subscales (body fat and height); (c) for the selected pro-health and adaptive exercise motives, Cluster 4 had higher levels on all subscales. **Conclusions**: Our results show that holding views in line with positive body image is also beneficial for the functioning of adult men. However, further research needs to be conducted in this area to determine whether the content in the interventions and prevention activities for both sexes should be the same and what factors should be taken into account in order to influence excessive fixation on a muscularity.

Keywords: body appreciation; body attitudes; body mass index; body positivity; exercise motives; men; muscle dysmorphia

1. Introduction

Body positivity (most often marked on social media as #BodyPositive/#BoPo) is a social movement focusing on the topic of body acceptance, regardless of differences between people in this context (concerning, among others, body size and shape, skin tone, gender and physical abilities) [1–3]. It is a social movement that challenges the modern pressure to achieve commonly promoted "standards" of beauty. The main ideas of this movement focus on appreciating the functionality and health of the human body, instead of focusing excessively on physical appearance [1–3]. Research shows that these attitudes may be associated with healthier eating behaviors and a more adaptive attitude to one's own body [1,4,5]. Content related to #BodyPositivity also refers to taking care of the body through physical activity, which is based on the assumption that exercise is a form of taking care of physical and mental health, and the chosen type of activity is a source of pleasure [6–9].

A questionnaire that seems to reflect well some selected aspects of the attitudes related to #BodyPostivity is the Body Appreciation Scale 2 [10]. This measure is related to the attitude towards the body—body appreciation—that we wanted to measure. After reviewing the literature, we identified that this measure more strongly reflects certain selected views related to #BodyPostivity; it should be emphasized, however, that it does not directly measure all views related to the mentioned social movement, and the concepts of body positivity and positive body image are not identical.

As mentioned above, #BodyPostivity aims to encourage adopting an attitude towards the body that will be associated with respect for one's own body, avoiding constantly making harmful comparisons with others; it encourages having positive beliefs about one's body and undertaking adaptive behaviors that will be associated with the desire to take care of one's physical and mental health [1,2,5,6,9]. This social movement is designed to influence various components of the attitude towards the body, including cognitive aspects (body-related beliefs and thoughts—i.e., my body is unattractive/too fat), emotional aspects (body-related feelings and emotions—i.e., shame, fear, blame) and behavioral aspects (body-related actions and behaviors—e.g., physical activity, body grooming) [11]. #BodyPostivity also encourages us to be aware of the commonly existing pressure to change the figure and/or shape of one's body according to the applicable "standard", referring mainly to the phenomena of fat shaming or fatphobia (anti-fat bias which is related to prejudicial assumptions concerning people with overweight or obesity, and the mechanism of shaming this group) [12]. Earlier research in this area shows that there is a negative relationship between body appreciation and various dimensions related to attitudes towards the body (e.g., subscales of Sociocultural Attitudes Towards Appearance Questionnaire 4R [13]). However, according to the authors' knowledge, there are no studies evaluating the relationship between the intensity of body appreciation and variables related to body attitudes in men measured using the Male Body Attitude Scale (especially studies that also refer to beliefs related to the muscularity of the body and the desire to change in this regard).

Another important aspect of the attitude towards one's own body is muscle dysmorphia. According to DSM V, muscle dysmorphia (MD) is a subtype of body dysmorphic disorder related to the preoccupation with the idea and beliefs that one's body is not sufficiently muscular and lean [14–21]. It is associated with a strong dependence of one's self-esteem on physical appearance, with people with MD perceiving their body as small and/or weak, even if their build is average or when they have developed musculature. Therefore, it contributes to taking actions that enable the individual to achieve the desired ideal figure according to their thinking. Importantly, however, the behaviors that people with MD engage in are often compulsive and include, but are not limited to, rigid diet plans, calculation of macro-nutritional values of every item of consumed food, excessive exercise, excessive use of dietary supplements and other substances that may affect the shape of the figure (e.g., anabolic-androgenic steroids). The compulsiveness of the behaviors undertaken is also related to the fact that these people do not give up these activities, even if they see negative consequences for their physical and mental health and their social, sexual, and professional functioning, rest, recreation, etc. People with MD have strong anxiety that their body is not muscular and lean enough, which may be associated with obsessive thoughts about the body and a tendency to avoid situations where their body is exposed to others who may evaluate their appearance [14,15,17–21]. With reference to the above information and the relationship between MD and body appreciation, the only study known to the authors that concerns this relationship is the findings obtained in a group of Lebanese adolescents that indicate a negative relationship between these variables [22]. Studies on adult men seem to be lacking in this context.

In the above information, it is worth noting that the variable associated with the topic of body image is physical activity. Much of the available research, research reviews, and meta-analyses focus on assessing how physical activity is related to a more adaptive body attitude and/or how physical activity interventions can be used to shape a more positive body image [23]. As is well known, motivation for exercise can vary, with many factors influencing this motivation, and one such factor may be our attitude towards our bodies [23–27]. In this context, only a few studies have been conducted so far on the relationship between body appreciation and exercise motives [26–28], with these studies showing that there is a positive correlation between body appreciation and functional motives for exercise, for example, health, enjoyment, and challenging oneself [27]. Moreover, a systematic review indicated that there is a positive correlation between the above-mentioned (pro-health and adaptive) types of motivation for exercise and health-oriented exercises and positive body image and healthy eating behaviors, while exercise for reasons related to appearance has a negative correlation with the last two mentioned variables [28]. It is, therefore, worth investigating whether adult men having views in line with those presented in the #BodyPositivity social movement are associated with such motives for exercise that are mentioned in many sources related to #BoPo—that is, pleasure and the desire to take care of the health and functionality of one's body (often expressed as "nimbleness").

To sum up, although knowledge about body image, muscle dysmorphia and physical activity is extensive in diverse populations e.g., [16,23,28], research and knowledge on positive body image and muscle dysmorphia, body attitudes and exercise motives in Polish men remain limited. Polish studies published so far have concentrated mainly on the relationship between negative body image and other variables [29,30] or were limited to only women [31] (and as we know, on the one hand, many studies show that women are characterized by a more negative attitude towards their bodies, both in the cognitive, emotional and behavioral aspects, compared to men; on the other hand, these data are often different in relation to the drive for muscularity, e.g., [11,13,17]). Other studies were based on strictly homogeneous samples (e.g., athletes [32]; gym users [33]). In general, there are few studies in the world assessing the importance of the approach to one's body based on beliefs related to #BodyPositivity for their adaptive functioning in men (including beliefs directly related to muscle dysmorphia, body attitudes and exercise motives). Given the research on women or students regarding the numerous benefits of having a belief-based attitude from the #BodyPositivity [23–28], it is vital to develop a fuller understanding of this issue in a sample of adult males. Clarity on this issue is essential to ensure that appropriate interventions are made to improve the functioning of Polish men. When undertaking research in this area, it should also be remembered that many previous analyses indicate that body mass index (BMI)/weight status according to BMI may be important both for body image, muscle dysmorphia and exercise motives and (despite actions related to a #BodyPositivity social movement), people with excessive body weight may still feel stronger pressure to change their physical appearance [16,30,34,35]. Therefore, this work has the following aims: (1) classify different conditions associated with body appreciation and weight status (body mass index; BMI); and (2) analyze and compare the severity of muscle dysmorphia, body attitudes, and exercise motives. We hypothesized (our main hypothesis) that men with high body appreciation and healthy (normal) weight would have significantly lower levels of muscle dysmorphia and the non-adaptive (negative) multiple dimensions of body attitudes, as well as a greater level of the selected pro-health and adaptive exercise motives than men with low body appreciation and excess body weight. Moreover (as part of further analyses), additional comparisons were also made in the above-mentioned areas between the two groups of men already mentioned (men with high body appreciation and healthy weight and men with low body appreciation and excess weight) and the other two groups (men with low body appreciation and healthy weight and men with high body appreciation and excess weight).

2. Materials and Methods

2.1. Participants and Procedures

Our study was approved by the Ethics Committee (no. 2021/3/4E/5) and all procedures were conducted under the Declaration of Helsinki. The data used in the current analysis were collected from May 2021 to April 2023. Participants were recruited online (e.g., via social media such as Facebook, Instagram) and by on-site flyers (universities and workplace locations). The recruitment strategy was based on using general advertisements and flyers in an academic setting and in general public areas (no inclusion/exclusion criteria beyond BMI considerations—were used). Prior to data collection, all men were informed of the study's aim and anonymity. Informed consent was sought prior to their participation. (This included assurances that participants could withdraw from the study at any time without incurring any penalties and that the outcomes would only be utilized for research purposes). Next, participants completed our online survey (using Google Forms). Completing the survey took approximately 15–20 min. The participation was voluntary (without remuneration).

Four hundred men volunteered for the study. For the purpose of this analysis, we established a dichotomous variable describing BMI according to the recommendations of the World Health Organization: healthy (normal) vs. excess body weight. Therefore, people with underweight were removed from the database ($N = 26$). Our final sample included 374 Polish men who ranged in age from 18 to 58 years ($M = 28.96$, $SD = 8.52$) and in self-reported body mass index (BMI) from 18.52 to 43.83 kg/m^2 ($M = 25.55$, $SD = 3.75$). In terms of relationship status, 183 (48.93%) were single, 98 (26.20%) were partnered but not married, 78 (20.86%) were married, and 15 (4.01%) had some other status. In terms of education, 10 (2.67%) had completed primary school, 23 (6.15%) vocational school, 176 (47.06%) secondary school, and 165 (44.12%) had completed an undergraduate degree or completed a Master's degree.

2.2. Measures

2.2.1. The Body Appreciation Scale-2

To measure body appreciation, the participants completed the Body Appreciation Scale-2 (BAS-2) [10]. It consists of 10 items in total, giving a mean score reflecting body appreciation. Participants respond on a 5-point scale (from strongly disagree to strongly agree; example item: I am comfortable in my body). The higher the score, the higher body appreciation. Previous studies indicate that this measure has adequate validity and reliability [10,36]. In our analysis, McDonald's ω was 0.95.

2.2.2. The Muscle Dysmorphic Disorder Inventory

Muscle dysmorphia was measured using the Muscle Dysmorphic Disorder Inventory (MDDI) [37]. It includes 13 items which, when summed up, give a total score and three subscales: (a) drive for size (example item: I think my chest is too small), (b) appearance intolerance (example item: I wear loose clothing so that people cannot see my body), and (c) functional impairment (example item: I pass up social activities (e.g., watching football games, eating dinner, going to see a movie, etc.) with friends because of my workout schedule). Participants rate statements on a 5-point scale from 1 (never) to 5 (always). The higher the score, the higher the muscle dysmorphia symptoms. Previous studies indicate that this measure has adequate construct and factorial validity and reliability [37,38]. In our analysis, we used total scores and all subscales. The McDonald's ω values were as follows: $\omega_{total} = 0.85$, $\omega_{drive\ for\ size} = 0.87$, $\omega_{appearance\ intolerance} = 0.80$, and $\omega_{functional\ impairment} = 0.85$.

2.2.3. The Male Body Attitude Scale

The non-adaptive (negative) multiple dimensions of body attitudes were assessed with the Male Body Attitude Scale (MBAS) [39]. It includes 24 items, providing a total score and three subscales: (a) muscularity (example item: I think I have too little muscle on my body), (b) body fat (example item: I am concerned that my stomach is too flabby), and (c) height (example item: I wish I were taller). Each item is responded to on a 6-point scale from 1 (never) to 5 (always). Mean scores are used with higher scores representing more non-adaptive (negative) body attitudes. Previous studies indicate that this measure has adequate construct and factorial validity and reliability [39]. In our analysis, we used total scores and all subscales. The McDonald's ω values were as follows: $\omega_{total} = 0.93$, $\omega_{muscularity} = 0.91$, $\omega_{body\ fat} = 0.90$, and $\omega_{height} = 0.80$.

2.2.4. The Exercise Motivations Inventory-2

To measure exercise motives, participants completed the Exercise Motivations Inventory–2 (EMI-2) [24]. It consists of 51 items, giving 14 subscales (mean score). For each item, a 6-point Likert scale is used, ranging from 0 (not at all true for me) to 5 (very true for me). The higher the score, the stronger the intensity of the selected type of motivation to exercise. In our analysis, we selected three subscales (pro-health and adaptive exercise motives): (a) enjoyment (example item: Because I enjoy the feeling of exerting myself), (b) positive health (example item: Because I want to maintain good health), and (c) nimbleness (example item: To stay/become more agile). Previous studies indicate that this measure has adequate validity and reliability [24,25,40]. The McDonald's ω values were as follows: $\omega_{enjoyment} = 0.93$, $\omega_{positive\ health} = 0.92$, and $\omega_{nimbleness} = 0.91$.

2.2.5. The Demographic Survey

Participants also provided the following information: age, relationship status, educational qualification, weight, and height. Weight status (body mass index; BMI) was calculated based on self-reported data. Using the basic recommendations of the World Health Organization [41], participants were divided into two groups: (a) healthy (normal) weight, $\leq 18.50 \leq \text{BMI} \leq 24.99\ \text{kg/m}^2$; and (b) excess weight (pre-obesity and obesity), $\text{BMI} \geq 25.00\ \text{kg/m}^2$.

2.3. *Statistical Analysis*

All analyses were conducted using IBM SPSS Statistic version 28. Firstly, to identify clusters (based on body appreciation and weight status), we used a two-step cluster analysis (with Schwarz's Bayesian criterion). This analysis was chosen as it is appropriate for samples of $N > 200$ and both categorical and continuous variables [42]. Secondly, a multivariate analysis of variance (MANOVA) was used to assess differences between the clusters with regard to muscle dysmorphia, body attitudes and exercise motives. A 5% significance level was used, and (to correct for multiple comparisons) the Bonferroni corrected/adjusted p-value was introduced.

3. Results

3.1. Cluster Analysis of Body Appreciation and Body Mass Index

Four clusters were labeled and characterized as follows: (a) Cluster 1 (N = 70), low body appreciation (M = 2.59) and healthy (normal) weight (100% participants $18.50 \leq \text{BMI} \leq 24.99$ kg/m^2); (b) Cluster 2 (N = 130), high body appreciation (M = 3.99) and excess weight (100% participants BMI ≥ 25.00 kg/m^2); (c) Cluster 3 (N = 58), low body appreciation (M = 2.42) and excess weight (100% participants BMI ≥ 25.00 kg/m^2); and (d) Cluster 4 (N = 116), high body appreciation (M = 4.25) and healthy weight (100% participants $18.50 \leq \text{BMI} \leq 24.99$ kg/m^2). Table 1 shows the demographic characteristics of these clusters.

Table 1. Demographic characteristics of the four clusters.

	Cluster 1 (N = 70): Low Body Appreciation and Healthy Weight	**Cluster 2 (N = 130): High Body Appreciation and Excess Weight**	**Cluster 3 (N = 58): Low Body Appreciation and Excess Weight**	**Cluster 4 (N = 116): High Body Appreciation and Healthy Weight**	
	M (SD)				*F*
Age	25.94 (6.86) ^{aB}	31.06 (9.45) ^{aC}	30.48 (8.30) ^{B}	27.67 (7.71) ^{C}	$F(3, 370) = 7.43$, $p < 0.001$
	N (%)				χ^2 and Cramer's V
Educational qualification					
Primary school	4 (5.71)	2 (1.54)	2 (3.45)	2 (1.72)	$\chi^2_{(9)} = 11.23$, Cramer's $V = 10$ ^{NS}
Vocational school	3 (4.29)	9 (6.92)	6 (10.34)	5 (4.31)	
Secondary school	38 (54.29)	53 (40.77)	26 (44.83)	59 (50.87)	
Undergraduate degree or completed a Master's degree	25 (35.71)	66 (50.77)	24 (41.38)	50 (43.10)	
Relationship status					
Single	43 (61.43)	54 (41.54)	30 (51.73)	56 (48.28)	$\chi^2_{(15)} = 30.08$, Cramer's $V = 0.16$ *
Partnered but not married	21 (30.00)	30 (23.08)	12 (20.69)	35 (30.17)	
Married	4 (5.71)	38 (29.23)	15 (25.86)	21 (18.10)	
Other status	2 (2.86)	8 (6.15)	1 (1.72)	4 (3.45)	

^{a}—significant differences between the groups with $p < 0.001$; ^{B,C}—significant differences between the groups with $p < 0.01$; ^{NS}—a non-significant ($p > 0.05$); * $p < 0.05$.

3.2. Comparison of the Four Clusters for Muscle Dysmorphia, Body Attitudes and Exercise Motives

MANOVA (using Pillai's trace) indicated a significant effect of clusters on (a) muscle dysmorphia, (I) V = 0.91, F(3, 368) = 1294.81, $p < 0.001$; (b) non-adaptive (negative) body attitudes, V = 0.94, F(3, 367) = 1453.38, $p < 0.001$; and (c) selected pro-health and adaptive exercise motives, V = 0.86, F(3, 368) = 729.82, $p < 0.001$. Tables 2–4 show results with more information about outcomes with Bonferroni's adjustment for multiple comparisons.

With reference to muscle dysmorphia, our results indicated that Clusters 3 and 4 were significantly different from each other in terms of total score and the subscale for appearance intolerance (lower level of symptoms in the latter Cluster). Cluster 1 and Cluster 2 (with lower levels of symptoms in the latter cluster), as well as Cluster 1 and Cluster 4 (with lower levels of symptoms in the latter cluster) also differed in the same aspects of muscle dysmorphia. In the context of appearance intolerance, Cluster 2 had significantly lower levels than Cluster 3 and higher levels than Cluster 4. In the drive for size subscale, a significant difference was found only between Cluster 1 and 2 (with lower levels of symptoms in the latter cluster). Regarding the other comparisons, no significant differences were found.

Table 2. Separate univariate ANOVAs on muscle dysmorphia.

	Cluster 1 (N = 70): Low Body Appreciation and Healthy Weight	Cluster 2 (N =130): High Body Appreciation and Excess Weight	Cluster 3 (N = 58): Low Body Appreciation and Excess Weight	Cluster 4 (N = 116): High Body Appreciation and Healthy Weight	
		M (SD)			*Post hoc*
		Muscle Dysmorphic Disorder Inventory			
		$F(3, 370) = 6.71, p < 0.001, \eta_p^2 = 0.05$			
Total score	34.66 (9.92)	30.70 (9.47)	34.38 (10.06)	29.08 (10.04)	1 vs. 2 * 1 vs. 3 1 vs. 4 ** 2 vs. 3 2 vs. 4 3 vs. 4 **
		$F(3, 370) = 2.71, p < 0.05, \eta_p^2 = 0.02$			
Subscale: drive for size	14.67 (4.85)	12.54 (5.00)	12.78 (5.37)	13.13 (5.48)	1 vs. 2 * 1 vs. 3 1 vs. 4 2 vs. 3 2 vs. 4 3 vs. 4
		$F(3, 370) = 37.00, p < 0.001, \eta_p^2 = 0.23$			
Subscale: appearance intolerance	10.47 (3.49)	8.49 (3.06)	11.97 (3.55)	6.96 (3.17)	1 vs. 2 *** 1 vs. 3 1 vs. 4 *** 2 vs. 3 *** 2 vs. 4 ** 3 vs. 4 ***
		$F(3, 370) = 0.63, p > 0.05, \eta_p^2 = 0.001$			
Subscale: functional impairment	9.51 (4.15)	9.67 (3.95)	9.64 (3.79)	8.99 (4.56)	1 vs. 2 1 vs. 3 1 vs. 4 2 vs. 3 2 vs. 4 3 vs. 4

* $p < 0.05$, ** $p < 0.01$, *** $p < 0.001$.

With regard to non-adaptive (negative) body attitudes, Cluster 4 had significantly lower levels of total score, body fat and height than Cluster 3. In terms of the same dimensions of negative body attitudes, Cluster 4 also presented significantly lower outcomes than Cluster 1. In terms of total score and the body fat subscale, Cluster 4 also had lower results than Cluster 2, and Cluster 2 was significantly different from Cluster 3 (worse functioning in the second of the mentioned clusters). The last significant difference was between Cluster 1 and Cluster 3 regarding body fat (worse functioning in the second of the mentioned clusters). Regarding the other comparisons, no significant differences were found.

Table 3. Separate univariate ANOVAs on non-adaptive (negative) body attitudes.

	Cluster 1 (*N* = 70): Low Body Appreciation and Healthy Weight	Cluster 2 (*N* =130): High Body Appreciation and Excess Weight	Cluster 3 (*N* = 58): Low Body Appreciation and Excess Weight	Cluster 4 (*N* = 116): High Body Appreciation and Healthy Weight	
		M (SD)			*Post hoc*
		Male Body Attitude Scale			
		$F(3, 370) = 18.18, p < 0.001, \eta_p{}^2 = 0.13$			
Total score	3.42 (1.03)	3.09 (0.94)	3.80 (1.06)	2.73 (0.90)	1 vs. 2 1 vs. 3 1 vs. 4 *** 2 vs. 3 *** 2 vs. 4 * 3 vs. 4 ***
		$F(3, 370) = 3.20, p < 0.05, \eta_p{}^2 = 0.03$			
Subscale: muscularity	3.59 (1.29)	3.14 (1.19)	3.51 (1.18)	3.15 (1.21)	1 vs. 2 1 vs. 3 1 vs. 4 2 vs. 3 2 vs. 4 3 vs. 4
		$F(3, 370) = 29.97, p < 0.001, \eta_p{}^2 = 0.20$			
Subscale: body fat	3.18 (1.19)	3.26 (1.13)	4.14 (1.28)	2.45 (1.00)	1 vs. 2 1 vs. 3 *** 1 vs. 4 *** 2 vs. 3 *** 2 vs. 4 *** 3 vs. 4 ***
		$F(3, 370) = 9.27, p < 0.001, \eta_p{}^2 = 0.07$			
Subscale: height	2.71 (1.11)	2.39 (0.90)	2.74 (0.92)	2.09 (0.87)	1 vs. 2 1 vs. 3 1 vs. 4 *** 2 vs. 3 2 vs. 4 3 vs. 4 ***

* $p < 0.05$, *** $p < 0.001$.

In relation to selected pro-health and adaptive exercise motives, Cluster 4 had higher levels on all subscales than Cluster 3. Similar results were found between Cluster 2 and 3 (worse functioning in the second of the mentioned clusters). In terms of enjoyment and positive health subscales, Cluster 4 also differed significantly from Cluster 1 (worse functioning in the second of the mentioned clusters). The last significant difference was between Cluster 1 and 2 in terms of the enjoyment subscale (worse functioning of the first of the mentioned clusters). With regard to the other comparisons, no significant differences were found.

Table 4. Separate univariate ANOVAs on selected pro-health and adaptive exercise motives.

	Cluster 1 (N = 70): Low Body Appreciation and Healthy Weight	Cluster 2 (N =130): High Body Appreciation and Excess Weight	Cluster 3 (N = 58): Low Body Appreciation and Excess Weight	Cluster 4 (N = 116): High Body Appreciation and Healthy Weight	
			M (SD)		*Post hoc*
			Exercise Motivations Inventory-2		
			$F(3, 370) = 11.09, p < 0.001, \eta_p^2 = 0.08$		
Subscale: enjoyment	2.52 (1.60)	3.42 (1.44)	2.37 (1.49)	3.33 (1.46)	1 vs. 2 *** 1 vs. 3 1 vs. 4 ** 2 vs. 3 *** 2 vs. 4 3 vs. 4 ***
			$F(3, 370) = 6.58, p < 0.001, \eta_p^2 = 0.05$		
Subscale: positive health	3.28 (1.58)	3.77 (1.33)	3.03 (1.38)	3.86 (1.33)	1 vs. 2 1 vs. 3 1 vs. 4 * 2 vs. 3 ** 2 vs. 4 3 vs. 4 **
			$F(3, 370) = 5.31, p < 0.01, \eta_p^2 = 0.04$		
Subscale: nimbleness	2.71 (1.56)	3.16 (1.54)	2.24 (1.38)	2.97 (1.52)	1 vs. 2 1 vs. 3 1 vs. 4 2 vs. 3 ** 2 vs. 4 3 vs. 4 *

* $p < 0.05$, ** $p < 0.01$, *** $p < 0.001$.

Overall, our results partially support our hypothesis, as lower levels of some symptoms of muscle dysmorphia and negative body attitudes, as well as higher levels of pro-health and adaptive exercise motives were observed in men with high body appreciation and healthy (normal) weight as compared with men with low body appreciation and excess body weight.

4. Discussion

This study aimed to investigate the clusters associated with body appreciation and weight status and compare them in the context of muscle dysmorphia, body attitudes, and exercise motives. The main hypothesis was that men with high body appreciation and healthy (normal) weight would have significantly lower levels of muscle dysmorphia and the non-adaptive (negative) multiple dimensions of body attitudes, as well as greater levels of the selected pro-health and adaptive exercise motives than those of low body appreciation and excess body weight. Four clusters were identified (Cluster 1—low body appreciation and healthy weight; Cluster 2—high body appreciation and excess weight; Cluster 3—low body appreciation and excess weight; Cluster 4—high body appreciation and healthy weight). By analyzing the most important findings, significant differences (in terms of most of the assessed scale/subscales) were found between men who had high body appreciation and healthy weight (Cluster 4) and men with low body appreciation and excess body weight (Cluster 3).

Considering the above-mentioned findings, results consistent with our hypothesis were obtained in terms of muscle dysmorphia on the total score (generally all symptoms expressed by responses to all items) and on one subscale (appearance intolerance). This may mean that men with high body appreciation and healthy weight (compared to those with low body appreciation and excess body weight) were characterized by a lower intensity of the general level of various symptoms of muscle dysmorphia, and (in the context of an appearance intolerance subscale) a lower level of this aspect of muscle dysmorphia, which is related to negative beliefs about body and appearance anxiety or body exposure avoidance. This is expressed by people wearing baggy clothes to the beach and a belief that their body is distasteful and ugly [37].

Outcomes consistent with our hypothesis were not obtained for the other two subscales of the Muscle Dysmorphic Disorder Inventory—drive for size and functional impairment. This might mean that Cluster 4 and Cluster 3 function similarly in these two areas related to muscular dysmorphia. For these subscales, individuals in these clusters would have a similar intensity of thoughts of being smaller/less muscular/weaker, and have similar wishes to increase strength and size. They would have similar desires to smoke and/or have negative emotions in situations that disturb the exercise routine. They would take various harmful actions that are supposed to "protect" against skipping these exercises, even if harmful, for example, to social functioning [18,37]. Interestingly, our results seem to be consistent with recent results in a group of Lebanese adolescents, which show that there is a negative correlation between body appreciation and overall muscle dysmorphic score, and that body appreciation is not significantly related to exercise addiction [22]. Summarizing our outcomes on muscle dysmorphia, one explanation for the findings in this study may be that for men, sharing the views of a #BodyPostivity social movement is protective for men in terms of the general (average) trend associated with this disorder. In particular, this sharing can be important for that aspect of muscle dysmorphia involving fear and body embarrassment, which is related to body fat and avoidance behaviors to hide an "imperfect" physique. This protective effect of posture associated with views overlapping with a #BodyPositivity social movement has not been reported for those aspects of muscle dysmorphia that are related to compulsiveness towards the development of muscle tissue and performing exercise.

Our results partially support our hypothesis also in the context of non-adaptive dimensions of body attitudes because Cluster 4 (compared to Cluster 3) was characterized by lower scores on the general scale and two subscales of the Male Body Attitude Scale—body fat and height. These results (as well as those presented above) indicate that men with high body appreciation and healthy weight (compared to those of low body appreciation and excess body weight) had lower levels of symptoms related to overall negative body attitude and (in relation to the subscales) had lower levels of such aspects of negative body attitudes which are associated with body fat and height (but not muscularity). To the best of the authors' knowledge, there are no studies analyzing the relationship between body appreciation and the results of the Male Body Attitude Scale. However, other studies (partly relating to similar relationships) show that there is a negative correlation between body appreciation and negative body attitude in both sexes, e.g., [13,43]. Once again, this indicates that views associated with a #BodyPositivity social movement refer to shaping a more adaptive attitude towards the body, but only in relation to general body dissatisfaction and perception of body fat and body weight, but not musculature and potentially harmful behaviors that can be undertaken to develop it.

Importantly, the results obtained in terms of the motives for undertaking exercise confirm the more adaptive and pro-health functioning of Cluster 4 compared to Cluster 3. More specifically, this could mean that exercise by the men in the sample with high body appreciation and health is strongly motivated by enjoyment, a positive attitude towards health, and a desire to be nimble. This is an interesting discovery, because on the one hand, in many places promoting the idea of #BodyPositivity, there is a reference to the fact that physical activity is an important element of taking care of physical and mental health, as well as life comfort; it is suggested that one should look for types of exercises that are pleasant and observe how they change one's capabilities, e.g., in this context, agility (and not compulsively focus on how body size or weight changes) [5–7,9,44,45].

Moreover, the scoping review shows that some studies indicate that a positive body image is associated with greater participation in physical activity and sports [23]. On the other hand, some studies conclude that much of the #BodyPositivity material does not refer to exercise at all. (Cohen et al. [46] indicated that building a positive body image did not include exercise, because this topic appeared only in 4% of the posts in their study.) Moreover, in another study analyzing 141 posts about physical activity with hashtags #BodyPositivity, it was found that half of the posts were about body changes, i.e., the history of how the body shape/weight changed, how hard the person worked for it and what they do to maintain their current appearance [47]. Much of the content analyzed did not seem to be directly related to the above-mentioned movements because the content indicating that a positive attitude towards the body was achieved by disciplining it with strict physical exercises and striving for "standards" of a slim figure. Other posts were related to advertising various products and services (unfortunately, often incompatible with #BodyPositivity). Only five out of all the posts analyzed concerned the enjoyment of doing physical activity itself, rather than doing it only to change the weight and/or shape of the body [47].

Selected additional comparisons between other clusters in terms of muscle dysmorphia and negative body attitudes are reported as follows: (a) Cluster 2 (high body appreciation and excess weight) and Cluster 4 (high body appreciation and healthy weight) achieved similar (not statistically significant) results in five out of eight comparative analyses in the analyzed subscales/scales; (b) Cluster 1 (low body appreciation and healthy weight) and Cluster 4 (high body appreciation and healthy weight) were statistically significantly different in five out of eight statistical analyses (with lower levels of selected aspects of muscle dysmorphia and negative body posture in Cluster 4). Moreover, in terms of pro-health and adaptive exercise motives, we report the following findings: (a) Clusters 2 and 4 did not differ significantly in any of the three comparisons, (b) Cluster 2 and 4 differed in two out of three comparative analyses (higher level of motivation based on enjoyment and positive health in Cluster 4).

Considering the above findings for these additional comparisons between clusters, it can be concluded that the level of body appreciation (i.e., beliefs consistent with a #BodyPostivity) is the key protective factor for the development and/or maintenance of most symptoms related to muscle dysmorphia and a negative attitude towards the body. The level of body appreciation is also the key for building pro-health and adaptive motivation for physical activity, while body weight is less important. However, further analyses should be carried out in this context to look closely at which variables not included in this study could help explain the discrepancies in the results obtained and examine more closely the relationship between the beliefs of the #BodyPostivity movement and the compulsive drive to develop muscle tissue (which seems to be as dangerous as the compulsive pursuit of thinness).

Finally, it should be added that some limitations are present in this study: (1)tThe study was based on self-reported questionnaires and data (note that reliance on self-reported height and weight for BMI calculation may introduce bias leading to underestimation or overestimation of body weight. Note also that BMI does not distinguish body fat from muscularity, which is important to consider when assessing muscle dysmorphia); (2) despite good parameters for validity and reliability in this sample, not all the scales used in this study have been validated in Poland, and when analyzing the results, it must be remembered that a very high value of McDonald's omega (ω) coefficient might also suggest redundancy in the items (rather than merely acceptable internal consistency); (3) the study is cross-sectional (it is not possible to draw causal relationships; (4) volunteers participated in the study (non-probability sampling); (5) residual confounding bias is possible due to some important mediators/moderators (e.g., body acceptance by others, [27]; eating disorders, [22]), which were not included in the study; (6) the Body Appreciation Scale-2 was not directly designed to assess beliefs related to #BodyPostivity. It should be remembered that body appreciation is only one of the concepts discussed within the body positivity movement and only one of the constructs relating to the assessment of a positive body image. Likewise, body positivity as a social movement and positive body image are not the same, i.e., they are not "substitutes" [48]. Finally, a suggestion for future research may be that in studies similar to ours, other statistical methods such as path analysis to reach a model can be appropriate. Additionally, it may be also worth verifying whether participants were previously exposed to #BodyPositivity content (and if so, to what extent).

5. Conclusions

Our results are mostly consistent with the assumed hypothesis because they confirm that (in terms of most of the assessed scale/subscales) men with high body appreciation and healthy (normal) weight have significantly lower levels of muscle dysmorphia and the non-adaptive (negative) multiple dimensions of body attitudes, as well as higher levels of the selected pro-health and adaptive exercise motives, than participants of low body appreciation and excess body weight. These findings show that holding views in line with positive body image is also beneficial for the functioning of adult men, which can be used in interventions and prevention in this group, including activities using social media. An important step may be intervention programs, public health initiatives, or mental health strategies to support men struggling with body image and other concerns in relation to eating disorders, body image dysmorphia, obesity and other mental and physical issues. In this area, the content from #BodyPositivity may be used to create educational materials on men's body image, with content focusing more on the functionality of our body and the positive components of body attitudes, as well as positive motivations for physical activity (related to feelings of success and enjoyment). However, further research needs to be conducted in this area to determine whether the content in these interventions and prevention activities for both sexes should be the same and what factors should be taken into account so that it is also possible to influence excessive fixation on muscularity.

Author Contributions: Conceptualization, K.C.-B., A.M. and J.M.; Data curation, K.C.-B.; Funding acquisition, K.C.-B.; Investigation, K.C.-B., A.M. and J.M.; Methodology, K.C.-B., A.M. and J.M.; Writing—original draft, K.C.-B., A.M. and J.M.; Writing—review and editing, K.C.-B., A.M. and J.M. All authors have read and agreed to the published version of the manuscript.

Funding: The publication is partially financed by Medical University of Silesia.

Institutional Review Board Statement: The study was conducted according to the guidelines of the Declaration of Helsinki and approved by the Ethics Committee from the University of Bielsko-Biala (no. 2021/3/4E/5, approved on 31 March 2021).

Informed Consent Statement: Informed consent was obtained from all subjects involved in the study.

Data Availability Statement: The datasets generated and/or analyzed during the current study are not publicly available due to ethical issues involving participants' data and privacy but are available from the corresponding author on reasonable request.

Conflicts of Interest: No potential conflict of interests are reported by the authors.

Abbreviations

The following abbreviations are used in this manuscript:

BMI	index
M	mean
SD	standard deviation
MD	muscle dysmorphia
N	total number of individuals
V, F	statistics for MANOVA (using Pillai's trace)
P	*p*-value
vs.	versus
η_p^2	effect size
BAS-2	Body Appreciation Scale-2
MDDI	Muscle Dysmorphic Disorder Inventory
MBAS	Male Body Attitude Scale
EMI-2	Exercise Motivations Inventory–2
MANOVA	multivariate analysis of variance

References

1. Chiat, A. Body Positivity Movement: Influence of Beauty Standards on Body Image. Available online: https://sophia.stkate.edu/cgi/viewcontent.cgi?article=1051&context=shas_honors (accessed on 13 January 2025).
2. Leboeuf, C. What Is Body Positivity? The Path from Shame to Pride. *Philos. Top.* **2019**, *47*, 113–127.
3. Sastre, A. Towards a Radical Body Positive. *Fem. Media Stud.* **2014**, *14*, 929–943. [CrossRef]
4. Carels, R.A.; Hlavka, R.; Selensky, J.C.; Solar, C.; Rossi, J.; Miller, J.C. A daily diary study of internalised weight bias and its psychological, eating and exercise correlates. *Psychol. Health* **2019**, *34*, 306–320. [CrossRef]
5. Tylka, T.L. Body appreciation. In *Handbook of Positive Body Image and Embodiment: Constructs, Protective Factors, and Interventions*; Tylka, T.L., Piran, N., Eds.; Oxford University Press: New York, NY, USA, 2019; pp. 22–32. [CrossRef]
6. Bahr, N. #Effyourbeautystandards: Message Construction in the Body Positivity Movement on Instagram. Available online: https://core.ac.uk/download/pdf/286998998.pdf (accessed on 13 January 2025).
7. Kite, L.; Kite, L. Body Image Resilience Program. Available online: https://courses.beautyredefined.org/courses/body-image-resilience-program (accessed on 13 January 2025).
8. Markula, P. Exploring the Body Positivity Movement. Psychology Today. Available online: https://www.psychologytoday.com/gb/blog/fit-femininity/202211/exploring-the-body-positivity-movement (accessed on 13 January 2025).
9. University Coaching for Activity and Nutrition. 10 Self Care Activities for Body Positivity and Self-Love. Available online: https://in.nau.edu/ucan/10-self-care-activities-for-body-positivity-and-self-love/ (accessed on 13 January 2025).
10. Tylka, T.L.; Wood-Barcalow, N.L. The Body Appreciation Scale-2: Item refinement and psychometric evaluation. *Body Image* **2015**, *12*, 53–67. [CrossRef]
11. Cash, T.F.; Smolak, L. *Body Image: A Handbook of Science, Practice, and Prevention*, 2nd ed.; The Guilford Press: New York, NY, USA, 2011.
12. Puhl, R.; Brownell, K.D. Bias, discrimination, and obesity. *Obes. Res.* **2001**, *9*, 788–805. [CrossRef]
13. Sundgot-Borgen, C.; Sundgot-Borgen, J.; Bratland-Sanda, S.; Kolle, E.; Klungland Torstveit, M.; Svantorp-Tveiten, K.M.E.; Mathisen, T.F. Body appreciation and body appearance pressure in Norwegian university students comparing exercise science students and other students. *BMC Public Health* **2021**, *21*, 532. [CrossRef]
14. American Psychiatric Association. *Diagnostic and Statistical Manual of Mental Disorders: DSM-5*; American Psychiatric Association: Washington, DC, USA, 2013.
15. Cerea, S.; Bottesi, G.; Pacelli, Q.F.; Paoli, A.; Ghisi, M. Muscle Dysmorphia and its Associated Psychological Features in Three Groups of Recreational Athletes. *Sci. Rep.* **2018**, *8*, 8877. [CrossRef]

16. Cooper, M.; Eddy, K.T.; Thomas, J.J.; Franko, D.L.; Carron-Arthur, B.; Keshishian, A.C.; Griffiths, K.M. Muscle dysmorphi A systematic and meta-analytic review of the literature to assess diagnostic validity. *Int. J. Eat. Disord.* **2020**, *53*, 1583–160 [CrossRef]
17. Murray, S.B.; Rieger, E.; Touyz, S.W.; De la Garza García Lic, Y. Muscle dysmorphia and the DSM-V conundrum: Where does belong? A review paper. *Int. J. Eat. Disord.* **2010**, *43*, 483–491. [CrossRef]
18. Pope, H.G.; Gruber, A.J.; Choi, P.; Olivardia, R.; Phillips, K.A. Muscle Dysmorphia. An underrecognised form of body dysmorph disorder. *Psychosomatics* **1997**, *38*, 548–557. [CrossRef]
19. Pope, H.G., Jr.; Phillips, K.A.; Olivardia, R. *The Adonis Complex: The Secret Crisis of Male Body Obsession*; Simon and Schuster: Ne York, NY, USA, 2000.
20. Olivardia, R. Mirror, mirror on the wall, who's the largest of them all? The features and phenomenology of muscle dysmorphi *Harv. Rev. Psychiatry* **2001**, *9*, 254–259. [CrossRef]
21. Phillips, K.A.; O'Sullivan, R.L.; Pope, H.G., Jr. Muscle dysmorphia. *J. Clin. Psychiatry* **1997**, *58*, 361. [CrossRef]
22. Rahme, D.; Dabbous, M.; Malaeb, D.; Hallit, S.; Obeid, S. The mediating effect of body appreciation between muscle dysmorphi and bulimia nervosa among Lebanese adolescents. *BMC Psychiatry* **2023**, *23*, 275. [CrossRef]
23. Sabiston, C.M.; Pila, E.; Vani, M.; Thogersen-Ntoumani, C. Body image, physical activity, and sport: A scoping review. *Psych Sport Exerc.* **2019**, *42*, 48–57. [CrossRef]
24. Markland, D.; Ingledew, D.K. The measurement of exercise motives: Factorial validity and invariance across gender of a revise Exercise Motivations Inventory. *Br. J. Health Psychol.* **1997**, *2*, 361–376. [CrossRef]
25. Ingledew, D.K.; Markland, D.; Medley, A.R. Exercise motives and stages of change. *J. Health Psychol.* **1998**, *3*, 477–489. [CrossRe
26. Homan, K.J.; Tylka, T.L. Appearance-based exercise motivation moderates the relationship between exercise frequency an positive body image. *Body Image* **2014**, *11*, 101–108. [CrossRef]
27. Tylka, T.L.; Homan, K.J. Exercise motives and positive body image in physically active college women and men: Exploring a expanded acceptance model of intuitive eating. *Body Image* **2015**, *15*, 90–97. [CrossRef]
28. Panão, I.; Carraçam, E.V. Effects of exercise motivations on body image and eating habits/behaviours: A systematic review. *Nu Diet.* **2020**, *77*, 41–59. [CrossRef]
29. Zarzycki, M.Z.; Słyk, S.; Price, S.; Flaga-Łuczkiewicz, M. Men's Muscularity Image—The Role among Polish Young Populatio *Men Masculinities* **2019**, *22*, 404–411. [CrossRef]
30. Gruszka, W.; Owczarek, A.J.; Glinianowicz, M.; Bąk-Sosnowska, M.; Chudek, J.; Olszanecka-Glinianowicz, M. Perception of bod size and body dissatisfaction in adults. *Sci. Rep.* **2022**, *12*, 1159. [CrossRef] [PubMed]
31. Izydorczyk, B.; Głomb, K.; Bętkowska-Korpała, B.; Yablonska, T.; Bulatevych, N.; Opałka, R.; Lizińczyk, S.; Sitnik-Warchulska, K Radtke, B.M.; Sajewicz-Radtke, U.; et al. Internalization of athletic body ideal as a mediating variable between family influenc and body image of young women. A cross-cultural study of polish, Italian, and Ukrainian women. *Front. Psychiatry* **2023**, *1* 1136079. [CrossRef] [PubMed]
32. Budzisz, A.; Sas-Nowosielski, K. Positive body image among Polish elite athletes. *Balt. J. Health Phys. Act.* **2021**, *13*, 9–1 [CrossRef]
33. Wiśniewska-Nogaj, L. Symptoms of muscle dysmorphia in male gym users. *J. Psychiatry Clin. Psychol.* **2019**, *19*, 129–14 [CrossRef]
34. Antony, V.C.; Azeem, K. Association of physical activity on exercise motivation and body mass index among university student *Phys. Educ. Stud.* **2021**, *25*, 129–135. [CrossRef]
35. Wilson, S.; Mehak, A.; Racine, S.E. Exposure to thin and non-thin bodies elicits 'feeling fat': Validation of a novel state measur *Eat. Behav.* **2023**, *48*, 101700. [CrossRef]
36. Razmus, M.; Razmus, W. Evaluating the psychometric properties of the Polish version of the Body Appreciation Scale-2. *Bod Image* **2017**, *23*, 45–49. [CrossRef]
37. Hildebrandt, T.; Langenbucher, J.; Schlundt, D.G. Muscularity concerns among men: Development of attitudinal and perceptua measures. *Body Image* **2004**, *1*, 169–181. [CrossRef]
38. Compte, E.J.; Cattle, C.J.; Lavender, J.M.; Murray, S.B.; Brown, T.A.; Capriotti, M.R.; Flentje, A.; Lubensky, M.E.; Obedin-Malive J.; Lunn, M.R.; et al. Psychometric evaluation of the muscle dysmorphic disorder inventory (MDDI) among cisgender gay me and cisgender lesbian women. *Body Image* **2021**, *38*, 241–250. [CrossRef]
39. Tylka, T.L.; Bergeron, D.; Schwartz, J.P. Development and psychometric evaluation of the Male Body Attitudes Scale (MBAS *Body Image* **2005**, *2*, 161–175. [CrossRef]
40. Sas-Nowosielski, K.; Nowicka, M.; Kowalczyk, A. Age-related Differences in Motives for and Barriers to Exercise Among Wome Exercising in Fitness Centers. *New Educ. Rev.* **2017**, *49*, 30–39. [CrossRef]
41. World Health Organization. A Healthy Lifestyle—WHO Recommendations. Available online: https://www.who.int/europe news-room/fact-sheets/item/a-healthy-lifestyle---who-recommendations (accessed on 13 January 2025).

42. Bittmann, R.M.; Gelbard, R.M. Decision-making method using a visual approach for cluster analysis problems; indicative classification algorithms and grouping scope. *Expert. Syst.* **2007**, *24*, 171–187. [CrossRef]
43. Tobin, L.N.; Barron, A.H.; Sears, C.R.; von Ranson, K.M. Greater body appreciation moderates the association between maladaptive attentional biases and body dissatisfaction in undergraduate women. *J. Exp. Psychopathol.* **2019**, *10*, 2043808719838937. [CrossRef]
44. Kite, L. Are Body Positivity and Fitness Compatible? Available online: https://www.morethanabody.org/body-positive-fitness/ (accessed on 13 January 2025).
45. Santos, J.D. 15 Body Positivity Activities: Love Your Body Unconditionally. Available online: https://butfirstjoy.com/body-positivity-activities/ (accessed on 13 January 2025).
46. Cohen, R.; Irwin, L.; Newton-John, T.; Slater, A. #bodypositivity: A content analysis of body positive accounts on Instagram. *Body Image* **2019**, *29*, 47–57. [CrossRef]
47. Griffin, M.; Bailey, K.A.; Lopez, K.J. #BodyPositive? A critical exploration of the body positive movement within physical cultures taking an intersectionality approach. *Front. Sports Act. Living* **2022**, *4*, 908580. [CrossRef]
48. Wood-Barcalow, N.L.; Alleva, J.M.; Tylka, T.L. Revisiting positive body image to demonstrate how body neutrality is not new. *Body Image* **2024**, *50*, 101741. [CrossRef]

nutrients MDPI

Article

Parents of Adolescents with Anorexia Nervosa and Parents of Adult Women with Anorexia Nervosa

Federico Amianto [1,*], Giulia Dell'Oca [1], Daniele Marcotulli [2], Chiara Davico [2] and Andrea Martinuzzi [2]

1 Neurosciences Department, University of Torino, Via Cherasco 15, 10126 Torino, Italy; giulia.delloca@edu.unito.it
2 Section of Child and Adolescent Neuropsychiatry, Department of Public Health and Pediatric Sciences, University of Turin, 10126 Torino, Italy; daniele.marcotulli@unito.it (D.M.); chiara.davico@unito.it (C.D.); andrea.martinuzzi@unito.it (A.M.)
* Correspondence: federico.amianto@unito.it; Tel.: +39-011-3135248; Fax: +39-011-3135439

Abstract: Background: Anorexia nervosa (AN) remains a severe psychiatric disorder with multifactorial pathogenesis and an uncertain prognosis. It is essential to identify any factors that may contribute to its onset in order to improve the targeting of preventive and therapeutic interventions. The present study explores the characteristics of parents of daughters with AN, comparing those with different ages of onset and ages at intake, in order to identify potential contributing factors from the parental side. **Methods:** The study recruited 69 adolescents and 56 adults diagnosed with AN, along with 73 healthy controls (HC). The 80 mothers and 69 fathers of the participants were compared to controls in terms of the age of onset and age at intake of their daughters. Self-administered instruments were used to assess personality (TCI), eating behaviors (EDI-2), general psychopathology (BDI), and family functioning (FAD). **Results:** The analysis revealed that several personality and psychopathological traits distinguished the parents of AN participants from the HC group in both conditions. Both mothers of adolescent- and adult-onset AN participants with any age at intake displayed greater harm avoidance and lower self-directedness facets, as well as greater inadequacy and social insecurity than controls. Fathers were less disordered and more self-indulgent and compassionate, but lower in role definition. Specifically, mothers of daughters with adolescent-onset AN and younger age at intake were more prone to depression. In contrast, mothers of daughters with an adult age at intake showed lower resourcefulness and higher levels of perceived inadequacy. **Conclusions:** Higher resourcefulness and a lower sense of ineffectiveness may help mothers facilitate earlier therapeutic intervention for their daughters. On the other hand, maternal depressive symptoms may play a significant role in the earlier onset of and intake for AN in their daughters. Supporting assertive qualities in mothers through preventive interventions is recommended, while maternal depression should be appropriately treated to prevent an early psychopathological onset in daughters.

Keywords: AN adolescents; age of onset; age of intake; mothers; resourcefulness; inadequacy; depression

1. Introduction

Anorexia nervosa is a severe mental disorder that typically begins in adolescence or early adulthood but often persists or recurs later in life (DSM-5). It displays a complex and multifactorial pathogenesis that remains largely unknown [1]. However, it is widely believed that the family environment and its relational dynamics play a key role in the onset, development, and persistence of eating disorders (EDs) [2,3].

Recent research has shifted focus from exploring parental traits as risk factors for the onset of anorexia nervosa (AN) in daughters and sons. This is partly because it has been clearly established that no single specific parental profile can be definitively linked to the disorder [4]. Moreover, the correlation between parents' personality traits and the psychopathology of daughters with AN is complex, making it difficult to draw definitive conclusions about the pathogenic role of parents [5]. Nevertheless, research on risk factors related to parental features is still of interest to facilitate family interventions.

In fact, research supports the importance of family involvement in therapeutic programs for AN [6]. Family involvement can include encouraging parents to restore their parenting roles with the support of the therapeutic team [7]. It may also involve parental counseling to enhance empathy and address dysfunctional family dynamics, which can improve therapeutic outcomes [8]; for instance, low levels of care from both parental figures have been linked to poorer therapeutic outcomes in patients with AN [9].

Parents' personality traits interact with those of their daughters, forming the foundation of family dynamics which, in turn, influences the personality traits and eating psychopathology of daughters with AN [10]. This relationship is often nonlinear, involving complex interactions, as parental personality traits do not exert a singular and direct effect on their daughters' psychopathology [5]. On one hand, the complexity of family dynamics is responsible for the inconclusive results of previous research. On the other hand, there is a call for caution when conducting and interpreting research on parents' personality traits. Investigating these traits and their correlations with clinical and psychopathological features in daughters may inform counseling, family therapy, or even preventive interventions. For example, early studies using the Temperament and Character Inventory [10–12] showed that, compared to controls, mothers and fathers of patients with anorexia exhibit distinctive temperament and character traits. Fathers of patients with AN scored higher on harm avoidance (HA) and reward dependence (RD) and lower on persistence (P) and self-directedness (SD), while mothers scored higher on HA and lower on SD. These results were based on small samples and require replication, underscoring the need for more in-depth research [4,10]. Nevertheless, they show a relationship between parental personality profiles and the psychopathological features of daughters with AN [5].

Berking [13] recently underlined that psychopathology during adolescence may be conceived as a maladaptive strategy to cope with undesired affective states, and Ratcliffe [14] presented evidence that external "scaffolding" of emotions may be used by adolescents for emotional regulation, in particular when the regulatory structure is lost. Thus, parents represent a resource for emotional regulation that may be lost when psychopathology emerges in children. Family interventions based on counseling [8] or family therapy [15,16] are crucial to improve emotional regulation among adolescents affected with anorexia nervosa; this is even more relevant when parents display any kind of psychopathology [17].

Some studies examining the age of onset of AN have found that earlier therapeutic intervention during adolescence leads to a better prognosis than intervention in adulthood. Specifically, targeted psychotherapeutic and pharmacological treatments can reduce the risk of chronicity of this disorder's severe psychopathological aspects [18,19]. However, an earlier age of onset may have different effects on the psycho-endocrine state [20] and the development of personality traits [21], and has been associated with worse long-term outcomes in terms of both psychiatric comorbidities and BMI [22]. Therefore, the age of onset and the timing of therapeutic intervention for AN appear to be important clinical indicators when choosing the most appropriate therapeutic approach [23].

Nevertheless, to the best of our knowledge, no study has explored the relationship between parental characteristics and the age of onset or intake for the treatment of AN. Thus, it remains unclear whether parents' personality or psychopathological traits are related to the age of onset or intake for the treatment of AN in their daughters.

This study aimed to investigate the personality and psychopathological traits of parents of adolescent or adult daughters with AN. The first aim was to confirm previous findings on the specific personality and psychopathological traits that characterize parents of daughters with AN in these two distinct age groups and to compare these two groups of parents with healthy controls. The second aim was to explore whether these traits relate to the age of onset or intake for the treatment of AN among daughters. Given the effectiveness of family involvement in the therapeutic process of AN, linking the age of onset to parental features may have significant implications for preventive and therapeutic strategies [24,25].

2. Materials and Methods

2.1. Sample Description

The initial sample consisted of 118 female adolescents diagnosed with an ED who were referred to the outpatient services for EDs at the Child Neuropsychiatry Department of the Regina Margherita Children's Hospital (OIRM), which is part of the City of Health and Science in Turin.

The inclusion criteria for parent–patient pairs were as follows: (1) a diagnosis of anorexia nervosa (AN) according to the DSM-5 (Diagnostic and Statistical Manual of Mental Disorders, Fifth Edition) criteria; (2) age under 18 years; (3) willingness of at least one parent to participate in the study; (4) the ability and willingness of both parent and adolescent to comprehend and complete self-administered tests; and (5) completion of the administered psychometric tests.

Based on these criteria, the following participants were excluded from the study: 13 individuals with binge eating disorder (BED), including 4 participants who also had obesity; 16 individuals with bulimia nervosa (BN); 6 individuals with obesity; 5 individuals with Otherwise Specified Feeding and ED (OSFED) who did not meet the criteria for atypical anorexia nervosa; 5 individuals with somatoform disorders; and 12 individuals with other diagnoses. Additionally, among the parents of the included participants, one mother and five fathers who were unavailable or who declined participation were excluded.

Thus, the final sample for this study consisted of parents (80 mothers and 69 fathers) of 80 adolescents with AN (Table 1). Two control groups of parents were recruited: 56 pairs of parents of adult participants with AN (56 mothers and 54 fathers) and 63 parents of healthy controls from the database of the Neuroscience Department of the University of Turin.

2.2. Procedure

The diagnoses of AN and atypical AN were established by an experienced neuropsychiatrist (FA) through a structured clinical interview (K-SADS) based on the DSM-5 criteria.

The severity of the disorder was assessed by the clinician using the Clinical Global Impression (CGI) scale at T0 (patient intake).

Parents of adolescent participants with AN completed the following battery of self-administered questionnaires: the Temperament and Character Inventory (TCI), the Eating Disorder Inventory-2 (EDI-2), the Beck Depression Inventory-II (BDI-II), and the Family Assessment Device (FAD).

2.3. Measures

2.3.1. Clinical Global Impression [26]

The CGI Severity Scale is a scale which clinicians use to provide an estimate of the severity of a patient's illness and psychopathology. The score is assigned by a psychiatrist-trained specialist, taking into consideration various aspects of the patient and their pathology: BMI, frequency and severity of binge eating and purging behaviors, overall functioning, and duration of illness.

2.3.2. Temperament and Character Inventory [27]

The TCI is a self-report questionnaire based on the assumptions of the biosocial theory of personality developed by Cloninger [28]. It consists of 240 true/false items that evaluate personality features. Of these, 116 assess temperamental traits (novelty seeking [NS], HA, RD, and P); 119 evaluate three character traits (SD, cooperativeness [C], and self-transcendence [ST]), and 5 evaluate the presence of personality disorders (PDs).

2.3.3. Eating Disorder Inventory-2 [29]

The EDI-2 test is a self-administered questionnaire that comprehensively assesses the salient features of psychopathology in ED. It consists of 91 items divided into 11 subscales: 3 subscales measure eating behavior (drive for thinness, bulimia, body dissatisfaction), while the other 8 subscales measure the psychopathological traits most frequently associated with ED (inadequacy, perfectionism, interpersonal distrust, interoceptive awareness, maturity fear, asceticism, impulsivity, and social insecurity).

2.3.4. Beck Depression Inventory (BDI) [30]

The BDI is a self-administered questionnaire with 13 items that has been used extensively to assess the severity of depressive symptoms.

2.3.5. Family Assessment Device [31]

The FAD is a self-administered questionnaire that assesses overall family functioning based on the perceptions of family members.

It is an assessment tool consisting of 60 items that investigate 7 different dimensions of family functioning: problem solving, communication, family roles, emotional resonance, emotional involvement, control behavior, and general operation.

2.4. Ethical Issues

This study was conducted in accordance with the Declaration of Helsinki as revised by the 75th World Medical Association General Assembly in October 2024, and in compliance with Good Clinical Practice (GCP) and current regulatory provisions. It was approved by the Intercompany Review Board of Torino (CEI) (protocol 00107/2019; protocol number 0099307).

2.5. Statistical Analysis

Although this was a retrospective study based on a convenience sample, we made certain our sample size would be adequate for hypothesis testing. Using the R package pwr, we computed the statistical power with an average group size of 55 participants to detect a medium effect size (Cohen's $f = 0.25$) at a p-value of 0.05. The resulting power was 82%.

Statistical analyses were conducted using the advanced statistical software, Statistical Package for the Social Sciences (SPSS) version 28.0.1.0.

The personality and psychopathological traits of mothers and fathers of daughters with AN with adolescent onset/intake and those with adult onset/intake were compared with parents of healthy controls using the ANOVA test. These comparisons were conducted separately for parents based on their daughters' age of onset and intake into therapeutic treatment. Due to the high number of comparisons, Bonferroni correction was applied, with the significance threshold set at $p < 0.001$.

3. Results

Table 1 displays the sociodemographic data of the adolescent participants.

Table 1. Comparison of demographic and clinical data.

		Adolescent Patients (N = 69)	Adult Patients (N = 56)
Age of onset of AN (years)	mn ± sd	12.9 ± 2.9	17.9 ± 3.37
BMI at intake	mn ± sd	17.8 ± 2.8	16.9 ± 2.3
CGI	mn ± sd	4.4 ± 0.8	3.9 ± 1.2

BMI = body mass index, CGI = clinical global impression.

3.1. Differences in Parents' Traits Based on Age of Onset of AN in Daughters

3.1.1. Mothers

Table 2 shows the ANOVA comparison between the mothers of daughters with AN onset in adolescence or adulthood and healthy controls.

Table 2. ANOVA comparison of mothers based on age of onset of daughters' AN.

	Adolescent Onset AN (a, n = 105) Mean ± sd	Adult Onset AN (b, n = 31) Mean ± sd	Healthy Controls (c, n = 63) Mean ± sd	F	p	η^2	Post Hoc Analysis
Fear of uncertainty (HA2)	5.2 ± 1.4	5.1 ± 1.7	3.9 ± 1.9	13.244	0.001	0.122	b, a > c
Harm avoidance (HA)	18.4 ± 5.8	18.8 ± 7.1	14.5 ± 5.9	10.082	0.001	0.095	b, a > c
Maturity (SD1)	5.6 ± 1.7	5.1 ± 2.0	6.9 ± 1.5	18.681	0.001	0.164	b, a < c
Purposefulness (SD2)	5.1 ± 1.9	4.7 ± 2.0	6.2 ± 1.4	11.810	0.001	0.110	b, a < c
Resourcefulness (SD3)	3.7 ± 1.5	2.9 ± 1.9	4.3 ± 1.0	11.017	0.001	0.103	b, a < c
Self-directedness (SD)	29.9 ± 7.6	27.9 ± 9.6	33.7 ± 7.6	8.647	0.001	0.083	b, a < c
Inadequacy (IN)	3.5 ± 4.4	4.8 ± 4.5	1.7 ± 3.0	7.133	0.001	0.076	b, a > c
Social insecurity (IS)	3.8 ± 3.9	4.5 ± 4.2	2.0 ± 2.5	7.611	0.001	0.081	b, a > c
Beck Depression Inventory (BDI)	9.0 ± 7.2	7.2 ± 6.1	3.9 ± 6.7	10.775	0.001	0.104	a > c

a = Adolescent-Onset AN; b = Adult-Onset AN; c = Healthy Controls.

The mothers of participants with adolescent and adult onset of AN showed higher levels of HA, particularly higher levels of fear of uncertainty (HA2), and lower levels of SD, particularly lower levels of maturity (SD1), resourcefulness (SD2), and purposefulness (SD3) ($p < 0.001$). They also displayed higher levels of social insecurity (IS) and inadequacy (IN) than healthy controls ($p < 0.001$).

The mothers of participants with AN onset in adolescence showed higher levels of depression (BDI) than healthy controls ($p < 0.001$).

3.1.2. Fathers

Table 3 shows the ANOVA comparison between the fathers of daughters with AN onset in adolescence or adulthood and the fathers of healthy controls.

The fathers of participants with AN onset in adolescence or adulthood showed higher levels of self-acceptance (SD4) and compassion (C4) and lower levels of disorder (NS4) than the fathers of healthy controls ($p < 0.001$). They also displayed higher levels of role definition (FAD3) than the fathers of healthy controls ($p < 0.001$).

Table 3. ANOVA comparison of fathers based on age of onset of daughters' AN.

	Adolescent Onset AN (a, n = 91) Mean ± sd	Adult Onset AN (b, n = 32) Mean ± sd	Healthy Controls (c, n = 57) Mean ± sd	F	p	η^2	Post Hoc Analysis
Disorder (NS4)	3.6 ± 1.9	3.4 ± 1.9	5.1 ± 2.2	11.880	0.001	0.123	a, b < c
Self-acceptance (SD4)	7.5 ± 2.7	7.9 ± 5.8	5.4 ± 3.2	12.572	0.001	0.121	a, b > c
Compassion (C4)	7.5 ± 2.0	8.4 ± 3.2	6.2 ± 2.8	8.816	0.001	0.087	a, b > c
Role definition (FAD3)	2.1 ± 0.4	2.2 ± 0.4	1.8 ± 0.6	7.779	0.001	0.005	a, b > c

a = Adolescent-Onset AN; b = Adult-Onset AN; c = Healthy Controls.

3.2. *Comparison of Personality Traits of Parents of Daughters with AN Based on Age at Treatment Intake*

Table 4 shows the ANOVA comparison of the personality traits of mothers of participants with AN, grouped according to their daughters' age at treatment intake.

Table 4. ANOVA comparison of mothers based on age of intake of daughters' AN.

	Adolescent Intake (a, n = 80) Mean ± sd	Adult Intake (b, n = 56) Mean ± sd	Healthy Controls (c, n = 63) Mean ± sd	F	p	η^2	Post Hoc Analysis
Fear of uncertainty (HA2)	5.1 ± 1.4	5.2 ± 1.6	3.9 ± 1.9	13.236	0.001	0.122	b, a > c
Harm avoidance (HA)	18.6 ± 6.0	18.5 ± 6.4	14.5 ± 5.9	10.034	0.001	0.095	b, a > c
Maturity (SD1)	5.7 ± 1.6	5.1 ± 2.0	6.9 ± 1.5	19.894	0.001	0.172	b, a < c
Purposefulness (SD2)	5.2 ± 1.7	4.8 ± 2.1	6.2 ± 1.4	12.267	0.001	0.114	b, a > c
Resourcefulness (SD3)	3.7 ± 1.4	3.0 ± 1.8	4.3 ± 1.0	12.750	0.001	0.118	b < a, c
Self-directedness (SD)	30.4 ± 6.9	28.3 ± 9.4	33.7 ± 5.9	9.031	0.001	0.086	b, a < c
Inadequacy (IN)	3.4 ± 4.0	4.5 ± 4.9	1.7 ± 3.0	7.318	0.001	0.078	b > c
Social insecurity (IS)	3.7 ± 3.4	4.4 ± 4.6	2.0 ± 2.5	7.954	0.001	0.084	b, a > c
Beck Depression Inventory (BDI)	9.9 ± 7.7	6.9 ± 5.7	3.9 ± 6.7	13.059	0.001	0.123	a > c

a = Adolescent-Onset AN; b = Adult-Onset AN; c = Healthy Controls.

The mothers of adult participants at treatment intake showed higher levels of inadequacy (IN, $p < 0.001$) than the healthy controls, and higher levels of SD3 ($p < 0.001$) than both the healthy controls and those of adolescent participants at treatment intake.

In contrast, the mothers of adolescent participants at treatment intake showed higher BDI scores than the healthy controls ($p < 0.001$).

Both the mothers of adolescent participants and those of adult participants at treatment intake showed higher fear of uncertainty (HA2) and HA scores and lower SD1, SD2, and SD scores than the healthy controls ($p < 0.001$). They also displayed higher levels of IS than the healthy controls ($p < 0.001$).

Table 5 shows the ANOVA comparison of the personality traits of fathers of participants with AN, grouped according to their daughters' age at treatment intake.

In particular, the fathers of adult participants at treatment intake showed higher levels of affective involvement (FAD5) than the fathers of healthy controls ($p < 0.001$). Both the fathers of adolescent participants and those of adult participants at treatment intake showed higher levels of SD4 and C4 and lower levels of NS4 than the fathers of healthy controls. They also displayed higher levels of FAD3 than the fathers of healthy controls ($p < 0.001$).

Table 5. ANOVA comparison of fathers based on intake of onset of daughters' AN.

	Adolescent Intake (a, n = 69) Mean ± sd	Adult Intake (b, n = 54) Mean ± sd	Healthy Controls (c, n = 57) Mean ± sd	F	p	η^2	Post Hoc Analysis
Disorder (NS4)	3.6 ± 1.8	3.4 ± 2.0	5.1 ± 2.2	12.080	0.001	0.124	b, a < c
Self-acceptance (SD4)	7.2 ± 2.7	8.0 ± 2.6	5.4 ± 3.2	13.545	0.001	0.129	b, a > c
Compassion (C4)	7.4 ± 2.1	8.2 ± 2.6	6.2 ± 2.8	9.122	0.001	0.090	b, a > c
Role definition (FAD3)	2.1 ± 0.4	2.2 ± 0.3	1.8 ± 0.6	8.210	0.001	0.083	b, a > c
Affective involvement (FAD5)	1.9 ± 0.5	2.1 ± 0.3	1.7 ± 0.6	6.957	0.001	0.071	b > c

a = Adolescent-Onset AN; b = Adult-Onset AN; c = Healthy Controls.

4. Discussion

The present study aimed to compare the personality and psychopathological traits of mothers and fathers of adolescents and young women affected by AN, grouped based on the age of onset of their daughters' disorder and the age at intake to an outpatient service. Due to the cross-sectional nature of this study, no causal relationships can be established. Nevertheless, the data obtained can provide insights to support parental counseling for the prevention and treatment of this disorder [8].

In general, several differences in personality traits were found between the parents of participants with AN and the parents of healthy controls, confirming previous findings on this topic, which was the first aim of the study [10–12,32,33]. Mothers of participants with AN were characterized by high levels of harm avoidance and low levels of self-directedness in terms of personality traits, as well as a greater sense of inadequacy and social insecurity related to eating psychopathology. Moreover, most of these differences were common across subgroups of parents whose daughters were adolescents or adults at the onset of AN or at intake for treatment of AN.

Regarding the second aim of the study, few differences specifically distinguished the parents of participants with AN and the parents of healthy controls based on the age of onset of the disorder. Three differences emerged among mothers, while only one was observed among fathers. This may highlight the relatively greater influence of mothers on the onset of the disorder [34], but also potentially suggests fathers' lower engagement in managing their daughters' health problems, especially in consideration of the lower participation of fathers in this research.

The mothers of adolescent participants at treatment intake exhibited higher levels of resourcefulness than the mothers of adult participants at treatment intake. This may indicate greater problem solving ability, meaning they are better equipped to acquire the tools necessary to address challenges in their daughters' upbringing [35]. In the general population, high levels of resourcefulness—a subdimension of self-directedness—are associated with a lower incidence of depressive [36] and other mental disorders [4]. The present study suggests that, while resourcefulness may not be protective against the onset of AN in daughters, it characterizes mothers who are more proactive and prepared to handle problematic situations, facilitating earlier intake to treatment services. Previous research suggests that early treatment intake is a positive prognostic factor for AN [19,37]. Thus, promoting positive attitudes towards treatment services among mothers may lead to better outcomes for their daughters.

Compared to the healthy controls, only the mothers of adult participants at treatment intake exhibited higher levels of inadequacy (EDI). The initiation of treatment for AN in adulthood may sometimes result from diagnostic delays [19,38], which could lead to feelings of guilt among mothers for failing to recognize the disorder in their daughters earlier, contributing to their sense of inadequacy [39]. Alternatively, perceived inadequacy may be associated with lower levels of resourcefulness in this group of mothers, potentially delaying their daughters' treatment due to their lack of confidence in managing the issue [7]. Encouraging mothers to take the initiative in addressing their daughters' illness through psychoeducation, promoting greater awareness of available therapeutic resources, and providing support in decision-making may help mitigate feelings of inadequacy and improve secondary prevention strategies [6,40,41].

The mothers of participants who were adolescents at the onset of AN or at treatment intake exhibited higher levels of depressive symptoms than the mothers of the control group. Various studies have highlighted that parental psychopathology, particularly in mothers, is strongly linked to the risk of EDs in daughters [42,43]. Elevated maternal depressive symptoms may, therefore, be considered a risk factor for earlier onset and, consequently, earlier treatment intake of AN in daughters. Increased maternal depression can negatively affect the entire family environment, increasing the stress and emotional burden felt by daughters with AN [44]. As evidenced by the literature on anxiety and depressive disorders, parents' depression may impair the developmental trajectory of children before adulthood and represents a strong risk factor that may be associated with unfavorable parental behaviors [45,46].

Concerning fathers, no significant differences were found between subgroups based on the age of onset of AN or the age at treatment intake. While the existing literature indicates the role of fathers in the onset of AN [10,12,32,33], their influence may be less relevant to the age of onset of this disorder or the age at treatment intake compared to mothers.

In this study, fathers exhibited fewer personality differences compared with mothers. Fathers tend to be more disorganized, which may negatively impact daughters with obsessive–compulsive personality traits [47]. This temperamental trait may contribute to a weaker role definition within the family, potentially leading to dysfunctional family dynamics [10]. However, in this study, the fathers of participants with AN also displayed higher levels of self-acceptance and compassion compared to the fathers of healthy controls, which could serve as protective factors against the development of mental disorders [48].

The fathers of adult participants at treatment intake reported lower levels of emotional involvement compared to those of healthy controls, suggesting reduced participation in family activities and interests [49]. Previous studies have indicated that paternal parenting attitudes may predict daughters' eating psychopathology [33,50]. A disengaged and passive father who demonstrates little involvement in his daughter's life may contribute to an earlier onset of eating disorder symptoms [49–51].

Given the cross-sectional nature of this study and the relatively small cohort of families with daughters affected by AN, further research using prospective study designs is needed to explore the causal links between parental characteristics and AN onset and outcomes in daughters.

Additionally, due to the complexity and heterogeneity of families affected by AN in terms of clinical severity and treatment pathways, larger sample sizes are necessary to yield more generalizable results and make more specific inferences regarding different parental subgroups.

Despite the detailed assessment conducted by the neuropsychiatrist and the reliability of the diagnostic criteria used, a potential limitation of this study is the difficulty in retrospectively identifying the exact age of onset of the disorder with sufficient accuracy.

Finally, due to the small number of participants with binge/purging AN in the sample, this study did not separately analyze the two diagnostic subtypes, which may be associated with distinct parental characteristics.

5. Conclusions

As established in previous research, the parents of participants with AN exhibited distinct personality traits compared with the parents of healthy controls, with certain characteristics differentiating mothers of adolescent participants versus those of adult participants at the onset of AN or at treatment intake.

The mothers of adolescent participants at treatment intake for AN demonstrated higher levels of resourcefulness and lower levels of inadequacy, which potentially facilitated their earlier recognition of their daughters' problems. According to the literature, promoting resourcefulness and feelings of adequacy through preventive psychoeducational interventions may improve the prognosis and treatment efficacy for daughters with AN. Conversely, raising awareness among mothers, general practitioners, and mental health professionals about early treatment for maternal depressive symptoms may help prevent the onset of AN in adolescents.

Although fathers were less differentiated in terms of personality traits compared with mothers when grouped based on the age of onset of AN and the age at treatment intake, they exhibited lower levels of emotional involvement. Targeted interventions should aim to enhance fathers' affective involvement to increase their awareness of their daughters' distress and needs.

Future studies should focus on the prospective assessment of parental personality's influence on psychopathology, eating disorder severity, and treatment outcomes in daughters with AN. Additionally, research should explore interactions between parental personality and other aspects of family functioning, such as family history, socioeconomic factors, couple dynamics, and parent–daughter relationships. Finally, future investigations should differentiate participants based on AN diagnostic subtypes, specifically distinguishing between the restrictive subtype, the binge-eating/purging subtype, and atypical forms.

Author Contributions: Conceptualization, F.A.; methodology, F.A., C.D. and A.M.; software, F.A. and D.M.; validation, F.A., G.D., D.M. and C.D.; formal analysis, F.A. and D.M.; investigation, F.A., G.D. and D.M.; resources, F.A. and A.M.; data curation, F.A., G.D. and D.M.; writing—original draft preparation, F.A. and G.D.; writing—review and editing, F.A., G.D., D.M., C.D. and A.M.; supervision, F.A. and A.M.; project administration, F.A.; funding acquisition, F.A. All authors have read and agreed to the published version of the manuscript.

Funding: The authors wish to thank Fondazione Cassa di Risparmio di Torino for its contribution in funding the present research (Grant CRT Erogazioni Ordinarie; Protocol number: 2022.AI1398.U1598; 7 December 2022, RF = 2022.1832).

Institutional Review Board Statement: The study was conducted in accordance with the Declaration of Helsinki as revised by the 75th World Medical Association General Assembly in October, 2024 and in compliance with Good Clinical Practice (GCP) and current regulatory provisions, and approved by the Intercompany Review Board of Torino (CEI) approved this study (protocol 00107/2019; protocol number 0099307) date: 7 October 2019.

Informed Consent Statement: Written informed consent was obtained from all subjects involved in the study.

Data Availability Statement: Raw data of the study are available upon reasonable request to the corresponding author.

Acknowledgments: The authors wish to express their gratitude to the medical and nursing staff of the inpatient service at the Child Neuropsychiatry Department of Regina Margherita Children's Hospital.

Conflicts of Interest: The authors declare no conflicts of interest.

Abbreviations

The following abbreviations are used in this manuscript:

AN	Anorexia Nervosa
VS	versus
CEI	Intercompany Review Board of Torino
HC	healthy controls
TCI	Temperament and Character Inventory
EDI-2	Eating Disorder Inventory 2
BDI	Beck Depression Inventory
FAD	Family Assessment Device
DSM-5	Diagnostic and Statistical Manual 5
OIRM	Regina Margherita Children's Hospital
BED	Binge Eating Disorder
BN	Bulimia Nervosa
OSFED	Otherwise Specified Feeding and Eating Disorders
GCP	Good Clinical Practice
K-SADS	Kiddie Schedule for Affective Disorders and Schizophrenia
CGI	Clinical Global Improvement
ANOVA	Analysis of the Variance
HA	Harm Avoidance
HA2	Fear Of Uncertainty
SD	Self-Directedness
SD1	Maturity
SD2	Resourcefulness
SD3	Purposefulness
IS	Social Insecurity
IN	Inadequacy
SD4	Self-acceptance
C4	Compassion
NS4	Disorder
FAD3	Role Definition
HA2	Fear of Uncertainty
FAD5	Affective Involvement

References

1. Strober, M.; Johnson, C. The need for complex ideas in anorexia nervosa: Why biology, environment, and psyche all matter, why therapists make mistakes, and why clinical benchmarks are needed for managing weight correction. *Int. J. Eat. Disord.* **2012**, *45*, 155–178. [CrossRef] [PubMed]
2. Siqueira, A.B.R.; dos Santos, M.A.; Leonidas, C. Confluências das relações familiares e transtornos alimentares: Revisão integrativa da literatura. *Psicol. Clín.* **2020**, *32*, 123–149.
3. Treasure, J.; Schmidt, U. The cognitive-interpersonal maintenance model of anorexia nervosa revisited: A summary of the evidence for cognitive, socio-emotional and interpersonal predisposing and perpetuating factors. *J. Eat. Disord.* **2013**, *1*, 13. [CrossRef] [PubMed]
4. Amianto, F.; Abbate Daga, G.; Bertorello, A.; Fassino, S. Exploring personality clusters among parents of ED subjects. Relationship with parents' psychopathology, attachment, and family dynamics. *Compr. Psychiatry* **2013**, *54*, 797–811. [CrossRef]
5. Amianto, F.; Ercole, R.; Marzola, E.; Abbate Daga, G.; Fassino, S. Parents' personality clusters and eating disordered daughters' personality and psychopathology. *Psychiatry Res.* **2015**, *230*, 19–27. [CrossRef]
6. Treasure, J.; Parker, S.; Oyeleye, O.; Harrison, A. The value of including families in the treatment of anorexia nervosa. *Eur. Eat. Disord. Rev. Prof. J. Eat. Disord. Assoc.* **2021**, *29*, 393–401. [CrossRef]
7. Robinson, A.L.; Strahan, E.; Girz, L.; Wilson, A.; Boachie, A. "I know I can help you": Parental self-efficacy predicts adolescent outcomes in family-based therapy for eating disorders. *Eur. Eat. Disord. Rev. Prof. J. Eat. Disord. Assoc.* **2013**, *21*, 108–114. [CrossRef]

8. Amianto, F.; Bertorello, A.; Spalatro, A.; Milazzo, M.; Signa, C.; Cavarero, S.; Abbate Daga, G.; Fassino, S. Adlerian Parent Counseling in Eating Disorders: Preliminary data of a controlled clinical trial. *Eat. Weight. Disord. Stud. Anorex. Bulim. Obes.* **201** *19*, 303–314. [CrossRef]
9. Swanson, H.; Power, K.; Collin, P.; Deas, S.; Paterson, G.; Grierson, D.; Yellowlees, A.; Park, K.; Taylor, L. The relationship betwee parental bonding, social problem solving and eating pathology in an anorexic inpatient sample. *Eur. Eat. Disord. Rev. Prof. J. E Disord. Assoc.* **2010**, *18*, 22–32. [CrossRef]
10. Fassino, S.; Amianto, F.; Abbate-Daga, G. The dynamic relationship of parental personality traits with the personality an psychopathology traits of anorectic and bulimic daughters. *Compr. Psychiatry* **2009**, *50*, 232–239. [CrossRef]
11. Fassino, S.; Abbate-Daga, G.; Amianto, F.; Leombruni, P.; Boggio, S.; Rovera, G.G. Temperament and character profi of eating disorders: A controlled study with the Temperament and Character Inventory. *Int. J. Eat. Disord.* **2002**, *3* 412–425. [CrossRef] [PubMed]
12. Fassino, S.; Svrakic, D.; Abbate-Daga, G.; Leombruni, P.; Amianto, F.; Stanic, S.; Rovera, G.G. Anorectic family dynamic Temperament and character data. *Compr. Psychiatry* **2002**, *43*, 114–120. [CrossRef] [PubMed]
13. Berking, M. Emotion regulation and mental health: Current evidence and beyond. *World Psychiatry* **2024**, *23*, 438–439. [CrossRe
14. Ratcliffe, M. Emotion regulation, scaffolding and psychiatry. *World Psychiatry* **2024**, *23*, 439–440. [CrossRef]
15. Adambegan, M.; Wagner, G.; Nader, I.W.; Fernandez-Aranda, F.; Treasure, J.; Karwautz, A. Internalizing and externalizin behaviour problems in childhood contribute to the development of anorexia and bulimia nervosa-a study comparing sister pai *Eur. Eat. Disord. Rev.* **2012**, *20*, 116–120. [CrossRef]
16. Rhind, C.; Salerno, L.; Hibbs, R. The Objective and Subjective Caregiving Burden and Caregiving Behaviours of Parents c Adolescents with Anorexia Nervosa. *Eur. Eat. Disord. Rev.* **2016**, *24*, 310–319. [CrossRef]
17. Zitzmann, J.; Rombold-George, L.; Rosenbach, C.; Renneberg, B. Emotion Regulation, Parenting, and Psychopatholog A Systematic Review. *Clin. Child. Fam. Psychol. Rev.* **2024**, *27*, 1–22. [CrossRef]
18. Abbate-Daga, G.; Pierò, A.; Rigardetto, R.; Gandione, M.; Gramaglia, C.; Fassino, S. Clinical, psychological and personalit features related to age of onset of anorexia nervosa. *Psychopathology* **2007**, *40*, 261–268. [CrossRef]
19. Piñar-Gutiérrez, A.; Dios-Fuentes, E.; Remón-Ruiz, P.; Del Can-Sánchez, D.; Vázquez-Morejón, A.; López-Narbona, M.; Dasti Rodríguez de Guzmán, J.; Venegas-Moreno, E.; Soto-Moreno, A. Description of characteristics and outcomes of a cohort c patients with severe and enduring eating disorders (SE-ED). *J. Eat. Disord.* **2021**, *9*, 135. [CrossRef]
20. DeSocio, J.E. The neurobiology of risk and pre-emptive interventions for anorexia nervosa. *J. Child Adolesc. Psychiatr. Nurs.* **201** *26*, 16–22. [CrossRef]
21. van Noort, B.M.; Lohmar, S.K.; Pfeiffer, E.; Lehmkuhl, U.; Winter, S.M.; Kappel, V. Clinical characteristics of early onset anorexi nervosa. *Eur. Eat. Disord. Rev. Prof. J. Eat. Disord. Assoc.* **2018**, *26*, 519–525. [CrossRef]
22. Herpertz-Dahlmann, B.; Dempfle, A.; Egberts, K.M.; Kappel, V.; Konrad, K.; Vloet, J.A.; Bühren, K. Outcome of childhoo anorexia nervosa-The results of a five- to ten-year follow-up study. *Int. J. Eat. Disord.* **2018**, *51*, 295–304. [CrossRef] [PubMed]
23. Jenkins, Z.M.; Chait, L.M.; Cistullo, L.; Castle, D.J. A comparison of eating disorder symptomatology, psychological distress an psychosocial function between early, typical and later onset anorexia nervosa. *J. Eat. Disord.* **2020**, *8*, 56. [CrossRef] [PubMed]
24. Le Grange, D.; Lock, J.; Loeb, K.; Nicholls, D. Academy for eating disorders position paper: The role of the family in eatin disorders. *Int. J. Eat. Disord.* **2009**, *1*, 1–5. [CrossRef]
25. Monteleone, A.M.; Mereu, A.; Cascino, G.; Castiglioni, M.C.; Marchetto, C.; Grasso, M.; Pontillo, M.; Pisano, T.; Vicari, S.; Zann V. Coping with Adolescents Affected by Anorexia Nervosa: The Role of Parental Personality Traits. *Front. Psychol.* **2021**, *1* 678745. [CrossRef]
26. Busner, J.; Targum, S.D. The Clinical Global Impressions Scale: Applying a research tool in clinical practice. *Psychiatry* **2007**, *4*, 28–37
27. Cloninger, C.R. Temperament and personality. *Curr. Opin. Neurobiol.* **1994**, *4*, 266–273. [CrossRef]
28. Cloninger, C.R. A systematic method for clinical description and classification of personality variants: A proposal. *Arch. Ge Psychiatry* **1987**, *44*, 573–588. [CrossRef]
29. Garner, D.M.; Rizzardi, M.; Trombini, E.; Trombini, G. *EDI 2: Eating Disorder Inventory 2: Manuale*; Giunti Organizzazioni Special Florence, Italy, 1995.
30. Beck, A.T.; Brown, G.; Steer, R.A.; Eidelson, J.I.; Riskind, J.H. Differentiating anxiety and depression: A test of the cognitiv content-specificity hypothesis. *J. Abnorm. Psychol.* **1987**, *96*, 179–183.
31. Epstein, N.B.; Ryan, C.E.; Bishop, D.S.; Miller, I.W.; Keitner, G.I. *The McMaster Model: A View of Healthy Family Functioning* The Guilford Press: New York, NY, USA, 2003; pp. 581–607.
32. Amianto, F.; Northoff, G.; Abbate Daga, G.; Fassino, S.; Tasca, G.A. Is Anorexia Nervosa a Disorder of the Self? A Psychologica Approach. *Front. Psychol.* **2016**, *7*, 849. [CrossRef]
33. Amianto, F.; Spalatro, A.V.; Rainis, M.; Andriulli, C.; Lavagnino, L.; Abbate-Daga, G.; Fassino, S. Childhood emotional abus and neglect in obese patients with and without binge eating disorder: Personality and psychopathology correlates in adulthoo *Psychiatry Res.* **2018**, *269*, 692–699. [CrossRef] [PubMed]

34. Skårderud, F. Bruch Revisited and Revised. *Eur. Eat. Disord. Rev.* **2009**, *17*, 83. [CrossRef] [PubMed]
35. Li, X.; Theisen, A.; Seo, C.; Sibley, D.S. Resourcefulness: Current Insights and Future Directions for Family Scholars and Clinicians. *Fam. J.* **2018**, *26*, 433–443. [CrossRef]
36. Mochcovitch, M.D.; Nardi, A.E.; Cardoso, A. Temperament and character dimensions and their relationship to major depression and panic disorder. *Braz. J. Psychiatry* **2012**, *34*, 342–351. [CrossRef]
37. Ambwani, S.; Cardi, V.; Albano, G.; Cao, L.; Crosby, R.D.; Macdonald, P.; Schmidt, U.; Treasure, J. A multicenter audit of outpatient care for adult anorexia nervosa: Symptom trajectory, service use, and evidence in support of "early stage" versus "severe and enduring" classification. *Int. J. Eat. Disord.* **2020**, *53*, 1337–1348. [CrossRef]
38. Mairs, R.; Nicholls, D. Assessment and treatment of eating disorders in children and adolescents. *Arch. Dis. Child.* **2016**, *101*, 1168–1175. [CrossRef]
39. Boduszek, D.; Debowska, A. Feelings of Inadequacy Scale. In *Encyclopedia of Personality and Individual Differences*; Zeigler-Hill, V., Shackelford, T.K., Eds.; Springer International Publishing: Cham, Switzerland, 2017; pp. 1–3. ISBN 978-3-319-28099-8.
40. Ciao, A.; Pascual, S.; Hodges, G. The Role of Parents and Other Caregivers in the Early Detection of Eating Disorders. In *Eating Disorders*; Patel, V.B., Preedy, V.R., Eds.; Springer International Publishing: Cham, Switzerland, 2023; pp. 283–312. ISBN 978-3-031-16691-4.
41. Jacobi, C.; Hütter, K.; Völker, U.; Möbius, K.; Richter, R.; Trockel, M.; Jones Bell, M.; Lock, J.; Taylor, C.B. Efficacy of a Parent-Based, Indicated Prevention for Anorexia Nervosa: Randomized Controlled Trial. *J. Med. Internet Res.* **2018**, *20*, e296. [CrossRef]
42. Cerniglia, L.; Muratori, P.; Milone, A.; Paciello, M.; Ruglioni, L.; Cimino, S.; Levantini, V.; Tambelli, R. Paternal psychopathological risk and psychological functioning in children with eating disorders and Disruptive Behavior Disorder. *Psychiatry Res.* **2017**, *254*, 60–66. [CrossRef]
43. Hirshfeld-Becker, D.R.; Micco, J.A.; Henin, A.; Petty, C.; Faraone, S.V.; Mazursky, H.; Bruett, L.; Rosenbaum, J.F.; Biederman, J. Psychopathology in Adolescent Offspring of Parents with Panic Disorder, Major Depression, or Both: A 10-Year Follow-Up. *Am. J. Psychiatry* **2012**, *169*, 1175–1184. [CrossRef]
44. Natsuaki, M.; Shaw, D.; Neiderhiser, J.; Ganiban, J.; Harold, G.; Reiss, D.; Leve, L. Raised by Depressed Parents: Is it an Environmental Risk? *Clin. Child. Fam. Psychol. Rev.* **2014**, *17*, 357–367. [CrossRef]
45. Franzoi, D.; Bockting, C.; Bennett, K.F.; Odom, A.; Lucassen, P.J.; Pathania, A.; Lee, A.; Brouwer, M.; Van de Schoot, R.; Wiers, R.; et al. Which individual, social, and urban factors in early childhood predict psychopathology in later childhood, adolescence and young adulthood? A systematic review. *SSM-Popul. Health* **2023**, *25*, 101575. [CrossRef]
46. Powell, V.; Lennon, J.; Jones, R.B.; Stephens, A.; Weavers, B.; Osborn, D.; Allardyce, J.; Potter, R.; Thapar, A.; Collishaw, S.; et al. Following the children of depressed parents from childhood to adult life: A focus on mood and anxiety disorders. *JCPP Adv.* **2023**, *3*, e12182. [CrossRef] [PubMed]
47. Liu, L.; Liu, C.; Zhao, X. Mapping the Paths from Styles of Anger Experience and Expression to Obsessive-Compulsive Symptoms: The Moderating Roles of Family Cohesion and Adaptability. *Front. Psychol.* **2017**, *8*, 671. [CrossRef] [PubMed]
48. Germer, C.K.; Neff, K.D. Self-Compassion in Clinical Practice. *J. Clin. Psychol.* **2013**, *69*, 856–867. [CrossRef] [PubMed]
49. Geraldo, R.P.; Lange, E.S.N. O Declínio da Função Paterna na Anorexia Feminina. *Rev. Subjetividades* **2016**, *16*, 34–45. [CrossRef]
50. Jones, C.J.; Leung, N.; Harris, G. Father-daughter relationship and eating psychopathology: The mediating role of core beliefs. *Br. J. Clin. Psychol.* **2010**, *45*, 319–330. [CrossRef]
51. Salafia, E.H.; Schaefer, M.K.; Haugen, E.C. Connections Between Marital Conflict and Adolescent Girls' Disordered Eating: Parent–Adolescent Relationship Quality as a Mediator. *J. Child. Fam. Stud.* **2014**, *23*, 1128–1138. [CrossRef]

nutrients

MDPI

Article

The Additive Psychosocial Effects of Binge Eating and Food Insecurity Among Midlife and Older Women

Lisa Smith Kilpela [1,2,*], Taylur Loera [1], Salomé Adelia Wilfred [1], Jessica Salinas [1], Sabrina E. Cuauro [3] and Carolyn Black Becker [3]

1 Center for Research to Advance Community Health (ReACH Center), Department of Medicine, University of Texas Health Science Center at San Antonio, San Antonio, TX 78229, USA; loerat@uthscsa.edu (T.L.); wilfred@uthscsa.edu (S.A.W.); salinasj11@uthscsa.edu (J.S.)
2 South Texas Veterans Healthcare System, Geriatric Research Education and Clinical Center (GRECC), San Antonio, TX 78229, USA
3 Department of Psychology, Trinity University, San Antonio, TX 78212, USA; sc235@rice.edu (S.E.C.); cbecker@trinity.edu (C.B.B.)
* Correspondence: kilpela@uthscsa.edu

Abstract: Background/Objectives: Evidence suggests that food insecurity (FI) is a risk factor for eating disorder (ED) symptoms, especially binge eating (BE), yet research focusing on the psychosocial effects among midlife/older women is lacking. Midlife/older women living with FI experience intersectional disadvantage, thus highlighting the need for an independent investigation of the cultural and contextual factors of this population. The current study examined the difference in psychological health and quality of life (QOL) among women living with BE and FI (BE + FI) versus FI without BE. **Method**: Female clients of a food bank, aged 50+ (N = 295; M age = 62.1 years, SD = 8.2) living with FI completed measures of BE and psychosocial comorbidities. The measures were provided in English and Spanish. **Results**: A multivariate analysis of covariance compared women living with BE and FI (BE + FI) versus FI without BE on outcomes related to mental health and wellbeing. Covarying for age, FI severity, and ethnicity, the results indicated that women living with BE + FI reported worsened anxiety, depression, ED-related psychosocial impairment, internalized weight stigma, and QOL versus women living with FI without BE (all $ps < 0.001$). Effect sizes ranged from small to medium to large. **Conclusions**: Midlife/older women living with BE + FI report poorer psychological health and QOL than those living with FI without BE, demonstrating a critical need for mental healthcare in this population. Innovative solutions—and likely a portfolio of interventional approaches with various entry points and delivery modalities—are warranted, if we are to make significant strides in addressing ED symptoms in this population.

Keywords: binge eating; food insecurity; psychological comorbidity; older adults

1. Introduction

Food insecurity (FI) is defined as a household-level condition marked by an inability to consistently access nutritional and safe foods in socially acceptable ways [1,2]. The severity of FI is considered to be a spectrum in which households may range from high food security (i.e., regular access to sufficient food) to very low food security (i.e., disrupted eating patterns and extremely reduced food intake) [2]. FI is a worldwide health issue that impacts low-, middle-, and high-income nations like the United States [3]. In 2020, at least 60 million Americans (one in every five Americans) were recorded visiting food pantries, food banks, and other community food initiatives [4].

FI represents a significant social determinant of health (SDoH) barrier that negatively impacts physical health, mental health, wellbeing, and school/work [5–7]. Additionally, bourgeoning research has identified FI as a potential risk factor for eating disorder (ED) symptoms [8]. EDs are serious psychiatric illnesses that carry risks for significant health commodities such as osteoporosis, cardiac arrhythmia, and electrolyte abnormalities [9,10]. Claiming the lives of over 10,000 Americans every year, EDs have the second highest mortality rate of all mental health disorders [11,12]. Importantly, findings indicate that FI may comprise a risk factor for EDs, which challenges previously held stereotypes about who is at risk for EDs (i.e., thin, young, white, affluent, women/girls) [13]. The limited research conducted to date indicates that FI may be a risk for ED pathology via multiple etiological pathways.

For instance, individuals living with FI experience dietary restraint secondary to limited food availability in the home [14]. Notably, dietary restraint as a construct has been widely recognized to increase the risk for EDs among food-secure populations [15,16]. In FI populations, research indicates that ED risk from dietary restraint may be particularly elevated in the case of parents restricting their own food intake even when food is available so as to reserve food for children in the home [14].

Cyclical periods of more and less severe FI also can result in discrete and alternating periods of heightened food scarcity and availability. This, in turn, may result in periods of elevated consumption—even resembling or representing binge eating—when more food is available in the home, especially when subsequent meals are not guaranteed [17]. Indeed, research supports the association between FI and binge-eating (BE) severity and frequency, greater loss of control, and elevated rates of binge-eating disorder (BED) among adolescents and adults living with FI [18–24]. Thus, mounting data indicate that living with FI, including the cyclical patterns of scarcity/availability, likely increases the risk for ED behaviors.

FI and BE are also linked by a number of systemic issues that contribute to worsened health outcomes, including geographical barriers to healthy eating, and decreased healthcare access [25,26]. For instance, many FI households have limited access to high-quality grocery stores that sell affordable nutritious food (i.e., conditions found in food deserts [27–29]). FI households also often are located in "food swamps", which are associated with easy access to food retailers (e.g., fast food restaurants, convenience stores) selling low-cost and highly palatable food (HPF; i.e., processed food high in salt, sugar, and fat [29]. Research investigating BE with animal models suggests that consumption of HPF can contribute to the development of BE. For instance, Boggiano and colleagues [30] found that some rats begin to BE when HPF is introduced into their diet even though they consumed normal amounts of food when their diet consisted of rat chow. HPF also has been linked to behaviors associated with BE, such as intense cravings and loss of control over consumption [31]. Thus, research supports that those who frequently consume these foods are at a higher risk of ED pathology.

Additionally, low-income individuals living with FI often lack regular access to healthcare. The luxury of preventive treatment, dietary education, and mental healthcare is not available to those who cannot afford to visit the doctor. Without access to mental health resources, individuals may turn to engaging in unhealthy coping mechanisms, such as BE [32]. Although engaging in such behaviors can offer a temporary sense of relief from stress, it ultimately leads to worse health outcomes over time.

To date, the majority of FI/ED research has focused on adolescents and younger adults, thus neglecting the potential risks related to ED symptoms for individuals in mid- or later life living with FI. Importantly, midlife may be a window of vulnerability for developing EDs, as women face a series of physical, hormonal, and psychosocial transitions. Menopause-related hormonal changes can trigger fluctuations in body shape, weight, and metabolism, which contributes to body dissatisfaction and unhealthy eating patterns. Furthermore, women in midlife often experience psychosocial transitions, such as becoming part of the "sandwich generation", where they simultaneously care for aging parents and children in the home. These transitions can compound added stress and anxiety, leading to unhealthy coping mechanisms (e.g., emotional eating). Data show that 12–26% of midlife/older women engage in at least weekly BE (consuming an abnormally large amount of food in one sitting while simultaneously feeling out of control [33–38], meeting the frequency criterion for (BED). In the limited data examining ED pathology among midlife and older adults living with FI, BED was the most common ED behavior endorsed, and a more severe FI was correlated with a greater risk for BE [38]. Among these prior studies examining the frequency of ED behaviors among midlife and older women living with FI, 17–20% of women reported BE on at least a weekly basis [37,38]. Hooper and colleagues reported that 44.5% of midlife and older adults (68.5% female) reported BE in the past month, with no gender differences in the rates of reporting BE during this time frame [38].

As data are starting to emerge regarding the prevalence and frequencies of ED behaviors among midlife and older women living with FI and other significant SDoH barriers, gaps remain regarding the full clinical picture of individuals living with both BE and FI. In particular, gaps remain regarding the potential differential health burden of living with BE and FI, versus FI alone, in older populations living with intersectional disadvantage (older age, female gender, limited financial resources, minority ethnoracial identity [39]. Among younger, majority, and non-food insecure populations, BED is associated with myriad health consequences, including worse mental health status and quality of life (QOL). Limited data exist, however, on the psychosocial health correlates of BED when living with significant SDoH, such as FI. Thus, the purpose of the current study is to examine the differences in psychosocial health indices and quality of life (QOL) among midlife/older women living with BE and FI (BE + FI) versus FI without BE while controlling for specific established ED risk factors (age, racioethnic identity, and severity of FI). This comparison allows us to evaluate the potential additive effect of BE in the context of living with FI and other significant SDoH barriers (e.g., limited financial resources, lower levels of education), which comprise risk factors for health disparities broadly. We hypothesized that women living with BE + FI would report worse psychosocial health compared to those living with FI without BE.

2. Materials and Methods

2.1. Participants

The participants included women (N = 313) aged 50+ years (M = 62.1 years, SD = 8.2; range 50–94 years) who sought assistance at the San Antonio Food Bank (SAFB). Of note, the SAFB's language regarding the people it serves has changed in recent years from "clients" to "neighbors" (i.e., the SAFB serves neighbors). As such, we use this terminology to reflect the preferred language of the SAFB. All women in this study identified as living with FI. The majority of participants (80%) self-identified their ethnicity as Hispanic/Latina. Most neighbors (66%) reported an annual household income of ≤USD 12,000; 31.2% reported graduating from high school. Additionally, over a third of individuals reported living with a disability (31%). See Table 1 for a breakdown of the sociodemographics by group.

Table 1. Participant sociodemographic data.

Demographics	FI Only n = 250 M (SD) or N (%)	FI + BE n = 63 M (SD) or N (%)
Age	62.2 (8.1)	61.5 (9.1)
Ethnicity		
Latino/Hispanic	203 (81.2%)	46 (73%)
Black/African American	8 (3.2%)	3 (4.8%)
White/Caucasian	28 (11.2%)	11 (17.5%)
Other/Multiple *	11 (4.4%)	3 (4.8%)
Primary language spoken		
English	139 (55.8%)	38 (60.3%)
Spanish	73 (29.3%)	17 (27%)
English and Spanish	37 (14.9%)	8 (12.7%)
Food Insecurity		
Not food insecure	17 (6.8%)	---
Household FI	26 (10.4%)	1 (1.6%)
Individual FI	145 (58%)	41 (65.1%)
Child hunger	62 (24.8%)	21 (33.3%)
Education		
No or some grade school	30 (12%)	9 (14.2%)
Finished grade school	16 (6.4%)	5 (7.9%)
Some high school	52 (20.8%)	11 (17.5%)
High school/GED	80 (32%)	18 (28.6%)
Some college or technical	54 (21.6%)	16 (25.4%)
Bachelor+	18 (7.2%)	4 (6.4%)
Annual household income		
<USD 10,000	108 (45.8%)	30 (49.2%)
USD 10,000–USD 35,000	112 (47.6%)	30 (49.2%)
USD 35,000–USD 90,000	15 (6.2%)	---
USD 90,000+	1 (0.4%)	1 (1.6%)
Marital status		
Single	66 (26.4%)	12 (19%)
Married/living with partner	66 (26.4%)	18 (28.6%)
Divorced or separated	68 (27.2%)	22 (34.9%)
Widowed	50 (20%)	11 (17.5%)
Children under 18 in the household	70 (28%)	17 (27%)
Living with disability	78 (31.2%)	24 (38.1%)
Diabetes	131 (52.4%)	36 (57.1%)

Notes. * Some racioethnic groups were collapsed into 'other' due to small sample sizes, including Native American (n = 1) and multiple races.

2.2. Procedure

This study was conducted in collaboration with the SAFB and approved by the Trinity University Institutional Review Board (IRB). The SAFB provides service to 29 counties in Texas and serves over 100,000 neighbors per week. Locally, the child FI rate at the SAFB is 22.2%; data from the U.S. Department of Agriculture show that 15.5% of households in Texas are food insecure. Approximately 20% of people residing in San Antonio live below the official poverty line (U.S. Census Bureau, 2023) [40].

While food distribution is the main duty of the SAFB, the SAFB is also partnered with Workforce Solutions and Alamo Neighbor Services to assist with employment opportunities and federal benefits. Research assistants (RAs) approached individuals at the SAFB who were waiting for these services; wait times for services average around 30–50 min, which meant that interested neighbors could participate in the study without any disruption to their access to services at the SAFB. We note that we intentionally recruited individuals who were not waiting to receive food. RAs used standardized recruitment scripts (provided in both English and Spanish to accommodate neighbors' language preferences) to inquire about a neighbor's interest in study participation. Interested neighbors were given more detailed information. RAs followed the informed consent process and provided interested neighbors with a consent form; they had the choice to read this form independently or have a summary of each section read aloud by RAs.

After providing informed consent, the participants completed a self-report survey. Since literacy rates are lower among individuals with FI, all materials were altered to match a sixth-grade reading level. Given the high frequency of Spanish speakers in San Antonio, all scripts and measures were provided in English and Spanish. Any measures that were not already available in Spanish were translated into Spanish by two bilingual members of the research team. To verify that the meaning of each question remained the same in both English and Spanish, two other bilingual members of the research team back-translated all materials. A bilingual individual who grew up in San Antonio then reviewed the Spanish version and made small changes to reflect the local Spanish dialect spoken in San Antonio (see Becker et al. 2017, 2023 [18,41], for full details regarding measures modifications for reading level and Spanish language). Spanish-speaking RAs were also on-site throughout the entire data collection period.

Based on individual preference, participants were given the choice of either a paper or tablet version of the survey. For any participants who experienced difficulty reading the questionnaire, RAs read aloud survey items and response options. The survey took an average of 25 min to complete. In order to protect neighbor anonymity, all questionnaires were numerically coded in advance to organize the data without collecting identifying information. To further maintain confidentiality, the participants were asked not to include their names or any identifying information on the survey. Upon completion of the self-report survey, participants signed for a USD 8 gift card to the largest grocery store in the area. Afterward, RAs had the opportunity to debrief each participant and give them a copy of the consent form along with a list of free or low-cost mental health services.

Demographics

Participants self-reported their age, race and ethnicity, primary language spoken, annual household income, highest level of education, marital status, employment status, children in the household, disability status, and medical history. While waiting for services on-site, the participants also completed measures of FI, ED pathology, anxiety, depression, QOL, ED-related psychosocial impairment, internalized weight stigma, and body shame (see Table 2 for descriptives). We have conducted 3 previous studies in collaboration with the SAFB ($N > 2000$ participants since 2016) and found that this population has very low access to physicians and/or scales (which are a luxury item). As such, many neighbors have no way of knowing their weight. Thus, we opted to remove questions about height and weight out of data validity concerns.

Table 2. Descriptive statistics for dependent variables.

Measures	FI Only *M* (SD)	FI + BED *M* (SD)
Depression (PHQ-9)	7.6 (6.4)	11.7 (5.8)
Quality of Life	0.34 (0.58)	0.79 (0.78)
Internalized Weight Stigma (WSSQ)	25.7 (5.8)	21.7 (5)
Clinical Impairment (CIAQ)	21.6 (10.2)	27.2 (11.5)
Body Image (BISS)	6.9 (10.8)	19.4 (14.5)
Anxiety (GAD-7)	12 (15.9)	30.4 (16.8)

2.3. Food Insecurity (FI)

The Radimer/Cornell Food Insecurity Measure (RCFIM [42,43]) was used. To assess FI, we used the 13-item RCFIM. Items in this measure are scored on a 3-point Likert scale (0 = not true; 1 = sometimes true; 2 = always true). A sample item includes "I worry about whether my food will run out before I get money to buy more". Using responses from the RCFIM, the participants are classified into one of the following groups: (1) household FI, which is linked to food scarcity but not hunger; (2) individual FI, which involves an inability to obtain enough food for every member of the household because of insufficient resources; and (3) child-hunger household FI, where adults report having hungry children at home [43]. Child hunger in the home is considered the most severe level of FI because adults will generally try to protect children from hunger. Thus, the adults in the household are likely hungrier than the children. We reclassified the least severe group as "not food insecure" (NFI) rather than "food secure". Despite some participants not meeting the full criteria for FI, all participants in this study are utilizing resources at the SAFB, indicating that they are living with some degree of FI. Kendall and colleagues [42] reported that the RCFIM has strong internal consistency. The internal consistency in our current sample was high (Cronbach's $\alpha = 0.92$).

2.4. Eating Disorder Pathology

The Eating Disorder-15 (ED-15 [44]) was used. We assessed ED pathology using the ED-15. This 15-item questionnaire measures the frequency of ED symptoms during the last week. Items are scored on a 7-point Likert scale (0 = not at all to 6 = all of the time). This measure includes two subscales, 'Weight & Shape Concerns' and 'Eating Concerns'. The first ten items of the ED-15 measure eating attitudes; a sample item is 'Over the past week, how often have I been preoccupied with thoughts of food and eating'. The last five items require open-ended responses and are only answered if participants have partaken in dysregulated behaviors, such as binge eating. We used self-reported BE episodes on the ED-15 for group categorization (i.e., BE + FI versus FI without FI). The ED-15 has been shown to have good clinical validity and reliability (current sample $\alpha = 0.95$; [44]).

2.5. Anxiety

The Generalized Anxiety Disorder questionnaire (GAD-7 [45]) was used. We used the seven-item GAD-7 to assess the frequency of anxiety symptoms. This questionnaire asked participants to reflect on the preceding two weeks and rate their anxiety on a 4-point Likert scale (0 = not at all to 3 = nearly every day); higher scores indicate more significant anxiety symptoms. The GAD-7 is a well-validated and reliable measure of anxiety ($\alpha = 0.92$). Internal consistency within our sample was excellent ($\alpha = 0.94$).

2.6. Depression

The Personal Health Questionnaire Depression Scale (PHQ-8 [46]) was used. We employed the 8-item version of the PHQ to screen for depressive symptoms over the past 2 weeks. Participants were asked to rate how often they were bothered by problems such as feeling hopeless or depressed. Responses were rated on a 4-point Likert scale (0 = not at all to 4 = nearly every day), and higher scores indicate greater depressive symptoms. Research suggests that the PHQ-8 is a valid and reliable measure of depression (Cronbach's $\alpha = 0.88$). We used the PHQ-8 instead of the 9-item version (PHQ-9) because the PHQ-8 excludes the item inquiring about suicidal ideation ("Thoughts that you would be better off dead, or of hurting yourself"). The PHQ-8 and the PHQ-9 are highly correlated ($r = 0.997$) and have similar sensitivity [47]. Within our sample, internal consistency for the PHQ-8 was excellent ($\alpha = 0.92$).

2.7. *Quality of Life (QOL)*

The EUROHIS-QOL-8 was used [48]. QOL was measured using the 8-item EUROHIS-QOL-8, which is adapted from the World Health Organization Quality of Life Scale (WHOQOL-BREF). We selected this measure to capture QOL, as it is significantly briefer than many QOL measures and, therefore, minimizes participant burden. Items on this scale measure the overall quality of life, energy, general health, self-esteem, daily living activity, finances, living conditions, and social relationships over the past two weeks. Items are scored on a 5-point Likert scale, with higher scores indicating better QOL. Internal consistency in the current sample was good ($\alpha = 0.85$).

2.8. *Eating-Related Psychosocial Impairment*

The Clinical Impairment Assessment Questionnaire (CIAQ [49]) was used. We administered the CIAQ to measure ED-related psychosocial impairment over the past month. This 16-item questionnaire asks about the impact of exercising, eating habits, and feelings about weight/shape on various aspects of life (e.g., cognitive functioning, social engagement, and work performance) using a 4-point Likert scale (0 = not at all to 3 = a lot). The CIAQ score is summed; higher scores indicate greater impairment. The CIAQ has very good internal consistency and construct validity [49]; internal consistency in the current sample was excellent (current $\alpha = 0.98$).

2.9. *Weight Stigma*

The Weight Self-Stigma Questionnaire (WSSQ [50]) was used. We used the WSSQ to measure internalized weight stigma. The WSSQ consists of 10 items on a 5-point Likert scale (1 = completely disagree to 5 = completely agree). For this study, we used the total score; higher scores indicate greater weight self-stigma. Similar to our previous studies with populations living with FI [18,19], we modified questions to improve comprehension for individuals with lower reading levels. Two items from the original measure (twelve items) were removed due to the complexity of the questions, and we changed the wording of "weight problems" and "overweight" to "fat" (e.g., "People discriminate against me because I'm fat"). This modified measure has had excellent internal validity in prior work ($\alpha = 0.94$ [41]); internal consistency in our sample was high ($\alpha = 0.94$).

2.10. *Body Shame*

The Body Image Shame Scale (BISS [51]) was used. We used the BISS global score to assess the overall body shame experienced by participants. The BISS is comprised of 14 items, which can be divided into 2 subscales (internalized and externalized body shame). Factor analyses have demonstrated that the BISS can be scored as a global factor or as separate subscales representing distinct factors that underlie this higher-order global factor on body image shame. Psychometric properties for both the global score and the subscales are strong [51]. Thus, to minimize the number of tests, we used the global score to capture body shame in this sample. Global internal consistency was high in the current sample ($\alpha = 0.98$).

Analytic Strategy

Descriptive statistics captured sociodemographic variability, including established ED-risk variables of FI severity, age, and ethnicity. Groups were split based on the frequency of BE episodes over the past week; those who reported a $\geq$1 BE over the past week on the ED-15 ($n = 57$; 20.1%) were categorized in the BED + FI group, while those who denied any BE in the past week on the ED-15 ($n = 227$; 79.9%) were categorized as the FI group. To examine potential between-group differences in all of the health indices while accounting for multiple dependent variables, we conducted a multivariate analysis of covariance (MANCOVA), covarying for participant age, race/ethnicity, and FI severity. Levene's test of equality of error variances examined the error variance of the dependent variable across groups. Box's M Test and Pillai's Trace statistics were used to assess the variance–covariance matrices and account for unequal matrices when evaluating assumptions.

3. Results

Levene's test of equality of error variances indicated that all dependent variables were of equal variances across groups, except the CIAQ, which measures ED-related impairment. Box's M Test of equality of covariance matrices (including intercept + age + ethnoracial group + FI severity + BE group) was significant ($p = 0.001$), suggesting that there may be unequal covariance matrices. Because Box's M is oversensitive in large samples, such as ours, we examined Pillai's Trace as a more robust test of true between-group differences. Pillai's Trace was significant for our independent variable ($p < 0.001$), suggesting a true difference between the BE + FI and FI groups.

Overall, women living with BE + FI reported higher anxiety ($p < 0.001$) and depressive symptoms ($p < 0.001$), greater ED-related psychosocial impairment ($p < 0.001$), poorer QOL ($p < 0.001$), higher internalized weight stigma ($p = 0.001$), and greater body image shame ($p < 0.001$) than women living with FI without BE when covarying for age, ethnicity, and FI severity. Between-group effect sizes ranged from small to medium to large. Regarding covariates, older age was significantly related to lower anxiety ($p < 0.001$) and depression symptoms ($p = 0.023$), less ED-related impairment ($p < 0.001$), and lower body image shame ($p = 0.006$). Greater severity of FI was related to higher anxiety ($p < 0.001$) and depressive symptoms ($p < 0.001$), poorer QOL ($p < 0.001$), and more ED-related impairment ($p = 0.028$) and body shame ($p = 0.031$). Ethnicity was not significantly related to any of the outcome variables. See Table 3 for results.

Table 3. MANCOVA Results.

		Measures	F	Sig.	Partial Eta Squared
Covariates	Age	Anxiety	15.860	<0.001	0.053
		Quality of Life	1.027	0.312	0.004
		Internalized Weight Stigma	2.232	0.136	0.008
		Depression	5.218	0.023	0.018
		Clinical Impairment	12.527	<0.001	0.042
		Body Image	7.564	0.006	0.026
	Ethnicity	Anxiety	0.204	0.652	0.001
		Quality of Life	0.072	0.788	0.000
		Internalized Weight Stigma	0.018	0.893	0.000
		Depression	0.157	0.692	0.001
		Clinical Impairment	0.011	0.917	0.000
		Body Image	0.456	0.500	0.002
	FI Severity	Anxiety	15.769	<0.001	0.053
		Quality of Life	38.883	<0.001	0.120
		Internalized Weight Stigma	0.091	0.763	0.000
		Depression	19.158	<0.001	0.063
		Clinical Impairment	4.900	0.028	0.017
		Body Image	4.693	0.031	0.016
Fixed Factor	BED + FI vs. FI	Anxiety	14.060	<0.001	0.047
		Quality of Life	15.260	<0.001	0.051
		Internalized Weight Stigma	10.834	0.001	0.037
		Depression	24.141	<0.001	0.078
		Clinical Impairment	48.859	<0.001	0.147
		Body Image	53.932	<0.001	0.160

4. Discussion

The purpose of this study was to investigate the potential additive psychosocial comorbidity of living with BE in the context of FI (BE + FI) versus FI without BE among older women. Importantly, *all* women in the study reported significant SDoH barriers in addition to living with FI (e.g., low annual household income, lower levels of education) that did not differ between groups. As such, the primary aim of this study was to begin identifying the potential additive psychosocial burden that living with BE contributes by comparing women with similar SDoH barriers and sociodemographic characteristics.

The results indicated that approximately 20% of older adult women (aged 50+) living with FI reported BE on at least a weekly basis. Consistent with our hypotheses, older women living with BE + FI reported greater anxiety and depressive symptoms, ED-related impairment, internalized weight stigma, and body shame, as well as poorer QOL when covarying for age, racioethnic identity, and FI severity. Thus, living with BE in the context of FI is associated with elevated psychosocial comorbidity, above and beyond that experienced by older women who experience similar and significant SDoH barriers. These results shed light on factors relevant to BE and SDoH in two primary ways: (1) the additive psychosocial burden of BE and FI, compared to that of living with FI in the absence of BE, and (2) the cultural and contextual considerations needed for developing and expanding services for older women living with this complex clinical picture in an environment without easy access to care.

First, the results highlight the psychosocial burden faced by women living with FI and BE, demonstrating a multifaceted need for mental healthcare in this population. Notably, given the intersectional disadvantage of women in our sample (i.e., female, older age, minoritized ethnicity, living with FI, living with lower financial resources, and education), it is critical that we first consider the important cultural and social factors potentially amplifying these additive psychosocial burdens of living with BE in the context of FI, including but not limited to, systematic forms of oppression. For example, due to new Texas laws targeting those who are undocumented, individuals may experience heightened levels of emotional distress and may be more hesitant to go to places offering services, further exacerbating their emotional distress. This exacerbated emotional distress may then interact with financially based dietary restraint to make undocumented individuals and their loved ones even more susceptible to engaging in BE behaviors [52] and the additive psychosocial burden of BE in the context of FI, as seen in this sample. Building on this example of cultural and contextual relevance in identifying risk factors for diverse populations, future research is needed to better disentangle the nuances of living with FI and ED pathology so as to advance the field in ways that promote inclusivity and expand our conceptualizations of those who are at risk for EDs and how and why. This is especially important when considering the context of systemic oppression and historical discrimination in the medical system, which has resulted in earned medical mistrust by many minoritized and marginalized populations.

Second, we need a deepened understanding of the potential harms of living with ED pathology (e.g., BE) in the context of facing significant SDoH barriers to recovery in order to formulate innovative approaches for improving health equity. In recognizing that many of these factors are maintained on the institutional level, it is imperative that we conceptualize, develop, build, and advocate for multi-level interventions, which will very likely involve advocacy work in health and resource policy. Innovative solutions—and likely a portfolio of multi-level interventional approaches with various entry points and delivery modalities—are warranted if we are to make significant strides in improving mental health equity. Specifically, target system-level interventions to not isolate or target the individual living with significant SDoH barriers. In other words, it is important that we conceptualize these psychosocial burdens differently than we do for individuals living with sufficient resources. It is also critical to approach our conceptualization of psychopathology through a lens of understanding the lives of individuals facing SDoH barriers to health equity, as some behaviors historically seen as disordered in the context of privilege may serve as survival behaviors in the context of poverty (e.g., food restriction). Ultimately, this mindset is needed to ensure that we do not pathologize living with SDoH barriers by putting the onus on the individual rather than the systems of oppression in which they are living. This new conceptualization will, in turn, pave the way for better and more inclusive interventions.

Longitudinal research that evaluates the prospective impacts of living with BE and FI using a multi-method assessment is also urgently needed if we are to identify and understand causal pathways. Further, the use of mixed-methods research would assist in examining and better understanding systematic, cultural, and individual barriers and facilitators to diagnosis and treatment, as well as how these various factors interact. Longitudinal mix-methods research is critical if we want to understand the bidirectional relationships that undoubtedly need to be investigated. For instance, BE may trigger depression, particularly if out-of-control eating worsens FI. Yet, depression may lead to a search for emotion regulation strategies, which may include BE. These two relationships might exist in the same person, again creating a cascade of psychosocial distress.

Future research will additionally need to be focused on understanding stigma and how stigma impacts the chronicity of BE and other psychosocial comorbidities among older women living with FI. We will likely need to develop system-level interventions, with consideration for cultural and contextual factors, such as environmental circumstances that impede or promote remission of BE in the context of living with FI. Future research also will need to investigate preventive programming at the system level (i.e., not exclusively targeting the individual living with FI for treatment without considering the lived environment, which reflects a longstanding history of systems of oppression).

Not everyone who lives with FI goes on to develop BE. Recent research suggests that temperamental factors may influence the emergence of various mental health concerns, including EDs [53]. Longitudinal research will also play a much-needed role in determining how temperament interacts with SDoH so that targeted interventions for individuals can also be developed, given that systemic-level interventions can take time to implement, particularly when government is resistant to this level of intervention.

Although further research is critically needed to inform both policies and clinical practice, a few common-sense suggestions are in order. Those working with older women living with FI should screen for BE, as older women with BE have reported feeling their distress about their eating is both invisible and unheard [34]. De-stigmatizing pathological eating behaviors and offering validation and empathy are critical first steps in providing support. For those who treat EDs, all patients should be screened for FI, since patients can experience shame around FI and fail to voluntarily disclose their difficulty procuring adequate food. Asking about FI normalizes it and makes it easier for patients to discuss their challenges. Given the critical role of dietary restraint in the onset and maintenance of EDs, all providers also should have plans in place (e.g., supplements; food; gift cards to buy food; and resources for facilitating access to food banks) to help patients living with FI become more food secure.

Limitations

The limitations of the current study include its cross-sectional design, which uses self-report data. Ideally, future research should capture BE symptoms and psychosocial comorbidities using multi-faceted assessments and longitudinal designs. Given the cross-sectional nature of this study, we cannot infer the chronology of psychosocial symptom onset or maintenance. It could be that living with BE and FI increases the risk for other mental health symptoms. Alternatively, facing psychological symptoms, such as depression, increases the likelihood of developing BE symptoms. Future research is needed to disentangle the risk profile of living with FI for older populations to identify potential avenues for preventive, multi-level interventions. The ED-15, while brief and minimizing participant burden, only captures BE in the past week. Given the cyclical nature of food insecurity in some populations, this could correspond to cyclical patterns of ED symptom fluctuation. Participants in this study, however, were not presenting to the food pantries (i.e., for food distribution) but to Neighbor Services (e.g., applying for or renewing federal benefits). Thus, they were not presenting for food distribution at the time of study participation. The prevalence of BE over the past week in this study (20%) matches past studies that capture BE frequency over longer periods of time (e.g., [37], suggesting that this may reflect a more longstanding frequency of BE behaviors. Additionally, because we included all older women presenting for services at the SAFB, this resulted in unequal sample sizes between the BE + FI and FI groups. The use of multivariate analyses with covariate adjustments reduces the potential influence of unequal sample sizes; Pillai's Trace further supported the interpretation that differences between groups existed. Future research using selective sampling strategies could remedy sample size limitations.

5. Conclusions

Living with FI is associated with an increased risk for myriad mental health symptoms, including ED pathology [18,19,24]. This study demonstrates that living with BE in the presence of FI worsens the psychosocial burden experienced by older women above and beyond that associated with FI and related SDoH. Mixed-methods longitudinal research is critically needed to understand causal pathways and to begin to create the foundational knowledge that will be crucial to the development of both system-level and individual-level preventative and treatment interventions. Given the role of SDoH in mental health disparities, innovative approaches with multi-level interventions will likely be needed in order to improve health equity for populations living with FI and ED pathology, including BE. Ultimately, it is time to overcome the notion that EDs are disorders of wealth. Instead, we need to recognize the intersecting nature of EDs and SDoH and strive for more inclusivity and health equity considerations in our research and intervention development (e.g., multi-level interventions).

Author Contributions: Study design—C.B.B. and L.S.K.; Data collection—S.E.C.; Original Writing—L.S.K., T.L., C.B.B., J.S. and S.A.W.; Editing—S.A.W. and J.S.; Conceptualization of current study/analyses—C.B.B. and L.S.K.; Analysis or interpretation of the data—L.S.K., T.L. and J.S. All authors have read and agreed to the published version of the manuscript.

Funding: This work was supported by the National Institute on Aging (NIA) [K76AG060003] and the National Institute of Health [R01AG086777].

Institutional Review Board Statement: This study was deemed exempt by the Trinity University IRB (#169816 approved on 14 March 2022).

Informed Consent Statement: Informed consent was obtained from all subjects involved in this study.

Data Availability Statement: The dataset generated and/or analyzed during the current study is not publicly available but is available from the corresponding author upon reasonable request.

Acknowledgments: We thank the San Antonio Food Bank for their assistance in this research and the H-E-B grocery company, the McNairs Scholars Program, and the Murchison Summer Undergraduate Research Fellowship Program for financial support.

Conflicts of Interest: The authors declare no conflicts of interest.

Abbreviations

BE	Binge eating
BED	Binge-eating Disorder
ED	Eating Disorder
ED	15-Item Eating Disorder Pathology Questionnaire
FI	Food Insecurity
NFI	Not Food insecure
IRB	Institutional Review Board
QOL	Quality of Life
RCFIM	Radimer/Cornell Food Insecurity Measure
GAD-7	7-Item Generalized Anxiety Disorder Questionnaire
PHQ-8	8-Item Personal Health Questionnaire
EUROHIS-QOL-8	8-Item European Health Interview Survey-Quality of Life
CIAQ	Clinical Impairment Assessment Questionnaire
WSSQ	Weight Self-Stigma Questionnaire
BISS	Body Image Shame Scale
MANCOVA	Multivariate Analysis of Covariance
SDoH	Social Determinants of Health

References

1. Anderson, S.A. Core indicators of nutritional state for difficult-to-sample populations. *J. Nutr.* **1990**, *120*, 1555–1598. [CrossRef] [PubMed]
2. Economic Research Service. Food Security in the U.S.—Definitions of Food Security 2025. Available online: https://www.ers.usda.gov/topics/food-nutrition-assistance/food-security-in-the-us/definitions-of-food-security (accessed on 10 January 2025).
3. Jones, A.D. Food insecurity and mental health status: A global analysis of 149 countries. *Am. J. Prev. Med.* **2017**, *53*, 264–273. [CrossRef] [PubMed]
4. Feeding America. How We Measure Hunger in the U.S. 2021. Available online: https://www.feedingamerica.org/hunger-blog/how-we-measure-hunger-america (accessed on 10 January 2025).
5. Leung, C.W.; Tester, J.M. The association between food insecurity and diet quality varies by race/ethnicity: An analysis of national health and nutrition examination survey 2011–2014 results. *J. Acad. Nutr. Diet.* **2019**, *119*, 1676–1686. [CrossRef]
6. Liu, Y.; Njai, R.S.; Greenlund, K.J.; Chapman, D.P.; Croft, J.B. Relationships between housing and food insecurity, frequent mental distress, and insufficient sleep among adults in 12 US States, 2009. *Prev. Chronic Dis.* **2014**, *11*, 130334. [CrossRef] [PubMed]
7. Van Woerden, I.; Hruschka, D.; Bruening, M. Food insecurity negatively impacts academic performance. *J. Public Aff.* **2019**, *19*, e1864. [CrossRef]
8. Hazzard, V.M.; Loth, K.A.; Hooper, L.; Becker, C.B. Food insecurity and eating disorders: A review of emerging evidence. *Curr. Psychiatry Rep.* **2020**, *22*, 74. [CrossRef]
9. Sato, Y.; Fukudo, S. Gastrointestinal symptoms and disorders in patients with eating disorders. *Clin. J. Gastroenterol.* **2015**, *8*, 255–263. [CrossRef]
10. Sidiropoulos, M. Anorexia nervosa: The physiological consequences of starvation and the need for primary prevention efforts. *McGill J. Med.* **2007**, *10*, 20. [CrossRef]
11. Arcelus, J.; Mitchell, A.J.; Wales, J.; Nielsen, S. Mortality rates in patients with anorexia nervosa and other eating disorders: A meta-analysis of 36 studies. *Arch. Gen. Psychiatry* **2011**, *68*, 724–731. [CrossRef]
12. Deloitte Access Economics. The Social and Economic Cost of Eating Disorders in the United States of America: A Report for the Strategic Training Initiative for the Prevention of Eating Disorders and the Academy for Eating Disorders. 2020. Available online: https://www.hsph.harvard.edu/striped/report-economic-costs-of-eating-disorders/ (accessed on 10 January 2025).
13. Capodilupo, C.M. One size does not fit all: Using variables other than the thin ideal to understand Black women's body image. *Cult. Divers. Ethn. Minor. Psychol.* **2015**, *21*, 268. [CrossRef]
14. Middlemass, K.M.; Cruz, J.; Gamboa, A.; Johnson, C.; Taylor, B.; Gomez, F.; Becker, C.B. Food insecurity & dietary restraint in a diverse urban population. *Eat. Disord.* **2021**, *29*, 616–629. [PubMed]
15. Keys, A.; Brožek, J.; Henschel, A.; Mickelsen, O.; Taylor, H.L. *The Biology of Human Starvation*; University of Minnesota Press: Minneapolis, MN, USA, 1950; Volume 2.

16. Jacobi, C.; Hayward, C.; de Zwaan, M.; Kraemer, H.C.; Agras, W.S. Coming to terms with risk factors for eating disorders: Application of risk terminology and suggestions for a general taxonomy. *Psychol. Bull.* **2004**, *130*, 19. [CrossRef] [PubMed]
17. Tester, J.M.; Lang, T.C.; Laraia, B.A. Disordered eating behaviours and food insecurity: A qualitative study about children with obesity in low-income households. *Obes. Res. Clin. Pract.* **2016**, *10*, 544–552. [CrossRef] [PubMed]
18. Becker, C.B.; Middlemass, K.; Taylor, B.; Johnson, C.; Gomez, F. Food insecurity and eating disorder pathology. *Int. J. Eat. Disord.* **2017**, *50*, 1031–1040. [CrossRef]
19. Becker, C.B.; Middlemass, K.M.; Gomez, F.; Martinez-Abrego, A. Eating disorder pathology among individuals living with food insecurity: A replication study. *Clin. Psychol. Sci.* **2019**, *7*, 1144–1158. [CrossRef]
20. Rasmusson, G.; Lydecker, J.A.; Coffino, J.A.; White, M.A.; Grilo, C.M. Household food insecurity is associated with binge-eating disorder and obesity. *Int. J. Eat. Disord.* **2019**, *52*, 28–35. [CrossRef]
21. Stinson, E.J.; Votruba, S.B.; Venti, C.; Perez, M.; Krakoff, J.; Gluck, M.E. Food insecurity is associated with maladaptive eating behaviors and objectively measured overeating. *Obesity* **2018**, *26*, 1841–1848. [CrossRef]
22. Kim, B.H.; Ranzenhofer, L.; Stadterman, J.; Karvay, Y.G.; Burke, N.L. Food insecurity and eating pathology in adolescents. *Int. J. Environ. Res. Public Health* **2021**, *18*, 9155. [CrossRef]
23. West, C.E.; Darling, K.E.; Ruzicka, E.B.; Sato, A.F. Household income and loss of control eating in adolescence: Examining the role of food insecurity. *Appetite* **2021**, *165*, 105291. [CrossRef]
24. Hazzard, V.M.; Hooper, L.; Larson, N.; Loth, K.A.; Wall, M.M.; Neumark-Sztainer, D. Associations between severe food insecurity and disordered eating behaviors from adolescence to young adulthood: Findings from a 10-year longitudinal study. *Prev. Med.* **2022**, *154*, 106895. [CrossRef]
25. Sarlio-Lähteenkorva, S.; Lahelma, E. Food insecurity is associated with past and present economic disadvantage and body mass index. *J. Nutr.* **2001**, *131*, 2880–2884. [CrossRef] [PubMed]
26. Marques, L.; Alegria, M.; Becker, A.E.; Chen, C.N.; Fang, A.; Chosak, A.; Diniz, J.B. Comparative prevalence, correlates of impairment, and service utilization for eating disorders across US ethnic groups: Implications for reducing ethnic disparities in health care access for eating disorders. *Int. J. Eat. Disord.* **2011**, *44*, 412–420. [CrossRef] [PubMed]
27. Cummins, S.; Macintyre, S. "Food deserts"—Evidence and assumption in health policy making. *BMJ* **2002**, *325*, 436–438. [CrossRef] [PubMed]
28. Dutko, P.; Ver Ploeg, M.; Farrigan, T. *Characteristics and Influential Factors of Food Deserts*; USDA: Washington, DC, USA, 2012.
29. Kato, Y.; Irvin, C. Flow of Food and People across the City: An Examination of Local Food Access in a New Orleans Food Desert. *Spaces Flows Int. J. Urban Extra Urban Stud.* **2013**, *3*, 45–56. [CrossRef]
30. Boggiano, M.M.; Artiga, A.I.; Pritchett, C.E.; Chandler-Laney, P.C.; Smith, M.L.; Eldridge, A.J. High intake of palatable food predicts binge-eating independent of susceptibility to obesity: An animal model of lean vs obese binge-eating and obesity with and without binge-eating. *Int. J. Obes.* **2007**, *31*, 1357–1367. [CrossRef]
31. Ayton, A.; Ibrahim, A.; Dugan, J.; Galvin, E.; Wright, O.W. Ultra-processed foods and binge eating: A retrospective observational study. *Nutrition* **2021**, *84*, 111023. [CrossRef]
32. Dave, J.M.; Thompson, D.I.; Svendsen-Sanchez, A.; Cullen, K.W. Perspectives on barriers to eating healthy among food pantry clients. *Health Equity* **2017**, *1*, 28–33. [CrossRef]
33. American Psychiatric Association. *Diagnostic and Statistical Manual of Mental Disorders (DSM-5®)*; American Psychiatric Association: Washington, DC, USA, 2013.
34. Kilpela, L.S.; Marshall, V.B.; Keel, P.K.; LaCroix, A.Z.; Espinoza, S.E.; Hooper, S.C.; Musi, N. The clinical significance of binge eating among older adult women: An investigation into health correlates, psychological wellbeing, and quality of life. *J. Eat Disord.* **2022**, *10*, 97. [CrossRef]
35. Marcus, M.D.; Bromberger, J.T.; Wei, H.-L.; Brown, C.; Kravitz, H.M. Prevalence and selected correlates of eating disorder symptoms among a multiethnic community sample of midlife women. *Ann. Behav. Med.* **2007**, *33*, 269–277. [CrossRef]
36. Thompson, K.A.; Bardone-Cone, A.M. Disordered eating behaviors and attitudes and their correlates among a community sample of older women. *Eat. Behav.* **2019**, *34*, 101301. [CrossRef]
37. Wilfred, S.A.; Becker, C.B.; Kanzler, K.E.; Musi, N.; Espinoza, S.E.; Kilpela, L.S. Binge eating among older women: Prevalence rates and health correlates across three independent samples. *J. Eat. Disord.* **2021**, *9*, 1–10. [CrossRef] [PubMed]
38. Hooper, S.C.; Kilpela, L.S.; Gomez, F.; Middlemass, K.M.; Becker, C.B. Eating disorder pathology in a sample of midlife and older adults experiencing food insecurity. *Eat. Behav.* **2023**, *49*, 101742. [CrossRef]
39. Crenshaw, K. *On Intersectionality: Essential Writings*; New Press: New York, NY, USA, 2019.
40. U.S. Census Bureau. 2023. Available online: https://data.census.gov/profile/San_Antonio_city,_Texas?g=160XX00US4865000 (accessed on 8 January 2025).
41. Cuauro, S.E.; Santos, N.; Andrade, E.; Dani, A.W.; Sanchious, S.N.; Hooper, S.C.; Becker, C.B. Internalized Weight Stigma and Weight Discrimination: Associations with Quality of Life and Psychosocial Impairment in a Sample Living with Food Insecurity. *Int. J. Environ. Res. Public Health* **2023**, *20*, 7147. [CrossRef]

2. Kendall, A.; Olson, C.M.; Frongillo, E.A., Jr. Validation of the Radimer/Cornell measures of hunger and food insecurity. *J. Nutr.* **1995**, *125*, 2793–2801. [CrossRef]
3. Radimer, K.L.; Olson, C.M.; Greene, J.C.; Campbell, C.C.; Habicht, J.-P. Understanding hunger and developing indicators to assess it in women and children. *J. Nutr. Educ.* **1992**, *24*, 36S–44S. [CrossRef]
4. Tatham, M.; Turner, H.; Mountford, V.A.; Tritt, A.; Dyas, R.; Waller, G. Development, psychometric properties and preliminary clinical validation of a brief, session-by-session measure of eating disorder cognitions and behaviors: The ED-15. *Int. J. Eat. Disord.* **2015**, *48*, 1005–1015. [CrossRef]
5. Spitzer, R.L.; Kroenke, K.; Williams, J.B.; Löwe, B. A brief measure for assessing generalized anxiety disorder: The GAD-7. *Arch. Intern. Med.* **2006**, *166*, 1092–1097. [CrossRef]
6. Kroenke, K.; Spitzer, R.L.; Williams, J.B.; Löwe, B. The patient health questionnaire somatic, anxiety, and depressive symptom scales: A systematic review. *Gen. Hosp. Psychiatry* **2010**, *32*, 345–359. [CrossRef]
7. Razykov, I.; Ziegelstein, R.C.; Whooley, M.A.; Thombs, B.D. The PHQ-9 versus the PHQ-8—Is item 9 useful for assessing suicide risk in coronary artery disease patients? Data from the Heart and Soul Study. *J. Psychosom. Res.* **2012**, *73*, 163–168. [CrossRef]
8. Pires, A.C.; Fleck, M.P.; Power, M.; da Rocha, N.S. Psychometric properties of the EUROHIS-QOL 8-item index (WHOQOL-8) in a Brazilian sample. *Rev. Bras. Psiquiatr.* **2018**, *40*, 249–255. [CrossRef]
9. Bohn, K.; Doll, H.A.; Cooper, Z.; O'Connor, M.; Palmer, R.L.; Fairburn, C.G. The measurement of impairment due to eating disorder psychopathology. *Behav. Res. Ther.* **2008**, *46*, 1105–1110. [CrossRef] [PubMed]
0. Lillis, J.; Luoma, J.B.; Levin, M.E.; Hayes, S.C. Measuring weight self-stigma: The weight self-stigma questionnaire. *Obesity* **2010**, *18*, 971–976. [CrossRef] [PubMed]
1. Duarte, C.; Pinto-Gouveia, J.; Ferreira, C.; Batista, D. Body image as a source of shame: A new measure for the assessment of the multifaceted nature of body image shame. *Clin. Psychol. Psychother.* **2015**, *22*, 656–666. [CrossRef] [PubMed]
2. Wilfred, S. "I Can't. I Just Can't Anymore!": Considering the Impact of Microaggressions and Discrimination on Binge Eating Behavior Among Black Women. Ph.D. Thesis, University of Missouri, Kansas City, MO, USA, 2024.
3. Favaretto, E.; Bedani, F.; Brancati, G.E.; De Berardis, D.; Giovannini, S.; Scarcella, L.; Martiadis, V.; Martini, A.; Pampaloni, I.; Perugi, G.; et al. Synthesising 30 years of clinical experience and scientific insight on affective temperaments in psychiatric disorders: State of the art. *J. Affect. Disord.* **2024**, *362*, 406–415. [CrossRef] [PubMed]

nutrients

MDPI

Article

Parental Perspectives on Eating Disorders of Their School-Age Children with ADHD in Hong Kong: A Qualitative Study

Shu-Cheng Chen [1], To Ming Stanley Wu [2], Han Li [3], Jia-Wen Shou [4], Jing Qin [1], Guo-Tao Wu [5,*], Wai-Yin Cheng [6] and Wing-Fai Yeung [3,7,8,*]

1 Centre for Smart Health, School of Nursing, The Hong Kong Polytechnic University, Hung Hom, Hong Kong, China; shucheng.chen@connect.polyu.hk (S.-C.C.)
2 Department of Rehabilitation Sciences, The Hong Kong Polytechnic University, Hong Kong, China
3 School of Nursing, The Hong Kong Polytechnic University, Hong Kong, China
4 Li Dak Sum Yip Yio Chin R&D Centre for Chinese Medicine, The Chinese University of Hong Kong, Hong Kong, China
5 Psychology Department, Southwest University, Chongqing 400715, China
6 Department of Food Science and Nutrition, The Hong Kong Polytechnic University, Hong Kong, China
7 Research Center for Chinese Medicine Innovation, The Hong Kong Polytechnic University, Hong Kong, China
8 Research Institute for Smart Ageing, The Hong Kong Polytechnic University, Hong Kong, China
* Correspondence: gtgtgtwu@163.com (G.-T.W.); jerry-wf.yeung@polyu.edu.hk (W.-F.Y.)

Abstract: Background: Children with attention deficit hyperactivity disorder (ADHD) frequently encounter eating problems. However, qualitative research on the eating problems of these children and the strategies employed by their parents to manage these issues remains limited. This study aimed to explore the eating problems of school-age children with ADHD and the coping strategies used by parents in urban settings like Hong Kong. **Methods:** A descriptive qualitative design was utilized, employing semi-structured focus group interviews. Purposive sampling was used to recruit 12 parents who voluntarily participated in five focus group sessions. The interviews were conducted in Cantonese, audio-recorded, and transcribed verbatim. Data were analyzed using template thematic analysis to identify key themes and subthemes. **Results:** Two major themes emerged: challenges affecting ADHD children's eating behaviors and parental coping strategies in Hong Kong. Children's eating difficulties stemmed from ADHD-specific behaviors, compounded by Hong Kong's demanding educational system and urban environmental constraints. In response, parents developed multifaceted coping approaches, ranging from dietary modifications and behavioral management strategies to healthcare resource utilization, while adapting their urban lifestyle to accommodate their children's needs. **Conclusions:** Children with ADHD face eating challenges that intersect with Hong Kong's sociocultural environment, where educational pressure, limited living spaces, and parents' work schedules influence their eating patterns. Parents adopt integrated Eastern–Western approaches, supported by Hong Kong's comprehensive healthcare resources spanning professional networks and community programs. Evidence-based dietary guidelines are essential to address ADHD-related nutritional misconceptions.

Keywords: ADHD; eating problems; parental strategies; qualitative research; school-age children; Hong Kong

1. Background

1.1. Attention Deficit Hyperactivity Disorder (ADHD)

ADHD is a neurodevelopmental disorder characterized by persistent patterns of inattention, hyperactivity, and impulsivity that interfere with functioning or development [1]. It is one of the most common mental disorders in children, with an estimated incidence rate of 5–8% globally [2–4]. The primary symptoms of ADHD include difficulty sustaining attention, excessive activity, and impulsive behavior [5]. ADHD frequently coexists with other psychiatric and developmental disorders, such as anxiety, depression, and learning disabilities, complicating its clinical presentation and management [6]. This disorder considerably influences not only the affected children, leading to challenges in academic performance and social relationships, but also their families, who often experience heightened stress and disruption in daily routines [7]. Conventional interventions for ADHD typically involve pharmacological treatments, such as stimulant medications, and behavioral therapies [8]. However, these interventions have limitations, including side effects, variability in individual response, and insufficient long-term efficacy in some cases [9].

1.2. Eating Problems of Children with ADHD

Children with ADHD frequently encounter considerable eating problems, which can present as irregular eating patterns, diminished appetite and overeating, and a tendency towards unhealthy food choices [10,11]. These patterns vary significantly among ADHD subtypes, with predominantly inattentive and combined types showing higher risk of overweight status, while the hyperactive type is often associated with a lower BMI [12]. For example, among children with ADHD, 29% were at risk of being overweight and 17.3% were classified as overweight [11], with a higher prevalence observed in the inattentive and combined subtypes [13]. These issues often include symptoms such as skipping meals, overeating, food selectivity, and a preference for high-sugar and high-fat foods [14,15]. Such eating problems can negatively affect physical health, leading to obesity, nutritional deficiencies, and poor growth patterns [16,17]. In school-age children, these eating problems can exacerbate ADHD symptoms, adversely affecting their cognitive function, energy levels, and overall academic performance [18,19]. The causes of eating problems in children with ADHD are multifaceted, involving a combination of genetic, neurobiological, and environmental factors [20]. Neurobiological factors include the dysregulation of dopamine pathways, which play a critical role in reward processing and appetite control [21]. The impulsivity and inattention characteristic of ADHD can hinder the development of healthy eating habits [22], particularly affecting those with the predominantly inattentive type through a decreased awareness of satiety cues [23]. ADHD medications, particularly stimulants, can contribute to eating problems by suppressing appetite, leading to reduced food intake and weight loss [24,25]. Without medication, children may demonstrate increased impulsive eating behaviors and difficulty in recognizing satiety signals [26]. Environmental influences, such as family mealtime dynamics and the availability of healthy food options, play a crucial role [27,28]. Addressing these eating problems is essential for improving the overall health and well-being of children with ADHD, necessitating a multidisciplinary approach that encompasses dietary management [29], behavioral strategies [30], and parental training and education [31,32].

1.3. Research Gap

Eating problems among children with ADHD are prevalent, and the effect these issues have on their health and development is considerable. However, most existing studies focus predominantly on the core and behavioral symptoms of ADHD, often overlooking the nuanced dietary challenges and parental feeding practices. A notable gap exists in the literature regarding the specific eating problems of school-age children with ADHD and the strategies employed by parents to manage these problems [10,18]. While some research has recognized the influence of ADHD interventions on appetite and eating patterns [24,33], qualitative data capturing the firsthand experiences and perspectives of children and their parents in real-world settings are limited. This gap is particularly pronounced in the context of densely populated urban environments, such as Hong Kong, where unique cultural, social, and environmental factors may influence dietary habits and parental strategies [34]. The present study aimed to address this gap by utilizing focus group interviews conducted in Hong Kong to delve into the eating habits of school-age children with ADHD, the specific dietary issues they face, and the coping strategies parents employ. The results could provide valuable insights into the multifaceted nature of eating problems in children with ADHD within a supercity context and inform more effective, tailored support to these families.

2. Methods

This study utilized a descriptive qualitative design [35], grounded in naturalistic inquiry, to achieve a comprehensive understanding of a specific event. The research findings were reported in alignment with the Consolidated Criteria for Reporting Qualitative Research [36].

2.1. Participants and Settings

Recruitment occurred in Hong Kong between February and March 2024, utilizing promotional posters on Facebook and invitations via WhatsApp (Meta Platforms, Inc., iOS Version 24.2.1). Parents of school-age children with ADHD were invited to participate. The participants joined the individual interviews to discuss their experiences and perspectives on their children's eating behavior and parental feeding strategies. Written information about the qualitative study was provided to potential participants to assess their interest in participation. The informed consent form comprehensively detailed the study's purpose, design, methodology, benefits, risks, and data privacy protocols and included contact information for further inquiries. The inclusion criteria specified that participants must be (1) parents of children aged 6–8 years with a documented ADHD diagnosis and (2) residents of Hong Kong who were fluent in Cantonese. The participants' preferred interview times were recorded, and mutually convenient schedules were arranged. Following a thorough explanation of the study's purpose, procedures, and importance, the participants provided a written informed consent. The participants were also informed about the use of audio recordings, assured of the confidentiality of their information, and apprised of their right to withdraw from the study at any time without penalty. Focus group interviews, a qualitative research method that gathers data through guided small-group discussions, were conducted on the campus of The Hong Kong Polytechnic University. This method was chosen because it enables researchers to collect rich data through participant interactions and group discussions. A sample size of approximately 12–24 participants was determined necessary to achieve thematic saturation—the point at which additional interviews no longer generate new themes or substantial insights about the research topic [37]. Thematic saturation helps ensure that sufficient data has been collected to comprehensively understand the phenomenon being studied. Purposive sampling was selected as the most appropriate approach for this study for several reasons. First, it allowed us to identify participants who could provide rich, detailed information about the specific feeding experiences of children with ADHD in Hong Kong. Second, this sampling method enabled us to efficiently recruit participants that met our precise inclusion criteria while managing resource constraints. To ensure participant relevance and minimize selection bias, we implemented a structured screening process requiring (1) a documented ADHD diagnosis from qualified healthcare providers, (2) verification of child's age within the specified range, and (3) confirmation of the parents' direct involvement in daily feeding activities. Participant selection was conducted by two researchers (SCC and HL) using these predetermined criteria to minimize subjective judgment.

2.2. Data Collection

The interview guide, comprising seven open-ended questions in Chinese (Table 1), was initially developed by the first author (SCC). This guide was subsequently revised by an experienced ADHD researcher (GTW) and a qualitative research expert (WFY). Semi-structured focus group interviews were conducted face-to-face by two moderators (SCC and LYP). While traditional focus groups often include 6–8 participants, we deliberately chose smaller groups of 2–3 participants for 3 specific reasons. First, given that ADHD has genetic components, some participating parents may also experience attention-related challenges, making smaller groups more conducive to sustained engagement. Second, the intimate setting of 2–3 participants provided a more confidential environment, particularly important given the stigma often associated with ADHD diagnoses. Third, this format enabled a more in-depth exploration of individual experiences and allowed each participant adequate time to fully articulate their thoughts about the learning platform. A pilot test was conducted with two participants from the first interview group to ensure the comprehensibility of all questions. All interviews were conducted in Cantonese. At the commencement of each session, the moderators introduced themselves, outlined the purpose and procedures of the interview, emphasized the importance of confidentiality, and addressed any questions from the participants. Data collection was halted when thematic saturation was achieved. All interviews were audio-recorded and transcribed verbatim in Chinese prior to data analysis. Participants were offered a cash incentive of HKD 200.

Table 1. Questions for the semi-structured interview.

For your child, what do you consider healthy eating habits?
Do you think your child has any eating problems? If yes, please describe the specific eating problems. If not, please describe your child's usual eating habits.
Does your child have allergic reactions due to improper diet or certain foods?
Have your child's eating problems caused any impact on you?
How do you view the impact of ADHD medication on your child's eating habits?
What factors determine or influence your choices and combinations of food for your child?
For your child's eating problems, what efforts or coping measures have you taken in caring and feeding your child? How effective are they?

2.3. Data Analysis

All interviews were recorded and transcribed verbatim in traditional Chinese prior to data analysis. Each individual was assigned a unique, randomly generated code to ensure participant confidentiality. Descriptive characteristics were employed to summarize the demographic data. Data analysis was conducted using template thematic analysis [38], which is a systematic method for identifying patterns and themes within qualitative data. This process involved developing a thematic code tree—a hierarchical structure that organizes the identified themes from broad categories to specific subthemes. Key quotations, which are representative verbatim excerpts from participants' responses, were extracted from the transcripts to illustrate and support each identified theme in our findings. Two researchers (SCC and HL) independently read each transcript multiple times to thoroughly familiarize themselves with the data, aiming to deeply understand the participants' perspectives on their children's eating habits and parental coping strategies. The researchers manually performed line-by-line coding, condensing the codes based on identified similarities and differences. Higher-level abstract codes were then extracted and organized into subthemes and main themes. Any disagreements between the researchers were resolved through discussion until consensus was reached. Finally, the identified themes and subthemes, along with their representative quotes, were translated into English.

2.4. Trustworthiness

Several procedures were implemented to ensure the trustworthiness of the qualitative data collected from focus groups on the basis of the criteria established by Lincoln: credibility, dependability, confirmability, and transferability [39,40]. For credibility, the focus group protocol was revised during two group meetings, and the discussion questions were pilot tested with two participants. Investigators were selected on the basis of their requisite knowledge and expertise in qualitative research, and purposive sampling techniques were employed to select focus group participants. Dependability was achieved through regular debriefing sessions with WFY, an expert in qualitative studies, and by providing participants with the findings, including the thematic code tree and key quotations, for comments and confirmation. The coding structure was validated by another researcher (GDW) and revalidated by the corresponding author (WFY) through a review of the original transcripts. Confirmability was ensured by returning transcripts to the participants for feedback, maintaining a critical and honest stance through self-scrutiny, and employing negative case analysis to enhance the validity of interpretations. Finally, transferability was addressed by applying the saturation theory to determine the richness of the data [41], with data collection continuing until new information was nearly exhausted by the third focus group session [42].

3. Results

The focus group interviews were conducted between March and April 2024. A total of 38 parents were invited to participate in the study, and 12 accepted the invitation. A total of five focus group interviews were conducted. The interviews had a mean duration of 53.4 min and ranged from 47 min to 59 min. The number of participants in each group ranged from two to three. The participants in each group were unfamiliar with one another. Data saturation was applied to guide the data collection [41], with themes and subthemes that were established in the third focus group interview session and enriched after the fifth focus group session.

3.1. Sample Profile

The twelve parents (ten females [83.3%] and two males [16.7%]) of children with an ADHD diagnosis attended the five sessions. The mean age of the parents was 40.1 years (SD = 3.7), and the mean age of their children was 6.9 years (SD = 0.9). The participants' demographic information is presented in Table 2.

Table 2. Demographic characteristics of the participants interviewed.

Characteristics	All Participants (n = 12)	Session 1 (n = 2)	Session 2 (n = 2)	Session 3 (n = 3)	Session 4 (n = 3)	Session 5 (n = 2)
Age, mean (SD)						
Parents	40.1 (3.7)	37.5 (0.7)	37 (2.8)	40 (3.0)	44.3 (3.2)	39.5 (3.5)
Child	6.9 (0.9)	7.5 (0.7)	6.5 (0.7)	6.3 (0.6)	7.3 (1.2)	7 (1.4)
Gender (parents), n (%)						
Male	2 (16.7)	0 (0)	0 (0)	1 (33.3)	0 (0)	1 (50)
Female	10 (83.3)	2 (100)	2 (100)	2 (66.7)	3 (100)	1 (50)
Gender (child), n (%)						
Male	10 (83.3)	2 (100)	2 (100)	2 (66.7)	3 (100)	1 (50)
Female	2 (16.7)	0 (0)	0 (0)	1 (33.3)	0 (0)	1 (50)

Table 2. *Cont.*

Characteristics	All Participants (n = 12)	Session 1 (n = 2)	Session 2 (n = 2)	Session 3 (n = 3)	Session 4 (n = 3)	Session 5 (n = 2)
Level of education (parents), n (%)						
Senior high school	4 (33.3)	1 (50)	1 (50)	2 (66.7)	0 (0)	0 (0)
College or above	8 (66.7)	1 (50)	1 (50)	1 (33.3)	3 (100)	2 (100)
Career (parents), n (%)						
Professional/Semi-professional	4 (33.3)	0 (0)	1 (50)	1 (33.3)	1 (33.3)	1 (50)
Unskilled worker	1 (8.3)	1 (50)	0 (0)	0 (0)	0 (0)	0 (0)
Homemaker	5 (41.7)	0 (0)	1 (50)	1 (33.3)	2 (66.7)	1 (50)
Others	2 (16.7)	1 (50)	0 (0)	1 (33.3)	0 (0)	0 (0)
Child's BMI, mean (SD)	14.3 (1.8)	13.7 (1.3)	14.1 (1.8)	13.7 (0.7)	16.1 (2.7)	13.2 (0.05)
Treatment for children's ADHD, n (%)						
Medicine	3 (25)	1 (50)	0 (0)	1 (33.3)	0 (0)	1 (50)
CBT	3 (25)	0 (0)	0 (0)	1 (33.3)	2 (66.7)	0 (0)
Others	1 (8.3)	0 (0)	0 (0)	1 (33.3)	0 (0)	0 (0)

Abbreviations: SD: standard deviation; ADHD: attention deficit hyperactivity disorder; CBT: cognitive behavioral therapy; BMI: body mass index.

3.2. Major Themes

In terms of the parents' expression of their children's eating problems and their parental coping strategies, two main themes were identified from the data: (1) challenges affecting ADHD children's eating behaviors in Hong Kong and (2) parents' coping strategies in Hong Kong. The specific subthemes under each theme were described, and Table 3 presents the code structure. Following the established thematic analysis methodology [43], our analysis focused on identifying meaningful patterns across the dataset. Our interpretations were shaped by our theoretical frameworks and research context, acknowledging that different researchers might develop varying interpretations recognized strength in qualitative inquiry. Through team discussions and reflexive practice, we ensured our interpretations remained grounded in the data. In selecting illustrative quotes, we considered: (1) how the quote captured the participants' lived experiences; (2) the richness and depth of expression in conveying the concept; and (3) how well it represented the essence of the identified theme. While we note when multiple participants ($\geq$4) expressed similar views, the significance of the themes was determined by their capacity to illuminate meaningful aspects of the phenomenon under study rather than quantitative prevalence.

3.2.1. Challenges Affecting ADHD Children's Eating Behaviors in Hong Kong

The challenges presented three subthemes: (a) ADHD-specific eating behaviors, (b) challenges related to the local educational system, and (c) challenges related to the urban environment.

ADHD-Specific Eating Behaviors

The participants reported various challenges regarding their children's eating problems, categorized into ADHD eating patterns, the impact of ADHD medication, and ADHD-related allergic reactions. The parents described mealtimes as particularly stressful when children exhibit impulsive and hyperactive behaviors; one parent noted, "Sometimes when his emotions flare up, he becomes very unreasonable. Mealtimes are always stressful. He can't sit still, keeps moving around, and needs constant supervision." (031). Another common issue was the erratic engagement with food, with children often leaving the table if not immediately interested in eating: "Most of the time, if he's not really hungry, he'll just walk away and do something else first." (024). The impact of ADHD medication further complicated eating behaviors, as it tended to significantly reduce appetite and can also affect sleep, growth, and emotional stability: "He already eats very little, and after his

ADHD medication, his appetite drops even more. He barely eats a few bites, and no matter what we offer, it seems useless." (015); "ADHD medication affected his sleep, reduced his appetite, impacted his height growth, and also caused emotional problems." (059). Additionally, ADHD-related allergies presented another layer of complexity, requiring parents to vigilantly monitor and adapt diets to manage sudden allergic reactions to common foods: "When he was young, he suddenly itched after eating salmon, then eggs... once he suddenly became allergic to beef, itching after eating it." (031); "He has respiratory issues when eating citrus, oranges, strawberries, and mangoes, so we have to be careful with his diet." (012).

Table 3. Code structures.

Themes	Subthemes	Code Units
• Challenges affecting ADHD children's eating behaviors in Hong Kong	• ADHD-specific eating behaviors	• Impulsive/hyperactive/attentive eating patterns • ADHD medication impact • ADHD-related allergic constitution impact
	• Challenges related to the local educational system	• School schedule impact (e.g., morning routine, course schedule) • Academic workload impact (e.g., homework culture) • Teacher–student interaction impact (e.g., children's emotional problems)
	• Challenges related to the urban environment	• Parents' extended working hours • Reliance on domestic helpers • Ubiquitous fast-food accessibility • Cramped living spaces
• Parents' coping strategies in Hong Kong	• ADHD dietary strategies	• General dietary adjustments (e.g., rice, sugar, yogurt) • Traditional Chinese dietary approaches (e.g., Chinese dietary soup)
	• Behavioral management	• Planning physical activity • Innovating eating approaches (e.g., incentives, tableware, cooking involvement) • Regulating children's emotion
	• Hong Kong healthcare resource utilization	• Dual alternative therapy options (traditional and modern approaches) • Health information resources (e.g., media, seminar) • Professional support networks (e.g., university research, open courses) • ADHD parent peer support • School–family collaboration
	• Urban lifestyle adaptation	• Fast-paced schedule management • Home environment adjustment (e.g., family member, dining space) • Home–outside eating balance • Domestic helper integration

Challenges related to the local educational system

Educational challenges were related to the school schedule, academic workload, and teacher–student interactions. School schedules in Hong Kong are particularly demanding, with early starts and long days that disrupt normal eating patterns, as one parent explained, "In the morning, I prepare breakfast for him, and even though he should be hungry, he often doesn't eat—perhaps waking up early affects his appetite." (001). The extended school hours also leave little time for other activities, further impacting children's well-being: "Hong Kong students' daily school schedules are really long—by the time they get home after school, there's basically no time left for other activities." (012). Additionally, the heavy academic workload exacerbates stress, with extensive homework that overwhelms these children and complicates time management: "In primary school, homework just piles up—that's his focus. Everything is laid out there, making it difficult to manage time." (043). Negative teacher–student interactions also profoundly affect these children, leading to emotional distress and decreased appetite: "He came home saying the teacher scolded him, which affected his mood completely. He barely had any appetite for dinner." (001); "His teacher treats him as if he has intellectual disabilities... these students already struggle to cope with regular classes—if teachers are also impatient with them, they simply cannot survive in school." (059).

Challenges related to the urban environment

This subtheme reflects key factors contributing to the difficulties of parents living in supercities like Hong Kong. Extended working hours for parents were a significant concern, with one parent noting, "There was a period when I was extremely busy and couldn't take care of him. Both his father and I leave early and return late from work." (001), indicating the limited parental supervision available due to job commitments. This often necessitates reliance on domestic helpers, which introduces its own set of challenges: "I believe healthy eating habits start with regular mealtimes and appropriate portions. Since I have to work, I rely on our domestic helper to take care of him. The domestic helper has limited authority—when she's watching the children, they will read while eating because they don't respect her." (031), highlighting issues of authority and adherence to structured eating practices. Additionally, the ubiquity of fast-food options poses a further obstacle, particularly in densely populated urban areas where convenience often overrides nutritional consideration: "When we lived in Ap Lei Chau, there was a McDonald's nearby. He would always insist on having the McChicken meal and refuse to eat anything else. He absolutely had to have McDonald's." (012), illustrating the temptation and ease of access to less healthy food choices in Hong Kong's compact residential districts. Cramped living conditions also exacerbate these challenges, as limited space can disrupt mealtime routines and behavior management: "When preparing dinner, because our home is small, we all eat together in the living room where space is limited. When he can't sit still and moves around, there's not much we can do." (024).

3.2.2. Parents' Coping Strategies in Hong Kong

Parents' strategies revealed four subthemes: (a) ADHD dietary strategies, (b) behavioral management, (c) Hong Kong healthcare resource utilization, and (d) urban lifestyle adaptation.

ADHD Dietary Strategies

Dietary adjustments have been adopted on several aspects. One approach was avoiding foods with artificial additives believed to affect emotional stability: "I know that foods with too many artificial colorings can affect emotional stability, so now I pay special attention to choosing healthy foods for my children and won't let them eat carelessly." (012). A parent eliminated white rice and sugar, substituting them with alternatives like cane or brown sugar to mitigate hyperactivity: "I heard that white rice isn't good for ADHD children, so our whole family stopped eating white rice... we also stopped using white sugar, switching to cane sugar or brown sugar because white sugar has many chemicals that make ADHD children more hyper." (043). Another said: "I mainly buy avocado, nuts, fish... telling him not to eat so many snacks, I saw a news report saying they affect attention." (013). Additionally, probiotic-rich foods were incorporated based on their potential benefits for gut health, which was linked to cognitive and emotional well-being: "After hearing a university study that certain probiotics are good for children's intestines, the body's second brain, I try to find these foods for him, like yogurt or Yakult." (012). Traditional Chinese dietary methods were also utilized, one said: "Because I have seen a Chinese medicine practitioner frequently sharing on social media about how to strengthen the spleen, discussing purple yam powder and black bean powder, and I prepare these drinks for my son." (052).

Behavioral Management

The parents employed several behavioral management strategies to improve eating habits, focusing on physical activity, innovative mealtime tactics, and emotional regulation. Physical exercises like orienteering are used to stimulate appetite, as one parent notes: "Inducing hunger makes him willing to eat... On Fridays he participated in orienteering, running for two hours, then going to school and coming back, he would actually ask for food" (012). Innovative eating elements include incentives and clever tableware adjustments; for example, parents use time-bound rewards to motivate their children: "Using rewards, for example, I tell my son if he eats earlier, then Dad will play with him for a while... if he finishes eating by 9, he'll have 15 min to play; if he's late, the playtime will be reduced." (004), and oversized bowls to visually reduce portion sizes: "My friend's child eats very little, so he humorously bought a large bowl to make the usual amount look small, making the child think they finished it in just two bites." (050). Involvement in food preparation also encourages eating: "She buys groceries himself or helps with cooking, and she eats more..." (015). Regulating emotions through enjoyable and timely meals is crucial; one parent describes how improving the mealtime environment positively impacted their child's appetite: "Because he has emotional issues, I put effort into making things he likes and make fun shapes in his lunchbox... Now he's in second grade, he has become quite chubby... Since he gets very irritable when hungry, dinner must always be on time." (031).

Hong Kong Healthcare Resource Utilization

The parents utilized a blend of healthcare resources in Hong Kong. Some parents explored non-pharmaceutical treatments to promote healthy development: "We're currently considering exercise therapy or acupuncture as treatment options for my child." (012); "I've tried non-pharmaceutical treatments on my child, such as acupuncture and *tuina*, to support their healthy development." (001). Health information resources also play a critical role, with parents frequently consulting medical columns in magazines and attending seminars to gain insights into ADHD management: "We read medical columns in magazines and newspapers where doctors share advice on what soups to drink and what foods can help boost a child's health and reduce frailty." (043); "I attended a talk by a psychiatrist at Heep Hong Society who mentioned that ADHD medications can reduce children's appetite, and long-term use of ADHD medications might lead to high blood pressure, high blood sugar, and high cholesterol." (012). Professional support networks are crucial, with parents engaging in university research and open courses that provide training and resources: "We joined a university study using pediatric *tuina* for ADHD. The practitioners analyzed the issues and taught us the techniques... They even sent me teaching videos afterward—it was excellent." (013); "Over these past few years, we've been regularly taking our son to various classes and different centers, and he has also participated in social skills groups." (004). Peer support among parents is another valuable resource, where sharing experiences and tips online helps in discovering new coping strategies: "I look up other ADHD mothers' suggestions online. For example, someone mentioned cooking partridge soup with Tiger's Milk mushroom and *Lingzhi*" (050); "I often read friends' shared experiences and online information, which consistently mention that ADHD medications affect appetite, so I keep reminding myself about this." (013). Lastly, school–family collaboration is emphasized to ensure a supportive educational environment without over-reliance on medication: "If he's not disrupting classroom order, there's no need for medication. Even now that he's in Primary 1 and 2, I regularly discuss with his class teachers." (012).

Urban Lifestyle Adaptation

Urban lifestyle adaptation plays a crucial role for ADHD families in Hong Kong. Parents adjusted their family routines to accommodate the needs of their children. A mother mentioned: "Lack of sleep affects his mood and eating habits... so we've adjusted to having dinner at 6 p.m. and bedtime at 8:30 p.m., allowing proper digestion before sleep." (031). Adjustments to the home environment are also significant. Some families preferred to limit the influence of extended family members, like grandparents, to maintain consistent discipline and routines. One said: "it's better that we don't live with the grandparents normally, as there's less intervention. They tend to be too permissive with their grandchild..." (012). Additionally, eating environment adjustments were implemented to improve focus and eating habits: "During his toddler years, he needed TV while eating. We transitioned from TV to children's songs, and finally to picture books during meals.", a parent mentioned (050). The balance between home-cooked and outside meals was carefully managed: "I think environmental factors are very important—eating out versus eating at home is different. When we're out, I allow them to eat less healthy foods... But at home, it must be healthy—home-cooked meals are never deep-fried, and we use less sugar and salt." (052). Furthermore, the integration of domestic helpers into the family's routine involved specific instructions to ensure that dietary guidelines are followed, enhancing consistency in the child's diet: "I remind our domestic helper how to feed my children, for example, serving the child enough portions of rice..." (031).

4. Discussion

4.1. Main Findings

This study aimed to explore the eating problems of school-age children diagnosed with ADHD and the coping strategies employed by their parents in urban areas like Hong Kong. The use of descriptive semi-structured, face-to-face focus group interviews facilitated rich, dynamic discussions that uncovered a wide range of parental strategies and challenges, enhancing the depth of the data collected [44]. This study is the first to specifically focus on the eating problems of school-age children with ADHD and the real-world coping strategies of their parents within the context of a developed and densely populated urban environment like Hong Kong. This unique cultural, social, and environmental context provided a rich backdrop for understanding the dynamics of eating problems in children with ADHD. The findings contribute valuable insights that could inform more effective, tailored interventions to support families dealing with ADHD in similar urban settings. Through a thematic analysis, two major themes emerged: (1) challenges affecting ADHD children's eating behaviors in Hong Kong and (2) parents' coping strategies in Hong Kong. The key findings revealed the multifaceted nature of eating challenges among children with ADHD, encompassing ADHD-specific eating problems, as well as Hong Kong's educational and environmental challenges. Furthermore, parents employed a range of strategies to manage their children's eating problems, including ADHD dietary approaches, behavioral management, Hong Kong healthcare resource utilization, and urban lifestyle adaption.

4.2. Comparison with Previous Studies

The findings of this study align with several observations from earlier research. First, the difficulties related to children's eating problems, such as slow eating, distraction, and picky eating, match those observed in earlier studies on children with ADHD [10]. These problems can exacerbate mealtime challenges and increase parental stress, as noted in previous literature. Second, the influence of ADHD symptoms on eating problems, such as hyperactivity and inattention, is in accord with recent studies that highlighted the role of neurobiological factors in disrupting regular eating patterns [45]. Lastly, the negative effect of ADHD medication on appetite and eating problems, such as reduced food intake and weight loss, has been consistently documented in prior studies [46–50]. The present study also highlighted considerable issues related to children's constitution, such as allergies and poor gastrointestinal function, which affect their eating problems. These findings suggest that the physiological challenges faced by children with ADHD are compounded by their eating issues, necessitating a comprehensive approach to dietary management that considers behavioral and medical factors. The literature indicates that children with ADHD often have comorbid conditions like gastrointestinal issues and food allergies, which can further complicate their eating problems [51,52]. The considerable effect of allergies and gastrointestinal issues on children's eating problems warrants further investigation. Our findings reveal the co-occurrence of allergic conditions among participants with ADHD, which aligns with growing evidence of this association in the literature. Recent meta-analyses have shown that individuals with ADHD have a significantly higher prevalence of allergic diseases compared to those without ADHD [53]. The biological mechanisms underlying this association may involve shared inflammatory pathways and neuroimmune interactions. Studies suggest that inflammatory mediators can affect dopamine and norepinephrine systems, which are implicated in ADHD pathophysiology [54]. Additionally, both conditions share common genetic risk factors and environmental triggers that may contribute to their co-occurrence [55]. This overlap highlights the importance of considering allergic conditions in ADHD clinical management and suggests potential shared pathophysiological mechanisms that warrant further investigation.

However, notable inconsistencies can be observed between the findings of the present study and those of earlier studies. Contrary to some research that suggests a minimal effect of family mealtime dynamics on children's eating behaviors [56], the results of the present study highlight considerable family conflicts and psychological stress associated with managing these eating problems. The possible explanation for this discrepancy may be the unique sociocultural context of Hong Kong, where family cohesion and parental expectations are particularly emphasized, potentially intensifying the stress experienced by parents [57]. Additionally, the narrow living spaces in Hong Kong [58], coupled with immense living pressures, may contribute to heightened family tensions and conflicts during mealtimes. While some studies have reported that educational interventions alone are sufficient to manage eating problems in children with ADHD [59], the findings of the present study suggest that a multifaceted approach, including dietary adjustments, environmental modifications, and physical activity, is more effective. The development of the city likely makes parents more focused on education and more patient with their children [60]. They have more channels through which to learn scientific methods for managing ADHD and access to more resources than those in less developed areas [61]. This increased access to information and resources enables parents to implement a broader range of strategies to effectively manage their children's eating problems. Additionally, while participants demonstrated BMI values within the normal range, parental reports indicated concerns about lean body composition and slower weight gain. This pattern aligns with the existing literature documenting differential weight presentations across ADHD subtypes.

Previous research has established that inattentive and combined subtypes tend toward a higher BMI [12], while predominantly hyperactive presentations often associate with normal to lower BMI ranges. In our interviews, parental concerns primarily centered on selective eating, nutritional adequacy, and maintaining adequate weight, rather than weight excess. This pattern may reflect several factors: first, our sample potentially included a higher proportion of hyperactive-type ADHD children; second, the low prevalence of medication use among participants may have influenced the observed eating behavior patterns; and third, the unique dietary culture and lifestyle patterns in Hong Kong may have contributed to these outcomes. These findings suggest the need for future research to systematically document and analyze ADHD subtype distribution, explore dietary behavioral variations across subtypes, and examine the impact of medication status on eating behaviors.

Some parents reported using innovative methods to encourage their children to eat, including using large bowls to create the illusion of smaller portions and using food coloring to make meals more appealing. These strategies highlight the parents' willingness to experiment with unconventional methods to overcome eating challenges. Previous research supports the idea that visual and sensory enhancements can improve children's eating behavior by making food more attractive and engaging [62]. Involving children in food preparation emerged as another effective strategy, with parents noting increased food intake when children participated in buying groceries or cooking. This approach fosters improved eating habits and a sense of responsibility and engagement, aligning with the concept of participatory education. Studies have shown that involving children in food preparation can increase their willingness to try new foods and improve their overall dietary habits [63,64]. The innovative eating methods suggest a need to explore creative, child-friendly strategies for managing eating problems in children with ADHD. Future studies could investigate the effects of playful techniques and the involvement of children in food preparation to managing ADHD-related eating problems.

Notably, Hong Kong possesses comprehensive healthcare resources and support systems, including professional networks, university research programs, and community health organizations that can be leveraged to develop and disseminate evidence-based dietary guidance, providing a foundation for implementing targeted nutritional education programs for ADHD families. However, the analysis of parental narratives revealed prevalent misconceptions regarding the dietary management of ADHD. Parents reported various dietary modifications and restrictions based on common beliefs about food impacts on ADHD symptoms. Many of these dietary interventions lack evidence support; particularly, the widely held belief about sugar inducing hyperactivity has been consistently disproven in controlled studies [65,66]. While elimination diets show limited efficacy in specific cases of food sensitivities, general food category restrictions remain unsupported by current evidence [67,68]. This disparity between parental practices and evidence-based recommendations underscores the need for professional dietary guidelines that bridge cultural beliefs and scientific evidence [12], particularly within Hong Kong's unique healthcare context.

4.3. Implications

This study has several implications across various domains. For ADHD researchers, the findings underscore the necessity of exploring the multifaceted nature of eating problems in children with ADHD. Further qualitative and quantitative studies are needed to capture the living experiences of families in diverse cultural and urban context, as well as develop a more comprehensive understanding of the challenges related to ADHD and eating problems. Further studies should explore the direct impact of ADHD-related impulsivity on eating behaviors to understand better the mechanisms that lead to eating disorders in this population. Longitudinal studies could track changes in eating behaviors over time, relating them to impulsivity levels and ADHD symptom management.

While our study provides valuable insights, we acknowledge potential sampling issues. Our participant pool included 66.7% (8/12) of parents with college education or above, which may not fully represent Hong Kong's general population. This high proportion of well-educated parents in our sample partially reflects Hong Kong's unique socio-educational context, where there is strong emphasis on academic achievement and high educational attainment. Hong Kong's competitive education system and cultural value placed on academic excellence may influence how parents approach their children's ADHD and eating issues. Well-educated parents might be more proactive in seeking medical attention and participating in research studies, which could explain their overrepresentation in our sample. Future studies should consider strategies to recruit participants from more diverse educational backgrounds to better represent the full spectrum of Hong Kong families.

For ADHD experts and pediatricians, a holistic approach should be adopted to manage ADHD in children, integrating specific eating problems, parental strategies, and behavioral and medical interventions. For ADHD families, parents and other caregivers of children could refer to the strategies identified in this study (e.g., using innovative methods to make meals more appealing) to improve children's eating habits. Moreover, creating structured and supervised eating environments might help manage the impulsive eating behaviors typically seen in children with ADHD. Integrating these strategies with general ADHD treatment could lead to more holistic care and better overall outcomes for affected children.

4.4. Limitations

This study has several limitations. First, the sample was limited to parents of children with ADHD in Hong Kong, predominantly representing those from higher educational backgrounds, which may limit generalizability to different cultural or socioeconomic contexts. Nevertheless, the findings may be applicable to other urban Chinese populations with similar educational and socioeconomic characteristics. Second, the study focused solely on parental perspectives and lacked input from children with ADHD themselves. Third, the high heritability of ADHD suggests that some participating parents may exhibit ADHD-related emotional characteristics, which may have led to the exaggeration of certain issues and emotions, especially in group dynamics. Finally, while our smaller focus groups (2–3 participants) differed from traditional sizes (6–8), this decision addressed the unique needs of our study population, offering better scheduling flexibility, sustained engagement, and privacy protection for ADHD parents. Through multiple small groups, we achieved thematic saturation while maintaining intimate peer discussions.

5. Conclusions

The findings reveal that children with ADHD face eating challenges uniquely shaped by Hong Kong's advanced metropolitan environment. The city's intense academic pressure, limited living spaces, and parents' demanding work schedules—characteristics typical of this developed society—significantly impact children's eating patterns. Parents have adapted by integrating Eastern and Western approaches, leveraging Hong Kong's world-class healthcare infrastructure of professional networks, alternative therapies, and community programs. These findings highlight the critical role of urban-specific healthcare support in addressing ADHD-related eating challenge. Evidence-based dietary guidelines are imperative to address parental misconceptions in ADHD management.

Author Contributions: S.-C.C.: Conceptualization, Methodology, Writing—original draft. T.M.S.W.: Conceptualization, Formal analysis. H.L.: Data Curation, Formal analysis. J.-W.S.: Writing—Review and Editing. J.Q.: Writing—Review and Editing. G.-T.W.: Conceptualization, Data Curation, Formal analysis. W.-Y.C.: Writing—Review and Editing. W.-F.Y.: Methodology, Formal analysis, Writing—Review and Editing. All authors approved the final manuscript. All authors have read and agreed to the published version of the manuscript.

Funding: This research received no external funding.

Institutional Review Board Statement: The study was conducted in accordance with the Declaration of Helsinki, and approved by the Institutional Review Board of the Hong Kong Polytechnic University (Ref. No.: HSEARS20230810005; 13 September 2023).

Informed Consent Statement: Informed consent was obtained from all subjects involved in the study.

Data Availability Statement: The research data are available from the corresponding author upon request, with personal information redacted to ensure privacy.

Conflicts of Interest: All authors declare that there are no potential conflict of interests.

References

1. American Psychiatric Association. *Diagnostic and Statistical Manual of Mental Disorders*, 5th ed.; American Psychiatric Publishing: Arlington, VA, USA, 2013.
2. Polanczyk, G.; de Lima, M.S.; Horta, B.L.; Biederman, J.; Rohde, L.A. The worldwide prevalence of ADHD: A systematic review and metaregression analysis. *Am. J. Psychiatry* **2007**, *164*, 942–948. [CrossRef] [PubMed]
3. Thomas, R.; Sanders, S.; Doust, J.; Beller, E.; Glasziou, P. Prevalence of attention-deficit/hyperactivity disorder: A systematic review and meta-analysis. *Pediatrics* **2015**, *135*, e994–e1001. [CrossRef] [PubMed]
4. Willcutt, E.G. The prevalence of DSM-IV attention-deficit/hyperactivity disorder: A meta-analytic review. *Neurotherapeutics* **2012**, *9*, 490–499. [CrossRef] [PubMed]
5. Barkley, R.A. *Attention-Deficit Hyperactivity Disorder: A Handbook for Diagnosis and Treatment*; Guilford Publications: New York, NY, USA, 2014.
6. Pliszka, S. Practice parameter for the assessment and treatment of children and adolescents with attention-deficit/hyperactivity disorder. *J. Am. Acad. Child. Adolesc. Psychiatry* **2007**, *46*, 894–921. [CrossRef]
7. Harpin, V.A. The effect of ADHD on the life of an individual, their family, and community from preschool to adult life. *Arch. Dis. Child.* **2005**, *90* (Suppl. S1), i2–i7. [CrossRef]
8. Dalrymple, R.A.; Maxwell, L.M.; Russell, S.; Duthie, J. NICE guideline review: Attention deficit hyperactivity disorder: Diagnosis and management (NG87). *Arch. Dis. Child. Educ. Pract.* **2020**, *105*, 289–293. [CrossRef]
9. Faraone, S.V.; Biederman, J.; Spencer, T.J.; Aleardi, M. Comparing the efficacy of medications for ADHD using meta-analysis. *MedGenMed* **2006**, *8*, 4.
10. Cortese, S.; Moreira-Maia, C.R.; St Fleur, D.; Morcillo-Peñalver, C.; Rohde, L.A.; Faraone, S.V. Association Between ADHD and Obesity: A Systematic Review and Meta-Analysis. *Am. J. Psychiatry* **2016**, *173*, 34–43. [CrossRef]
11. Curtin, C.; Bandini, L.G.; Perrin, E.C.; Tybor, D.J.; Must, A. Prevalence of overweight in children and adolescents with attention deficit hyperactivity disorder and autism spectrum disorders: A chart review. *BMC Pediatr.* **2005**, *5*, 48. [CrossRef]
12. Cortese, S.; Tessari, L. Attention-Deficit/Hyperactivity Disorder (ADHD) and Obesity: Update 2016. *Curr. Psychiatry Rep.* **2017**, *19*, 4. [CrossRef]
13. Ptacek, R.; Stefano, G.B.; Weissenberger, S.; Akotia, D.; Raboch, J.; Papezova, H.; Domkarova, L.; Stepankova, T.; Goetz, M. Attention deficit hyperactivity disorder and disordered eating behaviors: Links, risks, and challenges faced. *Neuropsychiatr. Dis. Treat.* **2016**, *12*, 571–579. [CrossRef] [PubMed]
14. Cortese, S.; Angriman, M.; Maffeis, C.; Isnard, P.; Konofal, E.; Lecendreux, M.; Purper-Ouakil, D.; Vincenzi, B.; Bernardina, B.D.; Mouren, M.C. Attention-deficit/hyperactivity disorder (ADHD) and obesity: A systematic review of the literature. *Crit. Rev. Food Sci. Nutr.* **2008**, *48*, 524–537. [CrossRef] [PubMed]
15. Holtkamp, K.; Konrad, K.; Müller, B.; Heussen, N.; Herpertz, S.; Herpertz-Dahlmann, B.; Hebebrand, J. Overweight and obesity in children with Attention-Deficit/Hyperactivity Disorder. *Int. J. Obes. Relat. Metab. Disord.* **2004**, *28*, 685–689. [CrossRef] [PubMed]
16. Waring, M.E.; Lapane, K.L. Overweight in children and adolescents in relation to attention-deficit/hyperactivity disorder: Results from a national sample. *Pediatrics* **2008**, *122*, e1–e6. [CrossRef]
17. Agranat-Meged, A.N.; Deitcher, C.; Goldzweig, G.; Leibenson, L.; Stein, M.; Galili-Weisstub, E. Childhood obesity and attention deficit/hyperactivity disorder: A newly described comorbidity in obese hospitalized children. *Int. J. Eat. Disord.* **2005**, *37*, 357–359. [CrossRef]
18. Kim, J.; Mutyala, B.; Agiovlasitis, S.; Fernhall, B. Health behaviors and obesity among US children with attention deficit hyperactivity disorder by gender and medication use. *Prev. Med.* **2011**, *52*, 218–222. [CrossRef]

19. Cortese, S.; Morcillo Peñalver, C. Comorbidity between ADHD and obesity: Exploring shared mechanisms and clinical implications. *Postgrad. Med.* **2010**, *122*, 88–96. [CrossRef]
20. Davis, C.; Levitan, R.D.; Smith, M.; Tweed, S.; Curtis, C. Associations among overeating, overweight, and attention deficit/hyperactivity disorder: A structural equation modelling approach. *Eat. Behav.* **2006**, *7*, 266–274. [CrossRef]
21. Volkow, N.D.; Chang, L.; Wang, G.J.; Fowler, J.S.; Leonido-Yee, M.; Franceschi, D.; Sedler, M.J.; Gatley, S.J.; Hitzemann, R.; Ding Y.S.; et al. Association of dopamine transporter reduction with psychomotor impairment in methamphetamine abusers. *Am. J. Psychiatry* **2001**, *158*, 377–382. [CrossRef]
22. Groppe, K.; Elsner, B. Executive function and food approach behavior in middle childhood. *Front. Psychol.* **2014**, *5*, 447. [CrossRef
23. Fleming, K.A.; Heintzelman, S.J.; Bartholow, B.D. Specifying Associations Between Conscientiousness and Executive Functioning Mental Set Shifting, Not Prepotent Response Inhibition or Working Memory Updating. *J. Pers.* **2016**, *84*, 348–360. [CrossRef [PubMed]
24. Swanson, J.; Arnold, L.E.; Kraemer, H.; Hechtman, L.; Molina, B.; Hinshaw, S.; Vitiello, B.; Jensen, P.; Steinhoff, K.; Lerner, M. et al. Evidence, interpretation, and qualification from multiple reports of long-term outcomes in the Multimodal Treatment Study of children with ADHD (MTA): Part II: Supporting details. *J. Atten. Disord.* **2008**, *12*, 15–43. [CrossRef] [PubMed]
25. Martyn-Nemeth, P.; Penckofer, S.; Gulanick, M.; Velsor-Friedrich, B.; Bryant, F.B. The relationships among self-esteem, stress coping, eating behavior, and depressive mood in adolescents. *Res. Nurs. Health* **2009**, *32*, 96–109. [CrossRef]
26. Kaisari, P.; Dourish, C.T.; Higgs, S. Attention Deficit Hyperactivity Disorder (ADHD) and disordered eating behaviour: A systematic review and a framework for future research. *Clin. Psychol. Rev.* **2017**, *53*, 109–121. [CrossRef] [PubMed]
27. Fulkerson, J.A.; Larson, N.; Horning, M.; Neumark-Sztainer, D. A review of associations between family or shared meal frequency and dietary and weight status outcomes across the lifespan. *J. Nutr. Educ. Behav.* **2014**, *46*, 2–19. [CrossRef]
28. Berge, J.M.; Wall, M.; Hsueh, T.-F.; Fulkerson, J.A.; Larson, N.; Neumark-Sztainer, D. The protective role of family meals for youth obesity: 10-year longitudinal associations. *J. Pediatr.* **2015**, *166*, 296–301. [CrossRef]
29. Howard, A.L.; Robinson, M.; Smith, G.J.; Ambrosini, G.L.; Piek, J.P.; Oddy, W.H. ADHD is associated with a "Western" dietary pattern in adolescents. *J. Atten. Disord.* **2011**, *15*, 403–411. [CrossRef]
30. Sonuga-Barke, E.J.; Brandeis, D.; Cortese, S.; Daley, D.; Ferrin, M.; Holtmann, M.; Stevenson, J.; Danckaerts, M.; van der Oord, S. Döpfner, M.; et al. Nonpharmacological interventions for ADHD: Systematic review and meta-analyses of randomized controlled trials of dietary and psychological treatments. *Am. J. Psychiatry* **2013**, *170*, 275–289. [CrossRef]
31. Chen, S.C.; Yu, J.; Wang, H.S.; Wang, D.D.; Sun, Y.; Cheng, H.L.; Suen, L.K.; Yeung, W.F. Parent-administered pediatric Tuina for attention deficit/hyperactivity disorder symptoms in preschool children: A pilot randomized controlled trial embedded with a process evaluation. *Phytomedicine* **2022**, *102*, 154191. [CrossRef]
32. Chen, S.C.; Lo, K.C.; Li, H.; Wong, P.M.; Pang, L.Y.; Qin, J.; Yeung, W.F. Parental experiences of administering pediatric tuina for sleep and appetite in early school-aged children with attention deficit hyperactivity disorder: A qualitative study in Hong Kong *JMIR Pediatr. Parent.* **2024**, *12*, 65471. [CrossRef]
33. Chen, S.C.; Cheng, H.L.; Wang, D.D.; Wang, S.; Yin, Y.H.; Suen, L.K.; Yeung, W.F. Experience of parents in delivering pediatric tuina to children with symptoms of attention deficit hyperactivity disorder during the COVID-19 pandemic: Qualitative findings from focus group interviews. *BMC Complement. Med. Ther.* **2023**, *23*, 53. [CrossRef] [PubMed]
34. Stevenson, D. *Cities and Urban Cultures*; McGraw-Hill Education: London, UK, 2003.
35. Sandelowski, M. Focus on research methods: Whatever happened to qualitative description? *Res. Nurs. Health* **2000**, *23*, 334–340 [CrossRef] [PubMed]
36. Tong, A.; Sainsbury, P.; Craig, J. Consolidated criteria for reporting qualitative research (COREQ): A 32-item checklist for interviews and focus groups. *Int. J. Qual. Health Care* **2007**, *19*, 349–357. [CrossRef] [PubMed]
37. Saunders, B.; Sim, J.; Kingstone, T.; Baker, S.; Waterfield, J.; Bartlam, B.; Burroughs, H.; Jinks, C. Saturation in qualitative research Exploring its conceptualization and operationalization. *Qual. Quant.* **2018**, *52*, 1893–1907. [CrossRef] [PubMed]
38. Brooks, J.; McCluskey, S.; Turley, E.; King, N. The Utility of Template Analysis in Qualitative Psychology Research. *Qual. Res Psychol.* **2015**, *12*, 202–222. [CrossRef]
39. Forero, R.; Nahidi, S.; De Costa, J.; Mohsin, M.; Fitzgerald, G.; Gibson, N.; McCarthy, S.; Aboagye-Sarfo, P. Application of four-dimension criteria to assess rigour of qualitative research in emergency medicine. *BMC Health Serv. Res.* **2018**, *18*, 120 [CrossRef]
40. Lincoln, Y.S.; Guba, E.G. *Naturalistic Inquiry*; Sage: Beverly Hills, CA, USA, 1985.
41. Anderson, G.; Arsenault, N. *Fundamentals of Educational Research*; Routledge: London, UK, 2005.
42. Morse, J.M. Critical Analysis of Strategies for Determining Rigor in Qualitative Inquiry. *Qual. Health Res.* **2015**, *25*, 1212–1222 [CrossRef]
43. Braun, V.; Clarke, V. Using thematic analysis in psychology. *Qual. Res. Psychol.* **2006**, *3*, 77–101. [CrossRef]
44. Krueger, R.A. *Focus Groups: A Practical Guide for Applied Research*; Sage Publications: Thousand Oaks, CA, USA, 2014.

35. Soutullo, C.A.; Babatope, T.T. Attention deficit hyperactivity disorder and eating disorders: An overlooked comorbidity? *An. Sist. Sanit. Navar.* **2022**, *45*, e0994. [CrossRef]
36. Paclt, I.; Ptáček, R.; Florián, J. *Hyperaktivita;* Vzdělávací Institut ochrany dětí: Prague, Czech Republic, 2006.
37. Paclt, I.; Florian, J. Attention deficit in hyperactive children. *Ceska A Slov. Psychiatr.* **1996**, *92*, 23–40.
38. Poulton, A. Growth on stimulant medication; clarifying the confusion: A review. *Arch. Dis. Child.* **2005**, *90*, 801–806. [CrossRef] [PubMed]
39. Friedmann, N.; Thomas, J.; Carr, R.; Elders, J.; Ringdahl, I.; Roche, A. Effect on growth in pemoline-treated children with attention deficit disorder. *Am. J. Dis. Child.* **1981**, *135*, 329–332. [CrossRef] [PubMed]
40. Ptacek, R.; Kuzelova, H.; Paclt, I.; Zukov, I.; Fischer, S. ADHD and growth: Anthropometric changes in medicated and non-medicated ADHD boys. *Med. Sci. Monit.* **2009**, *15*, Cr595–Cr599. [PubMed]
41. Xu, G.; Liu, B.; Yang, W.; Snetselaar, L.G.; Chen, M.; Bao, W.; Strathearn, L. Association of Food Allergy, Respiratory Allergy, and Skin Allergy with Attention Deficit/Hyperactivity Disorder among Children. *Nutrients* **2022**, *14*, 474. [CrossRef]
42. Pelsser, L.M.; Frankena, K.; Toorman, J.; Savelkoul, H.F.; Pereira, R.R.; Buitelaar, J.K. A randomised controlled trial into the effects of food on ADHD. *Eur. Child. Adolesc. Psychiatry* **2009**, *18*, 12–19. [CrossRef]
43. Schans, J.V.; Cicek, R.; de Vries, T.W.; Hak, E.; Hoekstra, P.J. Association of atopic diseases and attention-deficit/hyperactivity disorder: A systematic review and meta-analyses. *Neurosci. Biobehav. Rev.* **2017**, *74 Pt A*, 139–148. [CrossRef]
44. Kerekes, N.; Sanchéz-Pérez, A.M.; Landry, M. Neuroinflammation as a possible link between attention-deficit/hyperactivity disorder (ADHD) and pain. *Med. Hypotheses* **2021**, *157*, 110717. [CrossRef]
45. Zhang, X.; Zhang, R.; Zhang, Y.; Lu, T. Associations between attention-deficit/hyperactivity disorder and allergic diseases: A two-sample Mendelian randomization study. *Front. Psychiatry* **2023**, *14*, 1185088. [CrossRef]
46. Fiese, B.H.; Foley, K.P.; Spagnola, M. Routine and ritual elements in family mealtimes: Contexts for child well-being and family identity. *New Dir. Child. Adolesc. Dev.* **2006**, *111*, 67–89. [CrossRef]
47. Shek, D.T. Family functioning and psychological well-being, school adjustment, and problem behavior in chinese adolescents with and without economic disadvantage. *J. Genet. Psychol.* **2002**, *163*, 497–502. [CrossRef]
48. Ng, S.; Zhang, Y.; Ng, K.; Wong, H.; Lee, J. Living environment and quality of life in Hong Kong. *Asian Geogr.* **2018**, *35*, 35–51. [CrossRef]
49. Muratori, P.; Bertacchi, I.; Masi, G.; Milone, A.; Nocentini, A.; Powell, N.P.; Lochman, J.E.; Jones, S.; Kassing, F.; Romero, D. Effects of a universal prevention program on externalizing behaviors: Exploring the generalizability of findings across school and home settings. *J. Sch. Psychol.* **2019**, *77*, 13–23. [CrossRef] [PubMed]
50. Leung, C.; Leung, S.; Lee, F.; Lo, S. Socioeconomic Difference in Development Among Preschool Children. *Hong Kong J. Paediatr.* **2020**, *25*, 98–106.
51. Mao, W. Family socioeconomic status and young children's learning behaviors: The mediational role of parental expectation, home environment, and parental involvement. *Int. J. Chin. Educ.* **2022**, *11*, 2212585X221124155. [CrossRef]
52. Chu, Y.L.; Farmer, A.; Fung, C.; Kuhle, S.; Storey, K.E.; Veugelers, P.J. Involvement in home meal preparation is associated with food preference and self-efficacy among Canadian children. *Public Health Nutr.* **2013**, *16*, 108–112. [CrossRef]
53. van der Horst, K.; Ferrage, A.; Rytz, A. Involving children in meal preparation. *Effects on food intake. Appetite* **2014**, *79*, 18–24.
54. Spence, C. Breakfast: The most important meal of the day? *Int. J. Gastron. Food Sci.* **2017**, *8*, 1–6. [CrossRef]
55. Wolraich, M.L.; Hagan, J.F., Jr.; Allan, C.; Chan, E.; Davison, D.; Earls, M.; Evans, S.W.; Flinn, S.K.; Froehlich, T.; Frost, J.; et al. Clinical Practice Guideline for the Diagnosis, Evaluation, and Treatment of Attention-Deficit/Hyperactivity Disorder in Children and Adolescents. *Pediatrics* **2019**, *144*, e20192528. [CrossRef]
56. Johnson, R.J.; Gold, M.S.; Johnson, D.R.; Ishimoto, T.; Lanaspa, M.A.; Zahniser, N.R.; Avena, N.M. Attention-deficit/hyperactivity disorder: Is it time to reappraise the role of sugar consumption? *Postgrad. Med.* **2011**, *123*, 39–49. [CrossRef]
57. Pelsser, L.M.; Frankena, K.; Toorman, J.; Rodrigues Pereira, R. Diet and ADHD, Reviewing the Evidence: A Systematic Review of Meta-Analyses of Double-Blind Placebo-Controlled Trials Evaluating the Efficacy of Diet Interventions on the Behavior of Children with ADHD. *PLoS ONE* **2017**, *12*, e0169277. [CrossRef]
58. Stevenson, J.; Buitelaar, J.; Cortese, S.; Ferrin, M.; Konofal, E.; Lecendreux, M.; Simonoff, E.; Wong, I.C.; Sonuga-Barke, E. Research review: The role of diet in the treatment of attention-deficit/hyperactivity disorder—An appraisal of the evidence on efficacy and recommendations on the design of future studies. *J. Child. Psychol. Psychiatry* **2014**, *55*, 416–427. [CrossRef]

nutrients

MDPI

Article

Cognitive Functions in Adolescent Girls with Anorexia Nervosa during Nutritional Rehabilitation

Katarzyna Jowik-Krzemińska [1,2,*], Dagmara Dylewska [3], Aleksandra Pawlińska-Maćkowiak [3], Agnieszka Słopień [1,†] and Marta Tyszkiewicz-Nwafor [1,†]

1 Department of Child and Adolescent Psychiatry, Poznan University of Medical Sciences, 27/33 Szpitalna St., 61-572 Poznan, Poland; asrs@gmail.com (A.S.); malamt@gmail.com (M.T.-N.)
2 Poznan University of Medical Sciences Doctoral School, 61-701 Poznan, Poland
3 Department of Adult Psychiatry, Poznan University of Medical Sciences, 27/33 Szpitalna St., 61-572 Poznan, Poland; dagmaradylewska@gmail.com (D.D.); pawlinska.mackowiak@gmail.com (A.P.-M.)
* Correspondence: 71595@student.ump.edu.pl or katarzynajowikk@gmail.com
† These authors contributed equally to this work.

Abstract: Background: The present study aimed to evaluate cognitive function and laboratory parameters in adolescent girls with anorexia nervosa (AN) before and after nutritional rehabilitation (NR) compared to healthy female peers (CG). Methods: We evaluated 36 girls with AN at two-time points, during acute malnutrition (AN1) and after NR, in a partially normalized weight status (AN2). We compared their cognitive functions and laboratory parameters to 48 healthy CG subjects. Cognitive function was assessed using a Cognitive Assessment Battery (CAB) assessment, depressive symptom levels were assessed using a Beck Depression Inventory (BDI) assessment, and eating disorders were assessed using an Eating Attitude Test (EAT-26). Results: The AN1 group scored better in total cognition, attention, estimation, and spatial perception than the CG group ($p < 0.05$), with scores increasing in the AN2 group. Shifting and visual perception values did not differ between the study groups ($p = 0.677$, $p = 0.506$, respectively). Laboratory tests showed no significant abnormalities and did not differ significantly between groups ($p > 0.05$). There was a negative correlation for EAT-26 and CAB in the AN1 group (rho = −0.43, $p = 0.01$), but not for BDI. Conclusions: Cognitive function in adolescent girls with AN was better than CG and correlated with EAT-26 score. These results highlight the high compensatory capacity of the adolescent body to maintain cognitive function despite severe malnutrition. Our results suggest that although normalization of body weight is crucial, other factors can significantly influence improvements in cognitive function. Cognitive deficits and laboratory tests may not be biomarkers of early forms of AN.

Keywords: anorexia nervosa; cognition; eating disorders; adolescents

1. Introduction

Anorexia nervosa (AN) is a serious metabo-psychiatric condition characterized by disturbed body image, a strong fear of gaining weight, and dietary restrictions resulting in significant weight loss. Years ago, studies indicated a fairly stable incidence, but health professionals are seeing an increasing number of eating disorder (ED) patients receiving both outpatient and inpatient psychiatric care, especially during and after the COVID-19 pandemic [1–5]. The average age of onset of AN has steadily decreased over the past two decades: in the 1990s, it was 16–19 years, while in 2010, it was between 12 and 15 years. According to data from the UK, in children aged 10–14, the incidence of AN increased from 2.5 to 7.5 per 100,000 children. Similar trends have been observed in European countries, including Germany, Italy, and Portugal [6–9]. Among the reasons for this phenomenon is believed to be the growing influence of social media among young people, leading to increased comparison and the creation of unrealistic expectations about one's body, and the influence of movements promoting anorexia-related behavior (so-called "pro-ana") [10,11].

In parallel, there is a rise in social pressure to achieve success in the broadest sense and anxiety about the future [12], as well as an increase in morbidity and hospitalization due to AN during the geopolitical instability and lockdown situation of the COVID-19 period. The stress of armed conflict, social isolation, pandemic stress, health anxiety, and financial insecurity increase anxiety, which promotes the development of ED among adolescents [13–15].

The etiopathogenesis of AN is still unknown, and treatment results are unsatisfactory. It has been suggested that cognitive deficits may be a marker of the trait or endophenotype of the disorder, but reports on this subject are divergent [16–18]. Some researchers take the position that the axial symptoms of AN reflect neuropsychological dysfunction; for example, impaired assessment of body size has been described as a result of poor visuospatial abilities and cognitive and behavioral rigidity [19–22]. The above impairments can complicate the treatment process by hindering the implementation of new cognitive and behavioral skills. Previous literature highlights the unknown mechanism of cognitive deficits. It appears that they may be related to the somatic condition, as well as depressive symptoms [23]. Comorbid depression has attracted considerable research interest in the AN literature due to rates of comorbidity with this condition, ranging from 50 to 75 percent [24]. At the same time, cognitive impairment is a core feature of major depressive disorder. However, the scientific discourse lacks a clear answer to the question of the impact of depressive symptoms on the course of ED [25,26]. Furthermore, a poor somatic condition, manifesting in malnutrition, secondary hypothyroidism, and anemia, may also impair cognitive function [27,28]. Another vital reason for emphasizing cognitive functions in AN is the association between poorer neuropsychological functioning and poorer treatment outcomes [16,18–20,22]. Identifying such pathological, heritable, and condition-independent features is a potential key to developing highly effective therapeutic models based on an etiological pathway.

Nutrition plays a fundamental role in the treatment of AN, as it is essential for restoring average body weight, restoring micro- and macronutrient deficiencies, and improving the patient's overall health [29]. Early initiation of nutritional rehabilitation (NR) leads to faster improvement in patients' psychophysical state, which affects their ability to participate more fully in psychotherapy and other forms of treatment.

Therefore, the main objective of this study was to determine cognitive deficits in children with severe AN who required hospitalization in 24 h psychiatric wards. We hypothesized that children and adolescents with severe AN would have more profound cognitive deficits compared to their condition after NR and healthy peers. Including a group of recovered patients in the study allowed us to draw preliminary conclusions about whether the presumed cognitive impairment is an established trait after recovery from AN, one of the critical criteria that must be met for an agent to be considered an endophenotype. Based on clinical experience and intuitive understanding of AN, we assumed that patients should experience impairments in estimation, spatial perception, shifting, and all types of memory and show higher values in inhibition. In addition, we evaluated changes in serum laboratory profile (blood count, thyroid panel, vitamin D3 levels) at baseline and after NR. We hypothesized that after weight stabilization, the results of the parameters would improve significantly from the expected deviations from norms at the beginning of treatment. The evaluation also included correlations between cognitive test scores (CAB), changes in laboratory results, body weight, and depressive symptoms. We hypothesized that there would be a positive correlation between changes in cognitive domains and changes in body weight and a negative correlation with depression scales.

2. Methods

2.1. Participants

This prospective project was conducted between January 2021 and April 2024. Thirty-nine patients aged 10–18 years admitted to the child and adolescent psychiatry unit in the acute phase of AN participated in the study. All patients admitted to the hospital for

AN were female during the study period. The study sample was anthropologically and demographically homogeneous. Written consent to participate in the study was obtained from all participants and their legal guardians.

AN diagnosis was made according to DSM-5 criteria after an interview with a child and adolescent psychiatrist. Exclusion criteria included physical illness and laboratory abnormalities unrelated to long-term food restriction. Between days 1 and 3 of admission, patients (AN1) underwent cognitive and anthropometric assessment (height and weight), psychological testing, and blood sampling. The same procedures were repeated at a second-time point, after completion of NR or partial normalization of body weight, on the day of discharge from the psychiatric ward (AN2).

Admitted patients were immediately placed on a NR program. Daily calorie intake was initially 2000 kcal and was gradually increased to 3000–3500 kcal, depending on the duration of hospitalization, laboratory results, and the rate of weight gain (approximately 1.0 kg per week was expected). Stabilization of health status was defined as follows:

patient consumption of 2000–3500 kcal per day;
exclusion of critical organ failure based on test results;
achievement of the discharge BMI determined at the start of hospitalization (according to centile grids appropriate for age, sex, and height);
confirmation by the attending physician of medical stabilization regarding somatic and psychological status, allowing further therapy in the outpatient setting.

During the project, eleven patients (28%) were discharged from the hospital at the request of a parent, against medical advice, before their psychosomatic state was fully restored. In this group, three patients were discharged on request within a few days of admission, so only the first examination (AN1) was performed on them without repeating it. Finally, thirty-six patients who underwent NR and spent at least 28 days in the hospital completed the study.

The control group (CG) was recruited at one of the local secondary schools. Forty-eight age- and sex-matched girls were included. Exclusion criteria in the CG were chronic somatic illness and psychiatric or neurodevelopmental disorders, including a history of ADHD or ED. Analogous to AN1, written consents were obtained from the participants and their legal guardians.

Weight and height were measured using a certified medical scale with a height gauge by a nurse to minimize the risk of measurement error. Body mass index (BMI) was calculated according to the formula BMI = weight (in kg)/height^2 (in m^2) [30]. The percentage of ideal body weight (%IBW) was calculated according to the Lorentz formula (for women: (height − 100) − ((height − 150)/2)) [31].

The Bioethics Committee approved study protocol 476/20 of the University of Poznan Medical School (17 June 2020). All procedures were carried out following the 1964 Declaration of Helsinki.

2.2. Biochemical Analysis

Venous blood was collected in the morning from fasting AN1 patients (8 h after the last meal) and analyzed in the hospital laboratory. An analogous collection was performed after NR, 1–3 days before planned discharge. Blood serum collected from CG was analyzed in the same hospital laboratory. Blood counts (red blood cells (RBCs), hemoglobin (HGB) and hematocrit (HCT), white blood cells (WBCs) and platelets (PLTs)), glucose and insulin levels, thyrotropic hormone (TSH), free thyroxine (ft4), and vitamin D (1.25(OH)2D3) levels were examined. From the glucose and insulin results, the homeostatic insulin resistance assessment model index (HOMA-IR) was calculated: insulin (mU/mL) × glucose (mg/dL).

2.3. Cognitive Assessment

Cognitive functions were tested using the CogniFit Cognitive Assessment Battery (CAB), a set of computer-assessed neuropsychological tests commonly used in research protocols. According to the manufacturer, the FDA registration number is 3017544020*, and the EUDAMED (European Database on Medical Devices) UDI-DI registration is 00860009958104 [32]. The CAB includes experiments validated against various standardized neuropsychological tests, including the full automatic Cambridge Neuropsychological Test battery, Raven's Standard Progressive Matrices, Wisconsin Card Sorting Test, Continuous Performance Test, and STROOP Test. Tests of its reliability have been demonstrated in previous studies, yielding corresponding measures of good internal consistency (Cronbach's alpha = 0.85–0.88), and test–retest reliability (r = 0.69–0.92). The assessment uses clinical scales and tests validated for the age and gender of the patient or participant. The set of tasks is designed to assess 22 basic cognitive abilities divided into five main domains: CA—Perception (Auditory Perception, Estimation, Recognition, Spatial Perception, Visual Perception, Visual Scanning); CA—Attention (Divided Attention, Focus Attention, Inhibition, Updating); CA—Reasoning (Planning, Processing Speed, Shifting); CA—Memory (Phonological Short-Term Memory, Contextual Memory, Short-Term Memory, Non-Verbal Memory, Visual Short-Term Memory, Working Memory, Naming); CA—Coordination (Hand–Eye Coordination, Response Time).

This neuropsychological test takes 30–40 min and is conducted online. All participants took the test on a laptop in a separate room, using in-ear headphones to ensure comfort and maximum reduction in external distractions.

2.4. Psychometric Tests

All study participants completed anonymous tests—the Beck Depression Inventory (BDI), assessing the severity of depressive symptoms, and the Eating Attitudes Test (EAT-26), assessing eating attitudes [33,34]. Both questionnaires were validated in the Polish version, obtaining Cronbach's α indices of 0.90–0.92 and 0.90, respectively. In both questionnaires, the higher the score, the greater the severity of depressive symptoms or eating disorders, respectively, with presumed cut-off points of 11 in the BDI and 20 in the EAT-26. Patients with AN were assessed twice at inclusion and the end of the program, while the CG group was evaluated once.

2.5. Statistics

Analyses were conducted using statistical software R, version 4.1.2. The normality of distributions was checked with a Shapiro–Wilk's test, as well as with the values of skewness and kurtosis. Variance homogeneity was assessed using a Levene's test. Independent comparisons were conducted with a Student's t-test for independent groups, Welch's t-test for independent groups, Mann–Whitney's U test, or Pearson's Chi-square test, as appropriate. Paired comparisons were conducted with paired t-test or Wilcoxon test, as appropriate. Correction of p values due to multiple comparisons was implemented using Benjamini and Hochberg adjustment for each type of comparison. The effect size was calculated for each comparison with either Cohen's D or r for the Wilcoxon test (Z statistic divided by the square root of sample size), with 95% confidence intervals. Either an independent or paired version was applied, as appropriate. Spearman's rho coefficient was used for correlation analyses due to non-normal distributions of some variables. Linear regression models were fitted to understand the impact of selected predictors on CAB. After the initial selection of parameters for multivariate models, a stepwise procedure was employed for the final variables selection. All statistical calculations assumed alpha = 0.05. The tests comparing EAT-26, CAB, and BDI values between groups achieved test power, respectively: 100%, 59%, and 99.6%.

3. Results

3.1. Anthropometric Data

Table 1 compares demographic and clinical data between AN1, AN2, and CG. The mean age of onset of AN in patients was 14.5 years, while the mean age of CG was 15.5 years. Patients with acute malnutrition (AN1) had lower BMI, body weight, and %IBW than patients with partial normalization of body weight (AN2). At the same time, AN2 patients had lower scores in these parameters than the CG.

Table 1. Demographic characteristics of patients with anorexia nervosa. Anthropometric parameters in low body weight (AN1), after nutritional rehabilitation (AN2), and in the control group (CG).

Variable	Group M ± SD/Me (Q1; Q3)			AN1 vs. AN2		AN1 vs. CG		AN2 vs. CG	
	AN1 (n = 36)	AN2 (n = 36)	CG (n = 48)	Cohen's D/Wilcoxon Effect Size r (95% CI) *	Adj p	Cohen's D/Wilcoxon Effect Size r (95% CI) **	Adj p	Cohen's D/Wilcoxon Effect Size r (95% CI) **	Adj p
Age	14.53 ± 1.59	-	15.52 ± 0.97	-	-	−0.78 (−1.23; −0.33)	0.005 [2]	-	-
Height [m]	1.61 (1.56; 1.65)	-	1.65 (1.62; 1.69)	-	-	0.34 (0.15; 0.53)	0.0065	-	-
BMI [kg/m^2]	13.51 ± 1.40	16.89 ± 1.51	22.70 ± 2.31	−2.27 (−2.94; −1.59)	<0.001 [3]	−4.66 (−5.49; −3.83)	<0.001 [2]	−2.90 (−3.51; −2.28)	<0.001 [2]
Body weight [kg]	34.46 ± 5.51	43.16 ± 7.02	62.27 ± 6.61	−1.29 (−1.58; −0.99)	<0.001 [3]	−4.51 (−5.32; −3.69)	<0.001 [1]	−2.81 (−3.42; −2.20)	<0.001 [1]
IBW	55.50 (53.19; 57.62)	-	57.25 (56.00; 59.62)	-	-	0.34 (0.14; 0.54)	0.005	-	-
%IBW	0.63 ± 0.07	0.79 ± 0.08	1.08 ± 0.11	−2.04 (−2.62; −1.47)	<0.001 [3]	−4.82 (−5.67; −3.96)	<0.001 [2]	−3.01 (−3.64; −2.37)	<0.001 [1]

Data presented as M ± SD or Me (Q1; Q3), M ± SD was used when distribution in each group was normal, and difference between AN1 and AN2 had normal distribution, Me (Q1; Q3) was used otherwise. M—mean, SD—standard deviation, Me—median, Q1—first quartile, Q3—third quartile, CI—confidence interval. Comparisons were made with Student's t-test for independent samples [1], Welch t-test for independent samples [2], Mann–Whitney U test, paired t-test [3]. p values were corrected with Benjamini and Hochberg adjustment in each comparison type; this Table presents corrected p values (adj p). * Variants for paired tests.; ** Variants for independent tests.

The percentage of patients with menarche and a history of menstrual bleeding in the AN1 group was 69.4%, while the corresponding percentage among CG was 100.0%. All patients in the AN1 group did not menstruate during hospitalization and for at least three months before hospitalization, while the rate of menstruating patients in the CG group was 100.0%.

The average length of hospitalization of patients with AN was 68 days. Analysis of hospital records within two years of the first hospitalization (at the time of the aforementioned study) showed that 15 (38.5%) were readmitted to the ward due to exacerbation/recurrence of AN symptoms.

3.2. Cognitive–Psychological Functioning

Despite the malnutrition, the AN1 group had statistically significantly higher total scores in the CAB than the CG. Moreover, the scores increased with the normalization of body weight (AN2). The same statistically significant tendency was observed in the studied groups concerning CA—Perception and CA—Attention. In CA—Reasoning, the AN1 group had lower scores than the CG and normalized it with body weight gain ($p = 0.036$). In contrast, CA—Memory did not differ between AN1 and CG but improved statistically significantly with weight normalization and was higher in the AN2 group than in CG. The same tendency was observed for CA—Coordination. (Table 2). A significant difference in BDI values was observed between AN1 and CG ($p < 0.001$). At the same time, there was a significant decrease throughout treatment ($p < 0.001$). The outcome of the AN2 and CG groups did not differ statistically significantly. Regarding EAT-26, differences were statistically significant, with the highest scores in AN1 and the lowest in CG (Figure 1).

The detailed analysis of single cognitive functions presented in Table 3 showed that despite the malnutrition, AN1 scored significantly higher than CG in estimation, recognition, spatial perception, focus attention, planning, visual short-term memory, contextual memory, and short-term memory. During NR (AN1 vs. AN2), auditory perception, recognition, visual perception, visual scanning, focus attention, updating, processing speed, phonological short-term memory, naming, contextual memory, short-term memory, working memory, response time, and hand–eye coordination improved statistically significantly. Estimation, spatial perception, divided attention, inhibition, planning, visual short-term memory, and non-verbal memory did not change with increasing body weight and remained higher as in the health peers (AN2 vs. CG). The shift value did not change between the AN1 and AN2 groups and remained without statistical difference compared to CG (p = 0.634).

Table 2. Values of depression indices (Beck Depression Inventory, BDI), eating disorders (Eating Attitude Teat, EAT-26), and cognitive function parameters measured with the Cognitive Assessment Battery (CAB) in adolescents with anorexia nervosa at low body weight (AN1) and nutritional rehabilitation (AN2) and in a healthy control group (CG).

Variable	Group M ± SD/Me (Q1; Q3)			AN1 vs. AN2		AN1 vs. CG		AN2 vs. CG	
	AN1 (n = 36)	AN2 (n = 36)	CG (n = 48)	Cohen's D/Wilcoxon Effect Size r (95% CI) *	Adj p	Cohen's D/Wilcoxon Effect Size r (95% CI) **	Adj p	Cohen's D/Wilcoxon Effect Size r (95% CI) **	Adj p
CAB	550.34 (492.76; 616.50)	629.57 (582.94; 656.24)	483.02 (457.70; 555.48)	0.85 (0.77; 0.87) [2]	<0.001 [1]	0.27 (0.04; 0.48) [2]	0.037	0.59 (0.42; 0.72) [2]	<0.001
CA—Perception	634.00 (563.00; 705.75)	681.50 (640.00; 733.75)	488.33 (458.00; 543.50)	0.55 (0.26; 0.77) [2]	0.002 [1]	0.54 (0.33; 0.70) [2]	<0.001	0.70 (0.56; 0.81) [2]	<0.001
CA—Attention	612.50 (547.50; 650.00)	660.00 (602.25; 690.25)	531.00 (527.47; 605.50)	0.59 (0.32; 0.80) [2]	0.001 [1]	0.27 (0.06; 0.47) [2]	0.036	0.50 (0.29; 0.66) [2]	<0.001
CA—Reasoning	599.00 (556.25; 646.25)	654.00 (620.00; 686.75)	622.00 (620.60; 674.50)	0.73 (0.56; 0.85) [2]	<0.001 [1]	0.27 (0.05; 0.49) [2]	0.036	0.12 (0.01; 0.34) [2]	0.348
CA—Memory	512.50 (435.00; 587.50)	619.00 (568.75; 647.25)	460.60 (455.80; 592.00)	0.83 (0.73; 0.87) [2]	<0.001 [1]	0.10 (0.01; 0.34) [2]	0.468	0.46 (0.27; 0.64) [2]	<0.001
CA—Coordination	391.00 (307.00; 500.00)	528.00 (424.25; 608.50)	315.33 (307.00; 400.50)	0.78 (0.63; 0.87) [2]	<0.001 [1]	0.21 (0.02; 0.41) [2]	0.091	0.51 (0.32; 0.68) [2]	<0.001
EAT-26	40.00 (31.75; 46.25)	24.50 (10.00; 33.00)	13.00 (6.00; 22.50)	0.76 (0.57; 0.86)	<0.001 [1]	0.63 (0.46; 0.75)	<0.001	0.26 (0.04; 0.47)	0.033
BDI	30.00 (20.50; 41.00)	20.00 (11.00; 30.50)	16.00 (9.00; 26.50)	0.69 (0.47; 0.86)	<0.001 [1]	0.44 (0.26; 0.61) [2]	<0.001	0.12 (0.01; 0.34) [2]	0.351

Data presented as M ± SD or Me (Q1; Q3), M ± SD was used when distribution in each group was normal, and the difference between AN1 and AN2 had normal distribution; Me (Q1; Q3) was used otherwise. M—mean, SD—standard deviation, Me—median, Q1—first quartile, Q3—third quartile, CI—confidence interval. Comparisons were made with Wilcoxon test [1]. p values were corrected with Benjamini and Hochberg adjustment in each comparison type; this Table presents corrected p values (adj p). In the case of Mann–Whitney U test/Wilcoxon, the r effect size for Wilcoxon test [2] was given. * Variants for paired tests. ** Variants for independent tests.

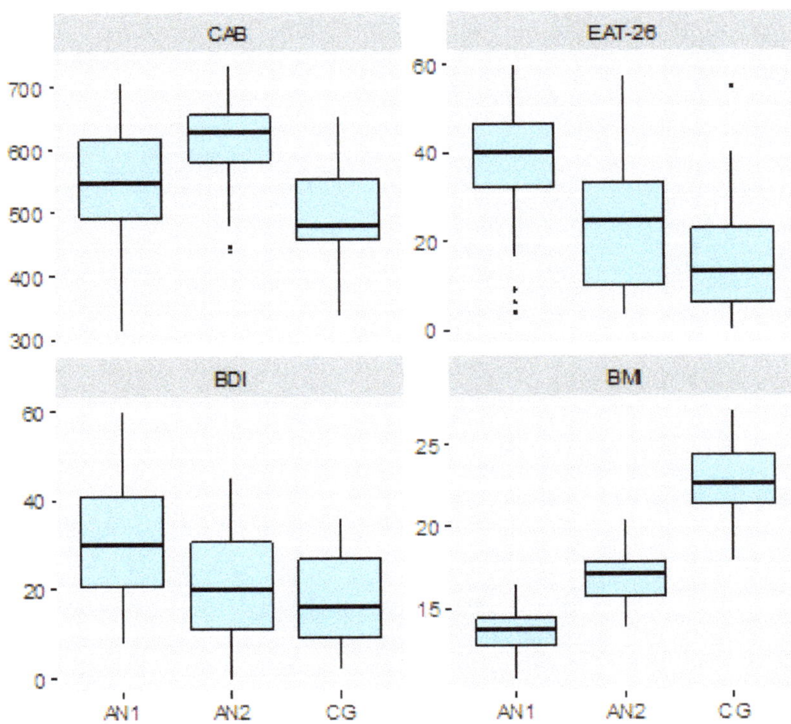

Figure 1. Boxplots presenting the distribution of selected parameters among patients with low body weight (AN1), after nutritional rehabilitation (AN2) and among the control group (CG).

Table 3. Values of single cognitive functions measured with the Cognitive Assessment Battery (CAB) in adolescents with anorexia nervosa at low body weight (AN1), after nutritional rehabilitation (AN2) and in a healthy control group (CG).

Main Variable	Variable	Group M ± SD/Me (Q1; Q3)			AN1 vs. AN2		AN1 vs. CG		AN2 vs. CG	
		AN1 (n = 36)	AN2 (n = 36)	CG (n = 48)	Cohen's D/Wilcoxon Effect Size r (95% CI) *	Adj p	Cohen's D/Wilcoxon Effect Size r (95% CI) **	Adj p	Cohen's D/Wilcoxon Effect Size r (95% CI) **	Adj p
CA—Perception	Auditory Perception	567.50 (447.25; 670.50)	688.50 (622.00; 742.25)	526.27 (523.63; 662.00)	0.73 (0.56; 0.84) [6]	<0.001 [4]	0.01 (0.00; 0.27) [6]	0.917	0.43 (0.22; 0.62) [6]	<0.001
	Estimation	619.50 (379.75; 696.75)	676.00 (505.50; 703.50)	514.87 (436.50; 573.50)	0.16 (0.01; 0.45) [6]	0.375 [4]	0.26 (0.04; 0.48) [6]	0.037	0.44 (0.21; 0.64) [6]	<0.001
	Recognition	561.00 (408.50; 634.75)	633.00 (577.50; 706.00)	387.87 (360.00; 545.00)	0.70 (0.49; 0.85) [6]	<0.001 [4]	0.27 (0.04; 0.48) [6]	0.036	0.57 (0.39; 0.72) [6]	<0.001
	Spatial Perception	613.00 (415.25; 647.25)	611.00 (308.00; 707.25)	258.47 (202.50; 317.00)	0.21 (0.01; 0.54) [6]	0.240 [4]	0.55 (0.36; 0.71) [6]	<0.001	0.50 (0.30; 0.67) [6]	<0.001
	Visual Perception	657.50 (589.25; 732.25)	694.50 (644.50; 737.25)	578.00 (577.13; 745.00)	0.47 (0.20; 0.68) [6]	0.007 [4]	0.09 (0.00; 0.32) [6]	0.506	0.26 (0.05; 0.48) [6]	0.034
	Visual Scanning	505.00 (263.50; 628.50)	599.50 (434.75; 631.00)	532.00 (496.50; 610.00)	0.52 (0.26; 0.75) [6]	0.003 [4]	0.18 (0.01; 0.41) [6]	0.156	0.07 (0.00; 0.29) [6]	0.634
CA—Attention	Divided Attention	787.50 (781.75; 800.00)	795.00 (787.50; 800.00)	785.87 (779.50; 795.50)	0.32 (0.03; 0.60) [6]	0.081 [4]	0.11 (0.01; 0.32) [6]	0.456	0.27 (0.05; 0.49) [6]	0.027
	Focus Attention	604.00 (436.00; 650.25)	629.00 (587.50; 680.25)	431.93 (399.00; 582.50)	0.63 (0.38; 0.81) [6]	<0.001 [4]	0.26 (0.05; 0.47) [6]	0.037	0.48 (0.28; 0.65) [6]	<0.001
	Updating	609.00 (411.00; 664.00)	696.50 (607.25; 736.75)	463.80 (457.90; 582.50)	0.82 (0.71; 0.87) [6]	<0.001 [4]	0.14 (0.01; 0.37) [6]	0.288	0.51 (0.33; 0.69) [6]	<0.001
	Inhibition	800.00 (220.50; 800.00)	800.00 (632.25; 800.00)	514.13 (513.07; 800.00)	0.27 (0.02; 0.55) [6]	0.089 [4]	0.09 (0.01; 0.32) [6]	0.522	0.28 (0.08; 0.49) [6]	0.023
CA—Reasoning	Planning	654.50 (524.25; 694.75)	663.50 (612.00; 737.75)	513.13 (511.57; 628.00)	0.30 (0.02; 0.58) [6]	0.099 [4]	0.30 (0.08; 0.50) [6]	0.022	0.45 (0.27; 0.63) [6]	<0.001
	Processing Speed	615.50 (515.50; 700.00)	675.50 (576.25; 710.75)	597.13 (585.50; 673.00)	0.52 (0.23; 0.74) [6]	0.003 [4]	0.01 (0.00; 0.26) [6]	0.917	0.20 (0.02; 0.42) [6]	0.108
	Shifting	769.50 (730.25; 788.50)	780.00 (745.00; 796.25)	754.00 (751.20; 794.00)	0.27 (0.02; 0.56) [6]	0.138 [4]	0.05 (0.00; 0.28) [6]	0.677	0.07 (0.00; 0.30) [6]	0.634
CA—Memory	Phonological Short-Term Memory	410.00 (270.75; 592.50)	511.50 (339.25; 648.50)	362.53 (324.50; 448.00)	0.47 (0.17; 0.71) [6]	0.007 [4]	0.10 (0.01; 0.32) [6]	0.468	0.27 (0.06; 0.49) [6]	0.028
	Visual Short-Term Memory	660.00 (509.00; 703.50)	655.50 (588.25; 715.25)	511.00 (508.47; 635.50)	0.06 (0.01; 0.39) [6]	0.747 [4]	0.26 (0.04; 0.47) [6]	0.037	0.31 (0.09; 0.52) [6]	0.011
	Naming	619.50 (472.25; 677.00)	669.00 (599.75; 722.25)	496.00 (485.27; 654.00)	0.45 (0.15; 0.70) [6]	0.009 [4]	0.14 (0.01; 0.37) [6]	0.284	0.32 (0.10; 0.51) [6]	0.010
	Contextual Memory	616.00 (518.50; 675.00)	707.50 (654.25; 736.25)	489.27 (476.13; 599.50)	0.78 (0.63; 0.86) [6]	<0.001 [4]	0.26 (0.05; 0.46) [6]	0.037	0.56 (0.39; 0.72) [6]	<0.001
	Short-Term Memory	609.50 (420.75; 661.50)	623.00 (517.50; 682.00)	410.93 (409.97; 553.00)	0.31 (0.03; 0.61) [6]	0.007 [4]	0.26 (0.04; 0.47) [6]	0.037	0.41 (0.19; 0.61) [6]	0.001
	Non-Verbal Memory	650.50 (474.00; 693.25)	670.50 (626.50; 722.25)	522.47 (504.73; 691.00)	0.31 (0.03; 0.57) [6]	0.083 [4]	0.16 (0.01; 0.39) [6]	0.228	0.38 (0.16; 0.55) [6]	0.002
	Working Memory	614.50 (464.50; 660.75)	666.50 (635.75; 719.00)	445.47 (445.47; 613.50)	0.82 (0.72; 0.87) [6]	<0.001 [4]	0.21 (0.02; 0.43) [6]	0.107	0.56 (0.39; 0.70) [6]	<0.001
CA—Coordination	Response Time	338.94 ± 164.63	395.72 ± 148.40	349.32 ± 124.31	−0.35 (−0.58; −0.13) [5]	0.005 [3]	−0.07 (−0.51; 0.37) [5]	0.790 [2]	0.34 (−0.11; 0.79) [5]	0.184 [1]
	Hand–Eye Coordination	229.50 (125.50; 498.25)	470.50 (215.00; 619.25)	198.07 (159.50; 241.50)	0.61 (0.38; 0.77) [6]	0.001 [4]	0.12 (0.01; 0.36) [6]	0.395	0.45 (0.22; 0.64) [6]	<0.001

Data presented as M ± SD or Me (Q1; Q3), M ± SD was used when distribution in each group was normal and the difference between AN1 and AN2 had normal distribution, Me (Q1; Q3) was used otherwise. M—mean, SD—standard deviation, Me—median, Q1—first quartile, Q3—third quartile, CI—confidence interval. Comparisons were made with Student's *t*-test for independent samples [1], Welch *t*-test for independent samples [2], Mann–Whitney U test, paired *t*-test [3], or Wilcoxon test [4]. *p* values were corrected with Benjamini and Hochberg adjustment in each comparison type; this Table presents corrected *p* values (adj *p*). In the case of *t*-tests, Cohen's D [5] was presented as the effect size; in case of Mann–Whitney U test/Wilcoxon, the r effect size for Wilcoxon test [6] was given. * Variants for paired tests. ** Variants for independent tests.

3.3. Biochemical Blood Results

In laboratory tests (Table 4), the mean level of 1.25(0H)2D in each group was below reference values but significantly higher in the AN1 than AN2 group. At the same time, the AN1 group was not statistically different from the CG ($p = 0.066$).

RBCs, HGB, and HCT in all three groups were within reference values. They did not change during weight rehabilitation (AN1 vs. AN2), and the results remained significantly lower than in CG after weight normalization.

Fasting glucose and insulin concentrations and HOMA-IR scores were significantly lower among patients in AN1 than in AN2. No statistically significant differences were observed between AN2 and CG. TSH values were not significantly different among all three groups. However, FT4 values were lower among patients in AN1 and AN2 than in CG with high strength of change as measured by the r effect size for the Wilcoxon test (AN1 vs. CG r = 0.57 CI 95 [0.39; 0.73] and AN2 vs. CG r = 0.75 Cl 95 [0.61; 0.83], respectively).

Table 4. Biochemical parameters in patients with low body weight (AN1), after nutritional rehabilitation (AN2), and control group (CG).

Variable	Group M ± SD/Me (Q1; Q3)			AN1 vs. AN2		AN1 vs. CG		AN2 vs. CG	
	AN1 (n = 36)	AN2 (n = 36)	CG (n = 48)	Cohen's D/Wilcoxon Effect Size r (95% CI) *	Adj p	Cohen's D/Wilcoxon Effect Size r (95% CI) **	Adj p	Cohen's D/Wilcoxon Effect Size r (95% CI) **	Adj p
1.25(0H)2D [ng/mL] (30.0–50.0)	24.85 (17.98; 35.00)	19.65 (11.05; 26.20)	19.30 (15.18; 25.77)	0.53 (0.27; 0.75) [6]	0.003 [4]	0.22 (0.03; 0.43) [6]	0.066	0.04 (0.00; 0.27) [6]	0.835
WBC [10^3/µL] (4.0–10.0)	4.35 (3.92; 5.03)	5.76 (5.06; 6.37)	6.65 (5.28; 7.46)	0.81 (0.68; 0.86) [6]	<0.001 [4]	0.60 (0.44; 0.72) [6]	<0.001	0.26 (0.05; 0.45) [6]	0.030
RBC [10^6/µL] (4.0–5.0)	4.39 ± 0.56	4.33 ± 0.40	4.66 ± 0.31	0.12 (−0.22; 0.46) [5]	0.523 [3]	−0.63 (−1.07; −0.18) [5]	0.030 [2]	−0.95 (−1.40; −0.49) [5]	<0.001 [1]
HGB [g/dL] (12.0–16.0)	13.45 (12.90; 14.30)	12.95 (12.28; 13.55)	13.65 (13.17; 14.03)	0.28 (0.02; 0.57) [6]	0.108 [4]	0.06 (0.00; 0.29) [6]	0.631	0.36 (0.17; 0.54) [6]	0.002
HCT [%]	39.30 (37.27; 41.10)	38.65 (36.72; 39.95)	39.55 (38.65; 40.85)	0.05 (0.01; 0.40) [6]	0.747 [4]	0.06 (0.00; 0.30) [6]	0.631	0.23 (0.03; 0.44) [6]	0.054
PLT [10^3/µL] (150–400)	226.94 ± 60.63	286.03 ± 51.03	290.35 ± 61.77	−1.03 (−1.55; −0.51) [5]	<0.001 [3]	−1.03 (−1.49; −0.57) [5]	<0.001 [1]	−0.08 (−0.51; 0.36) [5]	0.835 [1]
Glucose [mg/dL] (60–101)	73.17 ± 9.65	82.11 ± 5.87	84.81 ± 7.48	−1.08 (−1.61; −0.56) [5]	<0.001 [3]	−1.37 (−1.85; −0.89) [5]	<0.001 [1]	−0.40 (−0.83; 0.04) [5]	0.108 [1]
Insulin [mU/mL] (<15)	4.30 (2.80; 5.90)	6.15 (4.88; 9.48)	7.05 (5.30; 9.30)	0.61 (0.34; 0.83) [6]	0.001 [4]	0.53 (0.36; 0.67) [6]	<0.001	0.13 (0.01; 0.33) [6]	0.316
HOMA-IR	0.77 (0.54; 1.08)	1.23 (0.93; 2.05)	1.48 (1.13; 1.90)	0.67 (0.46; 0.83) [6]	<0.001 [4]	0.60 (0.46; 0.74) [6]	<0.001	0.15 (0.01; 0.35) [6]	0.237
TSH [mIU/L] (0.47–3.41)	2.02 ± 0.91	2.18 ± 0.99	2.14 ± 0.97	−0.17 (−0.51; 0.18) [5]	0.375 [3]	−0.13 (−0.57; 0.30) [5]	0.626 [1]	0.04 (−0.40; 0.47) [5]	0.945 [1]
FT4 [ng/dL] (0.86–1.37)	0.82 (0.77; 0.91)	0.79 (0.73; 0.85)	0.98 (0.93; 1.02)	0.43 (0.13; 0.68) [6]	0.013 [4]	0.57 (0.39; 0.73) [6]	<0.001	0.75 (0.61; 0.83) [6]	<0.001

Data presented as M ± SD or Me (Q1; Q3), M ± SD was used when distribution in each group was normal and the difference between AN1, and AN2 had normal distribution, Me (Q1; Q3) was used otherwise. M—mean, SD—standard deviation, Me—median, Q1—first quartile, Q3—third quartile, CI—confidence interval. Comparisons were made with Student's t-test for independent samples [1], Welch t-test for independent samples [2], Mann–Whitney U test, paired t-test [3], or Wilcoxon test [4]. p values were corrected with Benjamini and Hochberg adjustment in each comparison type; this Table presents corrected p values (adj p). In the case of t-tests, Cohen's D [5] was presented as the effect size; in the case of Mann–Whitney U test/Wilcoxon, the r effect size for Wilcoxon test [6] was given. * Variants for paired tests. ** Variants for independent tests.

3.4. Correlations between Cognitive Function Scores and Psychometric Variables

Correlations between CAB/CA parameters and BDI/EAT-26 were verified in patients with low body weight (AN1) and after partial normalization of body weight (AN2) and CG. A negative correlation was noted for EAT-26 and CAB in the AN1 group (rho = −0.43, p = 0.01) (Table 5).

Table 5. Correlation between CAB/CA parameters and selected variables for patients with low body weight (AN1), patients after nutritional rehabilitation (AN2), and control group (CG).

Variable	CAB		CA—Perception		CA—Attention		CA—Reasoning		CA—Memory		CA—Coordination	
	rho	p	rho	p	rho	p	rho	p	rho	p	rho	p
						AN1						
BDI	−0.18	0.286	−0.05	0.777	−0.18	0.290	−0.15	0.372	−0.15	0.382	−0.11	0.538
EAT-26	−0.43	0.010	−0.27	0.108	−0.29	0.090	−0.21	0.224	−0.34	0.040	−0.30	0.071
						AN2						
BDI	−0.14	0.414	−0.12	0.472	−0.08	0.652	−0.19	0.266	−0.09	0.593	−0.02	0.906
EAT-26	−0.31	0.063	−0.20	0.241	−0.18	0.296	−0.07	0.666	−0.26	0.133	−0.28	0.092
						CG						
BDI	−0.08	0.600	−0.10	0.532	−0.11	0.486	−0.02	0.914	−0.11	0.502	0.17	0.273
EAT-26	−0.16	0.299	−0.12	0.436	−0.35	0.024	−0.11	0.476	−0.25	0.110	0.11	0.505

rho—Spearman correlation coefficient.

3.5. Linear Regression

In univariate models of AN1, EAT-26, higher by 1, translated into CAB, lower by 2.77, β = −2.77 CI95 [−4.85; −0.69], p = 0.011 (Supplementary Materials—Table S1). The initial selection of variables for multivariate models was based on the magnitude of effect size for the difference between AN1 and AN2, p-value from univariate models, and clinical knowledge on potential predictors of CAB. Multivariate models in version 1 assumed the following variables: age, BMI, %IBW, glucose, HOMA-IR, EAT-26, and BDI. After utilizing the stepwise selection procedure, the final multivariate models comprised age, BMI, and EAT-26. EAT-26 impacted CAB statistically significantly in AN1. Its value, higher than 1, translated into CAB, lower by 2.34, β = −2.34 CI95 [−4.47; −0.21], p = 0.032. The impact of EAT-26 in AN2 on CAB was measured with a significance level of p = 0.053 (β = −1.49 CI95 [−3.00; 0.02], p = 0.053). Multivariate models in version 2 assumed the following variables: age, body weight, %IBW, glucose, HOMA-IR, EAT-26, and BDI. After utilizing the stepwise selection procedure, the final multivariate models consisted of body weight, glucose, and EAT-26. Body weight, higher by 1 kg, translated into CAB, lower by 5.83, β = −5.83 CI95 [−11.63; −0.03], p = 0.049 in AN1. In AN2, the impact of body weight and EAT-26 on CAB were measured with significance levels of p = 0.087 and p = 0.096, respectively (β = −2.85 CI95 [−6.14; 0.44], p = 0.087 and β = −1.27 CI95 [−2.77; 0.24], p = 0.096, respectively), Table 2. The model's fit in version 1 in a group with low body weight was assessed with R2 and adjusted R2, with the outcomes of 24.5% and 17.5%, respectively. The model's fit in version 2 in a group with low body weight assessed with R2 and adjusted R2 was 27.4% and 20.6%, respectively. Multicollinearity was assessed with VIF indicators, which was below 2.00 for all predictors and all multivariate models.

4. Discussion

The study presented here is the first part of a larger analysis of the psychophysical status of pediatric patients with AN and the dynamics of change during NR. Our initial hypothesis was that patients with severe AN would have cognitive deficits compared to patients after NR and the healthy population. We reasoned that reduced caloric and nutrient intake was crucial for the regression of cognitive functioning. Meanwhile, contrary to these expectations, the total mean CAB score and most studied cognitive parameters were higher in patients in the acute phase of AN and after NR than in healthy adolescents. At the same time, patients had significantly better cognitive performance after NR (AN2) than initially (AN1). However, some parameters, such as estimation, inhibition, planning, and spatial perception, did not change with weight gain, although they were higher than in the CG. Of the 22 studied cognitive functions, only shifting did not differ between groups. This is puzzling since the literature has divergently described the effects of ED on academic achievement and performance—both negatively [35,36] and positively [37]. However, this would be consistent with the fact that EDs are reported to be more common in individuals with high intelligence, perfectionism, or higher school achievement [38–41].

To our knowledge, short-term memory parameters have not yet been compared in adolescents with AN undergoing nutritional treatment. Our subjects had significantly better parameters despite the disease than CG, and these parameters still improved after NR. Meanwhile, Terhoeven et al. and Nikendei et al., in independent studies, argued that adult patients with AN showed worse results of this parameter than a healthy control group, and the deviations persisted despite restoration of normal body weight [42,43]. Our group differed significantly from those mentioned by age (<18 years old) and the fact of longitudinal follow-up, which allowed us to limit the influence of personal variables on the results after NR.

Inhibition, understood as the ability to control impulsive reactions, contributes to planning, goal-setting, and inhibition of automatic responses to stimuli and develops in early to middle adolescence. It has been hypothesized that the degree of proactive inhibition is related to how well an individual tolerates uncertainty and dominates reactive inhibition in patients with AN [44–46]. Shen et al. proved significant differences between intentional and reactive inhibition during adolescence, which integrate with age [47]. Both Suttkus' and Tenconi's work showed no differences between patients with AN and CG, but the studies included adolescents and young adults (mean age 19 in Tenconi's work, 26 in Suttkus' article) with a correspondingly long duration of illness (mean 24 months in Tenconi's) [48,49]. We show that adolescents in the acute phase of AN had similar inhibition scores as after NR, while not significantly different from healthy peers, which would confirm some independence of clinical and nutritional status. However, longitudinal evaluations are lacking in the literature, so we can only speculate that inhibition worsens with disease progression and duration.

Surprising results were obtained for the parameters of estimation and spatial perception, which, contrary to the intuitive assumption that they would be impaired due to the primary symptoms of ED (impaired perception of the shape and size of one's own body), are significantly better than in healthy subjects. Contrary to our initial assumptions, this is a significant difference, as earlier studies by Scarpin and Guardia confirmed impaired imaginal processes and spatial reference in AN compared to healthy subjects [50,51]. We do not know whether this mechanism is primary or secondary to the symptoms and consequences of AN, especially since the strength of the difference between AN and CG for estimation was moderate, and the values did not change during NR. This prompts us to extend further research on the mechanisms of impaired body representation in patients with high global spatial perception and to estimate and study the relationship and influence of factors other than body weight on the above variables.

AN is associated with poor cognitive flexibility, referring to the ability to change thoughts or actions according to situational demands. These findings are mostly observed in adults, and conclusions, including those of adolescents, are less consistent [20,52–55]. Our analysis showed that shifting did not change before and after treatment. We believe that adolescence, with its intense development of the central nervous system and cognitive abilities, influences the development of executive functions and protects against the neurodegenerative processes observed in adults with AN. This would be consistent with the lack of differences in working memory between AN1 and CG. Samanta Brooks et al. hypothesize that people with AN have an excessive and thus dysfunctional working memory, similar to other studies on the neural correlates of AN [56–58]. Some, however, indicate deficits [22,59] or no differences [42,60] between people with AN and overeaters or healthy individuals.

We examined a baseline biochemical panel from blood to better explore the relationship between cognitive functioning and its component parameters. Most clinicians, both pediatricians and psychiatrists, expect significant abnormalities in laboratory tests in patients with AN, especially as children have a lower percentage of body fat than adults, and the consequences of weight loss may be more severe because of this. In the course of AN, the typical changes described in the blood picture are anemia, leukopenia, and, less frequently, thrombocytopenia. Cell lineage changes are due to chronic malnutrition and bone marrow hypometabolism, myelosuppression, or reduced erythropoietin (EPO) or thrombopoietin (TPO) secretion [61,62]. Meanwhile, our patients, despite the need for hospital treatment due to their severe medical condition and severe malnutrition, did not show significant deviations in their blood biochemistry results. Both blood morphology parameters, such as red blood cell (RBC, HGB, HCT), WBC, and PLT lineage indices, did not exceed reference standards, indicating anemia, reduced cellular immunity or risk of pancytopenia. As shown in previous literature, the frequency and severity of hematological abnormalities associated with bone marrow hypoplasia may be related to disease duration and severity of malnutrition [51].

Similarly, despite extreme malnutrition, neither in the initial hospitalization nor subsequently did glucose and insulin levels deviate from laboratory norms and excluded morning hypoglycemia or insulin resistance (HOMA-IR < 2), which differs from previous literature reports of frequent hypoglycemia in patients [63].

Similarly, despite extreme malnutrition, neither in the initial hospitalization nor subsequently did glucose and insulin levels deviate from laboratory norms and excluded morning hypoglycemia or insulin resistance (HOMA-IR < 2), which differs from previous literature reports of frequent hypoglycemia in patients [64–66]. These significant differences between our study and prior literature may be due to the young age of the patients, the relatively short duration of the disease (first ED episode), and the high compensatory capacity of the adolescent body to maintain homeostasis despite a persistent negative energy balance. Moreover, this represents a very favorable prognostic factor, as hypoglycemic incidents and reduced liver volume are predictors of a severe and complicated course of the disease. Thyroid function tests in patients showed that both TSH and FT4 were normal in the AN1 and AN2 groups and CG. This is consistent with previous literature, which provides evidence that the pathology of the hypothalamic–pituitary–thyroid axis is not associated with menstrual retention [67].

In addition, our analysis assessed serum vitamin D3 levels. Although both AN and CG were deficient at the beginning of the study, the levels were nevertheless higher in female patients than in the healthy population. At the same time, the levels decreased during hospitalization and NR. We partly relate this to the lack of supplementation in the treatment protocol used and the conditions of stay (closed ward, limited outdoor and sun exposure). However, this is only a partial explanation for the above phenomenon: a review of the literature showed that, in most cases, a vitamin D deficit was observed in patients with AN compared to CG, even if their intake was the same, which was explained by reduced adipose tissue, reduced metabolic clearance and reduced vitamin D3 uptake by adipose tissue. This is important not only because of its association with the skeletal status of adolescent patients but also with the occurrence of depression and other psychiatric disorders [68–71]. We suggest that the relatively high levels, higher than in the healthy population, may be due to the claimed high attention to health and adequate vitamin and mineral supplementation in people with AN.

Malnutrition, secondary to AN, is a chronic condition in which metabolic and functional adaptive mechanisms develop to allow survival despite very low body weight and organ complications. We believe that in the course of AN in children and adolescents, despite low BMI, abnormalities in biochemical tests may not be clinically significant, reflect the severity of the disease, and may not be a reliable predictor of emergency conditions in the course of AN, such as cardiac arrhythmias or acute pancreatitis. This indicates a high adaptive capacity of the young organism.

We initially hypothesized that cognitive function would improve with normalization of body weight and restoring adequate nutrition and hydration, but our analyses did not yield the predicted conclusive result. As in the Hemmingsen et al. project, we did not confirm a positive correlation between BMI and improved cognitive function during NR. In our analysis, CAB level correlated negatively with body weight in the acute phase of AN [72]. At the same time, we did not show an association between depressive symptoms and CAB, although the severity of eating-disorder symptoms already correlated significantly with cognitive level. It can be speculated that other variables not included in the study have a significant impact on the improvement of cognitive performance after weight normalization. This could be, for example, the psychological well-being of the subject, which, due to illness and false beliefs or thought disorders, decreases with increasing body weight, as well as environmental factors or other pathophysiological variables. We link the refutation of the hypothesis of cognitive improvement depending on nutrition as measured by body weight and BMI to the clinical characteristics of individuals with AN, who are characterized by high levels of perfectionism, control, and obsessive–compulsive symptoms, which are manifested in the adolescent's daily life by regular and systematic study, high academic performance and sporting and artistic achievements. This is supported by a cohort study in which high school achievement and higher parental education were associated with increased ED risk [73].

The severity of depressive symptoms was significantly higher in AN1 patients than in CG and improved during AN treatment, reaching values similar to healthy peers. At the same time, we did not detect significant correlations between them and cognitive functions, despite the intuitive assumption that cognitive parameters would improve with a reduction in depressive symptoms. Interestingly, they improved with the withdrawal of eating disorder symptoms, once again indicating the enormous complexity of AN processes and mechanisms.

The main limitation of the presented study is the relatively small number of participants during the follow-up period, which may weaken the study's strength. However, the studies discussed above usually contain a similar group of subjects. Moreover, our study includes a very homogeneous group of patients regarding age, menstruation, number of episodes, and treatment method, which may improve its quality. Importantly, it is essential to remember that AN is a multifactorial disorder with a complex metabolic-psychiatric-social etiopathogenesis. In the present study, we focused on examining specific factors due to the breadth of the topic, omitting the influence of perfectionism level, anxiety, obsessive–compulsive symptoms, attachment style, or family functioning.

In the presented study, we did not include an analysis of sex hormone levels, although some studies described the link between hormonal and cognitive functioning in female patients with AN. Moreover, the CG was slightly older than AN by an average of 1 year, which could also be a potential factor for differences in maturation level and cognitive parameters. However, we believe the age difference was insignificant given the higher scores in the younger, sicker girls.

5. Conclusions

The main finding of this study is that the initially assumed cognitive impairment in adolescents with AN compared to healthy peers did not occur at all, and parameters continued to improve after NR treatment. These results suggest that some variables may be related to the patient's nutritional status. However, these are more complex correlations, and cognitive functioning must depend on many other factors not considered in previous studies. Adolescent patients with AN tend to have a shorter duration of illness, a shorter duration of hunger, and a higher rate of treatment-seeking (parental treatment seeking). The teenagers we studied required hospitalization for AN for the first time, indicating that this was their first acute episode of the disease. This probably explains the differences between our study and the literature. Years of malnutrition alter brain structure and function and cause permanent cognitive deficits analogous to scarring of brain structure. At the same time, morphological changes in brain structure take a different course, and the reduction in gray matter volume is more significant in adolescents than in adults. To date, there is no clear consensus in the literature about the effect of AN on neuropsychological function. Most studies have focused on adult patients with a long history of the disorder, leaving a gap in understanding adolescent patients with a shorter duration of AN and their experiences of starvation. Therefore, therapeutic interventions should be tailored to the duration of illness, degree of chronification, and associated neurocognitive deficits. The above study shows that cognitive deficits and laboratory tests may not be biomarkers of early-stage AN.

The results suggest that weight gain does not affect cognitive function. Investigating the dynamics of cognitive changes and the factors affecting them may be an essential target for future research. Neuropsychological functioning in the disease may be an important measure of prognosis, and a complete understanding of the cognitive function of patients with AN may provide more effective screening of disease risk groups, creating more tailored prevention and treatment programs.

Supplementary Materials: The following supporting information can be downloaded at: https://www.mdpi.com/article/10.3390/nu16203435/s1, Table S1: Linear regression outcomes for CAB in low body weight (AN1), after nutritional rehabilitation (AN2) and control group (CG).

Author Contributions: K.J.-K. participated in protocol development, data analysis, and manuscript writing. M.T.-N., D.D., A.P.-M. and A.S. participated in protocol development, literature search, writing, editing, and final manuscript approval. M.T.-N. and A.S. edited and approved the final manuscript. All authors have read and agreed to the published version of the manuscript.

Funding: The research was financed by a large research grant from statutory funding for young researchers, Poznan University of Medical Sciences Doctoral School (grant number 502-14-22193490-45055).

Institutional Review Board Statement: This article does not contain any studies with animals performed by any of the authors. The Bioethics Committee approved study protocol 476/20 of the University of Medicine in Poznan. All procedures involving human participants were in accordance with the ethical standards of the institutional and national research committee and with the 1964 Helsinki Declaration and its later amendments or comparable ethical standards.

Informed Consent Statement: Informed consent was obtained from all individual participants included in the study.

Data Availability Statement: The datasets used and analyzed during the current study are available from the corresponding author upon reasonable request.

Acknowledgments: The authors would like to thank all those who participated in this study for their enthusiastic involvement and hard work. They also thank the Poznan University of Medical Sciences for supporting the study. The funders had no role in the study design, data collection, and analysis; the decision to publish; or the preparation of this manuscript.

Conflicts of Interest: The authors declare no conflicts of interest.

Abbreviations

AN	anorexia nervosa
AN1	patients in the acute phase of anorexia nervosa
AN2	patients after partial normalization of body weight on the day of discharge
CA	cognitive abilities
CAB	Cognifit Assessment Battery
ED	eating disorders
FT4	thyroxine
HCT	hematocrit
HGB	hemoglobin concentration
NR	nutritional rehabilitation
PLT	platelet count
TSH	thyrotropic hormone
WBC	white blood cell
%IBW	percentage of ideal body weight

References

1. Wood, S.; Marchant, A.; Allsopp, M.; Wilkinson, K.; Bethel, J.; Jones, H.; John, A. Epidemiology of eating disorders in primary car in children and young people: A Clinical Practice Research Datalink study in England. *BMJ Open* **2019**, *9*, e026691. [CrossRef]
2. Petkova, H.; Simic, M.; Nicholls, D.; Ford, T.; Prina, A.M.; Stuart, R.; Livingstone, N.; Kelly, G.; MacDonald, G.; Eisler, I.; et a Incidence of anorexia nervosa in young people in the UK and Ireland: A national surveillance study. *BMJ Open* **2019**, *9*, e02733 [CrossRef]
3. Reas, D.L.; Rø, Ø. Time trends in healthcare-detected incidence of anorexia nervosa and bulimia nervosa in the Norwegia National Patient Register (2010–2016). *Int. J. Eat. Disord.* **2018**, *51*, 1144–1152. [CrossRef] [PubMed]
4. Agostino, H.; Burstein, B.; Moubayed, D.; Taddeo, D.; Grady, R.; Vyver, E.; Dimitropoulos, G.; Dominic, A.; Coelho, J.S. Trends i the Incidence of New-Onset Anorexia Nervosa and Atypical Anorexia Nervosa Among Youth During the COVID-19 Pandemic i Canada. *JAMA Netw. Open* **2021**, *4*, e2137395. [CrossRef]
5. Devoe, J.D.; Han, A.; Anderson, A.; Katzman, D.K.; Patten, S.B.; Soumbasis, A.; Flanagan, J.; Paslakis, G.; Vyver, E.; Marcou G.; et al. The impact of the COVID-19 pandemic on eating disorders: A systematic review. *Int. J. Eat. Disord.* **2023**, *56*, 5–2 [CrossRef] [PubMed]
6. Holland, J.; Hall, N.; Yeates, D.G.R.; Goldacre, M. Trends in hospital admission rates for anorexia nervosa in Oxford (1968–201 and England (1990–2011): Database studies. *J. R. Soc. Med.* **2016**, *109*, 59. [CrossRef] [PubMed]
7. Favaro, A.; Caregaro, L.; Tenconi, E.; Bosello, R.; Santonastaso, P. Time trends in age at onset of anorexia nervosa and bulimi nervosa. *J. Clin. Psychiatry* **2009**, *70*, 1715–1721. [CrossRef] [PubMed]
8. GBE—Gesundheitsberichterstattung des Bundes. Available online: https://www.gbe-bund.de/gbe/ (accessed on 18 March 2024
9. Cruz, A.M.; Gonçalves-Pinho, M.; Santos, J.V.; Coutinho, F.; Brandão, I.; Freitas, A. Eating disorders-Related hospitalizations i Portugal: A nationwide study from 2000 to 2014. *Int. J. Eat. Disord.* **2018**, *51*, 1201–1206. [CrossRef]
10. Fardouly, J.; Vartanian, L.R. Social Media and Body Image Concerns: Current Research and Future Directions. *Curr. Opin. Psych* **2016**, *9*, 1–5. [CrossRef]
11. Arseniev-Koehler, A.; Lee, H.; McCormick, T.; Moreno, M.A. #Proana: Pro-Eating Disorder Socialization on Twitter. *J. Adoles Health* **2016**, *58*, 659–664. [CrossRef]
12. Bills, E.; Greene, D.; Stackpole, R.; Egan, S.J. Perfectionism and eating disorders in children and adolescents: A systematic revie and meta-analysis. *Appetite* **2023**, *187*, 106586. [CrossRef]
13. Vostanis, P. Mental health provision for children affected by war and armed conflicts. *Eur. Child Adolesc. Psychiatry* **2024**, *3* 3293–3299. [CrossRef]
14. Gorrell, S.; Reilly, E.E.; Brosof, L.; Grange, D. Le Use of Telehealth in the Management of Adolescent Eating Disorders: Patien Perspectives and Future Directions Suggested from the COVID-19 Pandemic. *Adolesc. Health. Med. Ther.* **2022**, *13*, 45. [CrossRe

15. Muth, L.; Leven, K.H.; Moll, G.; Kratz, O.; Horndasch, S. Effects of the COVID-19 Restrictions on Eating Behaviour and Eating Disorder Symptomology in Female Adolescents. *Int. J. Environ. Res. Public Health* **2022**, *19*, 8480. [CrossRef]
16. Wang, S.B.; Gray, E.K.; Coniglio, K.A.; Murray, H.B.; Stone, M.; Becker, K.R.; Thomas, J.J.; Eddy, K.T. Cognitive rigidity and heightened attention to detail occur transdiagnostically in adolescents with eating disorders. *Eat. Disord.* **2021**, *29*, 408–420. [CrossRef] [PubMed]
17. Di Lodovico, L.; Versini, A.; Lachatre, M.; Marcheselli, J.; Ramoz, N.; Gorwood, P. Is decision-making impairment an endophenotype of anorexia nervosa? *Eur. Psychiatry* **2022**, *65*, e68. [CrossRef]
18. Smith, K.E.; Mason, T.B.; Johnson, J.S.; Lavender, J.M.; Wonderlich, S.A. A systematic review of reviews of neurocognitive functioning in eating disorders: The state-of-the-literature and future directions. *Int. J. Eat. Disord.* **2018**, *51*, 798–821. [CrossRef] [PubMed]
19. Lang, K.; Roberts, M.; Harrison, A.; Lopez, C.; Goddard, E.; Khondoker, M.; Treasure, J.; Tchanturia, K. Central Coherence in Eating Disorders: A Synthesis of Studies Using the Rey Osterrieth Complex Figure Test. *PLoS ONE* **2016**, *11*, e0165467. [CrossRef]
20. Fuglset, T.S. Is set-shifting and central coherence in anorexia nervosa influenced by body mass index, anxiety or depression? A systematic review. *BMC Psychiatry* **2021**, *21*, 137. [CrossRef]
21. Shott, M.E.; Filoteo, J.V.; Bhatnagar, K.A.C.; Peak, N.J.; Hagman, J.O.; Rockwell, R.; Kaye, W.H.; Frank, G.K.W. Cognitive Set-Shifting in Anorexia Nervosa. *Eur. Eat. Disord. Rev.* **2012**, *20*, 343. [CrossRef]
22. Weider, S.; Indredavik, M.S.; Lydersen, S.; Hestad, K. Neuropsychological function in patients with anorexia nervosa or bulimia nervosa. *Int. J. Eat. Disord.* **2015**, *48*, 397–405. [CrossRef] [PubMed]
23. Zacková, M.L.; Jáni, M.M.; Brázdil, M.; Nikolova, Y.S.; Marečková, K. Cognitive impairment and depression: Meta-analysis of structural magnetic resonance imaging studies. *NeuroImage Clin.* **2021**, *32*, 102830. [CrossRef] [PubMed]
24. American Psychiatric Association. *Diagnostic and Statistical Manual of Mental Disorders*; American Psychiatric Publishing: Washington, DC, USA, 2013. [CrossRef]
25. Hughes, E.K. Comorbid depression and anxiety in childhood and adolescent anorexia nervosa: Prevalence and implications for outcome. *Clin. Psychol.* **2012**, *16*, 15–24. [CrossRef]
26. Kahn, M.; Brunstein-Klomek, A.; Hadas, A.; Snir, A.; Fennig, S. Early changes in depression predict outcomes of inpatient adolescent anorexia nervosa. *Eat. Weight Disord.* **2020**, *25*, 777–785. [CrossRef]
27. Samson, K.L.I.; Fischer, J.A.J.; Roche, M.L. Iron Status, Anemia, and Iron Interventions and Their Associations with Cognitive and Academic Performance in Adolescents: A Systematic Review. *Nutrients* **2022**, *14*, 224. [CrossRef]
28. Przybylak, M.; Grabowski, J.; Bidzan, L. Cognitive functions and thyroid hormones secretion disorders. *Psychiatr. Pol.* **2021**, *55*, 309–321. [CrossRef]
29. Golden, N.H.; Cheng, J.; Kapphahn, C.J.; Buckelew, S.M.; Machen, V.I.; Kreiter, A.; Accurso, E.C.; Adams, S.H.; Le Grange, D.; Moscicki, A.-B.; et al. Higher-Calorie Refeeding in Anorexia Nervosa: 1-Year Outcomes from a Randomized Controlled Trial. *Pediatrics* **2021**, *147*, e2020037135. [CrossRef]
30. Weir, C.B.; Jan, A. BMI Classification Percentile and Cut Off Points. In *StatPearls [Internet]*; StatPearls Publishing: Treasure Island, FL, USA, 2024. [PubMed]
31. Nahler, G. Lorentz-formula. In *Dictionary of Pharmaceutical Medicine*; Springer: Vienna, Austria, 2009. [CrossRef]
32. Researchers Assessment Batteries Reliability and Validity Description of CogniFit Assessment Batteries. CogniFit Assessment Battery CogniFit © 2022. Available online: https://static.cognifit.com/customersupport/Validation+for+Researchers.pdf (accessed on 2 March 2024).
33. Rogoza, R.; Brytek-Matera, A.; Garner, D.M. Analysis of the EAT-26 in a non-clinical sample. *Arch. Psychiatry Psychother.* **2016**, *18*, 54–58. [CrossRef]
34. (PDF) Charakterystyka Psychometryczna Polskiej Adaptacji Kwestionariusza Depresji BDI-II Aarona T. Becka (Psychometric Properties of the Polish Version of the Aaron T. Beck's Depression Inventory BDI-II). Available online: https://www.researchgate.net/publication/269107443_Charakterystyka_psychometryczna_polskiej_adaptacji_Kwestionariusza_Depresji_BDI-II_Aarona_T_Becka_Psychometric_Properties_of_the_Polish_Version_of_the_Aaron_T_Beck%E2%80%99s_Depression_Inventory_BDI-II (accessed on 30 September 2024).
35. Yanover, T.; Thompson, J.K. Eating problems, body image disturbances, and academic achievement: Preliminary evaluation of the eating and body image disturbances academic interference scale. *Int. J. Eat. Disord.* **2008**, *41*, 184–187. [CrossRef]
36. Weider, S.; Indredavik, M.S.; Lydersen, S.; Hestad, K. Intellectual function in patients with anorexia nervosa and bulimia nervosa. *Eur. Eat. Disord. Rev.* **2014**, *22*, 15–24. [CrossRef]
37. Sundquist, J.; Ohlsson, H.; Winkleby, M.A.; Sundquist, K.; Crump, C. School Achievement and Risk of Eating Disorders in a Swedish National Cohort. *J. Am. Acad. Child Adolesc. Psychiatry* **2016**, *55*, 41. [CrossRef]
38. Ahrén, J.C.; Chiesa, F.; Koupil, I.; Magnusson, C.; Dalman, C.; Goodman, A. We are family—Parents, siblings, and eating disorders in a prospective total-population study of 250,000 Swedish males and females. *Int. J. Eat. Disord.* **2013**, *46*, 693–700. [CrossRef]
39. Ahrén-Moonga, J.; Silverwood, R.; Klinteberg, B.A.; Koupil, I. Association of higher parental and grandparental education and higher school grades with risk of hospitalization for eating disorders in females. *Am. J. Epidemiol.* **2009**, *170*, 566–575. [CrossRef]
40. Lopez, C.; Stahl, D.; Tchanturia, K. Estimated intelligence quotient in anorexia nervosa: A systematic review and meta-analysis of the literature. *Ann. Gen. Psychiatry* **2010**, *9*, 40. [CrossRef]

41. Forbush, K.; Heatherton, T.F.; Keel, P.K. Relationships between perfectionism and specific disordered eating behaviors. *Int. J. Eat. Disord.* **2007**, *40*, 37–41. [CrossRef]
42. Nikendei, C.; Funiok, C.; Pfüller, U.; Zastrow, A.; Aschenbrenner, S.; Weisbrod, M.; Herzog, W.; Friederich, H.C. Memory performance in acute and weight-restored anorexia nervosa patients. *Psychol. Med.* **2011**, *41*, 829–838. [CrossRef]
43. Terhoeven, V.; Kallen, U.; Ingenerf, K.; Aschenbrenner, S.; Weisbrod, M.; Herzog, W.; Brockmeyer, T.; Friederich, H.C.; Nikendei, C. Meaningful Memory in Acute Anorexia Nervosa Patients-Comparing Recall, Learning, and Recognition of Semantically Related and Semantically Unrelated Word Stimuli. *Eur. Eat. Disord. Rev.* **2017**, *25*, 89–97. [CrossRef]
44. Brown, M.; Robinson, L.; Campione, G.C.; Wuensch, K.; Hildebrandt, T.; Micali, N. Intolerance of Uncertainty in Eating Disorders: A Systematic Review and Meta-Analysis. *Eur. Eat. Disord. Rev.* **2017**, *25*, 329–343. [CrossRef]
45. Bartholdy, S.; Rennalls, S.J.; Jacques, C.; Danby, H.; Campbell, I.C.; Schmidt, U.; O'Daly, O.G. Proactive and reactive inhibitory control in eating disorders. *Psychiatry Res.* **2017**, *255*, 432–440. [CrossRef]
46. Fosco, W.D.; Hawk, L.W.; Colder, C.R.; Meisel, S.N.; Lengua, L.J. The development of inhibitory control in adolescence and prospective relations with delinquency. *J. Adolesc.* **2019**, *76*, 37. [CrossRef]
47. Shen, Y.; Zhao, H.; Zhu, J.; He, Y.; Zhang, X.; Liu, S.; Chen, J. Comparison of Intentional Inhibition and Reactive Inhibition in Adolescents and Adults: An ERP Study. *Dev. Neuropsychol.* **2020**, *45*, 66–78. [CrossRef]
48. Suttkus, S.; Schumann, A.; De la Cruz, F.; Bär, K.J. Attenuated neuronal and autonomic responses during error processing in anorexia nervosa. *Brain Behav.* **2021**, *11*, e2235. [CrossRef]
49. Tenconi, E.; Collantoni, E.; Meregalli, V.; Bonello, E.; Zanetti, T.; Veronese, A.; Meneguzzo, P.; Favaro, A. Clinical and Cognitive Functioning Changes After Partial Hospitalization in Patients with Anorexia Nervosa. *Front. Psychiatry* **2021**, *12*, 653506. [CrossRef]
50. Guardia, D.; Carey, A.; Cottencin, O.; Thomas, P.; Luyat, M. Disruption of Spatial Task Performance in Anorexia Nervosa. *PLoS ONE* **2013**, *8*, e54928. [CrossRef]
51. Federica, S.; Ilaria, B.; Valentina, V.; Leonardo, M.; Gianluca, C.; Alessandro, M.; Anna, S. Self-perception in anorexia nervosa: When the body becomes an object. *Neuropsychologia* **2022**, *166*, 108158. [CrossRef]
52. Dann, K.M.; Hay, P.; Touyz, S. Are poor set-shifting and central coherence associated with everyday function in anorexia nervosa? A systematic review. *J. Eat. Disord.* **2021**, *9*, 40. [CrossRef]
53. Lang, K.; Stahl, D.; Espie, J.; Treasure, J.; Tchanturia, K. Set shifting in children and adolescents with anorexia nervosa: An exploratory systematic review and meta-analysis. *Int. J. Eat. Disord.* **2014**, *47*, 394–399. [CrossRef]
54. Wu, M.; Brockmeyer, T.; Hartmann, M.; Skunde, M.; Herzog, W.; Friederich, H.C. Set-shifting ability across the spectrum of eating disorders and in overweight and obesity: A systematic review and meta-analysis. *Psychol. Med.* **2014**, *44*, 3365–3385. [CrossRef]
55. Hirst, R.B.; Beard, C.L.; Colby, K.A.; Quittner, Z.; Mills, B.M.; Lavender, J.M. Anorexia nervosa and bulimia nervosa: A meta-analysis of executive functioning. *Neurosci. Biobehav. Rev.* **2017**, *83*, 678–690. [CrossRef]
56. Brooks, S.J. A debate on working memory and cognitive control: Can we learn about the treatment of substance use disorders from the neural correlates of anorexia nervosa? *BMC Psychiatry* **2016**, *16*, 10. [CrossRef]
57. Brooks, S.J.; O'Daly, O.G.; Uher, R.; Schiöth, H.B.; Treasure, J.; Campbell, I.C. Subliminal food images compromise superior working memory performance in women with restricting anorexia nervosa. *Conscious. Cogn.* **2012**, *21*, 751–763. [CrossRef]
58. Israel, M.; Klein, M.; Pruessner, J.; Thaler, L.; Spilka, M.; Efanov, S.; Ouellette, A.S.; Berlim, M.; Ali, N.; Beaudry, T.; et al. *n*-back task performance and corresponding brain-activation patterns in women with restrictive and bulimic eating-disorder variants: Preliminary findings. *Psychiatry Res.* **2015**, *232*, 84–91. [CrossRef]
59. Seed, J.A.; McCue, P.M.; Wesnes, K.A.; Dahabra, S.; Young, A.H. Basal activity of the HPA axis and cognitive function in anorexia nervosa. *Int. J. Neuropsychopharmacol.* **2002**, *5*, 17–25. [CrossRef]
60. Lao-Kaim, N.P.; Giampietro, V.P.; Williams, S.C.R.; Simmons, A.; Tchanturia, K. Functional MRI investigation of verbal working memory in adults with anorexia nervosa. *Eur. Psychiatry* **2014**, *29*, 211–218. [CrossRef]
61. De Filippo, E.; Marra, M.; Alfinito, F.; Di Guglielmo, M.L.; Majorano, P.; Cerciello, G.; De Caprio, C.; Contaldo, F.; Pasanisi, F. Hematological complications in anorexia nervosa. *Eur. J. Clin. Nutr.* **2016**, *70*, 1305–1308. [CrossRef]
62. Mamou, G.; Sider, A.; Bouscary, D.; Moro, M.R.; Blanchet-Collet, C. Anemia in Anorexia Nervosa: The Best Way to Deal with it—An Overview of Literature. *J. Hum. Nutr. Food Sci.* **2016**, *4*, 1081.
63. Hütter, G.; Ganepola, S.; Hofmann, W.K. The hematology of anorexia nervosa. *Int. J. Eat. Disord.* **2009**, *42*, 293–300. [CrossRef]
64. Mehler, P.S.; Blalock, D.V.; Walden, K.; Kaur, S.; McBride, J.; Walsh, K.; Watts, J. Medical findings in 1026 consecutive adult inpatient-residential eating disordered patients. *Int. J. Eat. Disord.* **2018**, *51*, 305–313. [CrossRef]
65. Gibson, D.; Gibson, D.; Watters, A.; Watters, A.; Cost, J.; Cost, J.; Mascolo, M.; Mehler, P.S.; Mehler, P.S.; Mehler, P.S. Extreme anorexia nervosa: Medical findings, outcomes, and inferences from a retrospective cohort. *J. Eat. Disord.* **2020**, *8*, 25. [CrossRef]
66. Matsunaga, H.; Riku, K.; Shimizu, K.; Fujimi, S. Severe hypoglycemia with reduced liver volume as an indicator of end-stage malnutrition in patients with anorexia nervosa: A retrospective observational study. *J. Eat. Disord.* **2024**, *12*. [CrossRef]
67. Misra, M.; Klibanski, A. Neuroendocrine Consequences of Anorexia Nervosa in Adolescents. *Endocr. Dev.* **2010**, *17*, 197. [CrossRef] [PubMed]
68. DiVasta, A.D.; Feldman, H.A.; Brown, J.N.; Giancaterino, C.; Holick, M.F.; Gordon, C.M. Bioavailability of vitamin D in malnourished adolescents with anorexia nervosa. *J. Clin. Endocrinol. Metab.* **2011**, *96*, 2575–2580. [CrossRef] [PubMed]

9. Tasegian, A.; Curcio, F.; Dalla Ragione, L.; Rossetti, F.; Cataldi, S.; Codini, M.; Ambesi-Impiombato, F.S.; Beccari, T.; Albi, E. Hypovitaminosis D3, Leukopenia, and Human Serotonin Transporter Polymorphism in Anorexia Nervosa and Bulimia Nervosa. *Mediators Inflamm.* **2016**. [CrossRef] [PubMed]
0. Libuda, L.; Timmesfeld, N.; Antel, J.; Hirtz, R.; Bauer, J.; Führer, D.; Zwanziger, D.; Öztürk, D.; Langenbach, G.; Hahn, D.; et al. Effect of vitamin D deficiency on depressive symptoms in child and adolescent psychiatric patients: Results of a randomized controlled trial. *Eur. J. Nutr.* **2020**, *59*, 3415. [CrossRef]
1. Föcker, M.; Timmesfeld, N.; Bühlmeier, J.; Zwanziger, D.; Führer, D.; Grasemann, C.; Ehrlich, S.; Egberts, K.; Fleischhaker, C.; Wewetzer, C.; et al. Vitamin d level trajectories of adolescent patients with anorexia nervosa at inpatient admission, during treatment, and at one year follow up: Association with depressive symptoms. *Nutrients* **2021**, *13*, 2356. [CrossRef]
2. Hemmingsen, S.D.; Lichtenstein, M.B.; Hussain, A.A.; Sjögren, J.M.; Støving, R.K. Case report: Cognitive performance in an extreme case of anorexia nervosa with a body mass index of 7.7. *BMC Psychiatry* **2020**, *20*, 284. [CrossRef]
3. Laczkovics, C.; Czernin, K.; Carlitscheck, J.; Zeiler, M.; Schlund, P.; Wunram, H.L.; Lehmkuhl, G.; Krischer, M. Personality Disorder in Adolescent Patients with Anorexia Nervosa. *Psychopathology* **2023**, *56*, 268–275. [CrossRef]

nutrients

MDPI

Review

Natural Compounds and Their Potential in Eating-Related Aspects of Mental Health Disorders

Wenbin Ma [1,†], Ralf Regenthal [2,†] and Ute Krügel [3,*]

[1] School of Health and Rehabilitation, Chengdu University of Traditional Chinese Medicine, Chengdu 611137, China; mawenbin@cdutcm.edu.cn
[2] Division of Clinical Pharmacology, Rudolf Boehm Institute for Pharmacology and Toxicology, Leipzig University, 04107 Leipzig, Germany; ralf.regenthal@medizin.uni-leipzig.de
[3] Rudolf Boehm Institute for Pharmacology and Toxicology, Leipzig University, 04107 Leipzig, Germany
* Correspondence: ute.kruegel@medizin.uni-leipzig.de
† These authors contributed equally to this work.

Abstract

Background and Objectives: Mental health and healthy eating are inextricably linked by bi-directional interaction. As pharmacological interventions for eating disorders and mental illness have limited efficacy and are associated with significant side effects, natural compounds traditionally used in these fields represent an extremely rich source for potential future drugs. This review aims to summarise complex and/or specific pharmacological and clinical effects of mixed compositions and individual compounds derived from *Rosmarinus officinalis*, *Ginkgo biloba*, and *Bupleurum chinense* as well as from *Berberis vulgaris* and other berberine (BBR)-containing plants, which have been traditionally used for eating and mental health purposes. **Results and Conclusions:** The data on favoured natural compounds and main ingredients of compound mixtures presented here could provide new impetus for preventive or targeted supplementary treatment, potential drug development, and the design of new compound congeners with improved target spectrum and potency in mental health disorders and eating-related issues. Contemporary methodological development steps in this direction are then proposed.

Keywords: mental health disorders; eating disorders; *Rosmarinus officinalis*; *Ginkgo biloba*; *Bupleurum chinense*; berberine; gut-brain axis

1. Introduction

Living in an ever-changing world requires ongoing human–environmental and interpersonal interaction for subjective and physical well-being, including processes such as recognition, evaluation, and reorientation. Mental health and healthy eating are inextricably linked. Psychological well-being strongly influences the quality and quantity of food consumed, but nutrition can also influence mental health [1]. This bi-directional interaction is widely experienced and accepted. Therapeutic strategies in this field, especially pharmacological intervention are very limited and response rates in both, eating disorders (ED) and mental illness are still unsatisfactory.

Genetic risk factors and epigenetic modulation by multiple environmental and social impacts, which are not fully understood, may contribute to the etiopathogenesis and pathophysiology of mental health problems and altered eating behaviour. In addition, body dissatisfaction and dieting associated with personality disorders often precede ED, i.e., anorexia nervosa (AN), bulimia nervosa (BN), binge eating disorder (BED), avoidant restrictive food intake disorder (ARFID), pica, and rumination disorder (RD) [2]. Sociocultural distress provoked by idealised body images, mobbing, and humiliation may promote the development of anxiety, mood disorders and depressive episodes and thus act as a booster for ED. Such distress can also alter the reward system, leading to overeating resulting in obesity (OB) or substance abuse. Notably, OB and ED are phenomenologically opposite. However, in their development, both seem to share features ranging from ambivalent to disturbed perception and cognition. Today, the events in the individual development of either mental health problems or ED are poorly understood and even less so the relationship between both.

Not surprisingly, psychotherapeutic interventions are the mainstay of treatment for ED, as there are very limited psychopharmacological options for these disorders, e.g., fluoxetine and topiramate for BN, olanzapine for AN, lisdexamfetamine and topiramate for BED. However, like most of psychopharmacological active drugs, these medications have significant side effects, including those on eating behaviour itself. Moreover, olanzapine and topiramate have not yet received marketing authorization for use in ED.

Due to the limitations of drug treatment in ED, it is justified to search for more effective and safer treatment strategies also exploring natural products that are traditionally used for mental well-being without known safety concerns.

The aim of this narrative review is to provide a summary of complex and/or specific pharmacological effects of selected compositions or individual compounds derived from medicinal plants, here *Rosmarinus officinalis*, *Ginkgo biloba*, *Bupleurum chinense*, and *Berberis vulgaris*. The idea behind this is to provide new impetus for targeted supplementation and for potential drug development by different enhanced and standardised compositions and for the design of new compound congeners with improved target spectrum and binding affinity.

2. *Rosmarinus officinalis*

Rosmarinus officinalis, a member of the family Lamiaceae, is originally native to the Mediterranean region. Like several other kitchen spices, rosemary is used in traditional ethnic communities for a wide variety of health purposes as reviewed by Borges et al. [3]. These include gastrointestinal, digestive and appetite disturbances, circulatory and blood pressure problems, inflammation-related diseases (rheumatism, asthma bronchiale), and improvements in mental health like depressed mood, anxiety, or memory.

In addition to its use as an intensely aromatic spice, rosemary slows down the rancidification (oxidation) of oils rich in polyunsaturated fatty acids [4,5]. As an antimicrobial preservative, it inhibits the growth of bacteria that contribute to food spoilage [6]. Recognising this, rosemary extract is approved as antioxidant INS (E) No. 392. The aerial parts of the plant are used either as tea, tincture, or as essential oil (ISO 1342:2012) [7]. The latter is composed of more than 150 compounds and is particularly rich in volatile anti-inflammatory monoterpenes such as camphor [8], α-pinene [9], and 1,8-cineole (eucalyptol) [3,10]. More than 35 phenolic compounds were identified in rosemary extracts: phenolic diterpenes (e.g., carnosic acid, carnosol, rosmanol), flavonoids (e.g., gallic acid, catechin, hesperitin, quercetin, kaempferol, apigenin), and phenolic acids such as caffeoyl derivatives (e.g., caffeic acid and its ester, rosmarinic acid) [11,12], all of which have antioxidant activity in in vitro bioassays [13,14]. Pentacyclic triterpenes (sapogenins) of lupine, oleanane, and ursane structures are also found. Many of these identified compounds are also components of other herbs used for health purposes.

The potential pharmacological principles of individual compounds or required specific compositions of rosemary preparations relevant to body weight and metabolic regulation, circulation stimulation, and neuroprotection in mental health are only partially understood to date [15].

However, some common applications of rosemary are directly related to its anti-inflammatory biological activity, like asthma and rheumatic diseases. There is evidence that chronic low-grade inflammation by unbalanced production of pro- and anti-inflammatory (adipo)cytokines contributes to obesity-related insulin-resistance [16]. Likewise, in humans, mental disorders, such as anxiety, depression, or ED, and various types of dementia, bipolar disorder, and schizophrenia are partly linked to inflammatory processes, which makes rosemary preparations attractive to exploit [17–19].

Apparently mediated by carnosic acid, a potent inhibitor of prominent digestive enzymes like lipase, α-amylase, and α-glucosidase, body weight and insulin levels were reduced in lean and obese Zucker rats [20,21]. Furthermore, an improvement in metabolic disease-associated weight gain, inflammatory markers in the liver, pancreas, and brain was reported in a high-fat diet (HFD)-induced mouse model following oral administration of carnosic acid, as evidenced by a decrease in pro-inflammatory cytokines [22]. In particular, the inflammatory response to HFD in mouse brain was associated with an activation of the nuclear factor kappa B (NF-κB) signalling pathway, which was attenuated by carnosic acid treatment. Similar observations were made for limonene, which counteracted elevated apoptosis, inflammation, and oxidative stress in mouse brain after HFD [23].

However, in a double-blind, randomised, placebo-controlled clinical trial (RCT) in which patients with non-alcoholic fatty liver disease were treated with rosemary leaf powder (4 g per day) or placebo as part of a weight-loss diet for eight weeks, no additional beneficial effect on primary and secondary outcomes were detected [24]. In another cross-over RCT in overweight men, the postprandial inflammation caused by hyperglycaemia and hyperlipidaemia after oral ingestion of a high-saturated-fat, high-carbohydrate meal was attenuated by undefined amounts of rosemary in a mixture with various other spices [25].

Chronically restrained mice that developed hypercorticosteronemia and impaired insulin signalling, accompanied by cognitive impairment, were treated with another rosemary ingredient, the lipophilic pentacyclic triterpenoid ursolic acid [26]. This compound not only attenuated stress-induced reduction in body weight but also reduced corticosterone and tumour necrosis factor α (TNF-α) concentrations in plasma and parameters of oxidative stress in brain. In addition to an improved insulin sensitivity, the cognitive decline in the stressed mice was attenuated too. Although the underlying molecular mechanisms for ursolic acid-mediated anti-inflammatory effects are not enlightened so far, the suppression of the transcription factor NF-κB-regulated gene expression modulating cytokine production and cell survival in response to stress is documented in vitro and in vivo in a mouse model of graft-versus-host-disease [27]. Similarly, ursolic and rosmarinic acid were reported to prevent amyloid $A\beta_{1-42}$-induced deficits in cognition, synaptic regulation and adult hippocampal neurogenesis in mice [28]. Several other animal studies, although highly heterogeneous, confirmed beneficial effects of various preparations of rosemary in cognition and disease models [29].

The anti-inflammatory activity of mono- and diterpenes in rosemary is frequently reported [30]. Different but interacting pharmacological principles are proposed. One pathway involved is the inhibition of enzymes of the arachidonic acid cascade such as 5-lipoxigenase (5-LOX) and cyclooxygenases (COXs), which reduces the synthesis of inflammatory leukotrienes (LTB4) and prostaglandins (PGE2), e.g., by 1,8-cineole [31,32]. Another signalling pathway for some terpenes is the reduction in NF-κB activity. This attenuates the synthesis of the pro-inflammatory mediators TNF-α, interleukin-1β (IL-1β), and IL-6, of inflammatory enzymes (e.g., COX2, inducible nitric oxide synthase (iNOS)) and the expression of adhesion molecules and chemokines [33–35]. As a third mechanism, rosemary components, e.g., carnosol exert high antioxidant activity, thereby attenuating the harmful effects of reactive oxygen species (ROS) and lipid peroxidation [14].

These growing insights into the anti-inflammatory potential and the safe traditional use promote interest in rosemary for supportive application in mental disorders and ED. Preclinical observations in a mouse model of depression revealed an alleviated depression-like behaviour and a reduction in hippocampal oxidative stress by oral treatment with 1,8-cineole [36]. Preclinical mechanistic investigations on the central bioactivity of rosemary focused on neurotransmission. From behavioural studies with healthy mice fed acutely and sub-chronically with rosemary extract, Machado et al. (2009) predicted that rosemary's antidepressant-like effects were based on interaction with the monoaminergic system [37]. In particular, these acute effects were evoked in a dose-dependent manner by the rosemary constituent ursolic acid, which involved dopamine D1 and D2 receptors [38]. In agreement with responses of human patients to antidepressants, no psychostimulant effects were detected after acute oral administration of different rosemary preparations and for isolated carnosol in a similar behavioural approach in mice [39].

The described preclinical data are consistent with the observed antidepressant-like effects of single doses of rosmarinic and caffeic acid, which did not affect either monoamine uptake into synaptosomes or mitochondrial monoamine oxidase activity in mouse brain [40]. However, Lin et al. (2015) found evidence for a rosmarinic acid-mediated reduction in serotonin turnover in the rat hippocampus [41]. Moreover, both acids acutely induced a dose-dependent reduction in defensive freezing behaviour in mice exposed to conditioned fear stress [42]. Similarly, in healthy mice, isolated rosmanol, cirsimaritin, and salvigenin elicited antidepressant- and anxiolytic-like behaviour, attributed to modulation of GABA-A receptors [30]. In a recent study, systemically applied carnosic acid, a selective KCNQ3/5 potassium channel opener in parvalbumin-positive GABA neurons, reduced cell excitability and thereby diminished the cocaine reward in mice [43]. Finally, anxiolytic-like effects of rosemary in mice appear to involve the stimulation of oxytocinergic transmission [44]. This is remarkable as oxytocin is strongly involved in the control of stress responses and food intake and contributes to adaptive active coping in animals and humans [45].

Whereas behavioural effects of rosemary or of some integral components were reproducible in essence in preclinical research, data on rosemary from clinical studies on mental health are scare. In an RCT with healthy Iranian college students, rosemary (500 mg twice daily for one month) improved prospective and retrospective memory and sleep quality, and in addition reduced anxiety and depression [46]. In Japanese adult working men diagnosed with a poor mental health score, a four-week intervention with oral rosemary ameliorated mental energy and sleep quality [47]. Plasma analysis before and after consumption of rosemary tea (5 g dry weight once daily) by healthy volunteers for 10 days revealed significantly higher concentrations of a reliable biomarker of depression, the brain-derived neurotrophic factor (BDNF), an effect that may be related to its signalling through the neurotrophic tyrosine kinase receptor 2 (TRKB), which is essential for potential antidepressant actions [48,49].

In a small group of patients with newly diagnosed major depression, dried plant powder, which was administered as add-on to selective serotonin reuptake inhibitor (SSRI) therapy, reduced anxiety and depression scores significantly more effectively than SSRI alone [50]. Interestingly, some patients of the rosemary group reported increased appetite as side effect. Today, although appetising properties for rosemary are often mentioned, there is no sufficient evidence for that.

To the best of our knowledge, no clinical data about rosemary administration in eating disorders (ED) are available so far. However, ED is strongly linked to poor gut microbiome health, dysbiosis, and inflammation, as well as to impaired microbiome metabolite signalling involving short-chain fatty acids and tryptophan via vagus nerve innervation to the brain [51–54]. So, there is evidence that an impaired bi-directional communication along the microbiota–gut–brain axis and a malfunction of central pathways regulating food intake, motivation, and execution, as well as hedonic aspects of food intake or its restriction, contribute to the pathology of ED. Similarly, the conception of mental illness has been strongly associated with alterations in intestinal microbiome [55–59]. Therefore, the development of microbiome-based (supporting) therapies in ED could be promising. Such strategies are already in therapeutic use, possibly unintentionally, as multiple antidepressants have antimicrobial effects too, and as on the other hand some antibiotics may mediate antidepressant responses [60–62].

Rosemary and its components provide an example of natural products with multiple biological activities that also comprise antimicrobial properties beyond its effect as a preservative for food. In a preclinical model of chronically restrained mice with a depression-like outcome, Guo et al. (2018) found a significant intestinal dysbiosis rated as reduced Shannon index, enhanced community abundance of *Bacteroidetes* and *Proteobacteria*, and lowered *Firmicutes* and *Lactobacillus* spp., along with inflammatory responses in serum and the hippocampus [63]. The concomitant oral administration of a rosemary extract containing 60% carnosic acid in this study not only attenuated depression-like behaviour and inflammatory surrogate markers but also re-balanced the gut microbiota. To date, the link between the rosemary-mediated modification of gut microbiota and its supposed antidepressant potential seen in acute predictive models is only poorly understood.

Apart from direct effects on gut microbiome, the overall biological activity of rosemary relies on the bioavailability of its constituents. Romo Vaquero et al. (2013) [64] evidenced intestinal uptake and subsequent appearance of metabolites of carnosic acid, carnosol, and rosmanol in plasma in substantial concentrations for several hours in Zucker rats. Furthermore, small quantities of carnosic acid and carnosol (along with some of their metabolites) were detected in rat brain tissue [64]. Plasma levels of both were in a magnitude that correspond to their biological activity in a low micromolar range.

Analysis of different in vivo toxicity studies reveals that even high doses of rosemary extracts, carnosic, or ursolic acid fed over 90 days were safe [65]. In 2016, the Joint FAO/World Health Organisation (WHO) Expert Committee on Food Additives (JECFA) stated no safety concerns and established a temporary acceptable daily intake (ADI) for rosemary extract according to its specifications of 0–0.3 mg/kg body weight, expressed as carnosic acid plus carnosol content. This considered a no-observed-adverse-effect-level (NOAEL) of 64 mg/kg per day [66]. Importantly, in later studies on reproductive and developmental toxicity, according to the test guidelines of the Organisation for Economic Cooperation and Development's (OECD) and the specifications for food additives of the EU and JECFA, the NOAEL was doubled [67–69].

3. *Ginkgo biloba*

Ginkgo biloba L. is an endemic tree in China, grown worldwide today for nutrition, in particular the value of its seeds; for decoration; and also for health purposes. Its leaves, Ginkgo folium, are valued by the Anatomical Therapeutic Chemical/Defined Daily Dose Classification (ATC) of the WHO and the European Medicines Agency (EMA) as an antidementia drug (ATC N06DX02, Ginkgo folium) or as having "well-established use" for the improvement of (age-associated) cognitive impairment and of quality of life in mild dementia, respectively [70,71].

Evidence for the pharmacotherapeutic effects of natural products is frequently limited by their different phytochemical composition or product-by-process variations determining their pharmacokinetic and pharmacodynamic properties and therefore their clinical efficacy and safety.

A way to overcome these limitations was provided in case of *Ginkgo biloba* L. by strong defined growing and harvesting conditions and manufacturing processes providing standardised extracts, like EGb 761® and LI 1370, with enriched content of various ginkgo-specific flavonol glycosides and terpene trilactones (ginkgolides, bilobalide) considered to be the primary pharmacologically active components [72].

Today, the data situation regarding beneficial effects in Alzheimer's disease (AD) in clinical studies is still inconsistent. Whereas multiple studies reported beneficial effects of EGb 761® treatment in AD and vascular dementia [73,74], in other RCTs, this extract does not seem to reduce the risk for the progression of AD or its incidence, nor did it result in less cognitive decline in older adults with normal or mild cognitive decline [75–77]. A more recent analyses of efficacy and methodological challenges of the defined extract mixture EGb 761® in trials for mild-to moderate dementia did not consistently demonstrate its clinical utility for this indication [78,79]. Similarly, the National Center for Complementary and Integrative Health (NCCIH) of the National Institutes of Health (NIH) stated that there is no conclusive evidence that this defined *Ginkgo biloba* L. extract is helpful to improve or prevent cognitive decline [80]. Nonetheless, recognising overall data and focusing on beneficial effects on behavioural symptoms [81], EGb 761® was adopted in the dementia guidelines in Germany [82].

It should be considered that about 110 flavonoids, several terpenoids and nor-terpenoids, alkylphenols and alkylphenolic acid, carbonylic acids, lignans, polyanthocyanides, polyprenols, and polysaccharides, ingredients of ginkgo, might act in concert by broad pharmacological spectra [83]. Dependent on individual baseline sensitivity conditions, i.e., severity with respect to cognitive performance and social functioning, the observed effects in dementia should be valuated with care [84].

Apart from being used to treat or prevent cognitive decline, ginkgo extracts have been reported to have beneficial effects in psychiatric disorders, in particular on anxious mood or generalised anxiety disorders, as well as attention-deficit hyperactivity disorder (ADHD), and as an adjuvant to antipsychotics in schizophrenia, thought to be related in particular to the antioxidant properties of ginkgo components [85–87]. A recent meta-analysis of 21 trials preferentially from China compared the effects and safety of ginkgo extracts on patients with depression [88]. Here, the scores like the Hamilton depression scale (HAM) and the modified Barthel index (MBI) were significantly improved in ginkgo-treated patients. Furthermore, significantly elevated serum levels of BDNF and serotonin (5-HT) in these patients suggested that this natural product could lower depression symptoms. However, these observed beneficial characteristics of ginkgo extracts must be reproduced in clinical trials with a larger numbers of patients, also outside of China to avoid ethnic and genetic biases, with a highly standardised study design, particularly with regard to indication and disease status, to compound composition, to dose, and to treatment regime.

In addition to antioxidant activity decreasing ROS, ginkgo components are proposed to exert anti-inflammatory effects [89], to modulate enzymes responsible for degradation of neurotransmitters and formation of amyloid plaques [90,91], and to modulate BDNF expression in the hippocampus of stressed rats, a key player in the neuroplasticity hypothesis of depression [92].

So far, as the authors have researched, clinical studies on the effects of ginkgo extracts on eating behaviour in eating or mental disorders are not available, though this aspect attracts increasing interest.

Preclinical studies provide some preliminary hints that ginkgo extracts or selected components of them may modulate eating-related emotions, appetite, and food choice, as well as body weight regulation. As an example, in rats, in which the bacterial endotoxin lipopolysaccharide (LPS) induced symptoms of anhedonia, a 14-day pretreatment with EGb 761® prevented the decline of sucrose and food consumption and slightly alleviated the LPS-induced attenuation of dopamine in the reward-related nucleus accumbens [93,94]. Although the development of the animal's body weight under EGb 761® pretreatment alone is not reported, a comparatively higher food consumption of the EGb 761® group was in line with lower body weight loss 24 h after LPS-induced sickness behaviour.

In healthy mice, a seven-day treatment regime with ginkgo extract, and specifically with the terpenoid ginkgolide A, produced anxiolytic-like behaviour without alterations in body weight [95]. Other ingredients, the ginkgolides B, C, or bilobalide did not alter body weight or the behaviour in a predictive anxiety test. Likewise, the body weight of healthy rats was not affected after a 15 day-treatment with EGb 761® [96]. However, when rats with diet-induced obesity were treated with a ginkgo extract, the food intake and body adiposity were significantly reduced, whereas insulin sensitivity was increased, accompanied by a restored insulin-signalling cascade in muscle [97]. Compatibly, obese mice treated with a ginkgo extract expressed higher amounts of proteins associated with adipogenesis, carbon metabolism, and mitochondrial function and concomitantly showed a reduction in adipocyte hypertrophy in the visceral fat tissue. In parallel, parameters related to oxidative stress defence were also modulated, supporting the above-mentioned antioxidant activity [98]. Furthermore, in rats, a ginkgo extract improved the ovariectomy-induced resistance to serotonin-mediated hypophagia, at least in part through stimulation of the hypothalamic serotonergic activity [99]. The mechanisms by which ginkgo extract or its specific components may modulate energy homeostasis via the serotonergic system are only partly understood [100–102]. However, the induction of hypothalamic anorexigenic pro-opiomelanocortin (POMC), cocaine- and amphetamine-regulated transcript (CART), and 5-HT2C receptor gene expression, but not of orexigenic effectors in rats after a single ginkgo extract dose may suggest that components or specific compositions of this herb can act as rapid hypophagic appetite modulators [103].

These still small-scale preclinical results indicate that ginkgo extracts or isolated components may be biologically active in the regulation of metabolic and nutritional processes under certain conditions. However, this has to be further verified by systematic hypothesis-led and well-designed studies (model and disease conditions, compound compositions, dose levels, treatment regimes, and duration) in preclinical and clinical trials.

Advantageously, ginkgo extracts seem to be safe and well tolerated when moderate amounts, up to 240 mg per day, are ingested by humans [104]. The most commonly reported side effects are dizziness, gastrointestinal symptoms, and headache, but drug interactions with antithrombotic and non-steroidal anti-inflammatory drugs like clopidogrel and acetylsalicylic acid bear a minor bleeding risk [105].

4. *Bupleurum chinense*

Although little known outside Asia, the genus *Bupleurum*, especially the root of *B. chinense* (Radix bupleuri, Chai Hu) and that of many other subspecies, has been used for centuries for treatment of depression and other psychiatric disorders in China, Japan, South Korea, and other Asian countries. In traditional Chinese medicine (TCM), various formulas of Bupleurum in combination with other Chinese herbs, such as Chaihu–Shugan–San (CSS) and Xiao–Yao–San (XYS), have been widely applied for treatment of depression [106]. The China Food and Drug Administration (CFDA) has approved several of them [107]. However, no clinical studies using Radix bupleurum for mental health are listed in PubMed so far. Apart from this fact, few meta-analyses reported that herbal formulas containing *B. chinense*, either in combination with antidepressants or alone, can improve depressive symptoms and have low adverse effects. The remission rates were reported to be comparable or even higher than those achieved when antidepressants were used alone [108,109]. However, the robustness of the data is low. As rated by the authors themselves, the analysed studies were of high heterogeneity and low quality, not free from bias and partly without description of serious adverse events.

Despite this poor data situation, *B. chinense* is of interest in the search for drugs with a broad spectrum of activity contributing to mental health. As with other traditional herbal products, certain effects of Bupleurum-based formulations are attributed to a variety of bioactive ingredients. These mainly comprise terpenoids (triterpenoid and sterol saponins), phenols like flavonoids, phenylpropanoids with phenylpropionic acids (mainly caffeic acid) and lignans, mono- and sesquiterpens (essential oils), and many others. Many of these compounds have been shown to exert numerous synergistic pharmacological effects that could potentially be utilised in clinical applications [110].

Major components of the Bupleurum species are about 35 saponins, in particular saikosaponins A, C, and D (SSA, SSC, SSD), representing a group of glycosylated triterpenic oleanane and ursane derivatives. Preferably SSA, but also SSD, are considered as the main anti-inflammatory constituents of Bupleurum suppressing pro-inflammatory cytokines and associated proteins and thereby restricting the NF-κB pathway shown in vitro [111]. In addition, the inhibition of the mitogen-activated protein kinase (MAPK) pathway via reduction in phosphorylation of p38 MAPK, c-Jun *N*-terminal kinases (c-JNK), and extracellular signal-regulated kinases (ERK1/2) was repeatedly reported in vitro for both SSA and SSD [110]. Similarly, flavonoid aglycones like kaempferol and quercetin, preferentially abundant in plant's overground parts, exert anti-inflammatory activity in response to the bacterial toxin LPS, but have also a powerful antioxidative capacity by free radical scavenging in kinetic-based structure–activity analysis [112].

It should be noted that secondary plant substances, among them polyphenols, have restricted access to the brain [113]. Likewise, blood-to-brain passage is very different for triterpenoid saponins [114]. Therefore, and in view of manifold conceivable derivatives produced by microbiota, intestine, or liver, the origin of pharmacological effects on brain health is mostly unclear [115]. Irrespective of that, preparations of Bupleurum herb combinations are integral parts of traditional medicine, obviously unintentionally utilising a synergistic multi-target treatment for depression to enhance anti-inflammatory effects and neuroprotection and to keep side effects low. Therefore, preclinical research is aimed at scientific evidence for effectiveness of such treatments and their underlying mechanisms.

An example for such preclinical investigations is Chaihu-Shugan-San (CSS), composed of Bupleurum and six other herbs. CSS was fed for the last two weeks of four-week period of unpredictable mild stress to rats [116]. CSS improved body weight gain and food intake and reduced depression-like behaviour in rats. Interestingly, when CSS was decomposed to its two individual components, Shu Gan and Rou Gan, containing 4 or 3 herbs, respectively, and fed in the model, only the Shu Gan component exerted antidepressant effects. Proteomics comparison of rat's hippocampi revealed that complete CSS also altered the expression of proteins that were not regulated by these two components alone and vice versa. Further bioinformatics and protein analysis suggest that CSS modulated mainly antidepressant neurotransmitter pathways, most significant of GABA. Currently, there is no explanation for these complex interactions in target regulation by herb compositions.

In a similar preclinical chronic stress model in rats, one of the most accepted herbal pair formulations in TCM for antidepressant treatment, Chaihu–Baishao (radices of *B. chinense* and *Paeoniae lactiflora*) evoked superior synergistic antidepressant-like and anti-inflammatory activities compared to Bupleurum alone [117]. By subsequent network pharmacology with compound filtering, both herbs shared only one active compound out of 29. Furthermore, an average number of about 41 targets per compound and 6 compounds per target were calculated for the combination. From all identified targets, the MAPK pathway, as well as arachidonic acid and tryptophan metabolism, were most apparent, suggesting that this herb pair exerts combinatory effects on multiple depression-related signalling pathways in a comparable manner.

One reason for the improved effects of the herb combination of radices of Bupleurum and Paeoniae may be the enhanced bioavailability of several components including SSA, SSB2, and saikogenin derivatives in rats compared to administration of Bupleurum alone [118]. These data strongly argue for the importance of pharmacokinetic interaction of substance compositions, which subsequently may determine observable drug effects. Analogously, in an ex vivo rat model, SSA and SSD were poorly absorbed themselves, but they enhanced the intestinal wall passage of one of the most powerful antioxidant and anti-inflammatory active monoterpene glycosides of radix Paeoniae, paeoniflorin [119,120]. This is explained by the surfactant activity inherent in saponins that may increase the intestinal permeability by opening epithelial tight junctions. In addition, P-glycoprotein-mediated efflux and hydrolysis via glucosidases may interfere with the oral bioavailability of the manifold compounds in herb mixtures.

Furthermore, improved bioavailability of phytochemicals, when administered in combinations, was positively correlated with the appearance of their metabolites. The metabolites include picolinic acid, a by-product of the kynurenine pathway which is down-regulated in depression; itaconic acid, which inhibits the NLR family pyrin domain containing 3 (NLRP3) protein; and α-linolenic acid. These metabolites may substantiate the antidepressant properties of herbal combinations through a variety of synergistic neuroprotective, immunological, and anti-proliferative effects, as described in preclinical studies [118].

It is worth noting that radix Paeoniae reversed the dose-limiting hepatotoxicity of Bupleurum in rats, mediated by saikosaponin-induced inhibition of glutathione synthetase (GSS), subsequent oxidative stress, and activation of NF-κB/NLRP3 pathway. The chronic co-administration of both drugs not only evoked antidepressant-like effects in stressed rats, but it also may re-shape the hepatic redox balance, and inhibit inflammatory responses, possibly through the regulation of gut microbiota in favour of glucosidase activity to promote the conversion of saikosaponins into metabolites (saikogenins) without disturbing GSS-inhibiting properties [121].

Currently, modes of action of some individual Bupleurum active ingredients, prodrugs, or regulated endogenous metabolites are under preclinical investigation to further uncover their therapeutic potential [122]. Apart from antidepressant-like effects of Bupleurum extracts in stressed rats, components derived from their blood, like metabolites of SSA, SSB1, SSB2, SSC, and SSD; valerenic acid; glycyrrhetinic acid (enoloxone); and nootkatone individually improved reserpine-induced depression-like behaviour in the zebrafish. This behavioural adjustment was associated with increased 5-HT and lowered cortisol content [122]. Reproducible antidepressant-like effects of SSD in stressed rats were similarly associated with a reconstitution of plasma corticosterone and glucocorticoid receptor expression in the hippocampus [123]. These data suggest an SSD-mediated correction of the hypothalamic–pituitary–adrenal (HPA) axis dysfunction. Additionally, SSD improved hippocampal neurogenesis accompanied by a raise of phosphorylated cAMP response element-binding protein (p-CREB) and of BDNF levels, all essential for antidepressant-like effects.

The enhanced 5-HT in rodents and zebrafish after Bupleurum treatment may suggest that certain components might influence the regulation of appetite and weight, at least by stimulation of 5-HT2C receptors whose implication in depression is still under debate. In line with these findings, in structure–activity relationship studies, *B. chinense* extract and SSA itself exhibit strong 5-HT2C receptor agonistic activity [124]. In healthy rats, SSA elicited food intake suppression and weight gain inhibition, which is in agreement with the anorectic properties of 5-HT2C receptor agonists [124]. This raises the question of potential anti-obesity efficacy. This hypothesis is also supported by the dose-dependent effect of SSA to reduce the reinforcing and motivational properties of highly palatable, high caloric food or drugs and to suppress the cue-induced reinstatement of seeking behaviour, similar to the cannabinoid CB1 receptor antagonist/inverse agonist rimonabant, which was used as reference in this model [125,126]. The idea that SSA may have anorectic or anti-obesogenic effects should be pursued further using reproducible preclinical behavioural correlates by pharmacological intervention and with the observation of potential side effects.

It is likely that SSA may not only interfere with appetite-regulating neuronal mechanisms to suppress excessive food intake per se but also may dampen binge-like eating behaviour which also needs to be proven.

It is noteworthy that treatment of healthy mice for 34 days with a no further defined extract of *B. scorzonerifolium* Willd. by gavage did not affect the body weight gain [127]. The most likely explanation for this discrepancy is differences in the composition and content of saikosaponins in both plant subspecies. In particular, the amount of SSA is considerably higher in *B. chinense* [128,129]. This observation strongly points to the importance of well-defined standardised compositions and doses of natural products in terms of their target-orientated use in compromised individuals and evaluation of their potentially synergistic pharmacological basics.

5. *Berberis vulgaris, Coptis chinensis,* and Other Berberine-Containing Plants

Berberine (BBR) is one of the few alkaloids that are found not only in different genera of the same plant family, but also in plants of different families like *Berberidaceae* (*Berberis* spp.), *Ranunculaceae* (*Coptis* spp.), *Papaveraceae*, and *Caesalpineae*. Traditionally, plants containing BBR as a main active component, such as *Berberis vulgaris*, *Berberis aristata*, or *Coptis chinensis* (Huanglian), have been used to treat infections or diseases of skin or gastrointestinal tract. Nowadays, this isoquinoline alkaloid is also available by chemical synthesis.

Apart from current scientific interest in BBR to support glucose and lipid homeostasis and insulin sensitivity, it has become a social media hot-topic as a promoted dietary supplement with purported weight loss capabilities [130,131].

Indeed, a comprehensive systematic review and dose–response meta-analysis of clinical data found a significant reduction in body weight and body mass index (BMI) in adults by treatment with BBR [132]. Whereas BBR supplementation was mostly ineffective at normal BMI, in subgroups with impaired metabolic health, the effects of BBR on lipid profile, insulin resistance, and fasting glucose were significant, but required daily intake up to 1.8 g per day and at least a treatment duration of 40 weeks. The underlying data were reported to have a high risk of bias and inconsistent outcomes across individual trials. Therefore, there is still insufficient scientific evidence to conclude its clinical effectiveness.

In clinical practice, weight gain by psychotropic drugs with broad receptor profiles, e.g., the antipsychotic olanzapine or the antidepressant amitriptyline, is related to metabolic disorders and is one major reason for discontinuation of treatment [133]. A few preliminary clinical studies suggest that supplementation with BBR may alleviate this adverse effect. In one RCT, a small group of schizophrenic patients individually adjusted to one single antipsychotic was treated either with BBR (0.9 g daily, $n = 27$) or placebo ($n = 22$) [134].

Eight weeks after, the body weight was significantly lower in the BBR group, but limitations in study design, subject heterogeneity, and the lack of significance in the "before and after" within-group comparisons reduce the value of these data. In another RCT, mild metabolic alterations were induced by at least nine months of olanzapine treatment. Here, the BMI and other metabolic parameters were significantly improved after 12 weeks of accompanying treatment with BBR compared to placebo [135].

Preclinical studies revealed similar results. BBR (0.38 g/kg per day) and metformin (0.3 g/kg per day) were shown to prevent olanzapine-induced weight gain, white fat accumulation, and brown fat loss, responsible for thermogenesis in rats, but did not hinder the increased food intake [136]. This effect was explained by an increase in energy expenditure involving expression of the thermogenic AMP-activated protein kinase (AMPK) and uncoupling protein 3 (UCP3) genes, corresponding to reduced energy storage. Similarly, in mice, BBR and metformin lowered olanzapine-induced orexigenic signalling, obviously involving down-regulation of serum levels of ghrelin and leptin as well as reduced expression of orexigenic hypothalamic neuropeptides [137]. Interestingly, the olanzapine-induced hypothalamic expression of the transient receptor potential cation channels TRPV1/3, likely emerging targets in metabolic disorders, was attenuated by BBR.

Given that metformin may attenuate adverse metabolic effects of several psychotropic drugs and that common regulatory pathways are suggested for both, BBR may represent a justified alternative therapeutic strategy for mental health problems associated with metabolic or ED that needs to be systematically explored [133,138].

Patients with obesity often develop neuroinflammation accompanied by negative mood or depression, which is strongly associated with inadequate glucagon-like peptide-1 (GLP-1) signalling [139–141]. Therefore, direct or indirect stimulation of GLP-1 receptors is currently being discussed as a therapeutic option for BED, comorbid depression in obesity, or in psychopharmacological treatments associated with weight gain [142]. The latter has been demonstrated in four RCTs with weight loss outcomes following GLP-1 analogue treatment in patients with antipsychotic-induced weight gain [143,144].

It is therefore exciting that BBR increased the GLP-1 secretion in streptozotocin-induced diabetic rats and furthermore that antidiabetic-like effects (reduction in fasting glucose, increase in pancreatic insulin) and reduced food intake were observed in healthy rats after five weeks of 120 mg BBR/kg per day per os [145]. In a diabetic mouse model, BBR improved pancreatic islet β-cell function by activation of the GLP-1/GLP-1R/PKA signalling pathway in intestinal L-cells and in islet α-cells [146]. This item is further discussed below. Supporting these data, another animal study showed that BBR reduced HFD-induced weight gain in rats and suggested that BBR acts directly in the brain to counteract neuropeptide Y (NPY)-driven food intake [147].

While the appetite-suppressing effect of BBR may be appealing to patients with BED or with weight-related concerns, it could be dangerous when misused as it could exacerbate restrictive eating patterns or obsessive weight control behaviour. Therefore, the risk of its use in the context of such ED must be clarified.

On the other hand, although there is no robust evidence so far, the mild antidepressant and anxiolytic effects of BBR via serotonergic and dopaminergic pathways may improve mental health disturbances associated with ED. This is implied by preclinical studies in which BBR alleviates depressive-like behaviour induced by corticosterone administration or by chronic unpredictable mild stress (CUMS) in mice [148,149]. Improvements were related to anti-inflammatory processes, e.g., reduction in brain and peripheral cytokine levels and lower cerebral expression of NLRP3 inflammasome. Consistently, in two RCTs, BBR significantly improved negative symptoms and cognitive deficits in patients with schizophrenia [150,151]. These positive responses to BBR also appear to be associated with anti-inflammatory activity at the cytokine level.

In most studies, BBR was applied orally. However, its intestinal uptake is only approximate 0.5% due to its physicochemical properties, a high affinity to the efflux transporter P-glycoprotein and fast intestinal and hepatic first-pass metabolisation [152,153]. Consequently, mean achievable plasma concentrations of about 4 nM in animal models and humans, even after chronic administration, appear to be below the required concentrations for activation of AMPK for mitochondria function, for inhibition of acetylcholine esterase or for improvement of insulin resistance which all were reported to be in the µmolar range [154–157]. Pharmacokinetic studies in rats point to a ten-fold enrichment of BBR in liver compared to plasma, but only about 10% of plasma BBR seems to cross the blood–brain barrier (BBB) [152,153]. Furthermore, an improvement of viability of neuronal PC12 cells or of behaviour of 6-hydroxydopamine-treated zebrafish, both as models for neuroprotective effects of BBR, were observed only in concentrations above 0.1 µM [158].

All these uncertainties urgently call for systematic investigations of the relationship between BBR, its metabolites and supposed receptor binding affinities as well as consecutive target activities. Today, the manifold effects of BBR are only described at an observational level, but the molecular compound–target interactions necessary for these mechanisms remain largely unknown. Beyond that, questions arise as how such low plasma concentrations and limited access to the brain after oral BBR administration may mediate central effects on mental health in animal models and humans and whether such effects might also be attributable to the interaction of BBR with intestinal microbiome [159,160].

Apart from hepatic conversion into several active metabolites, gut microbiota reduces BBR to dihydroberberine, which has a five-fold higher absorption rate and is suggested to be re-oxidised in the intestine, thereby probably improving the parent compound bioavailability to the observed levels despite P-glycoprotein outward transport [157,161,162].

Not only the extent, but probably moreover the diversity of composition of the gut microbiome, is strongly related to psychiatric disorders such as anxiety and depression [163–165]. Simplified, even findings for alpha and beta diversity were inconsistent, higher abundance of pro-inflammatory species and lower short-chain fatty acid (SCFA) producing-bacteria seem to be related to intestinal, peripheral, and central inflammation.

In animal models of depression, BBR administration was shown to alter microbiota in favour of *Bacteroidetes* and *Lactobacilli* and *Bifidobacteria*, microbiota with anti-inflammatory and metabolic benefits, and to reduce *Firmicutes*. These changes were associated with an attenuation of gut-derived inflammation, the restoration of intestinal barrier integrity, and improvement of behavioural outcome [159,160,166]. SCFA, e.g., butyrate, propionate, and acetate, resulting from BBR-augmented carbohydrate fermentation increase the enteroendocrine activity, e.g., the release of GLP-1 and peptide YY from intestinal L cells as reviewed elsewhere [167]. Furthermore, they may enter the bloodstream as important signalling molecules within the gut–brain communication [166,168]. For example, SCFA affect the permeability of the blood–brain barrier and activate microglia [168]. Microbiota are also able to synthesise a range of major neurotransmitters such as biogenic amines, GABA or histamine. They may also alter the levels of neurotransmitters or other signalling molecules like peptides or steroids synthesised by the host. Thereby, the microbiome may communicate not only locally with the enteric nervous system but also contributes to the innervation of the vagus nerve or to the activity of the HPA axis [169]. Such a signalling might offer a plausible link between neuroinflammation, negative mood, and altered GLP-1 as outlined above.

Gut dysbiosis and reduced SCFA in faeces, intestine, and blood have repeatedly reported in ED, mainly for AN [170–173]. A strong case and progression sensitivity of microbiota alterations in AN was pointed out, which in future should be captured by longitudinal study designs considering clear diagnoses and self-reports. Most importantly, the composition of a "normal" microbiota, which differs dependent on geographic origin, eating habits, food choice, gender, age, and many other conditions, must be recognised to assess the effectiveness of clearly defined plant-derived products [174]. Even though data on the clinical use of BBR in ED and adjunctive therapies in AN are currently unavailable, the oral administration of BBR to address the restoration of intestinal microbiota and their fermentation products may be beneficial.

Having the low systemic bioavailability of BBR after oral administration in mind and looking for the missed junction to the observed effects of this compound, its interaction with gut microbiota and the restoration of their beneficial metabolic products such as SCFA or neurotransmitters may be an explanatory approach [175].

6. Summary and Future Implications

What important insights can be extracted from the above contemplations? Undoubtedly, there is some potential of the key ingredients discussed, particularly rosemary, Bupleurum, and Berberis, to positively influence physical and mental health.

For a large number of individual substances or extracts with different compositions, peripheral and in some cases also centrally mediated effects caused by interaction with certain pharmacological target structures have been demonstrated in vivo. Some of these effects could be of significance for the treatment of ED or body schema disorders associated with mental disorders.

Currently, favoured ingredients of plant products have primarily been investigated by mechanistic approaches in a fairly eclectic manner guided by traditional fields of application. Because of commonly used low or pharmaco-dynamically unclear doses of mixtures, no comprehensive dose–response profiles of specific substances in vivo and even less clear side-effect or toxicity profiles can be determined. Even though an often-favoured multi-target concept of low-dose substances with partly synergistic responses in the context of natural products may well have its justification, this does not necessarily lead to a conclusive theory of mechanisms of action. Thereby, several dose–effect relations remain unsolved which are mandatory for optimised use. Furthermore, studies with targeted combinations of biologically active compounds also have to scrutinise the relationship between synergistic efficacy and the resulting side effect profile.

As an important tool, the network pharmacology can help to complete the biological efficacy profile of a compound and to make synergistic principles more likely.

For effective exploitation of synergistic effects, however, the separate determination of the value and safety of the individual active ingredients in clearly defined pharmacodynamic study designs and dose–response relationships is essential.

The direct effects of rosemary's main compounds in ED are imaginable, but currently not very substantiated and at best of subordinate importance. So, rosemary extracts have not yet been specifically investigated in ED. However, the effects of rosemary ingredients that strengthen mental health via various central neuronal mechanisms, e.g., serotonin turnover and/or GABA receptor modulation, have been documented in preclinical approaches. The broad anti-inflammatory and antioxidant activity of many individual rosemary ingredients in vitro, such as 1,8-cineole or carnosic acid, may further support central mechanisms. As the anti-inflammatory effect of 1,8-cineole is not limited to rosemary, but is attributed to many other plants too, it forms part of a respective overall effect.

Following oral administration in humans, favoured rosemary ingredients like carnosic acid, carnosol, and rosmanol/rosmarinic acid were found in plasma and the brain—a prerequisite for direct peripheral and central effects. In sum, the collected data suggest that a secondary influence on eating behaviour is expectable.

More confusing are the preclinical and clinical data for *Bupleurum chinensis* because, with a few exceptions, in animal models, predominantly traditionally prepared mixtures or parts of mixtures were used. Nonetheless, there is preclinical evidence that triterpenoid saponins and their intestinal derived metabolites, which have very different access to circulation and brain, can mediate measurable central effects in multiple depression-related signalling pathways alone but strengthened in combinations. However, no clear dose–response relationships are known. If the reported 5HT2C agonistic receptor activity of SSA in healthy animals can be further utilised to solely establish an anorectic principle applicable in ED or body schema disorders or whether a CB1 receptor antagonistic effect contributes still remains unclear. An essential step forward to exploiting the potential benefits of Bupleurum is the determination of the biological fate and bioavailability of pure lead compounds and their main metabolites according to established pharmacokinetic guidelines. Based on this, associated receptors and their signalling pathways should be investigated in systematic dose–response relationship studies. This also applies to the effects of SSD in terms of re-balancing the HPA axis function and hippocampal neurogenesis in stress-induced depression-like behavioural symptoms, mechanisms which are possibly also associated with ED.

In European medicine, the multi-ingredient mixture of *Gingko biloba* leaves enriched with ginkgolides and bilobalides, even when used in standardised extracts, has gained limited value in early types of dementia like AD and is only recommended as a 'can'. Based on the current scientific literature, there is no evidence for an off-label medical use of ginkgo extracts in ED. Conceivable are only indirect effects on body weight due to modulation of central mechanisms involved in emotional regulation.

Forward-looking, this review refers to newer experimental data showing that a distinct ginkgo extract, when administered orally and subchronically to obese rats, reduced food intake, adiposity, and insulin resistance. Compatible with an induction of hypothalamic anorexigenic POMC, CART, and 5-HT2 gene expression in rats following one single dose of ginkgo extract only, components or compositions of this herb could potentially act as metabolic and hypophagic appetite modulators in future study approaches. However, these results must first be confirmed using defined extracts whose compositions have to be gradually minimised until individual key effects virtually disappear. Subsequent dose titrations with pure substances and recombination can provide further insight into the desired optimal effects.

For BBR, the review highlights some focal points of high interest for ED therapies. Firstly, preclinical and clinical studies, albeit with methodological weaknesses, indicate a beneficial effect comparable to metformin, but largely free of side effects that might be utilised in the future in antipsychotic-induced weight gain. The overall effect probably consists of an influence on fat thermogenesis, an increase in energy expenditure, and a reduction in orexigenic signalling. Secondly, in preclinical studies, BBR augments gastrointestinal carbohydrate fermentation associated with enhanced enteroendocrine activity. The GLP-1-like effects of BBR may be beneficial in pathological weight gain. However, given the low CNS levels that can be achieved, the direct contribution of BBR to central effects is questionable. Again, it follows that clarification of the pharmacokinetic fate of BBR in the human organism is an urgent task. Thirdly, gut dysbiosis is reported to be relevant in mental diseases as well as in ED, in particular in AN. As BBR is involved in the reorganisation of microbiome and its fermentation products, which probably serve as important systemic signalling molecules, it is worth being studied clinically in AN. Overall,

BBR opens a potential alternative therapeutic tool for mental health problems associated with metabolic or eating disorders.

Inspired by traditional uses of important plants and/or their value-determining main ingredients, the present analysis of scientific literature outlines the currently known spectrum of their effects and potential benefits in ED bi-directionally linked to mental health problems. However, the highly heterogeneous features of traditional extracts without standardised phytochemical profiling limit generalised statements on health effects in human.

Successful research strategies can only generate valid efficacy data provided that mixtures of plant substances are standardised to proposed marker compounds or separated into their individual components, which makes it possible to recognise and to verify the contribution of each individual substance and its targets. This paves the way to effectively utilise a multi-target concept in later research phases and, in the best case, to incorporate it into the development of an approved drug.

In parallel, it is essential to continue pharmacological research with pure substances or at least with very clearly standardised downscaled extracts on carefully predefined targets and downstream pharmacodynamic mechanisms. Based on a hypothesised mechanism of action, future clinical trials need to verify the positive effects in body schema disorders. This requires the determination of dose–response relationships of well-defined compounds, strict inclusion and exclusion criteria for study participants, and valid primary outcome measures, arranged at best in longitudinal study designs, all preconditions that are often neglected in investigations of natural products.

At this point, it must be emphasised that the absolute prerequisite for clinical studies is the clarification of the biological fate and pharmacokinetic behaviour of the parent substance and the most important metabolites in order to assign effects and dose–response relationships reliably. The often-limited availability of such data inevitably impedes the uncovering of their pharmacological effects. A challenge in this context is the quantitative and qualitative variability of metabolites produced in the intestine and liver. Therefore, isolated active metabolites or chemically synthesised analogues are well suited to prove their access to brain and their peripheral and central pharmacodynamics.

Contrary to the mostly only observational investigations of compound- or composition-induced phenomenological responses, research must also rely on hypotheses on relevant single or multiple target structures. The further exploration and validation of such hypotheses should include network pharmacology modelling as well as metabolomics-integrated pharmacokinetics to strengthen proposed mechanistic explanations and to identify candidate lead compounds. This could be another starting point for further structure–activity relationship studies. In preclinical-to-clinical translation, compounds identified in this way will add value when applied in experimental models, e.g., tissue cultures, blood–brain barrier systems, or relevant behavioural phenotypes up to patient-derived organoids.

An alternative expedient research strategy draws upon a clear pharmacological target structure and screens natural products, which are characterised and covered in drug banks for target efficacy, in in vitro assays, as successfully demonstrated by Tarrago et al. (2007) for the prolyl oligopeptidase found to be inhibited by BBR [176]. Here, the traditional fields of application may also guide the selection process of compounds, supported by defined algorithms. In addition, such an approach also may promote biology-orientated compound synthesis based on the plant-derived parent substance.

In those approaches, the traditional application may also determine the process for compound selection at best supported by algorithms of artificial intelligence.

Despite methodical shortcomings, there is growing experimental evidence for pharmacologically comprehensible and therapeutically useful effects of natural compounds or mixtures in mental illness, associated ED, or body schema disorders.

Author Contributions: Literature search and evaluation, W.M., R.R. and U.K.; writing or contribution to the writing, W.M., R.R. and U.K.; supervision and project administration, U.K. All authors have read and agreed to the published version of the manuscript.

Funding: This work was supported by the Sino-German Center (M-0679) and the Sichuan Science and Technology Program (2025YFHZ0121).

Acknowledgments: The authors gratefully acknowledge the excellent scientific support of Anne-Kathrin Krause (Leipzig) and Yong Tang (Chengdu).

Conflicts of Interest: The authors declare no conflicts of interest.

References

1. Polivy, J.; Herman, C.P. Mental health and eating behaviours: A bi-directional relation. *Can. J. Public Health* **2005**, *96* (Suppl. S3), S49–S53. [CrossRef]
2. Tan, E.J.; Raut, T.; Le, L.K.-D.; Hay, P.; Ananthapavan, J.; Lee, Y.Y.; Mihalopoulos, C. The Association between Eating Disorders and Mental Health: An Umbrella Review. *J. Eat. Disord.* **2023**, *11*, 51. [CrossRef] [PubMed]
3. Borges, R.S.; Ortiz, B.L.S.; Pereira, A.C.M.; Keita, H.; Carvalho, J.C.T. *Rosmarinus officinalis* Essential Oil: A Review of Its Phytochemistry, Anti-Inflammatory Activity, and Mechanisms of Action Involved. *J. Ethnopharmacol.* **2019**, *229*, 29–45. [CrossRef] [PubMed]
4. Quílez, M.; Ferreres, F.; López-Miranda, S.; Salazar, E.; Jordán, M.J. Seed Oil from Mediterranean Aromatic and Medicinal Plants of the Lamiaceae Family as a Source of Bioactive Components with Nutritional. *Antioxidants* **2020**, *9*, 510. [CrossRef] [PubMed]
5. Kitts, D.D.; Singh, A.; Fathordoobady, F.; Doi, B.; Pratap Singh, A. Plant Extracts Inhibit the Formation of Hydroperoxides and Help Maintain Vitamin E Levels and Omega-3 Fatty Acids During High Temperature Processing and Storage of Hempseed and Soybean Oils. *J. Food Sci.* **2019**, *84*, 3147–3155. [CrossRef] [PubMed]
6. Nieto, G.; Ros, G.; Castillo, J. Antioxidant and Antimicrobial Properties of Rosemary (*Rosmarinus officinalis*, L.): A Review. *Medicines* **2018**, *5*, 98. [CrossRef] [PubMed]
7. *ISO 1342:2012*; Essential Oil of Rosemary (*Rosmarinus officinalis* L.). International Organization for Standardization: Geneva, Switzerland, 2012. Available online: https://www.iso.org/standard/56521.html#lifecycle (accessed on 23 June 2025).
8. Silva-Filho, S.; De Souza Silva-Comar, F.; Wiirzler, L.; Do Pinho, R.; Grespan, R.; Bersani-Amado, C.; Cuman, R. Effect of Camphor on the Behavior of Leukocytes In Vitro and In Vivo in Acute Inflammatory Response. *Trop. J. Pharm. Res.* **2015**, *13*, 2031. [CrossRef]
9. Nam, S.-Y.; Chung, C.; Seo, J.-H.; Rah, S.-Y.; Kim, H.-M.; Jeong, H.-J. The Therapeutic Efficacy of α-Pinene in an Experimental Mouse Model of Allergic Rhinitis. *Int. Immunopharmacol.* **2014**, *23*, 273–282. [CrossRef] [PubMed]
10. Juhás, Š.; Bukovská, A.; Čikoš, Š.; Czikková, S.; Fabian, D.; Koppel, J. Anti-Inflammatory Effects of *Rosmarinus officinalis* Essential Oil in Mice. *Acta Vet. Brno* **2009**, *78*, 121–127. [CrossRef]
11. Vallverdú-Queralt, A.; Regueiro, J.; Martínez-Huélamo, M.; Rinaldi Alvarenga, J.F.; Leal, L.N.; Lamuela-Raventos, R.M. A Comprehensive Study on the Phenolic Profile of Widely Used Culinary Herbs and Spices: Rosemary, Thyme, Oregano, Cinnamon, Cumin and Bay. *Food Chem.* **2014**, *154*, 299–307. [CrossRef] [PubMed]
12. Del Baño, M.J.; Lorente, J.; Castillo, J.; Benavente-García, O.; Del Río, J.A.; Ortuño, A.; Quirin, K.-W.; Gerard, D. Phenolic Diterpenes, Flavones, and Rosmarinic Acid Distribution during the Development of Leaves, Flowers, Stems, and Roots of *Rosmarinus officinalis*. Antioxidant Activity. *J. Agric. Food Chem.* **2003**, *51*, 4247–4253. [CrossRef] [PubMed]
13. National Center for Biotechnology Information. PubChem Compound Summary for CID 5281792, Rosmarinic Acid. 2025. Available online: https://pubchem.ncbi.nlm.nih.gov/compound/Rosmarinic-acid (accessed on 23 June 2025).
14. Moreno, S.; Scheyer, T.; Romano, C.S.; Vojnov, A.A. Antioxidant and Antimicrobial Activities of Rosemary Extracts Linked to Their Polyphenol Composition. *Free Radic. Res.* **2006**, *40*, 223–231. [CrossRef] [PubMed]
15. De Oliveira, J.R.; Camargo, S.E.A.; De Oliveira, L.D. *Rosmarinus officinalis* L. (Rosemary) as Therapeutic and Prophylactic Agent. *J. Biomed. Sci.* **2019**, *26*, 5. [CrossRef] [PubMed]
16. Suganami, T.; Tanaka, M.; Ogawa, Y. Adipose Tissue Inflammation and Ectopic Lipid Accumulation. *Endocr. J.* **2012**, *59*, 849–857. [CrossRef] [PubMed]
17. Dani, C.; Tarchi, L.; Cassioli, E.; Rossi, E.; Merola, G.P.; Ficola, A.; Cordasco, V.Z.; Ricca, V.; Castellini, G. A Transdiagnostic and Diagnostic-Specific Approach on Inflammatory Biomarkers in Eating Disorders: A Meta-Analysis and Systematic Review. *Psychiatry Res.* **2024**, *340*, 116115. [CrossRef] [PubMed]
18. Jiao, W.; Lin, J.; Deng, Y.; Ji, Y.; Liang, C.; Wei, S.; Jing, X.; Yan, F. The Immunological Perspective of Major Depressive Disorder: Unveiling the Interactions between Central and Peripheral Immune Mechanisms. *J. Neuroinflamm.* **2025**, *22*, 10. [CrossRef] [PubMed]

19. Vallée, A. Neuroinflammation in Schizophrenia: The Key Role of the WNT/β-Catenin Pathway. *Int. J. Mol. Sci.* **2022**, *23*, 281 [CrossRef] [PubMed]
20. Ercan, P.; El, S.N. Bioaccessibility and inhibitory effects on digestive enzymes of carnosic acid in sage and rosemary. *Int. J. Bi Macromol.* **2018**, *115*, 933–939. [CrossRef] [PubMed]
21. Romo Vaquero, M.; Yáñez-Gascón, M.-J.; García Villalba, R.; Larrosa, M.; Fromentin, E.; Ibarra, A.; Roller, M.; Tomás-Barberá F.; Espín De Gea, J.C.; García-Conesa, M.-T. Inhibition of Gastric Lipase as a Mechanism for Body Weight and Plasma Lipic Reduction in Zucker Rats Fed a Rosemary Extract Rich in Carnosic Acid. *PLoS ONE* **2012**, *7*, e39773. [CrossRef] [PubMed]
22. Liu, Y.; Zhang, Y.; Hu, M.; Li, Y.; Cao, X. Carnosic Acid Alleviates Brain Injury through NF κB regulated Inflammation an Caspase 3 associated Apoptosis in High Fat induced Mouse Models. *Mol. Med. Rep.* **2019**, *20*, 495–504. [CrossRef] [PubMed]
23. Terzo, S.; Calvi, P.; Nuzzo, D.; Picone, P.; Allegra, M.; Mulè, F.; Amato, A. Long-Term Ingestion of Sicilian Black Bee Chestnu Honey and/or D-Limonene Counteracts Brain Damage Induced by High Fat-Diet in Obese Mice. *Int. J. Mol. Sci.* **2023**, *24*, 346 [CrossRef] [PubMed]
24. Akbari, S.; Sohouli, M.H.; Ebrahimzadeh, S.; Ghanaei, F.M.; Hosseini, A.F.; Aryaeian, N. Effect of Rosemary Leaf Powder wit Weight Loss Diet on Lipid Profile, Glycemic Status, and Liver Enzymes in Patients with Nonalcoholic Fatty Liver Disease: Randomized, Double-blind Clinical Trial. *Phytother. Res.* **2022**, *36*, 2186–2196. [CrossRef] [PubMed]
25. Oh, E.S.; Petersen, K.S.; Kris-Etherton, P.M.; Rogers, C.J. Spices in a High-Saturated-Fat, High-Carbohydrate Meal Reduc Postprandial Proinflammatory Cytokine Secretion in Men with Overweight or Obesity: A 3-Period, Crossover, Randomize Controlled Trial. *J. Nutr.* **2020**, *150*, 1600–1609. [CrossRef] [PubMed]
26. Mourya, A.; Akhtar, A.; Ahuja, S.; Sah, S.P.; Kumar, A. Synergistic Action of Ursolic Acid and Metformin in Experimental Mod of Insulin Resistance and Related Behavioral Alterations. *Eur. J. Pharmacol.* **2018**, *835*, 31–40. [CrossRef] [PubMed]
27. Checker, R.; Sandur, S.K.; Sharma, D.; Patwardhan, R.S.; Jayakumar, S.; Kohli, V.; Sethi, G.; Aggarwal, B.B.; Sainis, K.B. Poter Anti-Inflammatory Activity of Ursolic Acid, a Triterpenoid Antioxidant, Is Mediated through Suppression of NF-κB, AP-1 an NF-AT. *PLoS ONE* **2012**, *7*, e31318. [CrossRef] [PubMed]
28. Mirza, F.J.; Amber, S.; Sumera; Hassan, D.; Ahmed, T.; Zahid, S. Rosmarinic Acid and Ursolic Acid Alleviate Deficits i Cognition, Synaptic Regulation and Adult Hippocampal Neurogenesis in an Aβ1-42-Induced Mouse Model of Alzheimer' Disease. *Phytomedicine* **2021**, *83*, 153490. [CrossRef] [PubMed]
29. Hussain, S.M.; Syeda, A.F.; Alshammari, M.; Alnasser, S.; Alenzi, N.D.; Alanazi, S.T.; Nandakumar, K. Cognition Enhancing Effe of Rosemary (*Rosmarinus officinalis* L.) in Lab Animal Studies: A Systematic Review and Meta-Analysis. *Braz. J. Med. Biol. Re* **2022**, *55*, e11593. [CrossRef] [PubMed]
30. Abdelhalim, A.; Karim, N.; Chebib, M.; Aburjai, T.; Khan, I.; Johnston, G.A.R.; Hanrahan, J. Antidepressant, Anxiolytic an Antinociceptive Activities of Constituents from *Rosmarinus officinalis*. *J. Pharm. Pharm. Sci.* **2015**, *18*, 448. [CrossRef] [PubMed]
31. Juergens, U.R.; Stöber, M.; Vetter, H. Inhibition of Cytokine Production and Arachidonic Acid Metabolism by Eucalypt (1.8-Cineole) in Human Blood Monocytes in Vitro. *Eur. J. Med. Res.* **1998**, *3*, 508–510. [PubMed]
32. Takaki, I.; Bersani-Amado, L.E.; Vendruscolo, A.; Sartoretto, S.M.; Diniz, S.P.; Bersani-Amado, C.A.; Cuman, R.K.N. Ant Inflammatory and Antinociceptive Effects of *Rosmarinus officinalis* L. Essential Oil in Experimental Animal Models. *J. Med. Foo* **2008**, *11*, 741–746. [CrossRef] [PubMed]
33. Zhang, Q.; Lenardo, M.J.; Baltimore, D. 30 Years of NF-κB: A Blossoming of Relevance to Human Pathobiology. *Cell* **201** *168*, 37–57. [CrossRef] [PubMed]
34. Guo, Q.; Jin, Y.; Chen, X.; Ye, X.; Shen, X.; Lin, M.; Zeng, C.; Zhou, T.; Zhang, J. NF-κB in Biology and Targeted Therapy: Nev Insights and Translational Implications. *Signal Transduct. Target. Ther.* **2024**, *9*, 53. [CrossRef] [PubMed]
35. Pries, R.; Jeschke, S.; Leichtle, A.; Bruchhage, K.-L. Modes of Action of 1,8-Cineol in Infections and Inflammation. *Metabolites* **202** *13*, 751. [CrossRef] [PubMed]
36. Wu, W.; Wang, D.; Shi, Y.; Wang, Y.; Wu, Y.; Wu, X.; Shah, B.A.; Ye, G. 1,8-Cineole Alleviates Hippocampal Oxidative Stress i CUMS Mice via the PI3K/Akt/Nrf2 Pathway. *Nutrients* **2025**, *17*, 1027. [CrossRef] [PubMed]
37. Machado, D.G.; Bettio, L.E.B.; Cunha, M.P.; Capra, J.C.; Dalmarco, J.B.; Pizzolatti, M.G.; Rodrigues, A.L.S. Antidepressant-lik Effect of the Extract of *Rosmarinus officinalis* in Mice: Involvement of the Monoaminergic System. *Prog. Neuropsychopharmacol. Bio Psychiatry* **2009**, *33*, 642–650. [CrossRef] [PubMed]
38. Machado, D.G.; Neis, V.B.; Balen, G.O.; Colla, A.; Cunha, M.P.; Dalmarco, J.B.; Pizzolatti, M.G.; Prediger, R.D.; Rodrigues, A.L.S Antidepressant-like Effect of Ursolic Acid Isolated from *Rosmarinus officinalis* L. in Mice: Evidence for the Involvement of th Dopaminergic System. *Pharmacol. Biochem. Behav.* **2012**, *103*, 204–211. [CrossRef]
39. Machado, D.G.; Cunha, M.P.; Neis, V.B.; Balen, G.O.; Colla, A.; Bettio, L.E.B.; Oliveira, Á.; Pazini, F.L.; Dalmarco, J.B.; Simionatt E.L.; et al. Antidepressant-like Effects of Fractions, Essential Oil, Carnosol and Betulinic Acid Isolated from *Rosmarinus officinali* L. *Food Chem.* **2013**, *136*, 999–1005. [CrossRef] [PubMed]
40. Takeda, H.; Tsuji, M.; Inazu, M.; Egashira, T.; Matsumiya, T. Rosmarinic Acid and Caffeic Acid Produce Antidepressive-like Effec in the Forced Swimming Test in Mice. *Eur. J. Pharmacol.* **2002**, *449*, 261–267. [CrossRef] [PubMed]

41. Lin, S.-H.; Chou, M.-L.; Chen, W.-C.; Lai, Y.-S.; Lu, K.-H.; Hao, C.-W.; Sheen, L.-Y. A Medicinal Herb, *Melissa officinalis* L. Ameliorates Depressive-like Behavior of Rats in the Forced Swimming Test via Regulating the Serotonergic Neurotransmitter. *J. Ethnopharmacol.* **2015**, *175*, 266–272. [CrossRef] [PubMed]
42. Takeda, H.; Tsuji, M.; Miyamoto, J.; Matsumiya, T. Rosmarinic Acid and Caffeic Acid Reduce the Defensive Freezing Behavior of Mice Exposed to Conditioned Fear Stress. *Psychopharmacology* **2002**, *164*, 233–235. [CrossRef] [PubMed]
43. Tian, G.; Bartas, K.; Hui, M.; Chen, L.; Vasquez, J.J.; Azouz, G.; Derdeyn, P.; Manville, R.W.; Ho, E.L.; Fang, A.S.; et al. Molecular and Circuit Determinants in the Globus Pallidus Mediating Control of Cocaine-Induced Behavioral Plasticity. *Neuron* **2024**, *112*, 3470–3485.e12. [CrossRef] [PubMed]
44. Sasaki, K.; Ferdousi, F.; Fukumitsu, S.; Kuwata, H.; Isoda, H. Antidepressant- and Anxiolytic-like Activities of *Rosmarinus officinalis* Extract in Rodent Models: Involvement of Oxytocinergic System. *Biomed. Pharmacother.* **2021**, *144*, 112291. [CrossRef] [PubMed]
45. Onaka, T.; Takayanagi, Y. Role of Oxytocin in the Control of Stress and Food Intake. *J. Neuroendocrinol.* **2019**, *31*, e12700. [CrossRef] [PubMed]
46. Nematolahi, P.; Mehrabani, M.; Karami-Mohajeri, S.; Dabaghzadeh, F. Effects of *Rosmarinus officinalis* L. on Memory Performance, Anxiety, Depression, and Sleep Quality in University Students: A Randomized Clinical Trial. *Complement. Ther. Clin. Pract.* **2018**, *30*, 24–28. [CrossRef] [PubMed]
47. Araki, R.; Sasaki, K.; Onda, H.; Nakamura, S.; Kassai, M.; Kaneko, T.; Isoda, H.; Hashimoto, K. Effects of Continuous Intake of Rosemary Extracts on Mental Health in Working Generation Healthy Japanese Men: Post-Hoc Testing of a Randomized Controlled Trial. *Nutrients* **2020**, *12*, 3551. [CrossRef] [PubMed]
48. Achour, M.; Ben Salem, I.; Ferdousi, F.; Nouira, M.; Ben Fredj, M.; Mtiraoui, A.; Isoda, H.; Saguem, S. Rosemary Tea Consumption Alters Peripheral Anxiety and Depression Biomarkers: A Pilot Study in Limited Healthy Volunteers. *J. Am. Nutr. Assoc.* **2022**, *41*, 240–249. [CrossRef] [PubMed]
49. Casarotto, P.C.; Girych, M.; Fred, S.M.; Kovaleva, V.; Moliner, R.; Enkavi, G.; Biojone, C.; Cannarozzo, C.; Sahu, M.P.; Kaurinkoski, K.; et al. Antidepressant Drugs Act by Directly Binding to TRKB Neurotrophin Receptors. *Cell* **2021**, *184*, 1299–1313.e19. [CrossRef] [PubMed]
50. Azizi, S.; Mohamadi, N.; Sharififar, F.; Dehghannoudeh, G.; Jahanbakhsh, F.; Dabaghzadeh, F. Rosemary as an Adjunctive Treatment in Patients with Major Depressive Disorder: A Randomized, Double-blind, Placebo-controlled Trial. *Complement. Ther. Clin. Pract.* **2022**, *49*, 101685. [CrossRef] [PubMed]
51. Schneider, E.; Schmidt, R.; Cryan, J.F.; Hilbert, A. A Role for the Microbiota-Gut-Brain Axis in Avoidant/Restrictive Food Intake Disorder: A New Conceptual Model. *Int. J. Eat. Disord.* **2024**, *57*, 2321–2328. [CrossRef] [PubMed]
52. Helal, P.; Xia, W.; Sardar, P.; Conway-Morris, A.; Conway-Morris, A.; Pedicord, V.A.; Serfontein, J. Changes in the Firmicutes to Bacteriodetes Ratio in the Gut Microbiome in Individuals with Anorexia Nervosa Following Inpatient Treatment: A Systematic Review and a Case Series. *Brain Behav.* **2024**, *14*, e70014. [CrossRef] [PubMed]
53. Romeo, M.; Cavaliere, G.; Traina, G. Bulimia Nervosa and Depression, from the Brain to the Gut Microbiota and Back. *Front. Biosci.* **2024**, *29*, 277. [CrossRef] [PubMed]
54. Guo, W.; Xiong, W. From Gut Microbiota to Brain: Implications on Binge Eating Disorders. *Gut Microbes* **2024**, *16*, 2357177. [CrossRef] [PubMed]
55. Winter, G.; Hart, R.A.; Charlesworth, R.P.G.; Sharpley, C.F. Gut Microbiome and Depression: What We Know and What We Need to Know. *Rev. Neurosci.* **2018**, *29*, 629–643. [CrossRef] [PubMed]
56. Bogielski, B.; Michalczyk, K.; Głodek, P.; Tempka, B.; Gębski, W.; Stygar, D. Association between Small Intestine Bacterial Overgrowth and Psychiatric Disorders. *Front. Biosci.* **2024**, *15*, 1438066. [CrossRef] [PubMed]
57. Pisanu, C.; Squassina, A. We Are Not Alone in Our Body: Insights into the Involvement of Microbiota in the Etiopathogenesis and Pharmacology of Mental Illness. *Curr. Drug Metab.* **2018**, *19*, 688–694. [CrossRef] [PubMed]
58. Zheng, P.; Zeng, B.; Zhou, C.; Liu, M.; Fang, Z.; Xu, X.; Zeng, L.; Chen, J.; Fan, S.; Du, X.; et al. Gut Microbiome Remodeling Induces Depressive-like Behaviors through a Pathway Mediated by the Host's Metabolism. *Mol. Psychiatry* **2016**, *21*, 786–796. [CrossRef] [PubMed]
59. Pferschy-Wenzig, E.-M.; Pausan, M.R.; Ardjomand-Woelkart, K.; Röck, S.; Ammar, R.M.; Kelber, O.; Moissl-Eichinger, C.; Bauer, R. Medicinal Plants and Their Impact on the Gut Microbiome in Mental Health: A Systematic Review. *Nutrients* **2022**, *14*, 2111. [CrossRef] [PubMed]
60. Dinan, K.; Dinan, T. Antibiotics and Mental Health: The Good, the Bad and the Ugly. *J. Intern. Med.* **2022**, *292*, 858–869. [CrossRef] [PubMed]
61. Endo, T.H.; Santos, M.H.D.M.; Scandorieiro, S.; Gonçalves, B.C.; Vespero, E.C.; Perugini, M.R.E.; Pavanelli, W.R.; Nakazato, G.; Kobayashi, R.K.T. Selective Serotonin Reuptake Inhibitors: Antimicrobial Activity Against ESKAPEE Bacteria and Mechanisms of Action. *Antibiotics* **2025**, *14*, 51. [CrossRef] [PubMed]

62. Macedo, D.; Filho, A.J.M.C.; Soares De Sousa, C.N.; Quevedo, J.; Barichello, T.; Júnior, H.V.N.; Freitas De Lucena, D. Antidepressants, Antimicrobials or Both? Gut Microbiota Dysbiosis in Depression and Possible Implications of the Antimicrobial Effects of Antidepressant Drugs for Antidepressant Effectiveness. *J. Affect. Disord.* **2017**, *208*, 22–32. [CrossRef] [PubMed]
63. Guo, Y.; Xie, J.; Li, X.; Yuan, Y.; Zhang, L.; Hu, W.; Luo, H.; Yu, H.; Zhang, R. Antidepressant Effects of Rosemary Extracts Associate With Anti-Inflammatory Effect and Rebalance of Gut Microbiota. *Front. Pharmacol.* **2018**, *9*, 1126. [CrossRef] [PubMed]
64. Romo Vaquero, M.; García Villalba, R.; Larrosa, M.; Yáñez-Gascón, M.J.; Fromentin, E.; Flanagan, J.; Roller, M.; Tomás-Barberán, F.A.; Espín, J.C.; García-Conesa, M. Bioavailability of the Major Bioactive Diterpenoids in a Rosemary Extract: Metabolic Profile in the Intestine, Liver, Plasma, and Brain of Zucker Rats. *Mol. Nutr. Food Res.* **2013**, *57*, 1834–1846. [CrossRef] [PubMed]
65. Ghasemzadeh Rahbardar, M.; Hosseinzadeh, H. Toxicity and Safety of Rosemary (*Rosmarinus officinalis*): A Comprehensive Review. *Naunyn-Schmiedeberg's Arch. Pharmacol.* **2025**, *398*, 9–23. [CrossRef] [PubMed]
66. EFSA ANS Panel (EFSA Panel on Food Additives and Nutrient Sources added to Food); Younes, M.; Aggett, P.; Aguilar, F.; Crebelli, R.; Dusemund, B.; Filipič, M.; Frutos, M.J.; Galtier, P.; Gott, D.; et al. Scientific Opinion on the refined exposure assessment of extracts of rosemary (E 392) from its use as food additive. *EFSA J.* **2018**, *16*, e05373. [CrossRef] [PubMed]
67. Phipps, K.R.; Lozon, D.; Baldwin, N. Genotoxicity and Subchronic Toxicity Studies of Supercritical Carbon Dioxide and Acetone Extracts of Rosemary. *Regul. Toxicol. Pharmacol.* **2021**, *119*, 104826. [CrossRef] [PubMed]
68. WHO. *Safety Evaluation of Certain Food Additives: Prepared by the Eighty-Second Meeting of the Joint FAO/WHO Expert Committee on Food Additives (JECFA)*; WHO Food Additives Series 73; World Health Organization: Geneva, Switzerland, 2017; ISBN 978-92-4-166073-0.
69. Phipps, K.R.; Danielewska-Nikiel, B.; Mushonganono, J.; Baldwin, N. Reproductive and Developmental Toxicity Screening Study of an Acetone Extract of Rosemary. *Regul. Toxicol. Pharmacol.* **2021**, *120*, 104840. [CrossRef]
70. Norwegian Institute of Public Health, W.H.O. Collaborating Centre for Drug Statistics Methodology. Last Updated 27 December 2024. Available online: https://atcddd.fhi.no/atc_ddd_index/?code=N06DX02 (accessed on 21 June 2025).
71. European Union Herbal Monograph on *Ginkgo biloba* L., Folium EMA/HMPC/321097/2012. Available online: https://www.ema.europa.eu/en/documents/herbal-monograph/final-european-union-herbal-monograph-ginkgo-biloba-l-folium_en.pdf (accessed on 21 June 2025).
72. Kulić, Ž.; Lehner, M.D.; Dietz, G.P.H. *Ginkgo biloba* Leaf Extract EGb 761® as a Paragon of the Product by Process Concept. *Front. Pharmacol.* **2022**, *13*, 1007746. [CrossRef] [PubMed]
73. Napryeyenko, O.; Sonnik, G.; Tartakovsky, I. Efficacy and Tolerability of *Ginkgo biloba* Extract EGb 761® by Type of Dementia: Analyses of a Randomised Controlled Trial. *J. Neurol. Sci.* **2009**, *283*, 224–229. [CrossRef] [PubMed]
74. Kanowski, S.; Hoerr, R. *Ginkgo biloba* Extract EGb 761 in Dementia: Intent-to-Treat Analyses of a 24-Week, Multi-Center, Double-Blind, Placebo-Controlled, Randomized Trial. *Pharmacopsychiatry* **2003**, *36*, 297–303. [CrossRef] [PubMed]
75. Vellas, B.; Coley, N.; Ousset, P.-J.; Berrut, G.; Dartigues, J.-F.; Dubois, B.; Grandjean, H.; Pasquier, F.; Piette, F.; Robert, P.; et al. Long-Term Use of Standardised *Ginkgo biloba* Extract for the Prevention of Alzheimer's Disease (GuidAge): A Randomised Placebo-Controlled Trial. *Lancet Neurol.* **2012**, *11*, 851–859. [CrossRef] [PubMed]
76. Snitz, B.E.; O'Meara, E.S.; Carlson, M.C.; Arnold, A.M.; Ives, D.G.; Rapp, S.R.; Saxton, J.; Lopez, O.L.; Dunn, L.O.; Sink, K.M.; et al. *Ginkgo biloba* for Preventing Cognitive Decline in Older Adults: A Randomized Trial. *JAMA* **2009**, *302*, 2663–2670. [CrossRef] [PubMed]
77. DeKosky, S.T.; Williamson, J.D.; Fitzpatrick, A.L.; Kronmal, R.A.; Ives, D.G.; Saxton, J.A.; Lopez, O.L.; Burke, G.; Carlson, M.C.; Fried, L.P.; et al. *Ginkgo biloba* for Prevention of Dementia: A Randomized Controlled Trial. *JAMA* **2008**, *300*, 2253–2262. [CrossRef] [PubMed]
78. Necula, B.-R.; Necula, R.D.; Petric, P.S.; Ifteni, P.I.; Irimie, M.; Dima, L. EGb761 Trials for Mild-to-Moderate Dementia—What Have We Learned in the Past 18 Years? *Am. J. Ther.* **2024**, *31*, e645–e651. [CrossRef] [PubMed]
79. Birks, J.; Grimley Evans, J. *Ginkgo biloba* for Cognitive Impairment and Dementia. *Cochrane Database Syst. Rev.* **2009**. [CrossRef] [PubMed]
80. National Institutes of Health (NIH), National Center for Complementary and Integrative Health (NCCIH). Last Updated February 2025. Available online: https://www.nccih.nih.gov/health/ginkgo (accessed on 21 June 2025).
81. Savaskan, E.; Mueller, H.; Hoerr, R.; Von Gunten, A.; Gauthier, S. Treatment Effects of *Ginkgo biloba* Extract EGb 761® on the Spectrum of Behavioral and Psychological Symptoms of Dementia: Meta-Analysis of Randomized Controlled Trials. *Int. Psychogeriatr.* **2018**, *30*, 285–293. [CrossRef] [PubMed]
82. DGN e. V. & DGPPN e. V. (Hrsg.) S3-Leitlinie Demenzen—Living Guideline, Version 5.1, 28 March 2025. Available online: https://register.awmf.org/de/leitlinien/detail/038-013 (accessed on 21 June 2025).
83. Liu, L.; Wang, Y.; Zhang, J.; Wang, S. Advances in the Chemical Constituents and Chemical Analysis of *Ginkgo biloba* Leaf, Extract, and Phytopharmaceuticals. *J. Pharm. Biomed. Anal.* **2021**, *193*, 113704. [CrossRef] [PubMed]

84. Le Bars, P.L.; Velasco, F.M.; Ferguson, J.M.; Dessain, E.C.; Kieser, M.; Hoerr, R. Influence of the Severity of Cognitive Impairment on the Effect of the *Ginkgo biloba* Extract EGb 761® in Alzheimer's Disease. *Neuropsychobiology* **2002**, *45*, 19–26. [CrossRef] [PubMed]
85. Sarris, J. Herbal Medicines in the Treatment of Psychiatric Disorders: 10-year Updated Review. *Phytother. Res.* **2018**, *32*, 1147–1162. [CrossRef] [PubMed]
86. Nurzyńska-Wierdak, R. Plants with Potential Importance in Supporting the Treatment of Depression: Current Trends, and Research. *Pharmaceuticals* **2024**, *17*, 1489. [CrossRef] [PubMed]
87. Grosso, C.; Santos, M.; Barroso, M.F. From Plants to Psycho-Neurology: Unravelling the Therapeutic Benefits of Bioactive Compounds in Brain Disorders. *Antioxidants* **2023**, *12*, 1603. [CrossRef] [PubMed]
88. Lin, J.; Sun, X.; Yang, L. Effects and Safety of *Ginkgo biloba* on Depression: A Systematic Review and Meta-Analysis. *Front. Pharmacol.* **2024**, *15*, 1364030. [CrossRef] [PubMed]
89. Biernacka, P.; Adamska, I.; Felisiak, K. The Potential of *Ginkgo biloba* as a Source of Biologically Active Compounds—A Review of the Recent Literature and Patents. *Molecules* **2023**, *28*, 3993. [CrossRef] [PubMed]
90. Bogacz, A.; Karasiewicz, M.; Dziekan, K.; Procyk, D.; Górska-Paukszta, M.; Kowalska, A.; Mikołajczak, P.Ł.; Ożarowski, M.; Czerny, B. Impact of Panax Ginseng and *Ginkgo biloba* Extracts on Expression Level of Transcriptional Factors and Xenobiotic-Metabolizing Cytochrome P450 Enzymes. *Herba Pol.* **2016**, *62*, 42–54. [CrossRef]
91. Suárez-González, E.; Sandoval-Ramírez, J.; Flores-Hernández, J.; Carrasco-Carballo, A. *Ginkgo biloba*: Antioxidant Activity and In Silico Central Nervous System Potential. *Curr. Issues Mol. Biol.* **2023**, *45*, 9674–9691. [CrossRef] [PubMed]
92. Ayatollahi, S.A.; Khoshsirat, S.; Peyvandi, A.A.; Rezaei, O.; Mehrjardi, F.Z.; Nahavandi, A.; Niknazar, S. *Ginkgo biloba* modulates hippocampal BDNF expression in a rat model of chronic restraint stress-induced depression. *Physiol. Pharmacol.* **2020**, *24*, 285–297. [CrossRef]
93. Yeh, K.-Y.; Shou, S.-S.; Lin, Y.-X.; Chen, C.-C.; Chiang, C.-Y.; Yeh, C.-Y. Effect of *Ginkgo biloba* Extract on Lipopolysaccharide-Induced Anhedonic Depressive-like Behavior in Male Rats. *Phytother. Res.* **2015**, *29*, 260–266. [CrossRef] [PubMed]
94. Montes, P.; Ruiz-Sanchez, E.; Rojas, C.; Rojas, P. *Ginkgo biloba* Extract 761: A Review of Basic Studies and Potential Clinical Use in Psychiatric Disorders. *CNS Neurol. Disord. Drug Targets* **2015**, *14*, 132–149. [CrossRef] [PubMed]
95. Kuribara, H.; Weintraub, S.T.; Yoshihama, T.; Maruyama, Y. An Anxiolytic-Like Effect of *Ginkgo biloba* Extract and Its Constituent, Ginkgolide-A, in Mice. *J. Nat. Prod.* **2003**, *66*, 1333–1337. [CrossRef] [PubMed]
96. Rodriguez De Turco, E.B.; Droy-Lefaix, M.T.; Bazan, N.G. EGb 761 Inhibits Stress-Induced Polydipsia in Rats. *Physiol. Behav.* **1993**, *53*, 1001–1002. [CrossRef] [PubMed]
97. Banin, R.M.; Hirata, B.K.S.; Andrade, I.S.; Zemdegs, J.C.S.; Clemente, A.P.G.; Dornellas, A.P.S.; Boldarine, V.T.; Estadella, D.; Albuquerque, K.T.; Oyama, L.M.; et al. Beneficial Effects of *Ginkgo biloba* Extract on Insulin Signaling Cascade, Dyslipidemia, and Body Adiposity of Diet-Induced Obese Rats. *Braz. J. Med. Biol. Res.* **2014**, *47*, 780–788. [CrossRef] [PubMed]
98. Hirata, B.K.S.; Pedroso, A.P.; Machado, M.M.F.; Neto, N.I.P.; Perestrelo, B.O.; De Sá, R.D.C.C.; Alonso-Vale, M.I.C.; Nogueira, F.N.; Oyama, L.M.; Ribeiro, E.B.; et al. *Ginkgo biloba* Extract Modulates the Retroperitoneal Fat Depot Proteome and Reduces Oxidative Stress in Diet-Induced Obese Rats. *Front. Pharmacol.* **2019**, *10*, 686. [CrossRef] [PubMed]
99. Banin, R.M.; De Andrade, I.S.; Cerutti, S.M.; Oyama, L.M.; Telles, M.M.; Ribeiro, E.B. *Ginkgo biloba* Extract (GbE) Stimulates the Hypothalamic Serotonergic System and Attenuates Obesity in Ovariectomized Rats. *Front. Pharmacol.* **2017**, *8*, 605. [CrossRef] [PubMed]
100. Huguet, F.; Drieu, K.; Piriou, A. Decreased Cerebral 5-HT1A Receptors during Ageing: Reversal by *Ginkgo biloba* Extract (EGb 761). *J. Pharm. Pharmacol.* **1994**, *46*, 316–318. [CrossRef] [PubMed]
101. Bolaños-Jiménez, F.; De Castro, R.M.; Sarhan, H.; Prudhomme, N.; Drieu, K.; Fillion, G. Stress-induced 5-HT1A Receptor Desensitization: Protective Effects of *Ginkgo biloba* Extract (EGb 761). *Fundam. Clin. Pharmacol.* **1995**, *9*, 169–174. [CrossRef] [PubMed]
102. Sloley, B.D.; Urichuk, L.J.; Morley, P.; Durkin, J.; Shan, J.J.; Pang, P.K.T.; Coutts, R.T. Identification of Kaempferol as a Monoamine Oxidase Inhibitor and Potential Neuroprotectant in Extracts of *Ginkgo biloba* Leaves. *J. Pharm. Pharmacol.* **2000**, *52*, 451–459. [CrossRef] [PubMed]
103. Machado, M.M.F.; Pereira, J.P.; Hirata, B.K.S.; Júlio, V.S.; Banin, R.M.; Andrade, H.M.; Ribeiro, E.B.; Cerutti, S.M.; Telles, M.M. A Single Dose of *Ginkgo biloba* Extract Induces Gene Expression of Hypothalamic Anorexigenic Effectors in Male Rats. *Brain Sci.* **2021**, *11*, 1602. [CrossRef] [PubMed]
104. Unger, M. Pharmacokinetic Drug Interactions Involving *Ginkgo biloba*. *Drug Metab. Rev.* **2013**, *45*, 353–385. [CrossRef] [PubMed]
105. Mai, N.T.Q.; Hieu, N.V.; Ngan, T.T.; Van Anh, T.; Van Linh, P.; Thu Phuong, N.T. Impact of *Ginkgo biloba* Drug Interactions on Bleeding Risk and Coagulation Profiles: A Comprehensive Analysis. *PLoS ONE* **2025**, *20*, e0321804. [CrossRef] [PubMed]
106. Zeng, L.; Cao, Y.; Wang, L.; Dai, Y.; Hu, L.; Wang, Q.; Zhu, L.; Bao, W.; Zou, Y.; Chen, Y.; et al. Role of Medicinal Plants for Liver-Qi Regulation Adjuvant Therapy in Post-stroke Depression: A Systematic Review of Literature. *Phytother. Res.* **2017**, *31*, 40–52. [CrossRef] [PubMed]

107. National Medical Products Administration. Available online: https://english.nmpa.gov.cn/drugs.html (accessed o 21 June 2025).
108. Wang, Y.; Fan, R.; Huang, X. Meta-Analysis of the Clinical Effectiveness of Traditional Chinese Medicine Formula Chaihu-Shuga San in Depression. *J. Ethnopharmacol.* **2012**, *141*, 571–577. [CrossRef] [PubMed]
109. Yang, L.; Shergis, J.L.; Di, Y.M.; Zhang, A.L.; Lu, C.; Guo, X.; Fang, Z.; Xue, C.C.; Li, Y. Managing Depression with *Bupleuru chinense* Herbal Formula: A Systematic Review and Meta-Analysis of Randomized Controlled Trials. *J. Altern. Complement. Me* **2020**, *26*, 8–24. [CrossRef] [PubMed]
110. Teng, L.; Guo, X.; Ma, Y.; Xu, L.; Wei, J.; Xiao, P. A Comprehensive Review on Traditional and Modern Research of the Genu Bupleurum (*Bupleurum* L., *Apiaceae*) in Recent 10 Years. *J. Ethnopharmacol.* **2023**, *306*, 116129. [CrossRef] [PubMed]
111. Zhu, J.; Luo, C.; Wang, P.; He, Q.; Zhou, J.; Peng, H. Saikosaponin A Mediates the Inflammatory Response by Inhibiting th MAPK and NF-κB Pathways in LPS-Stimulated RAW 264.7 Cells. *Exp. Ther. Med.* **2013**, *5*, 1345–1350. [CrossRef] [PubMed]
112. Di Meo, F.; Lemaur, V.; Cornil, J.; Lazzaroni, R.; Duroux, J.-L.; Olivier, Y.; Trouillas, P. Free Radical Scavenging by Natura Polyphenols: Atom versus Electron Transfer. *J. Phys. Chem. A* **2013**, *117*, 2082–2092. [CrossRef] [PubMed]
113. Figueira, I.; Menezes, R.; Macedo, D.; Costa, I.; Dos Santos, C.N. Polyphenols Beyond Barriers: A Glimpse into the Brain. *Cur Neuropharmacol.* **2017**, *15*, 562–594. [CrossRef] [PubMed]
114. Stępnik, K. Biomimetic Chromatographic Studies Combined with the Computational Approach to Investigate the Ability c Triterpenoid Saponins of Plant Origin to Cross the Blood–Brain Barrier. *Int. J. Mol. Sci.* **2021**, *22*, 3573. [CrossRef] [PubMed]
115. Manach, C.; Scalbert, A.; Morand, C.; Rémésy, C.; Jiménez, L. Polyphenols: Food Sources and Bioavailability. *Am. J. Clin. Nut* **2004**, *79*, 727–747. [CrossRef] [PubMed]
116. Zhu, X.; Li, T.; Hu, E.; Duan, L.; Zhang, C.; Wang, Y.; Tang, T.; Yang, Z.; Fan, R. Proteomics Study Reveals the Anti-Depressiv Mechanisms and the Compatibility Advantage of Chaihu-Shugan-San in a Rat Model of Chronic Unpredictable Mild Stres *Front. Pharmacol.* **2022**, *12*, 791097. [CrossRef] [PubMed]
117. Li, X.; Qin, X.-M.; Tian, J.-S.; Gao, X.-X.; Du, G.-H.; Zhou, Y.-Z. Integrated Network Pharmacology and Metabolomics to Dissect th Combination Mechanisms of *Bupleurum chinense* DC-Paeonia Lactiflora Pall Herb Pair for Treating Depression. *J. Ethnopharmacc* **2021**, *264*, 113281. [CrossRef] [PubMed]
118. Chen, C.; Yin, Q.; Tian, J.; Gao, X.; Qin, X.; Du, G.; Zhou, Y. Studies on the Changes of Pharmacokinetics Behaviors c Phytochemicals and the Influence on Endogenous Metabolites After the Combination of Radix Bupleuri and Radix Paeonia Alba Based on Multi-Component Pharmacokinetics and Metabolomics. *Front. Pharmacol.* **2021**, *12*, 630970. [CrossRef] [PubMed]
119. Chen, Y.; Wang, J.; Yuan, L.; Zhou, L.; Jia, X.; Tan, X. Interaction of the Main Components from the Traditional Chinese Drug Pa Chaihu-Shaoyao Based on Rat Intestinal Absorption. *Molecules* **2011**, *16*, 9600–9610. [CrossRef] [PubMed]
120. He, D.-Y.; Dai, S.-M. Anti-Inflammatory and Immunomodulatory Effects of Paeonia Lactiflora Pall., a Traditional Chinese Herba Medicine. *Front. Pharmacol.* **2011**, *2*, 10. [CrossRef] [PubMed]
121. Chen, C.; Gong, W.; Tian, J.; Gao, X.; Qin, X.; Du, G.; Zhou, Y. Radix Paeoniae Alba Attenuates Radix Bupleuri-Induce Hepatotoxicity by Modulating Gut Microbiota to Alleviate the Inhibition of Saikosaponins on Glutathione Synthetase. *J. Pharn Anal.* **2023**, *13*, 640–659. [CrossRef] [PubMed]
122. Wu, S.; Li, H.-M.; Bing, Y.-F.; Zheng, Y.; Li, W.-L.; Zou, X.; Qu, Z.-Y. Bupleurum Scorzonerifolium: Systematic Research throug Pharmacodynamics and Serum Pharmacochemistry on Screening Antidepressant Q-Markers for Quality Control. *J. Pharn Biomed. Anal.* **2023**, *225*, 115202. [CrossRef] [PubMed]
123. Li, H.-Y.; Zhao, Y.-H.; Zeng, M.-J.; Fang, F.; Li, M.; Qin, T.-T.; Ye, L.-Y.; Li, H.-W.; Qu, R.; Ma, S.-P. Saikosaponin D Relieve Unpredictable Chronic Mild Stress Induced Depressive-like Behavior in Rats: Involvement of HPA Axis and Hippocampa Neurogenesis. *Psychopharmacology* **2017**, *234*, 3385–3394. [CrossRef] [PubMed]
124. Sun, C.-L.; Geng, C.-A.; Huang, X.-Y.; Ma, Y.-B.; Zheng, X.-H.; Yang, T.-H.; Chen, X.-L.; Yin, X.-J.; Zhang, X.-M.; Chen, J.- Bioassay-Guided Isolation of Saikosaponins with Agonistic Activity on 5-Hydroxytryptamine 2C Receptor from *Bupleurur chinense* and Their Potential Use for the Treatment of Obesity. *Chin. J. Nat. Med.* **2017**, *15*, 467–473. [CrossRef] [PubMed]
125. Maccioni, P.; Fara, F.; Gessa, G.L.; Carai, M.A.M.; Chin, Y.-W.; Lee, J.H.; Kwon, H.C.; Colombo, G. Reducing Effect of Saikosaponi A, an Active Ingredient of Bupleurum Falcatum, on Intake of Highly Palatable Food in a Rat Model of Overeating. *Fron Psychiatry* **2018**, *9*, 369. [CrossRef] [PubMed]
126. Maccioni, P.; Chin, Y.-W.; Corelli, F.; Kwon, H.C.; Colombo, G. Reducing Effect of Intragastrically Administered Saikosaponin A on Alcohol and Sucrose Self-Administration in Rats. *Nat. Prod. Res.* **2023**, *37*, 4256–4260. [CrossRef] [PubMed]
127. Bi, Y.; Li, M.; Wang, Y.; Yao, J.; Wang, Y.; Wang, S.; Zhuang, L.; Liu, S.; Li, Z.; Hao, Z.; et al. Saikosaponins from Bupleurun Scorzonerifolium Willd. Alleviates Microglial Pyroptosis in Depression by Binding and Inhibiting P2X7 Expression. *Phytomedicin* **2025**, *136*, 156240. [CrossRef] [PubMed]

128. Li, M.; Zhang, Q.; Zhu, T.; Liu, G.; Chen, W.; Chen, Y.; Bu, X.; Zhang, Z.; Zhang, Y. Broadly Targeted Metabolomics Analysis of Differential Metabolites Between *Bupleurum chinense* DC. and Bupleurum Scorzonerifolium Willd. *Metabolites* **2025**, *15*, 119. [CrossRef]
129. Wang, Z.; Tian, L.; Xiao, Y.; Zhao, M.; Chang, Y.; Zhou, Y.; Liu, S.; Zhao, H.; Xiu, Y. Quantitative and Differential Analysis between *Bupleurum chinense* DC. and Bupleurum scorzonerifolium Willd. Using HPLC-MS and GC-MS Coupled with Multivariate Statistical Analysis. *Molecules* **2023**, *28*, 5630. [CrossRef]
130. National Institutes of Health (NIH), National Center for Complementary and Integrative Health (NCCIH). Last Updated June 2023. Available online: https://www.nccih.nih.gov/health/in-the-news-berberine (accessed on 21 June 2025).
131. National Institutes of Health (NIH), National Center for Complementary and Integrative Health (NCCIH). Last Updated November 2023. Available online: https://www.nccih.nih.gov/health/berberine-and-weight-loss-what-you-need-to-know (accessed on 21 June 2025).
132. Zamani, M.; Zarei, M.; Nikbaf-Shandiz, M.; Hosseini, S.; Shiraseb, F.; Asbaghi, O. The Effects of Berberine Supplementation on Cardiovascular Risk Factors in Adults: A Systematic Review and Dose-Response Meta-Analysis. *Front. Nutr.* **2022**, *9*, 1013055. [CrossRef] [PubMed]
133. Miedlich, S.U.; Lamberti, J.S. Connecting the Dots: Understanding and Addressing the Metabolic Impact of Antipsychotic and Antidepressant Medications. *Ann. N. Y. Acad. Sci.* **2025**, *1546*, 35–57. [CrossRef] [PubMed]
134. Qiu, Y.; Li, M.; Zhang, Y.; Liu, Y.; Zhao, Y.; Zhang, J.; Jia, Q.; Li, J. Berberine Treatment for Weight Gain in Patients with Schizophrenia by Regulating Leptin Rather than Adiponectin. *Asian J. Psychiatry* **2022**, *67*, 102896. [CrossRef] [PubMed]
135. Pu, Z.; Sun, Y.; Jiang, H.; Hou, Q.; Yan, H.; Wen, H.; Li, G. Effects of Berberine on Gut Microbiota in Patients with Mild Metabolic Disorders Induced by Olanzapine. *Am. J. Chin. Med.* **2021**, *49*, 1949–1963. [CrossRef] [PubMed]
136. Hu, Y.; Young, A.J.; Ehli, E.A.; Nowotny, D.; Davies, P.S.; Droke, E.A.; Soundy, T.J.; Davies, G.E. Metformin and Berberine Prevent Olanzapine-Induced Weight Gain in Rats. *PLoS ONE* **2014**, *9*, e93310. [CrossRef] [PubMed]
137. Singh, R.; Bansal, Y.; Sodhi, R.K.; Singh, D.P.; Bishnoi, M.; Kondepudi, K.K.; Medhi, B.; Kuhad, A. Berberine Attenuated Olanzapine-Induced Metabolic Alterations in Mice: Targeting Transient Receptor Potential Vanilloid Type 1 and 3 Channels. *Life Sci.* **2020**, *247*, 117442. [CrossRef] [PubMed]
138. Moss, L.; Laudenslager, M.; Steffen, K.J.; Sockalingam, S.; Coughlin, J.W. Antidepressants and Weight Gain: An Update on the Evidence and Clinical Implications. *Curr. Obes. Rep.* **2025**, *14*, 2. [CrossRef] [PubMed]
139. Piątkowska-Chmiel, I.; Wicha-Komsta, K.; Pawłowski, K.; Syrytczyk, A.; Kocki, T.; Dudka, J.; Herbet, M. Beyond Diabetes: Semaglutide's Role in Modulating Mood Disorders through Neuroinflammation Pathways. *Cell. Mol. Neurobiol.* **2025**, *45*, 22. [CrossRef] [PubMed]
140. Yang, K.; Wu, Y.; He, Y.; Dai, J.; Luo, Y.; Xie, J.; Ding, W. GLP-1 and IL-6 Regulates Obesity in the Gut and Brain. *Life Sci.* **2025**, *362*, 123339. [CrossRef] [PubMed]
141. Shah, M.; Vella, A. Effects of GLP-1 on Appetite and Weight. *Rev. Endocr. Metab. Disord.* **2014**, *15*, 181–187. [CrossRef] [PubMed]
142. Himmerich, H.; McElroy, S.L. Glucagon-Like Peptide 1 Receptor Agonists in Psychiatry. *J. Clin. Psychopharmacol.* **2024**, *44*, 207–210. [CrossRef] [PubMed]
143. Trott, M.; Arnautovska, U.; Siskind, D. GLP-1 Receptor Agonists and Weight Loss in Schizophrenia—Past, Present, and Future. *Curr. Opin. Psychiatry* **2024**, *37*, 363–369. [CrossRef] [PubMed]
144. Chan, M.; Qin, Z.; Man, S.; Lam, M.; Lai, W.H.; Ng, R.M.K.; Lee, C.K.; Wong, T.L.; Lee, E.H.M.; Wong, H.K.; et al. Adjunctive Berberine Reduces antipsychotic-associated Weight Gain and Metabolic Syndrome in Patients with Schizophrenia: A Randomized Controlled Trial. *Psychiatry Clin. Neurosci.* **2022**, *76*, 77–85. [CrossRef] [PubMed]
145. Yu, Y.; Liu, L.; Wang, X.; Liu, X.; Liu, X.; Xie, L.; Wang, G. Modulation of Glucagon-like Peptide-1 Release by Berberine: In Vivo and in Vitro Studies. *Biochem. Pharmacol.* **2010**, *79*, 1000–1006. [CrossRef] [PubMed]
146. Wu, W.; Xia, Q.; Guo, Y.; Wang, H.; Dong, H.; Lu, F.; Yuan, F. Berberine Enhances the Function of Db/Db Mice Islet β Cell through GLP-1/GLP-1R/PKA Signaling Pathway in Intestinal L Cell and Islet α Cell. *Front. Pharmacol.* **2023**, *14*, 1228722. [CrossRef] [PubMed]
147. Park, H.-J.; Jung, E.; Shim, I. Berberine for Appetite Suppressant and Prevention of Obesity. *Biomed. Res. Int.* **2020**, *2020*, 3891806. [CrossRef] [PubMed]
148. Qin, Z.; Shi, D.-D.; Li, W.; Cheng, D.; Zhang, Y.-D.; Zhang, S.; Tsoi, B.; Zhao, J.; Wang, Z.; Zhang, Z.-J. Berberine Ameliorates Depression-like Behaviors in Mice via Inhibiting NLRP3 Inflammasome-Mediated Neuroinflammation and Preventing Neuroplasticity Disruption. *J. Neuroinflammation* **2023**, *20*, 54. [CrossRef] [PubMed]
149. Ge, P.; Qu, S.; Ni, S.; Yao, Z.; Qi, Y.; Zhao, X.; Guo, R.; Yang, N.; Zhang, Q.; Zhu, H. Berberine Ameliorates Depression-like Behavior in CUMS Mice by Activating TPH1 and Inhibiting IDO1 -associated with Tryptophan Metabolism. *Phytother. Res.* **2023**, *37*, 342–357. [CrossRef] [PubMed]

150. Pu, Z.; Wen, H.; Jiang, H.; Hou, Q.; Yan, H. Berberine Improves Negative Symptoms and Cognitive Function in Patients with Chronic Schizophrenia via Anti-Inflammatory Effect: A Randomized Clinical Trial. *Chin. Med.* **2023**, *18*, 41. [CrossRef] [PubMed]
151. Li, M.; Qiu, Y.; Zhang, J.; Zhang, Y.; Liu, Y.; Zhao, Y.; Jia, Q.; Fan, X.; Li, J. Improvement of Adjunctive Berberine Treatment on Negative Symptoms in Patients with Schizophrenia. *Eur. Arch. Psychiatry Clin. Neurosci.* **2022**, *272*, 633–642. [CrossRef] [PubMed]
152. Liu, Y.-T.; Hao, H.-P.; Xie, H.-G.; Lai, L.; Wang, Q.; Liu, C.-X.; Wang, G.-J. Extensive Intestinal First-Pass Elimination and Predominant Hepatic Distribution of Berberine Explain Its Low Plasma Levels in Rats. *Drug Metab. Dispos.* **2010**, *38*, 1779–1784. [CrossRef] [PubMed]
153. Tan, X.-S.; Ma, J.-Y.; Feng, R.; Ma, C.; Chen, W.-J.; Sun, Y.-P.; Fu, J.; Huang, M.; He, C.-Y.; Shou, J.-W.; et al. Tissue Distribution of Berberine and Its Metabolites after Oral Administration in Rats. *PLoS ONE* **2013**, *8*, e77969. [CrossRef] [PubMed]
154. Chen, W.; Miao, Y.-Q.; Fan, D.-J.; Yang, S.-S.; Lin, X.; Meng, L.-K.; Tang, X. Bioavailability Study of Berberine and the Enhancing Effects of TPGS on Intestinal Absorption in Rats. *AAPS PharmSciTech* **2011**, *12*, 705–711. [CrossRef] [PubMed]
155. Liu, C.-S.; Zheng, Y.-R.; Zhang, Y.-F.; Long, X.-Y. Research Progress on Berberine with a Special Focus on Its Oral Bioavailability. *Fitoterapia* **2016**, *109*, 274–282. [CrossRef] [PubMed]
156. Ji, H.-F.; Shen, L. Molecular Basis of Inhibitory Activities of Berberine against Pathogenic Enzymes in Alzheimer's Disease. *Sci. World J.* **2012**, *2012*, 1–4. [CrossRef] [PubMed]
157. Spinozzi, S.; Colliva, C.; Camborata, C.; Roberti, M.; Ianni, C.; Neri, F.; Calvarese, C.; Lisotti, A.; Mazzella, G.; Roda, A. Berberine and Its Metabolites: Relationship between Physicochemical Properties and Plasma Levels after Administration to Human Subjects. *J. Nat. Prod.* **2014**, *77*, 766–772. [CrossRef] [PubMed]
158. Zhang, C.; Li, C.; Chen, S.; Li, Z.; Jia, X.; Wang, K.; Bao, J.; Liang, Y.; Wang, X.; Chen, M.; et al. Berberine Protects against 6-OHDA-Induced Neurotoxicity in PC12 Cells and Zebrafish through Hormetic Mechanisms Involving PI3K/AKT/Bcl-2 and Nrf2/HO-1 Pathways. *Redox Biol.* **2017**, *11*, 1–11. [CrossRef] [PubMed]
159. Habtemariam, S. Berberine Pharmacology and the Gut Microbiota: A Hidden Therapeutic Link. *Pharmacol. Res.* **2020**, *155*, 104722. [CrossRef] [PubMed]
160. Chen, C.-Y.; Zhang, Y. Berberine: An Isoquinoline Alkaloid Targeting the Oxidative Stress and Gut-Brain Axis in the Models of Depression. *Eur. J. Med. Chem.* **2025**, *290*, 117475. [CrossRef] [PubMed]
161. Li, Y.; Ren, G.; Wang, Y.-X.; Kong, W.-J.; Yang, P.; Wang, Y.-M.; Li, Y.-H.; Yi, H.; Li, Z.-R.; Song, D.-Q.; et al. Bioactivities of Berberine Metabolites after Transformation through CYP450 Isoenzymes. *J. Transl. Med.* **2011**, *9*, 62. [CrossRef] [PubMed]
162. Feng, R.; Shou, J.-W.; Zhao, Z.-X.; He, C.-Y.; Ma, C.; Huang, M.; Fu, J.; Tan, X.-S.; Li, X.-Y.; Wen, B.-Y.; et al. Transforming Berberine into Its Intestine-Absorbable Form by the Gut Microbiota. *Sci. Rep.* **2015**, *5*, 12155. [CrossRef] [PubMed]
163. Simpson, C.A.; Diaz-Arteche, C.; Eliby, D.; Schwartz, O.S.; Simmons, J.G.; Cowan, C.S.M. The Gut Microbiota in Anxiety and Depression—A Systematic Review. *Clin. Psychol. Rev.* **2021**, *83*, 101943. [CrossRef] [PubMed]
164. Nikolova, V.L.; Smith, M.R.B.; Hall, L.J.; Cleare, A.J.; Stone, J.M.; Young, A.H. Perturbations in Gut Microbiota Composition in Psychiatric Disorders: A Review and Meta-Analysis. *JAMA Psychiatry* **2021**, *78*, 1343. [CrossRef] [PubMed]
165. Zhu, X.; Sun, Y.; Zhang, C.; Liu, H. Effects of Berberine on a Rat Model of Chronic Stress and Depression via Gastrointestinal Tract Pathology and Gastrointestinal Flora Profile Assays. *Mol. Med. Rep.* **2017**, *15*, 3161–3171. [CrossRef] [PubMed]
166. Huang, M.; He, Y.; Tian, L.; Yu, L.; Cheng, Q.; Li, Z.; Gao, L.; Gao, S.; Yu, C. Gut Microbiota-SCFAs-Brain Axis Associated with the Antidepressant Activity of Berberine in CUMS Rats. *J. Affect. Disord.* **2023**, *325*, 141–150. [CrossRef] [PubMed]
167. Zhang, L.; Wu, X.; Yang, R.; Chen, F.; Liao, Y.; Zhu, Z.; Wu, Z.; Sun, X.; Wang, L. Effects of Berberine on the Gastrointestinal Microbiota. *Front. Cell. Infect. Microbiol.* **2021**, *10*, 588517. [CrossRef] [PubMed]
168. Dalile, B.; Van Oudenhove, L.; Vervliet, B.; Verbeke, K. The Role of Short-Chain Fatty Acids in Microbiota–Gut–Brain Communication. *Nat. Rev. Gastroenterol. Hepatol.* **2019**, *16*, 461–478. [CrossRef] [PubMed]
169. Strandwitz, P. Neurotransmitter Modulation by the Gut Microbiota. *Brain Res.* **2018**, *1693*, 128–133. [CrossRef] [PubMed]
170. Morisaki, Y.; Miyata, N.; Nakashima, M.; Hata, T.; Takakura, S.; Yoshihara, K.; Suematsu, T.; Nomoto, K.; Miyazaki, K.; Tsuji, H.; et al. Persistence of Gut Dysbiosis in Individuals with Anorexia Nervosa. *PLoS ONE* **2023**, *18*, e0296037. [CrossRef] [PubMed]
171. Scala, M.; Tabone, M.; Paolini, M.; Salueña, A.; Iturra, R.A.; Ferreiro, V.R.; Alvarez-Mon, M.Á.; Serretti, A.; Soltero, M.D.R.G.; Rodriguez-Jimenez, R. Unlocking the Link Between Gut Microbiota and Psychopathological Insights in Anorexia Nervosa: A Systematic Review. *Eur. Eat. Disord. Rev.* **2025**, *33*, 700–718. [CrossRef] [PubMed]
172. Zhao, W.; Kodancha, P.; Das, S. Gut Microbiome Changes in Anorexia Nervosa: A Comprehensive Review. *Pathophysiology* **2024**, *31*, 68–88. [CrossRef] [PubMed]
173. Prochazkova, P.; Roubalova, R.; Dvorak, J.; Kreisinger, J.; Hill, M.; Tlaskalova-Hogenova, H.; Tomasova, P.; Pelantova, H.; Cermakova, M.; Kuzma, M.; et al. The Intestinal Microbiota and Metabolites in Patients with Anorexia Nervosa. *Gut Microbes* **2021**, *13*, 1902771. [CrossRef] [PubMed]
174. Carbone, E.A.; D'Amato, P.; Vicchio, G.; De Fazio, P.; Segura-Garcia, C. A Systematic Review on the Role of Microbiota in the Pathogenesis and Treatment of Eating Disorders. *Eur. Psychiatry* **2020**, *64*, e2. [CrossRef] [PubMed]

75. Wang, Y.; Tong, Q.; Ma, S.-R.; Zhao, Z.-X.; Pan, L.-B.; Cong, L.; Han, P.; Peng, R.; Yu, H.; Lin, Y.; et al. Oral Berberine Improves Brain Dopa/Dopamine Levels to Ameliorate Parkinson's Disease by Regulating Gut Microbiota. *Signal Transduct. Target. Ther.* **2021**, *6*, 77. [CrossRef] [PubMed]
76. Tarrago, T.; Kichik, N.; Seguí, J.; Giralt, E. The Natural Product Berberine is a Human Prolyl Oligopeptidase Inhibitor. *ChemMedChem* **2007**, *2*, 354–359. [CrossRef] [PubMed]

nutrients

MDPI

Review

Association Between Orthorexia and Plant-Based Diets—Is There a Vicious Cycle?

Patrycja Szulc, Kaja Willich and Patrycja Gogga *

Division of Food Commodity Science, Department of Clinical Nutrition, Faculty of Health Sciences, Medical University of Gdańsk, ul. Dębinki 7, 80-211 Gdańsk, Poland; patkaszulc@gumed.edu.pl (P.S.); kaja.willich@gumed.edu.pl (K.W.)

* Correspondence: patrycja.gogga@gumed.edu.pl

Abstract: Nowadays, social media and rapidly changing dietary trends encourage people to constantly—often excessively—control their diet, which leads to an increased risk of developing eating disorders, including orthorexia nervosa (ON). At the same time, more and more people reduce or give up consumption of meat and other animal products, adopting different types of plant-based (vegetarian) diets. The following paper aimed to demonstrate the significant similarities between orthorexia and plant-based diets and to highlight the necessity of developing new or adapting existing diagnostic tools for orthorexia considering the lifestyle characteristics of vegetarians, especially vegans. It remains unclear whether vegetarianism increases the risk of developing ON or whether the development of ON increases the chances of switching to a plant-based diet. However, based on the available literature, a positive association can be shown between the two. On the one hand, a vegetarian diet may be a cover for ON, but on the other, vegetarians, as a group avoiding specific food products, may be wrongly perceived as disordered. Thus, it is important to distinguish ON from the so-called healthy orthorexia (HO), which is a non-pathological interest in healthy eating, to avoid overdiagnosis and stigmatization of people using healthy alternative diets, including plant-based diets, since the mere fact of following them does not constitute evidence of orthorexia.

Keywords: plant-based diets; vegan; vegetarian; orthorexia nervosa; healthy orthorexia; eating disorders

1. Introduction

People's appearance affects their sense of self-worth. There is a belief that having a certain figure can make them fulfilled and happy human beings. The canons of beauty have changed over time. For instance, in the past, boyish, curvy, or athletic figures were desired in women. Currently, slim figures of women and athletic and muscular bodies of men are glorified. A "perfect" appearance has become a necessity, a feature that determines intelligence and control over life [1]. The pursuit of a desired body image is etiologically related to the pressure of society, which results from contemporary standards of beauty. Unachievable perfection increases criticism of one's own body image and the risk of certain triggers, such as depression or undertaking restrictive diets, contributing to the development of eating disorders [2].

Eating disorders are behavioral states characterized by serious and persistent disturbances of eating practices that affect physical, mental, and social health [3]. They are influenced by many factors: biological, personal, family, and socio-economic [2]. Nowadays, social media and wellness culture encourage people to constantly analyze their diet, often resulting in a worsening of one's relationship with food. Giving up specific food products and so-called clean eating—consuming only foods regarded as healthy, e.g., primarily unprocessed [4]—usually begins as an attempt to achieve optimal health through attention to diet but may lead to various eating disorders, including orthorexia nervosa (ON), and ultimately to malnutrition and low quality of life [5].

ON is the ideology of eating "only the right food". It involves counting calories, eliminating "fattening" products, and generally consuming a very modest group of foods. It can manifest itself with obsessive thoughts about food and constant meal planning, and people struggling with this disorder do not take pleasure in eating because they are afraid of it. Possible health consequences of ON are mineral and vitamin deficiencies, and—as a consequence—osteoporosis, hypertension, and anemia [6].

Limiting or excluding meat and other animal products is becoming increasingly popular, especially among young people. Despite the documented health benefits of adopting such dietary patterns, studies show a significant relationship between them and eating disorders—more than half of patients with eating disorders report that they began following various types of vegetarian diets after the onset of their disordered eating [7].

The following review aimed, firstly, to explore the hypothesis that ON and plant-based diets are interrelated and, secondly, to show that diagnostic tools currently used for ON are not applicable to vegetarians regarding their specific eating habits. Particular attention was also paid to the distinction between orthorexia and a non-pathological interest in healthy eating.

2. Methodological Approach and Search Strategy

The following paper is a narrative review. A literature search on the relationship between plant-based diets and orthorexia was conducted in PubMed and Google Scholar using the following keywords: "orthorexia nervosa", "plant-based diets", "vegetarianism", "veganism", and "eating disorders". After an initial screening of the abstracts, only studies closely related to the topic were chosen, i.e., assessing the incidence of ON among vegetarians and discussing the possible link between this eating disorder and plant-based diets. Basically, studies published between 2015 and 2024 in English and Polish were included; however, literature addressing definitions and the validation of questionnaires used as diagnostic tools as well as papers published earlier were excluded.

3. Plant-Based Diets

More and more people are deciding to give up meat and other animal products. There is a wide range of plant-based (vegetarian) diets—from less to more restrictive: lacto-ovo-vegetarianism (excludes meat and fish), ovo-vegetarianism (excludes meat, fish, and dairy), lacto-vegetarianism (excludes meat, fish, and eggs), pescetarianism (excludes only meat), and veganism (excludes all animal products). There are also so-called pseudo-vegetarian diets, namely semi-vegetarianism and flexitarianism, in which meat consumption is partially limited [8].

According to the largest dietetic associations (Academy of Nutrition and Dietetics, Dietitians of Canada, British Dietetic Association), properly balanced vegetarian diets (including vegan) are healthy and can be an appropriate choice for any stage of life (during pregnancy and lactation, in children, and in the elderly) and in athletes [9]. Additionally, the use of plant-based diets can bring numerous health benefits. Compared to meat eaters, vegetarians (especially vegans) have lower body mass and BMI [10]. Furthermore, plant-based diets can reduce the risk of diet-related diseases, including hypertension, type 2 diabetes, or some cancers [8]. However, followers of these diets are prone to deficiency of certain nutrients, namely vitamin B_{12} (supplementation of which is essential in a strict plant-based diet), vitamin D, calcium, iodine, iron, zinc, selenium, vitamin A, omega-3 fatty acids, and protein [9–11].

Usually, adopting a plant-based diet is an attempt to modify eating habits, during which animal-based foods and highly processed foods are replaced—whenever possible—with raw, unprocessed, or minimally processed plant-based products. There are several reasons for switching to a vegetarian diet, including health, ethical, or environmental motives [12].

4. Similarities Between Plant-Based Diets and Orthorexia Nervosa

ON shares several features and dieting behaviors with vegetarianism, such as restricting food intake according to specific dietary rules and an inability to be flexible in one's eating habits (Figure 1) [13]. Thus, adhering to these diets involves restrictions resembling cognitive restraint—the intention to continually, consciously control food intake to maintain or lose weight [14]—often used as an indicator of pathological eating behaviors [15]. However, it may not be applicable to vegetarians (especially vegans), as their avoidance of animal products is not necessarily indicative of disordered eating [16]. In fact, a study on vegetarians and vegans showed that both groups had lower cognitive restraint, emotional eating, and uncontrolled eating compared to omnivores, but on the other hand, they exhibited more behaviors associated with ON, such as a stronger focus on healthy eating, greater knowledge of it, and a heightened sense of wellbeing related to healthy food choices [15].

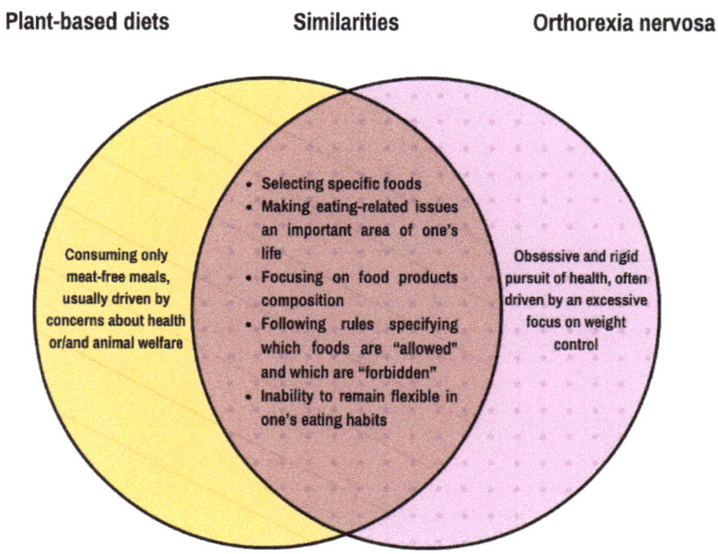

Figure 1. Similarities between plant-based diets and orthorexia nervosa. Based on [13].

Nevertheless, recent studies suggest that ON is associated with impaired cognitive functions, and plant-based diets could be a contributing factor [13]. Consequently, obsessive thoughts of food—a key feature of ON—appear to be more prevalent among vegetarians than non-vegetarians [17], potentially putting them at a higher risk of developing orthorexic tendencies or the disorder itself [15,18,19].

5. Healthy Orthorexia

Some studies suggest that orthorexia may also be a non-pathological interest in healthy eating, which is called a healthy orthorexia (HO) [20]. The bidimensional concept of orthorexia includes both pathological (ON) and non-pathological (HO) aspects of interest in healthy eating, which appear to vary significantly (Figure 2). In the case of ON, the motive showing the strongest association is weight control. Health content shows negligible and statistically insignificant relationship with ON. In the case of HO, the strongest association is observed with health content, followed by weight control and socio-political reasons [21]. It should be emphasized, though, that constant reductions in acceptable foods, resulting in a diet that includes only a small number of products considered edible, may not necessarily lead to a decrease in overall calories intake, which—in fact—may even be increased in subjects with ON [22]. Moreover, despite their apparent preoccupation with healthy eating, individuals with ON often exhibit relatively unhealthy eating habits and other undesirable lifestyle behaviors, such as increased screen time or increased smoking and alcohol consumption compared to healthy subjects [23].

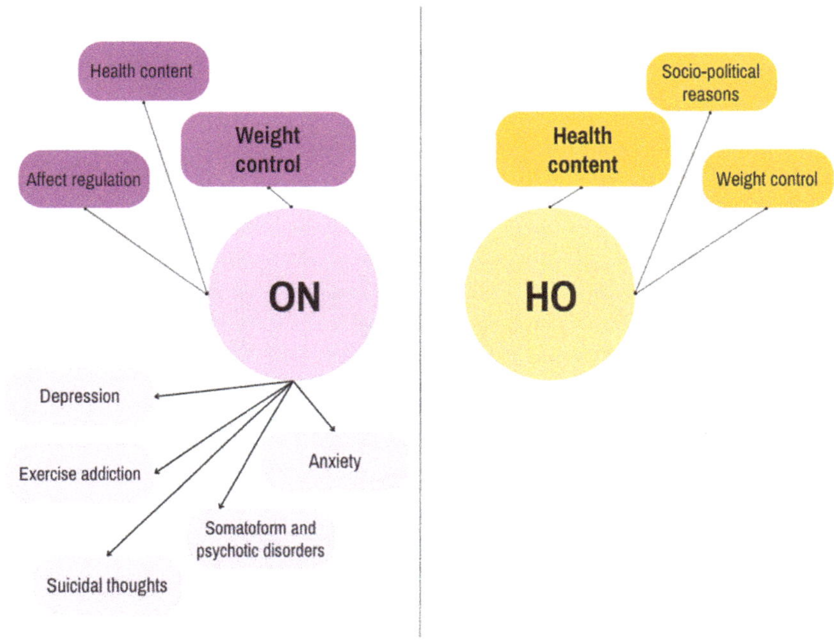

Figure 2. Motives for food choices and their psychopathological consequences in two types of orthorexia. Bigger font size indicates predominant motives. ON—orthorexia nervosa; HO—healthy orthorexia. Based on [21,24].

6. Diagnostic Criteria for Orthorexia Nervosa

ON is a relatively newly described eating disorder, and despite the constantly increasing awareness and public interest in this issue, it cannot be clearly classified as an eating disorder or a mental disorder. The available literature discusses whether ON should be considered a separate disorder, a variation on other disorders, or a cultural attitude [25–27]. It should be emphasized that ON is not included in the current Diagnostic Criteria for Mental Disorders (DSM-5-TR) or in the International Statistical Classification of Diseases and Related Health Problems (ICD-11) [25–27]. In addition, diagnosing ON may be difficult due to the lack of standard diagnostic criteria in the main psychiatric classification systems. It is also important to distinguish ON from other eating disorders (e.g., symptoms and behaviors typical for ON may also be characteristic for anorexia nervosa). Finally, it is crucial to differentiate between HO and ON to recognize where a care of one's diet quality ends and a pathological obsession—potentially leading to suffering and health damage—begins [26,27] and to avoid overdiagnosis and stigmatization of all alternative healthy diets (including plant-based diets) [26]. Nevertheless, the mere fact of reducing meat for ethical reasons should not be a diagnostic criterion for ON [28].

At the moment, despite many proposals for diagnostic criteria for ON, no uniform standard or consensus has been established [27]. However, proposed criteria for ON usually include the following features:

- Obsessive focus on healthy eating (rigid rules and restrictions, excessive attention to the nutritional value of meals, as well as the quality and purity of food) worsening everyday functioning;
- Emotional disorders (e.g., anxiety, fear, etc.) resulting from failure to follow the rigorous dietary rules imposed on oneself;
- Psychosocial problems in various areas of life (e.g., work- or school-related);
- Malnutrition and weight loss [26,27].

Selected psychometric tools for diagnosing ON are presented in Table 1. The most used are the ORTO-15 questionnaire and the Bratman Orthorexia Test (BOT) [27].

Table 1. The most frequently used and best described questionnaires for diagnosing orthorexia nervosa.

Name	Structure	Comment
EDE-Q (Eating Disorder Examination Questionnaire)	• 28 items. • Four subscales quantifying: "restraint", "eating concerns", "weight concerns", and "shape concerns" [29].	• Reliable and valid measure of eating disorders in diverse samples [29]. • Validated in studies of omnivores, weight-motivated vegetarians, and non-weight-motivated vegetarians [30]. • Brief three-factor model (7 items) validated in vegans and omnivores [31].
DEBQ (Dutch Eating Behavior Questionnaire)	• 33 items and three subscales. • Uses a 5-point Likert scale ranging from never (1) to very often (5). A mean score is calculated for each subscale. Higher scores on each subscale reflect higher levels of restrained, emotional, and external eating, respectively [32].	• A tool designed to assess restraint, emotions, and response to external factors of eating. Good psychometric properties of eating disorder scales in vegans [33].
ORTO-15	• 15 items. • Answers indicating the risk of orthorexia behavior receive 1 point, while those corresponding to a correct attitude to food receive 4 points. • The cut-off point is 40 points. Obtaining a lower number of points indicates a tendency toward ON. • This test and its adaptations are most often used in scientific research [34].	• Does not detect true pathological eating behaviors but rather normal dietary adherence in the vegetarian/vegan populations [35]. • Overestimates the prevalence of ON. • Poor psychometric properties. • Probably cannot distinguish between ON and HO [36].
TFEQ (Three-Factor Eating Questionnaire)	• 18 items. • Assesses three cognitive and behavioral domains of eating: restrained eating, binge eating, and emotional eating. • There is no universally used cut-off point [37].	• Suitable rather for describing eating habits than for diagnosing eating disorders [37].

Table 1. *Cont.*

Name	Structure	Comment
EAT (Eating Attitudes Test)	• 40 items. • 6-point Likert-type self-rating scale. • Individuals with a total score of 30 or higher are considered to have disordered eating [38].	• Poor psychometric properties in vegans [38].
EHQ (Eating Habits Questionnaire)	• 21 items. • Based on the 4-point Likert-type scale (from "false, not at all true" to "very true"). • The areas included in the questionnaire are knowledge about healthy eating, problems related to healthy eating, and positive attitudes towards healthy eating [39].	• Detects both ON and HO, with inability to distinguish between these separate constructs [40].
BOT (The Bratman Orthorexia Test)	• 10 items. • A score of 0–1 point means that the examined person does not suffer from ON, 2–3 points indicate a risk of this disorder, and 4 or more is diagnosed as ON [25].	• Not a psychometric test [25].
DOS (Düsseldorf Orthorexia Scale)	• 10 items. • Based on a 4-point Likert-type scale (from "this does not apply to me" to "this applies to me") [41]. • Cut-off point is 30, while scores ranging from 25 to 29 indicate a risk of ON [41].	• Inability to distinguish between patients suffering from anorexia and orthorexia [42]. • Detects both ON and HO, with inability to distinguish between these separate constructs [40].
TOS (Teruel Orthorexia Scale)	• Based on the 4-point Likert-type scale (from "does not concern you at all" to "completely affects you"). • Includes two subscales—TOS He (9 items) and TOS Ne (8 items)—for diagnosing HO and ON, respectively. • A higher score on both scales indicates a greater intensity of a given form of orthorexia [43].	• Extends the conceptualization of orthorexia beyond the problematic aspects of healthy eating to include non-problematic ones, i.e., HO. • Operates independently of any underlying psychopathology [42].

7. Two Sides of the Cycle

Half of patients with anorexia nervosa declare that they refuse to eat red meat because it is perceived as too caloric, distasteful, or anxiety-provoking. On the other hand, problematic eating behaviors developed after switching to a vegetarian diet, in the form of significant restrictions on the amount, frequency, or variety of food consumed, have also been observed [44]. Other studies indicate that 50% of anorexic patients follow a vegetarian diet [45], compared to 10% in the general population [46]. It remains unclear whether vegetarianism increases the risk of developing eating disorders or whether having an eating disorder increases the chances of choosing plant-based dietary pattern [47]. It cannot be ruled out that the pathology is perpetuated in a vicious cycle, in which restriction begets restriction [48] (Figure 3).

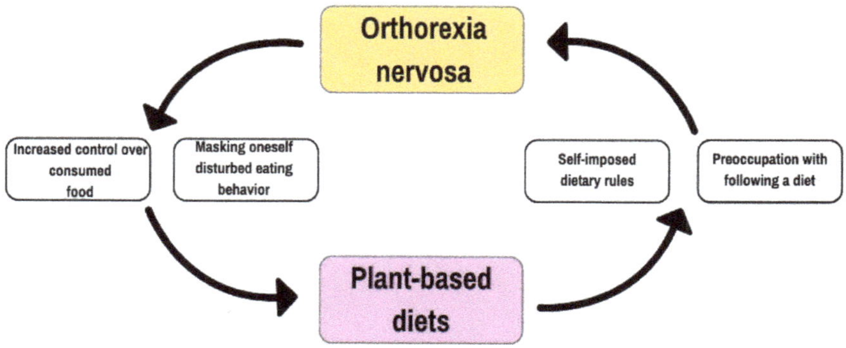

Figure 3. The vicious cycle of the relationship between orthorexia nervosa and plant-based diets. It is presumed that individuals preoccupied with strict dietary rules may develop orthorexic tendencies, while those with orthorexia may use plant-based diets to justify or mask abnormal eating behaviors. The cycle reinforces increased control over food intake and perpetuates dietary restrictions.

7.1. Plant-Based Diets as a Cover for Orthorexia Nervosa

Currently, there is an increased prevalence of vegetarianism (from 1% to 9%), especially in developed countries [45]. The reasons for choosing this dietary pattern vary depending on the study. One indicated that health/nutrition (37.5%) is the most common reason, followed by weight control (18.8%) and ethics towards animals (14.6%) [49]. In another study, the most common reasons were taste preferences (58.1%), followed by a healthier diet (19.4%) and weight control (9.6%) [50].

Conscious eating is associated with long-term health benefits but also with a sense of responsibility, which in some people can lead to an obsession with healthy eating, characterized by excessive control over food intake, forced behaviors, and self-control [51]. Some research suggested that use of the plant-based diets may be associated with a disturbed body image and complexes regarding body weight and figure that do not correspond to the contemporary canons of beauty [45]. Moreover, studies have shown that women who follow a vegetarian diet may be more likely to demonstrate disturbed eating attitudes and behaviors than women who follow an omnivore diet as well as men. It was also found that following certain diets or dietary rules, such as different types of vegetarian diets, is associated with orthorexic eating patterns [13].

Many people with disturbed eating habits and using (currently or in the past) a vegetarian diet admit that they adopted it because they wanted to increase control over the consumed food. In a patient with eating disorders and following a vegetarian diet, there is a high probability that the diet is a way of restricting one's food consumption as a part of the pathological eating behavior [52]. Vegetarianism may be a widely accepted way to limit food intake to control or reduce body weight while concealing pathological eating behaviors [53]. Since plant-based diets are characterized by a high intake of products such as vegetables, whole grains, legumes, and fruits, they have a positive effect on health, as they are high in fiber, bioactive compounds, and micro- and macro-elements and low in saturated fats and simple sugars [54]. This affects the perception of plant-based diets as low-calorie and low-fat, which on the one hand is good for general health [46] but on the other may be a strategy for avoiding food to control body weight [48]. It has been noted that eating disorders occurred more frequently in people who declared using a vegetarian diet for this very purpose [17].

With the right expertise and meal planning, there is no reason why a vegetarian—including vegan—diet cannot be well balanced and sufficient to meet the nutritional needs of any individual [55]. However, a person with ON exhibits inflexible eating behaviors, ranging from a focus on eating organic or raw foods to a complete avoidance of all foods perceived as unhealthy, which can lead to a disturbed relationship with food and malnutrition [45]. In one study, participants most frequently named plant-based foods (30%), organic/natural/non-GMO foods (18%), and protein foods (16%) as important components of "clean" diets [56]. Furthermore, two-thirds of people with a history of eating disorders reported that their choice of vegetarianism was associated with their eating disorders because it allowed them to reduce calorie intake and to increase their sense of control over consumed food [52].

Through avoidance and ritualization—perceiving vegan foods as healthy—people with ON experience temporary relief from anxiety while perpetuating intrusive thoughts about health and food [23].

The higher prevalence of eating disorders in vegetarians suggests that plant-based diets may be used to justify avoidance of food and to mask restrictive eating patterns used for weight control [13]. For a patient with an eating disorder, declaring being a vegetarian for animal rights reasons, for example, seems more socially acceptable and less uncomfortable than explicitly disclosing weight loss as a motive [48].

7.2. *Plant-Based Diets as a Path to Orthorexia Nervosa*

Although there is an increasing number of studies on vegetarianism, only few have examined the relationship between the use of these dietary patterns and a tendency to orthorexia disorders [13,28,47]. It has been suggested that vegetarianism may be a factor triggering and maintaining eating disorders, but the evidence supporting this thesis is ambiguous [53,57].

The results of studies assessing the incidence of ON among vegetarians are divergent—some have indicated a significant link between the use of plant-based diets and this disorder [28,47,58–60], while others have found no such association [36,61,62]. The discrepancy in results may be due to several reasons, including different definitions of types of vegetarianism or the use of different methods for diagnosing ON [28] and their not being adjusted to plant-based diets users; for obvious reasons, the dietary attitudes and behaviors of vegetarians differ from non-vegetarians, and this may be wrongly perceived as pathology [63].

Missbach et al. [58], in a sample of 1029 people, found that different vegetarian dietary patterns were associated with the occurrence of ON. Similarly, Kozik and Całyniuk [60], in a sample of 514 students from the First High School in Tychy, including 34 individuals following a vegetarian diet, found that while gender was not a significant risk factor for ON, adherence to a vegetarian diet was: more than a half of the vegetarians were at risk for ON compared to 30.2% of non-vegetarians [60]. Also, Dell'Osso et al. [64], in a sample of 2130 people from the academic community of the University of Pisa, found that vegetarians showed a significantly higher rate of ON symptoms than people on a typical diet. Moreover, women who obtained lower (more pathological) ORTO-15 scores were characterized by a lower BMI, were more often underweight, and were more often vegetarians [64].

Reynolds et al. [59] compared the tendency toward ON between vegans, vegetarians (using lacto-, ovo-, and lacto-ovo-vegetarian diets and different types of pseudovegetarian diets), and people who did not exclude any product groups. It was found that vegans and vegetarians had significantly more orthorexic tendencies than non-vegetarians. A particularly high incidence of ON was observed in the vegan group: 42.9% in dietary vegans and 30.8% in lifestyle and dietary vegans compared to 11.8% in omnivores. Furthermore, it was shown that people with greater orthorexic tendencies chose food for weight control and ethical reasons significantly more often than people with fewer orthorexic tendencies [59].

On the other hand, some studies do not support the thesis that plant-based diets and ON are related. Çiçekoğlu and Tunçay [61] examined the link between ON and dietary habits, comparing 31 vegans/vegetarians with 31 non-vegans/non-vegetarians. Using standardized questionaries (ORTO-11, EAT-40, and MOCI), researchers found no significant differences in ON tendencies or obsessive symptoms between the groups. Vegans/vegetarians adopted their diet primarily for ethical reasons and not due to a pathological focus on healthy eating. The authors concluded that neither vegetarianism nor veganism are inherently associated with ON and called for further research on that subject [61]. In a study investigating the relationship between social media usage and the risk of ON based on I-DOS score, Tarsitano et al. [62] found the highest prevalence of the disorder in individuals following an omnivorous diet (30.3%), followed by vegan or vegetarian diet followers (23.7%) and individuals adhering to other dietary patterns (20%) [62]. Corresponding observations were made by Dunn et al. [36]. In a group of 275 U.S. college students, authors investigated the prevalence of ON using the ORTO-15 questionnaire. The results showed that 71% of participants scored in the orthorexia range, but only 20% followed restrictive diets. In fact, participants who followed a vegan diet obtained the highest (least pathological) scores. However, it should be noted that this conclusion was drawn based on a very small sample—there were only 6 vegan subjects among 275 study participants [36].

An important aspect of diagnosing ON in vegetarians is the fact that they are more likely to have greater nutritional knowledge and pay more attention to the quality and composition of the products they choose. In a systematic review, in 9 of 12 analyzed studies, lacto-ovo-vegetarians or vegans had a 4.5–16.4-point higher HEI-2010 (Healthy Eating Index 2010) score than non-vegetarians [65]. Additionally, Brytek-Matera et al. [13] showed that vegans had greater knowledge of healthy eating compared to non-vegetarians and vegetarians excluding only meat from their diet.

Furthermore, the currently used diagnostic methods may not be adapted to vegans and other vegetarians for several reasons. Inherently, these diets require some level of dietary restraint to ensure that unacceptable foods are not consumed. Questionnaires may not be able to distinguish between underlying factors behind the restrictions—whether it is dietary restraint (e.g., plant-based diet) or cognitive restraint (e.g., weight control). In addition, they are likely unable to identify dietary behaviors unique to vegetarians, such as monitoring meal compositions when eating in public or reading food labels (Table 2). Therefore, it seems necessary to design a specific screening tool to assess eating disorder symptoms in individuals who follow plant-based diets. A validated self-report tool dedicated to this group would provide clinicians and researchers with a rapid, inexpensive, and effective way to identify individuals who may require in-depth assessment of dietary habits or intervention [53].

Recently, a method for diagnosing eating disorders dedicated to vegans and vegetarians—the Vegetarian Vegan Eating Disorder Screener (V-EDS)—was created. This is an 18-item self-report tool designed to assess eating disorders symptoms in vegetarians and vegans over the past 7 days. It was created based on the experience of vegetarians and vegans, the experience of people with a history of eating disorders, and the knowledge of psychologists and dietitians specializing in the field. The V-EDS was designed to distinguish the basic factors determining the increasing pathology of eating disorders (e.g., restricting food to affect body weight versus restricting food groups in vegetarian or vegan diets). The questionnaire is divided into two parts—the first one, consisting of 6 items, provides information on the respondent's diet, while the second, a 12-item part, refers to the respondent's behaviors and attitudes and examines the presence of pathology towards eating disorders. Both are assessed on a 5-point Likert scale, and the higher the obtained score, the more severe the eating disorder. An overall score of 18 is considered as the cut-off point for predicting clinical cases [53,66].

Table 2. Selected problematic and potentially misleading elements for vegetarians, with emphasis on vegans, in questionnaires for diagnosing orthorexia nervosa. Based on [47].

Name of Questionnaire	Problematic and Potentially Misleading Elements for Vegetarians with Comments
EDE-Q	Questions 3 and 4 on the restraint scale: **Have you tried to eliminate foods you like from your diet to affect your figure or weight?** **Have you tried to follow certain rules about food to affect your figure or weight?** Vegetarians exclude some or all animal products from their diet.
ORTO-15	Questions 2 and 8: **Do you feel confused when you go to the grocery store?** Vegans can often feel confused when reading the list of ingredients and assessing whether a product contains animal-derived ones. **Do you allow yourself any food-related transgressions?** Vegans usually do not allow themselves to consume animal products. However, it is important to remember that these limits are very individual.
TFEQ	Item 1 on the subscale of cognitive inhibition: **When I smell a sizzling steak or see a juicy piece of meat, I find it very difficult to stop eating, even if I have just finished a meal.** Vegetarians do not eat meat; thus this question seems inadequate and the answer unreliable.
EAT	Items 2, 19, 30, 32, and 33: **You prepare food for others, but you will not eat it yourself.** Vegans can often prepare dishes from animal products for others. **You like eating meat.** Vegetarians do not eat meat; thus this question seems to be inadequate and the answer unreliable. **You eat diet foods.** Products for vegetarians are often considered "diet" foods. **You show self-control when dealing with food.** Vegans must show self-control when dealing with foods containing animal products. **I feel that others put pressure on me to eat.** Vegans may feel pressured by family and friends to eat animal products because of a lack of understanding of their choices.
YFAS (Yale Food Addiction Scale)	Items 11 and 23 on the subscale of important social, work, or recreational activities that have been cut back or are being cut back: **There were times when I avoided work or social situations because I was unable to eat certain foods there.** Vegans may avoid work or social situations where vegan food options are limited. **I have tried to limit my consumption of certain foods.** Vegetarians limit some or all animal products. Item 24 on the subscale of persistent craving or repeated failed attempts to quit: **I have managed to limit or not eat these types of foods.** Vegetarians limit some or all animal products.

The V-EDS has the potential to serve as an accessible tool for the initial screening and ongoing monitoring of eating disorder symptoms progression among vegetarians and vegans. However, this tool has been only preliminarily validated in a small, mainly female sample. Future studies should aim to broaden the psychometric evaluation of the V-EDS by testing it with larger and more diverse populations and considering factors such as gender, age, cultural background, and history of eating disorders [66].

8. Conclusions

Based on the available literature, an association between ON and plant-based diets can be observed. However, the lack of consensus on the definition of ON and its diagnosis as well as the small number of studies involving people with a history of eating disorders who also adhere to plant-based diets makes it difficult to demonstrate a clear cause–effect relationship. Studies suggest that vegetarian diets may be chosen as an attempt to cover up orthorexic behaviors, while the dietary restrictions resulting from adopting these diets may potentially predispose individuals to disturbances in eating habits. Thus, it is important for specialists (including dietitians) to pay attention to the motives for choosing such diet types (health aspects vs. weight control) and their patients' general relationship with food. However, it is important to note that well-planned vegetarian diets can offer numerous health benefits, and the mere fact of adherence to these dietary patterns does not indicate orthorexia. Moreover, potential misinterpretation of the results obtained using existing diagnostic tools may lead to overdiagnosis and stigmatization of plant-based diets users; hence, it is necessary to develop new methods (or adapt current ones) that are more suitable for vegetarians, particularly vegans.

This narrative review has several limitations. It excluded non-English and non-Polish studies, and the overall scarcity of research on this subject hindered the interpretation of the results. Additionally, identifying studies that specifically investigated this issue was difficult; thus, the available literature provides only partial insights, failing to comprehensively explore this relatively new topic or offer definitive conclusions. Furthermore, as a non-systematic review, this study is more susceptible to bias and subjectivity due to the absence of a standardized methodology and a structured search strategy. Further research is needed to explore the relationship between ON and plant-based diets, including understanding of the cause and effect relationship, a clearer definition of ON, and the distinction between HO and ON. However, to our knowledge, this is the first study that offers a holistic perspective on the subject. Our work considers both the potential increased risk of orthorexia associated with plant-based diets and the risk of stigmatization of their adherents. By highlighting these two aspects, we underscore the need for a nuanced approach to assessing orthorexic tendencies in individuals following plant-based diets, ensuring that the diagnostic criteria are both sensitive and specific.

Author Contributions: P.S. and K.W., study design; P.S. and K.W., literature search; P.S., K.W. and P.G., manuscript preparation; P.G., primary responsibility for the final content. All authors have read and agreed to the published version of the manuscript.

Funding: This research received no external funding.

Conflicts of Interest: The authors declare no conflicts of interest.

References

1. Jasiński, M.; Dubelt, J.; Cybula-Misiurek, M.; Jasińska, E. Kult pięknej i szczupłej sylwetki a zagrożenia zdrowia młodzieży. In *Zagrożenie Życia i Zdrowia Człowieka*; Tatarczuk, J., Zboina, B., Dąbrowski, P., Eds.; Wydawnictwo Naukowe NeuroCentrum: Lublin, Poland, 2017; pp. 133–146.
2. Kochman, D.; Jaszczak, M. Zaburzenia odżywiania się-częsty problem współczesnej młodzieży Eating disorders-a common problem of modern youth. *Innow. Pielęgniarstwie Nauk. Zdrowiu* **2021**, *6*, 110–128. [CrossRef]
3. Padín, P.F.; González-Rodríguez, R.; Verde-Diego, C.; Vázquez-Pérez, R. Social media and eating disorder psychopathology: A systematic review. *Cyberpsychology J. Psychosoc. Res. Cyberspace* **2021**, *15*, 6. [CrossRef]
4. Cambridge University Press. (n.d.). Clean Eating. In Cambridge English Dictionary. Available online: https://dictionary.cambridge.org/dictionary/english/clean-eating (accessed on 27 February 2025).
5. Koven, N.; Abry, A. The clinical basis of orthorexia nervosa: Emerging perspectives. *Neuropsychiatr. Dis. Treat.* **2015**, *11*, 385–394. [CrossRef]

6. Możdżonek, P.; Antosik, K. Creating of dietary trends in the media and their influence on the development of eating disorders. *Nurs. Public Health.* **2017**, *7*, 159–164. [CrossRef]
7. Bardone-Cone, A.M.; Fitzsimmons-Craft, E.E.; Harney, M.B.; Maldonado, C.R.; Lawson, M.A.; Smith, R.; Robinson, D.P. The inter-relationships between vegetarianism and eating disorders among females. *J. Acad. Nutr. Diet.* **2012**, *112*, 1247–1252. [CrossRef]
8. Kent, G.; Kehoe, L.; Flynn, A.; Walton, J. Plant-based diets: A review of the definitions and nutritional role in the adult diet. *Proc. Nutr. Soc.* **2021**, *81*, 62–74. [CrossRef]
9. Melina, V.; Craig, W.; Levin, S. Position of the Academy of Nutrition and Dietetics: Vegetarian Diets. *J. Acad. Nutr. Diet.* **2016**, *116*, 1970–1980. [CrossRef] [PubMed]
10. Selinger, E.; Neuenschwander, M.; Koller, A.; Gojda, J.; Kühn, T.; Schwingshackl, L.; Barbaresko, J.; Schlesinger, S. Evidence of a vegan diet for health benefits and risks—An umbrella review of meta-analyses of observational and clinical studies. *Crit. Rev. Food Sci. Nutr.* **2023**, *63*, 9926–9936. [CrossRef]
11. Koeder, C.; Perez-Cueto, F.J.A. Vegan nutrition: A preliminary guide for health professionals. *Crit. Rev. Food Sci. Nutr.* **2022**, *64*, 670–707. [CrossRef]
12. Fehér, A.; Gazdecki, M.; Véha, M.; Szakály, M.; Szakály, Z. A Comprehensive Review of the Benefits of and the Barriers to the Switch to a Plant-Based Diet. *Sustainability* **2020**, *12*, 4136. [CrossRef]
13. Brytek-Matera, A.; Czepczor-Bernat, K.; Jurzak, H.; Kornacka, M.; Kołodziejczyk, N. Strict health-oriented eating patterns (orthorexic eating behaviours) and their connection with a vegetarian and vegan diet. *Eat. Weight. Disord.-Stud. Anorex. Bulim. Obes.* **2019**, *24*, 441–452. [CrossRef] [PubMed]
14. Banna, J.C.; Panizza, C.E.; Boushey, C.J.; Delp, E.J.; Lim, E. Association between Cognitive Restraint, Uncontrolled Eating, Emotional Eating and BMI and the Amount of Food Wasted in Early Adolescent Girls. *Nutrients* **2018**, *10*, 1279. [CrossRef]
15. Brytek-Matera, A. Restrained Eating and Vegan, Vegetarian and Omnivore Dietary Intakes. *Nutrients* **2020**, *12*, 2133. [CrossRef] [PubMed]
16. Heiss, S.; Hormes, J.M.; Timko, C.A. Vegetarianism and eating disorders. In *Vegetarian and Plant-Based Diets in Health and Disease Prevention*; Academic Press: Cambridge, MA, USA, 2017; pp. 51–69.
17. Dittfeld, A.; Gwizdek, K.; Jagielski, P.; Brzęk, J.; Ziora, K. A Study on the relationship between orthorexia and vegetarianism using the BOT (Bratman Test for Orthorexia). *Psychiatr. Polska* **2017**, *51*, 1133–1144. [CrossRef] [PubMed]
18. Barthels, F.; Meyer, F.; Pietrowsky, R. Orthorexic and restrained eating behaviour in vegans, vegetarians, and individuals on a diet. *Eat. Weight. Disord.-Stud. Anorex. Bulim. Obes.* **2018**, *23*, 159–166. [CrossRef]
19. Curtis, M.J.; Comer, L.K. Vegetarianism, dietary restraint, and feminist identity. *Eat Behav.* **2006**, *7*, 91–104. [CrossRef]
20. Şentürk, E.; Şentürk, B.G.; Erus, S.; Geniş, B.; Coşar, B. Dietary patterns and eating behaviors on the border between healthy and pathological orthorexia. *Eat. Weight. Disord.-Stud. Anorex. Bulim. Obes.* **2022**, *27*, 3279–3288. [CrossRef]
21. Depa, J.; Barrada, J.R.; Roncero, M. Are the motives for food choices different in orthorexia nervosa and healthy orthorexia? *Nutrients* **2019**, *11*, 697. [CrossRef]
22. Grammatikopoulou, M.G.; Gkiouras, K.; Markaki, A.; Theodoridis, X.; Tsakiri, V.; Mavridis, P.; Dardavessis, T.; Chourdakis, M. Food addiction, orthorexia, and food-related stress among dietetics students. *Eat. Weight. Disord.-Stud. Anorex. Bulim. Obes.* **2018**, *23*, 459–467. [CrossRef]
23. Zickgraf, H.F.; Barrada, J.R. Orthorexia nervosa vs. healthy orthorexia: Relationships with disordered eating, eating behavior, and healthy lifestyle choices. *Eat. Weight. Disord.-Stud. Anorex. Bulim. Obes.* **2022**, *27*, 1313–1325. [CrossRef]
24. Yakın, E.; Obeid, S.; Fekih-Romdhane, F.; Soufia, M.; Sawma, T.; Samaha, S.; Mhanna, M.; Azzi, R.; Mina, A.; Hallit, S. "In-between orthorexia" profile: The co-occurrence of pathological and healthy orthorexia among male and female non-clinical adolescents. *J. Eat. Disord.* **2022**, *10*, 155. [CrossRef] [PubMed]
25. Gortat, M.; Samardakiewicz, M.; Perzyński, A. Orthorexia nervosa—A distorted approach to healthy eating. *Psychiatr. Polska* **2021**, *55*, 421–433. [CrossRef] [PubMed]
26. Horovitz, O.; Argyrides, M. Orthorexia and Orthorexia Nervosa: A Comprehensive Examination of Prevalence, Risk Factors, Diagnosis, and Treatment. *Nutrients* **2023**, *15*, 3851. [CrossRef] [PubMed]
27. Donini, L.M.; Barrada, J.R.; Barthels, F.; Dunn, T.M.; Babeau, C.; Brytek-Matera, A.; Cena, H.; Cerolini, S.; Cho, H.-H.; Coimbra, M.; et al. A consensus document on definition and diagnostic criteria for orthorexia nervosa. *Eat. Weight. Disord.-Stud. Anorex. Bulim. Obes.* **2022**, *27*, 3695–3711. [CrossRef]
28. Parra-Fernández, M.L.; Manzaneque-Cañadillas, M.; Onieva-Zafra, M.D.; Fernández-Martínez, E.; Fernández-Muñoz, J.J.; Prado-Laguna, M.d.C.; Brytek-Matera, A. Pathological preoccupation with healthy eating (Orthorexia nervosa) in a spanish sample with vegetarian, vegan, and non-vegetarian dietary patterns. *Nutrients* **2020**, *12*, 3907. [CrossRef]
29. Fairburn, C.G.; Beglin, S.J. Eating Disorder Examination Questionnaire (EDE-Q) [database record]. *APA PsycTests* **1994**. [CrossRef]

30. Zickgraf, H.F.; Hazzard, V.M.; O'Connor, S.M.; Simone, M.; Williams-Kerver, G.A.; Anderson, L.M.; Lipson, S.K. Examinin vegetarianism, weight motivations, and eating disorder psychopathology among college students. *Int. J. Eat. Disord.* **2020**, 5 1506–1514. [CrossRef]
31. Heiss, S.; Timko, C.A.; Hormes, J.M. Confirmatory factor analysis of the EDE-Q in vegans and omnivores: Support for the bri three factor model. *Eat. Behav.* **2020**, *39*, 101447. [CrossRef]
32. Fisak, B.; Peterson, R.D.; Tantleff-Dunn, S.; Molnar, J.M. Challenging previous conceptions of vegetarianism and eating disorde *Eat. Weight. Disord.-Stud. Anorex. Bulim. Obes.* **2006**, *11*, 195–200. [CrossRef]
33. Heiss, S.; Coffino, J.A.; Hormes, J.M. Eating and health behaviors in vegans compared to omnivores: Dispelling common myth *Appetite* **2017**, *118*, 129–135. [CrossRef]
34. Donini, L.M.; Marsili, D.; Graziani, M.P.; Imbriale, M.; Cannella, C. Orthorexia nervosa: A preliminary study with a proposal f diagnosis and an attempt to measure the dimension of the phenomenon. *Eat. Weight. Disord.-Stud. Anorex. Bulim. Obes.* **2005**, 151–157. [CrossRef] [PubMed]
35. Heiss, S.; Coffino, J.A.; Hormes, J.M. What does the ORTO-15 measure? Assessing the construct validity of a common orthorex nervosa questionnaire in a meat avoiding sample. *Appetite* **2019**, *135*, 93–99. [CrossRef] [PubMed]
36. Dunn, T.M.; Gibbs, J.; Whitney, N.; Starosta, A. Prevalence of orthorexia nervosa is less than 1%: Data from a US sample. *Ea Weight. Disord.-Stud. Anorex. Bulim. Obes.* **2017**, *22*, 185–192. [CrossRef] [PubMed]
37. Karlsson, J.; Persson, L.-O.; Sjöström, L.; Sullivan, M. Psychometric properties and factor structure of the Three-Factor Eatin Questionnaire (TFEQ) in obese men and women. Results from the Swedish Obese Subjects (SOS) study. *Int. J. Obes.* **2000**, 2 1715–1725. [CrossRef]
38. Garner, D.M.; Garfinkel, P.E. The Eating Attitudes Test: An index of the symptoms of anorexia nervosa. *Psychol. Med.* **1979**, 273–279. [CrossRef]
39. Ambwani, S. Measuring "Orthorexia": Development of the eating habits questionnaire. *Int. J.* **2013**, *12*, 2.
40. Hallit, S.; Barrada, J.R.; Salameh, P.; Sacre, H.; Roncero, M.; Obeid, S. The relation of orthorexia with lifestyle habits: Arabi versions of the Eating Habits Questionnaire and the Dusseldorf Orthorexia Scale. *J. Eat. Disord.* **2021**, *9*, 102. [CrossRef]
41. Barthels, F.; Meyer, F.; Pietrowsky, R. Die Düsseldorfer Orthorexie Skala–Konstruktion und Evaluation eines Fragebogens zu Erfassung ortho-rektischen Ernährungsverhaltens. *Z. Klin. Psychol. Psychother.* **2015**, *44*, 97–105. [CrossRef]
42. Barthels, F.; Meyer, F.; Huber, T.; Pietrowsky, R. Orthorexic eating behaviour as a coping strategy in patients with anorexi nervosa. *Eat. Weight. Disord.-Stud. Anorex. Bulim. Obes.* **2017**, *22*, 269–276. [CrossRef]
43. Barrada, J.R.; Roncero, M. Bidimensional Structure of the Orthorexia: Development and Initial Validation of a New Instrumen *An. Psicol.* **2018**, *34*, 283–291. [CrossRef]
44. Dorard, G.; Mathieu, S. Vegetarian and omnivorous diets: A cross-sectional study of motivation, eating disorders, and bod shape perception. *Appetite* **2021**, *156*, 104972. [CrossRef]
45. Kalika, E.; Egan, H.; Mantzios, M. Exploring the role of mindful eating and self-compassion on eating behaviours and orthorexi in people following a vegan diet. *Eat. Weight. Disord.-Stud. Anorex. Bulim. Obes.* **2022**, *27*, 2641–2651. [CrossRef] [PubMed]
46. Kamiński, M.; Skonieczna-Żydecka, K.; Nowak, J.K.; Stachowska, E. Global and local diet popularity rankings, their secula trends, and seasonal variation in Google Trends data. *Nutrition* **2020**, *79–80*, 110759. [CrossRef] [PubMed]
47. McLean, C.P.; Kulkarni, J.; Sharp, G. Disordered eating and the meat-avoidance spectrum: A systematic review and clinica implications. *Eat. Weight. Disord.-Stud. Anorex. Bulim. Obes.* **2022**, *27*, 2347–2375. [CrossRef] [PubMed]
48. Sergentanis, T.N.; Chelmi, M.-E.; Liampas, A.; Yfanti, C.-M.; Panagouli, E.; Vlachopapadopoulou, E.; Michalacos, S.; Bacopoulo F.; Psaltopoulou, T.; Tsitsika, A. Vegetarian Diets and Eating Disorders in Adolescents and Young Adults: A Systematic Revie *Children* **2020**, *8*, 12. [CrossRef]
49. Klopp, S.A.; Heiss, C.J.; Smith, H.S. Self-reported vegetarianism may be a marker for college women at risk for disordered eatin *J. Am. Diet. Assoc.* **2003**, *103*, 745–747. [CrossRef]
50. Baş, M.; Karabudak, E.; Kiziltan, G. Vegetarianism and eating disorders: Association between eating attitudes and othe psychological factors among Turkish adolescents. *Appetite* **2005**, *44*, 309–315. [CrossRef]
51. Valente, M.; Syurina, E.V.; Muftugil-Yalcin, S.; Cesuroglu, T. "Keep Yourself Alive": From Healthy Eating to Progression t Orthorexia Nervosa A Mixed Methods Study among Young Women in the Netherlands. *Ecol. Food Nutr.* **2020**, *59*, 578–59 [CrossRef]
52. Paslakis, G.; Richardson, C.; Nöhre, M.; Brähler, E.; Holzapfel, C.; Hilbert, A.; de Zwaan, M. Author Correction: Prevalenc and psychopathology of vegetarians and vegans—Results from a representative survey in Germany. *Sci. Rep.* **2020**, *10*, 1981 [CrossRef]
53. McLean, C.P.; Chen, Z.; Song, R.; Le, J.; Fielding, J.; Sharp, G. Development and preliminary validation of a novel eating disorde screening tool for vegetarians and vegans: The V-EDS. *J. Eat. Disord.* **2024**, *12*, 4. [CrossRef]

54. Gwioździk, W.; Krupa-Kotara, K.; Całyniuk, B.; Helisz, P.; Grajek, M.; Głogowska-Ligus, J. Traditional, Vegetarian, or Low FODMAP Diets and Their Relation to Symptoms of Eating Disorders: A Cross-Sectional Study among Young Women in Poland. *Nutrients* **2022**, *14*, 4125. [CrossRef]
55. Fuller, S.J.; Brown, A.; Rowley, J.; Elliott-Archer, J. Veganism and eating disorders: Assessment and management considerations. *Bjpsych Bull.* **2022**, *46*, 116–120. [CrossRef]
56. Ambwani, S.; Shippe, M.; Gao, Z.; Austin, S.B. Is #cleaneating a healthy or harmful dietary strategy? Perceptions of clean eating and associations with disordered eating among young adults. *J. Eat. Disord.* **2019**, *7*, 17. [CrossRef]
57. Strahler, J.; Hermann, A.; Walter, B.; Stark, R. Orthorexia nervosa: A behavioral complex or a psychological condition? *J. Behav. Addict.* **2018**, *7*, 1143–1156. [CrossRef] [PubMed]
58. Missbach, B.; Hinterbuchinger, B.; Dreiseitl, V.; Zellhofer, S.; Kurz, C.; König, J. When Eating Right, Is Measured Wrong! A Validation and Critical Examination of the ORTO-15 Questionnaire in German. *PLoS ONE* **2015**, *10*, e0135772. [CrossRef] [PubMed]
59. Reynolds, R.; McGowan, A.; Smith, S.; Rawstorne, P. Vegan and vegetarian males and females have higher orthorexic traits than omnivores, and are motivated in their food choice by factors including ethics and weight control. *Nutr. Health* **2023**. [CrossRef] [PubMed]
60. Kozik, K.; Całyniuk, B. Selected eating behaviors and the risk of orthorexia nervosa in a group of high school students. *Roczn Państw Zakł Hig.* **2024**, *75*, 247–254. [CrossRef]
61. Çiçekoğlu, P.; Tunçay, G.Y. A Comparison of Eating Attitudes Between Vegans/Vegetarians and Nonvegans/Nonvegetarians in Terms of Orthorexia Nervosa. *Arch. Psychiatr. Nurs.* **2018**, *32*, 200–205. [CrossRef]
62. Tarsitano, M.G.; Pujia, R.; Ferro, Y.; Mocini, E.; Proni, G.; Lenzi, F.R.; Pujia, A.; Giannetta, E. Symptoms of Orthorexia Nervosa are associated with time spent on social media: A web-based survey in an Italian population sample. *Eur. Rev. Med. Pharmacol. Sci.* **2022**, *26*, 9327–9335. [CrossRef]
63. McLean, C.P.; Kulkarni, J.; Sharp, G. The 26-Item Eating Attitudes Test (EAT-26): Psychometric Properties and Factor Structure in Vegetarians and Vegans. *Nutrients* **2023**, *15*, 297. [CrossRef]
64. Dell'Osso, L.; Abelli, M.; Carpita, B.; Massimetti, G.; Pini, S.; Rivetti, L.; Gorrasi, F.; Tognetti, R.; Ricca, V.; Carmassi, C. Orthorexia nervosa in a sample of Italian university population. *Riv. Psichiatr.* **2016**, *51*, 190–196. [CrossRef] [PubMed]
65. Parker, H.W.; Vadiveloo, M.K. Diet quality of vegetarian diets compared with nonvegetarian diets: A systematic review. *Nutr. Rev.* **2019**, *77*, 144–160. [CrossRef] [PubMed]
66. McLean, C.P.; Chen, Z.; Fielding, J.; Sharp, G. Preliminary identification of clinical cut-off of the vegetarian vegan eating disorder screener (V-EDS) in a community and self-reported clinical sample of vegetarians and vegans. *J. Eat. Disord.* **2024**, *12*, 17. [CrossRef] [PubMed]

nutrients

MDPI

Review

Autism, ADHD, and Their Traits in Adults with Obesity: A Scoping Review

Lauren Makin [1,2,3], Adia Meyer [4], Elisa Zesch [4], Valeria Mondelli [1,2] and Kate Tchanturia [1,3,4,5,*]

1 Department of Psychological Medicine, Institute of Psychiatry, Psychology & Neuroscience, King's College London, London SE5 8AF, UK; lauren.makin@kcl.ac.uk (L.M.); valeria.mondelli@kcl.ac.uk (V.M.)
2 National Institute for Health and Care Research (NIHR) Maudsley Biomedical Research Centre at South London and Maudsley NHS Foundation Trust and King's College London, London SE5 8AF, UK
3 Centre for Research in Eating and Weight Disorders (CREW), Department of Psychological Medicine, King's College London, London SE5 8AF, UK
4 Department of Eating Disorders, South London and Maudsley NHS Foundation Trust, London SE5 8AZ, UK; adia.meyer@slam.nhs.uk (A.M.); elisa.zesch@slam.nhs.uk (E.Z.)
5 Department of Psychology, Ilia State University, 0162 Tbilisi, Georgia
* Correspondence: kate.tchanturia@kcl.ac.uk

Abstract: Introduction: Autism and ADHD shape behaviours related to food, exercise, and body image, potentially influencing obesity treatment outcomes, as seen in eating disorder research. Resultantly, autistic and ADHD patients with obesity may have distinct experiences and differences compared to non-autistic and non-ADHD patients. This review maps existing literature on autism and ADHD in adults with obesity. **Methods:** Following PRISMA guidelines, six databases (Embase, MEDLINE, PsycINFO, Web of Science, CENTRAL, and Scopus) were searched for studies on autism and/or ADHD (diagnosed, probable, or traits) in adults with obesity. Screening and data extraction were conducted twice independently for each record. **Results:** Thirty-one studies were included, with 1,027,773 participants. Two case reports described successful use of weight loss drugs in autistic people with obesity. Eight prevalence studies suggested ADHD is overrepresented in obesity, regardless of binge eating status. Nineteen studies examined clinical profiles: ADHD patients had lower socioeconomic status, poorer health-related quality of life, increased impulsivity, cognitive inflexibility, and neuroticism, alongside lower agreeableness, conscientiousness, self-directedness, and cooperativeness. ADHD patients also exhibited higher psychopathology, problematic alcohol use, and disordered eating. Eight studies assessed treatment responses, noting poorer outcomes from behavioural programs and obesity pharmacotherapy, but similar post-surgical weight outcomes, despite increased complications. Two studies considered ADHD-specific treatment adaptions, one reporting a successful trial of ADHD medication for weight loss and the other reporting on switching to transdermal ADHD medications after bariatric surgery. **Conclusions:** This review underscores the need for more research on autism and obesity. For ADHD, findings suggest frequent co-occurrence with obesity, but lived experiences and tailored interventions remain underexplored.

Keywords: comorbidity; neurodiversity; prevalence; treatment; attention-deficit/hyperactivity disorder; obesity; autism-spectrum disorder

1. Introduction

Neurodevelopmental conditions, such as autism spectrum disorder (autism) and attention-deficit/hyperactivity disorder (ADHD), affect individuals' experiences of the world and their behaviours, including relationships to food, exercise, and their own body [1,2]. Resultantly, these conditions may present unique challenges in the clinical presentation and treatment of obesity [3,4]. Evidence from eating disorder (ED) research suggests that adult patients respond better to treatments when their neurodevelopmental conditions, specifically autism [5], are considered, and treatments are correspondingly adapted.

Autism is characterised by differences in social interaction, communication, sensory processing, and restrictive, repetitive behaviours [6], which can impact eating [7,8]. This paper uses identity-first language, referring to "Autistic individuals", in line with the preferences of the autistic community [9–11].

Research often examines autistic traits and "probable" autism alongside formal diagnoses to capture a broader understanding of autism and address practical constraints. Many individuals with significant autistic traits lack a formal diagnosis due to assessment barriers, late recognition, and disparities affecting minority groups such as women [12–14]. Diagnostic measures require more time, training, and financial resources, while screening tools offer a more accessible way to identify subclinical traits that impact cognition, behaviour, and health outcomes and thus still have clinical utility [15]. Screening measures also increase sample sizes and generalizability, reducing the risk of underestimating autism's impact. However, they can introduce biases, including false positives and self-report inaccuracies. In contrast, formal diagnoses provide greater specificity and reliability, ensuring observed differences are truly related to autism rather than overlapping conditions like ADHD or anxiety [16]. Since diagnosed individuals may differ from undiagnosed counterparts in demographic characteristics, healthcare access, or trait severity, including studies utilising both approaches offers a more comprehensive understanding of autism's role in health outcomes while mitigating biases inherent in each method. When discussing studies, we will make it clear how autism was assessed, but more generally we will use the terms autism and autistic to encompass individuals with both formal autism diagnoses and those presenting with high autistic traits.

Qualitative studies have been key in understanding how autism interacts with eating [2,7,17]. For example, Kinnaird and colleagues [7] found that autism continued to impact participants' eating into adulthood, particularly in areas of sensory sensitivity, executive functioning, and rigidity. This also leads to differences in clinical populations. Autistic individuals with EDs also show differences in clinical presentation, including increased illness severity, earlier onset, and longer duration compared to non-autistic individuals [18,19]. Furthermore, autistic patients with EDs often felt that their autism-related needs are often unmet by standard ED treatments [20], leading to increased use of intensive options [5,21,22]. These findings have informed a series of ED treatment adaptions, called the PEACE pathway (https://www.peacepathway.org/, accessed on 23 January 2025), which reduced admission lengths and costs for patients with Eds [5].

In our search for existing reviews on this topic, we found none exploring autism in patients with obesity. However, there have been two systematic reviews and meta-analyses looking at the prevalence of obesity in autistic people, which both found obesity rates to be elevated in this group compared to controls [23,24], with more recent studies supporting these findings [25]. Additionally, a systematic review by Gilmore and colleagues [26] found obesity to increase the risk of in-hospital mortality and some chronic conditions among autistic adults. These reviews suggest that autism is likely overrepresented—but understudied—in adult patients with obesity. Assessing what information does exist on this topic is key for informing future research and ensuring a strong evidence base is built up to inform development in this area.

ADHD is also likely to be relevant to the treatment of obesity and has been studied more extensively than autism in this area. ADHD is characterised by persistent patterns of inattention, hyperactivity, and impulsivity [6]. Impulsivity may contribute to binge eating or purging behaviours, while inattention could hinder awareness of hunger or satiety [27,28]. Emotional dysregulation may lead to emotional eating as a coping mechanism, and executive function challenges may cause irregular eating patterns [29]. Zwennes and Loth [1] interviewed adults with ADHD and binge eating, obesity, or overweight. These patients described how they felt their eating was underpinned by their ADHD and underdeveloped coping skills. Resultantly, they felt care should be more personalised to their comorbidities.

There is currently limited research on the language preferences of ADHD individuals. This paper uses identity-first language, as this is concordant with our approach to discussing autism. We acknowledge that this decision may not be optimal and recognise the need for further research into the preferences of this population regarding how they are referenced, discussed, and studied. This paper also includes both formally diagnosed individuals and those exhibiting high ADHD traits, as is already common within the literature.

Regarding ADHD and obesity, Cortese and colleagues have published multiple systematic and narrative reviews on the topic [3,4,30–35]. They report the prevalence of ADHD in patients with obesity to be elevated [34], as well as discussing mechanisms and clinical implications [3,4,32,35]. Additionally, a recent meta-analysis by Caci and colleagues [36] found the prevalence of ADHD to be elevated in adult candidates for metabolic and bariatric surgery, and two other systematic reviews found an increased prevalence of ADHD in patients with obesity compared to controls [37,38]. There have also been several other reviews discussing potential mechanisms [39–42], clinical management [43], and outcomes [44]. Thus, it seems that there is a significant amount of research on ADHD and obesity. However, much of this literature emphasises biological and genetic factors [41]. It is not clear how many studies can inform clinical practice or consider management options outside surgery for obesity and pharmacotherapy for ADHD. For example, a preliminary search found little qualitative work on the perspectives and experiences of adult ADHD patients with obesity or exploring psychotherapeutic treatment options or adaptions.

In summary, research in the ED field suggests consideration of autism and ADHD may be beneficial in managing and treating adults with obesity; however, it remains to be seen whether there is sufficient evidence within the obesity field to guide these treatment adaptions. To inform future research and practice, a scoping review was deemed appropriate to systematically map existing literature and identify knowledge gaps relevant to the following questions:

1. What is the relative prevalence of autism and ADHD in adults with obesity, compared to the general population and within varying classes of obesity (I, II, III, and IV)?
2. What are the experiences and perspectives of autistic and ADHD adults with obesity, their carers, and their clinicians?
3. What clinically relevant differences exist between autistic or ADHD and non-autistic or non-ADHD adults with obesity, including in clinical presentation and treatment responses?
4. What treatment adaptions or adjunct therapies exist for autistic and ADHD adults with obesity?

2. Materials and Methods

A search for any existing scoping or systematic reviews on this topic was conducted on the 6 March 2024 in Cochrane Database of Systematic Reviews, PROSPERO, Embase, OVID Medline, APA PsycINFO, and Web of Science. The search strategy used is recorded on the OSF (https://doi.org/10.17605/OSF.IO/S7ATF). Relevant reviews were integrated into this paper's introduction. None were deemed to fulfil the aims of this review.

The JBI Manual for Evidence Synthesis [45] guided the study protocol, which was pre-registered on the Open Science Framework (OSF; https://doi.org/10.17605/OSF.IO/3JB24). Initially, it included studies on binge-type EDs regardless of weight status, alongside obesity-focused research. However, due to an unexpectedly high yield of results, the protocol was revised to simplify screening, and binge-type ED results are reported in a separate review [46]. This separation allowed for a more in-depth discussion of each topic. Studies on obesity, which included binge-type ED samples, were retained, and vice versa. Eligibility criteria were also refined during screening, with all changes documented on the OSF. The PRISMA Extension for Scoping Reviews [47] was used as the reporting guideline.

2.1. Eligibility Criteria

Studies were included if they: (1) involved human adults (18+) with polygenic, non-syndromic obesity (BMI $\geq$ 30), with qualitative studies including carers, family members, healthcare professionals, or experts; (2) assessed or reported diagnosed or probable autism, ADHD, or autistic or ADHD traits. Studies were excluded if they involved only animals, children, non-obese samples (BMI < 30), monogenic or syndromic obesity or autism, aggregated samples, unidimensional traits of autism or ADHD, solely biological or genetic data, or had insufficient abstract information and non-English full text. Samples with other comorbidities were not excluded, and no restrictions were placed on sex, ethnicity, location, or publication year. Grey literature, including conference abstracts and dissertations, was not excluded. Full eligibility criteria are in Table S1.

2.2. Information Sources and Search Strategy

LM developed the search strategy in consultation with university librarians and reviewed it with all authors. Pilot searches informed the final strategy and eligibility criteria. Terms for obesity were combined with neurodevelopmental condition terms (e.g., "autism", "ADHD") using both keywords (e.g., "obes*") and database-specific indexing terms (e.g., MeSH descriptors), while excluding animal studies. Full search strategies for each database are in Table S2. Databases used were Embase, MEDLINE via Ovid, PsycINFO, Web of Science, CENTRAL, and Scopus. Reference lists from reviews that passed title-and-abstract screening were also searched. Initial searches were conducted on 28 March 2024 and final checks on 1 November 2024.

2.3. Study Selection and Screening

LM, AM, and EZ conducted screening, and LM and AM conducted paper selection. After removing duplicates, titles and abstracts were screened (stage 1). Records passing this stage moved to full-text screening (stage 2), followed by hand-searching review articles (stage 3). Discrepancies were discussed within the team and principal author. Interrater reliability was K = 0.76 indicating substantial agreement and crude agreement exceeded our pre-specified 80% threshold. A follow-up search was performed by LM to capture new publications.

2.4. Data Extraction

Data were extracted using a form developed for this review, available on the OSF (v2).
LM and AM independently extracted data from all reports. No major discrepancies were noted. No formal study quality appraisal, bias assessment, or synthesis methods were used, as this goes beyond the scope of this review.

3. Results

The initial search yielded 14,895 results, with 7628 duplicates, leaving 7267 articles for screening. Of these, 68 were assessed for eligibility, and 28 met the inclusion criteria.

Main exclusion reasons included aggregated or child data, absence of autism or ADHD assessment, and biological-only data. A follow-up search produced 1296 results, of which 677 were duplicates; 13 articles were assessed for eligibility, and two more met the inclusion criteria. A final article was identified through citation screening, meaning a total of 31 articles met inclusion criteria. Figure 1 shows the PRISMA flow chart for this study [48].

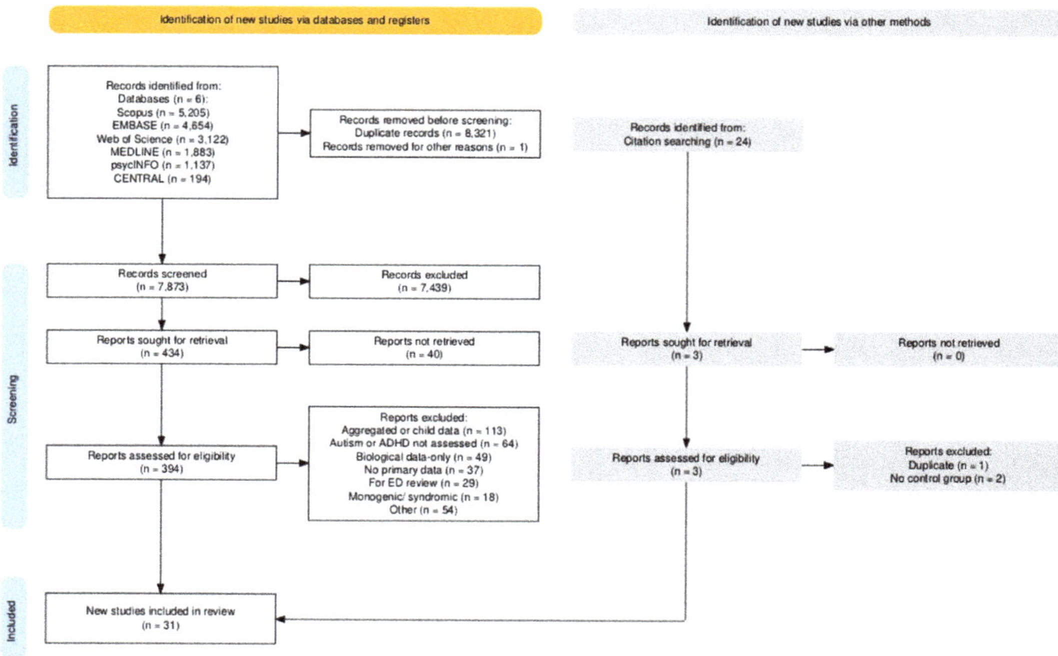

Figure 1. PRISMA flow chart for this review. ADHD = attention-deficit/hyperactivity disorder. ED = eating disorder.

3.1. Overview of Studies and Participant Characteristics

Table 1 summarises the characteristics of the 31 [49–79] studies included (more detailed participant characteristics are described in Tables S3–S6). These studies included 1,027,773 adult participants, mostly women (62.7%). Six studies reported the ethnicity of participants (total n = 997,618; white = 65%) [59–61,69,73,76]. Studies spanned 2002 to 2024 (Figure S1). Studies were mainly from Western Europe (n = 15; namely Sweden [50–52,67,77], Germany [65,72,75], Spain [62,63,71], France [57,64], Italy [55,56], and Finland [66]). Seven studies were from North America (USA [53,58,60,61,73] and Canada [59,68,76]), five were from the Middle East (Turkey [49,74,78,79] and Israel [54]), and two were from Brazil [69,70].

Table 1. Study characteristics and summary.

Study	Country, Design	Autism/ADHD	Medication Use	Sample Size, *n*	BMI Mean ± SD (Range)	Age, Years Mean ± SD (Range)	Sex Women, %	Ethnicity White, %	Relevance to Review
Akcan et al., (2021) [49]	Turkey, Case-control	Adult ADHD traits	No	200	(<25, 30+)	(18–65)	66.0	-	Prevalence
Alfonsson et al., (2012) [50]	Sweden, Cross-sectional	Probable adult ADHD	-	217	44.28 ± 6.02	41.04 ± 11.07	73.3	-	Clinical profiles
Alfonsson et al., (2013) [51]	Sweden, Cross-sectional	Probable adult ADHD	-	276	43.96 ± 5.82 (33.6–66.0)	42.38 ± 11.04	72.7	-	Clinical profiles
Alfonsson et al., (2014) [52]	Sweden, Longitudinal	Adult ADHD traits	-	129	42.8 ± 10.52	42.8 ± 10.52	78.3	-	Prevalence, Treatment responses
Altfas (2002) [53]	USA, Retrospective	Persistent ADHD diagnosis, traits	-	215	36.2 ± 8.2	43.4 ± 10.9	89.8	-	Prevalence, Treatment responses
Azran et al., (2017) [54]	Israel, Case report	ADHD diagnosis	Yes	1	-	52	0	-	Treatment options
Brancati et al., (2022) [55] †	Italy, Cross-sectional	Probable adult ADHD	-	110	(30+)	"Adults"	-	-	Clinical profiles
Brancati et al., (2024) [56]	Italy, Cross-sectional	Probable adult ADHD	-	260	46.27 ± 7.45 (31.95–76.95)	44.31 ± 10.71 (18–66)	71.9	-	Clinical profiles
Brunault et al., (2019) [57]	France, Cross-sectional	Persistent ADHD diagnosis	-	105	(35+)	46.5 ± 10.7	86.7	-	Clinical profiles,
Crowley et al., (2015) [58]	USA, Case report	Autism diagnosis	Yes	2	31.7, 33.1	19, 20	100.0	-	Treatment options
Davis et al., (2009) [59]	Canada, Case-double control	Persistent ADHD traits	-	181	Reported by group	Reported by group	Reported by group	Reported by group	Prevalence
Dempsey et al., (2010) [60]	USA, Cross-sectional	Probable adult ADHD	No	125	39.08 ± 6.33 (30–61.6)	43.7 ± 13.47 (21–74)	65.6	85.6	Clinical profiles
Dickinson et al., (2024) [61]	USA, Retrospective case-control cohort	ADHD diagnosis	Yes	996,929	Reported by group	Reported by group	Reported by group	Reported by group	Clinical profiles, Treatment responses
Docet et al., (2010) [62]	Spain, Case-control	ADHD diagnosis	No	243	(30+)	51 ± 13.4	75.9	-	Prevalence
Docet et al., (2012) [63]	Spain, Case-control	Probable adult ADHD	-	230	40.3 ± 5.7	42.3 ± 15.5	88.2	-	Clinical profiles
El Archi et al., (2021) [64]	France, Cross-sectional	Probable persistent ADHD	-	282	45.4 ± 7.7	43.1 ± 11.2	76.6	-	Clinical profiles
Gruss et al., (2012) [65]	Germany, Cross-sectional	Probable persistent ADHD	-	116	48.6 ± 8.1	38.6 ± 10.5	73.3	-	Clinical profiles
Jarvinen et al., (2019) [66]	Finland, Case report	Autism diagnosis	Yes	1	34.4	20	0.0	-	Treatment options
Laggeros et al., (2020) [67]	Sweden, Cohort	ADHD diagnosis	-	22,539	-	41.3 ± 11.0	75.3	-	Treatment responses
Levy et al., (2009) [68]	Canada	Persistent ADHD diagnosis	Yes	78	42.7	41.3	92.3	-	Treatment options
Marchesi et al., (2017) [69]	Brazil, Retrospective	Probable adult ADHD	No	40	43.9 ± 6.1	48.3 ± 10.2	93	25	Clinical profiles, Treatment responses
Nazar et al., (2016) [70]	Brazil, Cross-sectional	Persistent ADHD diagnosis	No	106	(30+)	38.99 ± 10.74 (18–59)	100.0	-	Prevalence, Clinical profiles

Table 1. *Cont.*

Study	Country, Design	Autism/ADHD	Medication Use	Sample Size, *n*	BMI Mean ± SD (Range)	Age, Years Mean ± SD (Range)	Sex Women, %	Ethnicity White, %	Relevance to Review
Nicolau et al., (2015) [71]	Spain, Case-control	Probable adult ADHD	-	60	48.35 ± 7.46	46.35 ± 9.9	78.3	-	Clinical profiles, Treatment responses
Nielsen et al., (2017) [72]	Germany, Comparative cross-sectional	Persistent ADHD probable, traits	-	248	48.3 ± 6.9	41.3 ± 11.0 (19–65)	79.0	-	Prevalence
Pagoto et al., (2010) [73]	USA, Cross-sectional	Probable adult ADHD	-	63	41.4 ± 6.8	50 ± 10	75	99	Clinical profiles, Treatment responses
Sahan et al., (2021) [74]	Turkey, Case-control	Persistent ADHD diagnosis	No	100	(35+)	(18–66)	Reported by group	-	Clinical profiles
Schafer et al., (2020) [75]	Germany, Cross-sectional	Probable adult ADHD	-	78	48.1 ± 8.3 (33.8–78.9)	42.9 ± 10.4 (24–69)	66.7	-	Clinical profiles
Stahel et al., (2019) [76]	Canada, cohort	ADHD diagnosis	Yes	280	Reported by group	Reported by group	Reported by group	Reported by group	Prevalence
Stenberg et al., (2023) [77]	Sweden, Cohort case-control	Medicated ADHD	Yes	4,293	Reported by group	Reported by group	76.2	-	Clinical profiles, Treatment responses
Taymur et al., (2015) [78] †	Turkey, Cross-sectional	Probable childhood ADHD	-	89	46.42 ± 5.34	34.84 ± 9.93	77.5	-	Clinical profiles
Taymur et al., (2016) [79]	Turkey, Cross-sectional	Probable childhood ADHD	-	177	(40+)	36.60 ± 8.46	80.8	-	Clinical profiles

† = abstract-only, sample may overlap with study directly below. ADHD = attention-deficit/hyperactivity disorder. BMI = Body Mass Index, kg/m^2. *n* = number of participants. SD = standard deviation. USA = United States of America.

Of the 31 studies included, only two studies, both case reports, examined autism in obesity [58,66]. These explored interventions for three patients with formal autism diagnoses and obesity. The other 29 studies investigated ADHD in obesity [49–57,59–65,67–79]. Eight examined the prevalence of ADHD in patients with obesity (*n* = 553) compared to those without obesity (*n* = 286) [49,53,59,62], within obesity classes (*n* = 556) [53,62,70,76], or before (*n* = 240) and after (*n* = 257) bariatric surgery [52,72]. Twenty-two studies considered clinical differences of ADHD patients with obesity compared to non-ADHD patients, with 19 considering pre-intervention differences (clinical profiles; ADHD patients, *n* = 55,595; non-ADHD patients, *n* = 948,000) [50,51,55–57,60,61,63–65,69–71,73–75,77–79], and eight considering differences post-intervention (treatment responses; ADHD patients, *n* = 5980; non-ADHD patients, *n* = 68,793) [52,53,61,67,69,71,73,77]. Two other studies explored ADHD-specific interventions for patients with obesity; one was a case report (*n* = 1) [54], and one was an intervention study (*n* = 78) [68]. No studies explored the experiences or perspectives of ADHD adults with obesity. Table 2 maps these papers.

Table 2. Mapping the number of papers investigating autism or ADHD in adults with obesity across the four topics of this review: prevalence, experiences and perspectives, clinical differences, and interventions.

		Relative Prevalence	Experiences and Perspectives	Clinical Differences		Targeted Interventions
				Clinical Profiles	Treatment Responses	
Autism	Traits	$n = 0$	$n = 0$	$n = 0$	$n = 0$	$n = 0$
	Screening	$n = 0$	$n = 0$	$n = 0$	$n = 0$	$n = 0$
	Diagnosis	$n = 0$	$n = 0$	$n = 0$	$n = 0$	$n = 2$ [58,66]
ADHD	Traits	$n = 5$ [49,52,53,59,72]	$n = 0$	$n = 0$	$n = 1$ [53]	$n = 0$
	Screening	$n = 1$ [72]	$n = 0$	$n = 14$ [50,51,55,56,60,63–65,69,71,73,75,78,79]	$n = 4$ [52,69,71,73]	$n = 0$
	Diagnosis	$n = 4$ [53,62,70,76]	$n = 0$	$n = 5$ [57,61,70,74,77]	$n = 4$ [53,61,67,77]	$n = 2$ [54,68]

ADHD = attention-deficit/hyperactivity disorder. n = number of studies. Red = <2 papers; Orange = 3–4 papers; Green = 5+ papers.

3.2. ADHD Measures

Table 3 outlines the ADHD measures used in the included papers [80–90]. Eleven studies used formal diagnoses of ADHD; seven of these used clinical interviews [53,57,62,68,70,74,76], mostly following the DSM-IV criteria. Four of these studies used structured interviews [57,70,74,76] and three supplemented interviews with screening measures [62,68,74]. Two studies used ICD-10 codes for ADHD diagnosis or prescription codes [61,67,77]. One study did not report how ADHD diagnosis was made [54]. Diagnosis of ADHD in adulthood requires that symptoms began in childhood, before age 12 [6]. However, not all studies confirmed that childhood symptoms had been considered when making the diagnosis.

Table 3. ADHD measures used.

Measure	Application	ADHD	Used by
AADHDS [81]	Self-report questionnaire	Probable adult ADHD	1 study [49]
ADHD-SCL-90-R [82]	Self-report questionnaire	Probable adult ADHD	2 studies [55,56]
ADHD-SR [83]	Self-report questionnaire	Probable adult ADHD	2 studies [65,75]
ASRS-v1.1 [84]	Self-report questionnaire	Probable adult ADHD	12 studies [50–52,60,62–64,68,69,71,73,74]
CAARS-SSV [85]	Self-report questionnaire	Probable adult ADHD	2 studies [59,72]
DIVA 2.0 [86]	Clinical interview	Diagnosed persistent ADHD	1 study [57]
ICD-10 F9.0	N/a	Diagnosed ADHD	2 studies [61,67]
ICD-10 N06BA	N/a	Medicated ADHD	1 study [77]
K-SADS-E [87,88]	Clinical interview	Diagnosed ADHD	1 study [70]
MINI [89]	Clinical interview	Diagnosed ADHD	1 study [76]
SCID-5 [90]	Clinical interview	Diagnosed ADHD	1 study [74]
WURS-25 [80]	Self-report questionnaire	Probable childhood ADHD	8 studies [59,64,65,68,72,74,78,79]

AADHDS = Adult ADHD Scale. ADHD = attention-deficit/hyperactivity disorder. ADHD-SCL-90-R = 16 ADHD-relevant items from the Symptom Checklist-90-Revised. ADHD-SR = the German ADHD Rating Scale. ASRS-v1.1 = Adult ADHD Self-Report Scale. CAARS-SSV = Self-report Screening Version of the Conners' Adult ADHD Rating Scale. DIVA 2.0 = 2nd version of the Diagnostic Interview for ADHD in adults. F9.0 = ICD-10 code denoting ADHD. ICD-10 = International Classification of Diseases, 10th Revision. K-SADS-E = Schedule for Affective Disorders and Schizophrenia module for ADHD, adapted for adults. MINI = Mini-International Neuropsychiatric Interview. N/a = not applicable. N06BA = ICD-10 code denoting Central Nervous System Stimulants, primarily medications used for ADHD, such as methylphenidate and amphetamine derivatives. SCID-5 = Structured Clinical Interview for DSM-5 Clinician Version. WURS-25 = short-version of the Wender Utah Rating Scale.

Sixteen studies screened for positive ADHD cases (probable ADHD) [50–52,55,56,60, 63–65,69,71–73,75,78,79], instead of making formal diagnoses. Eleven studies considered current symptoms in adults (adult ADHD) [50–52,55,56,60,63,69,71,73,75], two studies considered retrospective childhood symptoms (childhood ADHD) [78,79], and three studies considered both (persistent ADHD) [64,65,72]. Where it was unclear whether childhood traits had been considered, it was assumed that only current traits were counted. For one childhood measure, WURS-25 [80], different studies used differing cut-offs: three studies used a cut-off of 36 [74,78,79], whereas another study used 46 instead [64]. The two studies using the German version (WURS-k), which is slightly shorter, used a cut-off of 30 [65,72].

Five studies considered presence of ADHD traits without a cut-off (ADHD traits), three considering just adult traits [49,52,53] and two considering persistent traits [59,72].

3.3. *ADHD Medication*

Two case reports reported participants' full medication history [58,66], which included multiple medications that may be used for ADHD and/or affect eating and weight. The other case report described a patient on ADHD medication [54]. In two studies, ADHD medication was the intervention assessed [68] or was used as a proxy for ADHD diagnosis [77]. Two studies excluded participants with current use of any psychoactive medication [69,70], and two studies contained no participants who had received ADHD medication [62,74].

One study reported overall rates of antipsychotic and antidepressant medications [76], some of which are associated with weight gain, and another study included participants who had received obesity medication [61], which may have overlapped with ADHD medication. Two other studies excluded participants with current use of medications that affect weight [60] or if their obesity was secondary to medication use [49]. Otherwise, medication use was not reported by these studies. Eighteen studies did not comment on the medication status of their sample at all.

3.4. *Findings from Papers*

3.4.1. Prevalence of ADHD in Participants with vs. Without Obesity

Table S3 describes further study characteristics and findings of prevalence studies on ADHD in obesity. Docet and colleagues [62] found that participants with obesity (20.6%) were significantly more likely to receive an adult ADHD diagnosis than participants without obesity (6.8%; $p = 0.008$). Diagnosis was also significantly more likely in female participants with obesity (24%) compared to male participants with obesity (9.7%; $p < 0.05$ whereas there was no significant sex difference in participants without obesity (female: 7.7%; male: 4.8%; $p = 0.65$). Davis and colleagues [59] found significant differences in adult and childhood ADHD traits in patients with obesity, patients with binge eating, and patients with normal weight on adult ADHD traits ($p < 0.0001$). Adult and childhood ADHD traits were significantly higher in patients with binge eating (adult: 14.5 $\pm$ 6; childhood: 34.8 $\pm$ 20.6) than in patients with normal weight (adult: 9.3 $\pm$ 5.1; childhood: 18.1 $\pm$ 16.3; both: $p < 0.0001$), and there was no significant difference between patients with binge eating and those with obesity (adult: 13.4 $\pm$ 5.7, $p = 0.317$; childhood: 34.3 $\pm$ 19.9, $p = 907$). However, Akcan and colleagues [49] found no significant difference between mean adult ADHD traits in participants with obesity (31.69 $\pm$ 15.51) and without obesity (28.02 $\pm$ 16.93; $p = 0.11$). Altfas [53] did not find a significant difference in rate of adult ADHD diagnoses when comparing ADHD diagnoses in participants with obesity (I/II: 22.8%; III: 42.6%) against those with overweight (18.9%; $p = 0.11$).

3.4.2. Prevalence of ADHD Within Different Obesity Classes

Altfas [53] found that there was a significant difference in adult ADHD diagnosis, presence of 3–5 ADHD traits, and no diagnosis or traits across obesity-III, obesity-I/II, and overweight ($p < 0.025$). ADHD diagnoses were significantly more frequent amongst participants with obesity-III (42.6%) compared to those with obesity-I/II or overweight

(22.8% and 18.9%, respectively; $p = 0.002$). Two studies [62,70] did not find a significant difference between rates of adult or persistent ADHD diagnoses across participants with obesity-III (13.2–16.4%), those with obesity-II (9.4–27.3%), and those with obesity-I (5.7–18.7%; $p > 0.05$). Stahel and colleagues [76] found no significant differences in rates of adult ADHD diagnoses across patients with obesity-IV (2.7%) compared to those with obesity-II/III (0.8%; $p = 0.18$).

3.4.3. Prevalence of ADHD Before and After Bariatric Surgery

Alfonsson and colleagues [52] found that mean adult ADHD-hyperactivity traits significantly decreased after bariatric surgery (*pre:* 9.72 ± 4.51, *post:* 8.18 ± 5.92; $p < 0.001$). They found no significant difference between ADHD-attention traits before and after surgery (*pre:* 9.79 ± 4.88, *post:* 9.64 ± 6.5; $p = 0.38$). Nielsen and colleagues [72] found no significant differences in positive screening rates or average ADHD traits for adult, childhood, or persistent ADHD in patients with obesity measured pre-surgery compared to those who were measured post-surgery ($p > 0.05$).

3.4.4. Experiences and Perspectives

No studies looked at the experiences or perspectives of autistic or ADHD patients with obesity, nor the experiences or perspectives of other stakeholders.

3.4.5. Demographic Differences of ADHD and Non-ADHD Adults with Obesity

Table 4 summarises the demographic differences between ADHD and non-ADHD patients with obesity in the included studies (see Table S4 for further details on study characteristics and findings for all clinical profile papers). Eight studies compared demographics of ADHD and non-ADHD participants with obesity [56,57,60,61,64,65,70,77]. Six found no significant differences between participants with probable or diagnosed childhood, adult, or persistent ADHD and non-ADHD participants for age [56,57,60,64,65,70] or sex [56,57,65], but one found age, percentage of participants who were women, and percentage who were non-white to be lower in the diagnosed ADHD group [61]. Income and education were lower in the group diagnosed with, and medicated for, ADHD [77], and education and employment (versus unemployment) were lower in the group with probable persistent ADHD than in the group without ADHD [65].

Table 4. Summary of findings regarding differences in demographic outcomes between ADHD and non-ADHD participants with obesity.

Outcomes	Findings
Age	Mostly N.S [56,57,60,61,64,65,70]
Sex	Mostly N.S [56,57,61,65]
Ethnicity (% white)	↑ADHD [61]
Income	↓ADHD [77]
Education	↓ADHD [65,77]
Employment	↓ADHD [65]

N.S = no significant differences between ADHD and non-ADHD participants. ↑ ADHD = ADHD patients scored higher on the outcome than non-ADHD participants. ↓ ADHD = ADHD patients scored lower on the outcome than non-ADHD participants.

3.4.6. BMI Differences in ADHD and Non-ADHD Adults with Obesity

Table 5 summarises the obesity-related differences between ADHD and non-ADHD patients with obesity in the included studies. The age of onset of obesity did not significantly differ across the diagnosed childhood or adult ADHD group and the non-ADHD group [57].

Eleven studies compared BMI. Nine studies found no significant differences between current (pre- or no intervention) BMI between the participants with probable or diagnosed childhood, adult, or persistent ADHD and those without ADHD [51,56,57,60,64,65,70,71,73]. Five of these studies contained samples who went on to receive surgery [51,56,64,65,71]. However, one study found that BMI was significantly lower in the diagnosed ADHD group compared to the non-ADHD group when these groups were unmatched, and out of matched patients who went on to be treated with *pharmacotherapy* [61]. Two studies found BMI to be significantly higher in the diagnosed or probable adult ADHD group who went on to be treated by *surgery*, compared to the non-ADHD participants who also went on to receive surgery [61,69].

Table 5. Summary of findings regarding differences in obesity-related outcomes between ADHD and non-ADHD participants with obesity.

Study Outcomes	Findings
Bariatric measures	
Age of onset of obesity	N.S [57]
BMI (pre-/no intervention)	Mostly N.S [51,56,57,60,61,64,65,69–71,73]
Health-related Quality of Life	
Obesity-related problems (OP) [91]	↑ADHD [77]
Health-related quality of life (SF-36) [92]	↓ADHD [77]
Physical comorbidities	
Number of physical comorbidities	N.S [69]
Type 2 diabetes	N.S [73]
Sleep apnea	Mixed [57,77]
Weight loss attempts	
Attempts lasting <3 days	↑ADHD [73]
Attempts lasting >3 days	N.S [73]
Obesity interventions received	
Has/will received bariatric surgery	Mixed [57,61]
Surgery type	N.S [71]
Will receive pharmacotherapy	↑ADHD [61]

↑ADHD = ADHD patients scored higher on the outcome than non-ADHD participants. ↓ADHD = ADHD patients scored lower on the outcome than non-ADHD participants. BMI = Body Mass Index, kg/m^2. Mixed = findings from studies were conflicting. N.S = no significant differences between ADHD and non-ADHD participants. OP = Obesity-related Problems scale. SF-36 = Short Form Health Survey.

3.4.7. Health-Related Quality of Life and Physical Comorbidities Differences

On the Obesity-related Problems (OP) scale [91], health-related quality of life was significantly higher in the diagnosed and medicated ADHD group compared to the non-ADHD group [77], but was lower on the 36-item Short Form Health Survey (SF-36) [92]. The mean number of physical comorbidities [69] and rates of type 2 diabetes [73] did not significantly differ across the probable adult ADHD and the non-ADHD group. One study found significantly higher rates of sleep apnea in the group with diagnosed, and medicated, ADHD [77], but another study found no significant difference between sleep apnea rates in the diagnosed adult or childhood groups compared to the non-ADHD group [57].

3.4.8. Weight Loss Attempts and Interventions Received

The group with probable adult ADHD reported significantly more weight loss attempts lasting less than three days than the non-ADHD group [73]. There were no significant differences between the two groups on the number of weight loss attempts lasting more than three days [73]. The number of participants who had previously received bariatric surgery did not significantly differ across the diagnosed childhood or adult ADHD group and the non-ADHD group [57]. The diagnosed ADHD group were significantly more likely to receive obesity pharmacotherapy (any or specific) and receive obesity surgery (any or specific), compared to the non-ADHD group (matched or unmatched) [61]. There was no significant difference in the obesity surgery type used between the probable adult ADHD group and the non-ADHD group [71].

3.4.9. Differences in ADHD Traits in ADHD and Non-ADHD Adults with Obesity

Table 6 summarises the cognitive, personality, and temperament differences between ADHD and non-ADHD patients with obesity in the included studies. Using the DIVA 2.0, significantly more participants from the adult ADHD group were diagnosed with childhood ADHD, and significantly more participants from the childhood ADHD group were diagnosed with adult ADHD than in the non-ADHD groups [57]. The probable childhood ADHD group also had significantly more adult ADHD traits than the non-ADHD group [79]. Childhood ADHD traits were also significantly higher in the probable persistent ADHD group compared to the non-ADHD group [64].

Table 6. Summary of findings regarding differences in temperament outcomes between ADHD and non-ADHD participants with obesity.

Study Outcomes	Findings
Cognitive traits	
ADHD traits	↑ADHD [57,64,79]
Impulsivity (BIS-11) [93]	↑ADHD [60]
Flexibility (CLT) [75]	↓ADHD [75]
Inhibition (ST) [94]	N.S [60]
Personality (BFI) [95]	
Neuroticism	↑ADHD [64]
Agreeableness	↓ADHD [64]
Conscientiousness	↓ADHD [64]
Extraversion	N.S [64]
Openness	N.S [64]
Temperament and Character (TCI) [96]	
Self-directedness	↓ADHD [56]
Cooperativeness	↓ADHD [56]
Novelty seeking	N.S [56]
Reward dependence	N.S [56]
Persistence	N.S [56]
Self-transcendence	N.S [56]

↑ADHD = ADHD patients scored higher on the outcome than non-ADHD participants. ↓ADHD = ADHD patients scored lower on the outcome than non-ADHD participants. BFI = Big Five Inventory. BIS-11 = Barratt Impulsiveness Scale Version 11. CLT = Card and Lottery Task. N.S = no significant differences between ADHD and non-ADHD participants. ST = Stroop Test. TCI = Temperament and Character Inventory.

3.4.10. Impulsivity/Inhibition Differences in ADHD and Non-ADHD Adults with Obesity

On the Barratt Impulsiveness Scale Version 11 (BIS-11) [93], the group with probable adult ADHD scored significantly higher than the non-ADHD group [60], but scored lower on the Cards and Lottery Task (CLT), which measured flexible decision making regarding immediate and long-term consequences [75]. On the Stroop Test (ST), which measures response inhibition [94], there was no significant difference between the two groups [60].

3.4.11. Personality Differences in ADHD and Non-ADHD Adults with Obesity

When measured using the Big Five Inventory (BFI) [95], the group with probable persistent ADHD scored significantly higher in neuroticism and lower in agreeableness and conscientiousness than the non-ADHD group [64]. There was no significant difference between the two groups on extraversion or openness [64]. Using the Temperament and Character Inventory (TCI) [96], the group with probable adult ADHD was significantly lower on self-directedness and cooperativeness than the non-ADHD group [56]. There were no significant differences between the two groups for novelty seeking, reward dependence, persistence, or self-transcendence [56].

3.4.12. Psychopathological Differences in ADHD and Non-ADHD Adults with Obesity

Table 7 summarises the psychopathological differences between ADHD and non-ADHD patients with obesity in the included studies. Three studies used the SCL-90 to measure differences in psychopathology across participants with and without ADHD. Total scores were significantly higher in the groups with probable adult and childhood ADHD [56,79], but there were no significant differences on the somatization or anxiety sub-scales for the group with probable childhood ADHD compared to the non-ADHD group [78]. However, scores were higher for the group with diagnosed persistent ADHD on Beck's Anxiety Inventory (BAI) [74,97] and for the group with probable adult ADHD on the Hospital Anxiety and Depression Scale (HADS) [98] for both the anxiety and the depression sub-scales [50,51]. There were no significant differences between the group with diagnosed persistent ADHD and the non-ADHD group on anxiety scores [70], measured using the Portuguese version of the State-Trait Anxiety Inventory (STAI) [99] between the two groups.

Table 7. Summary of findings regarding differences in psychopathological outcomes between ADHD and non-ADHD participants with obesity.

Study Outcomes	Findings
Psychopathology measures	
Total psychopathology (SCL-90) [100]	↑ADHD [56,79]
Anxiety (BAI; HADS; SCL-90; STAI) [97–100]	Mostly ↑ADHD [50,51,70,74,78]
Depression (BDI; HADS) [98,101]	↑ADHD [50,51,65,70,71,74]
Somatization (SCL-90) [100]	N.S [78]
Emotional dysregulation (DERS-16) [102]	↑ADHD [64]
Alexithymia (TAS-20) [103]	↑ADHD [64]
Problematic alcohol use (AUDIT) [104]	↑ADHD [51]
Psychiatric disorders	
Any psychiatric disorder	N.S [65]
Anxiety or mood disorders	N.S [56]
Depressive disorders	N.S [65,73]
Panic disorder	N.S [56]
Any eating disorder	N.S [56]
Binge eating disorder	N.S [65]
Family history of anxiety or mood disorders	N.S [56]
Past psychotherapy	↑ADHD [65]

↑ADHD = ADHD patients scored higher on the outcome than non-ADHD participants. AUDIT = Alcohol Use Disorders Identification Test. BAI = Beck's Anxiety Inventory. BDI = Beck's Depression Inventory. DERS-16 = Difficulties in Emotion Regulation Scale. HADS = Hospital Anxiety and Depression Scale. N.S = no significant differences between ADHD and non-ADHD participants. SCL-90 = Symptom Checklist-90. STAI = State-Trait Anxiety Inventory. TAS-20 = Toronto Alexithymia Scale-20.

On Beck's Depression Inventory (BDI) [101], four studies found depression symptoms to be higher in the groups with diagnosed or probable persistent and adult ADHD compared to the non-ADHD group [65,70,71,74], including when combined with the Spanish version of the Revised Questionnaire of Eating and Weight patterns (EHQ-ES) [105]. Emotional dysregulation, measured by the French, 16-item version of the Difficulties in Emotion Regulation Scale (DERS-16) [102], and alexithymia measured by the French version of the Toronto Alexithymia Scale-20 (TAS-20) [103] were both significantly higher in the group with probable persistent ADHD [64]. The group with probable adult ADHD also scored significantly higher on the Alcohol Use Disorders Identification Test (AUDIT) [104] than the non-ADHD group [51].

3.4.13. Psychiatric Differences in ADHD and Non-ADHD Adults with Obesity

When assessed by clinicians, there were no significant differences in overall presence of psychiatric disorder [65], total rates of anxiety or mood disorders [56], depressive disorders [65], depression [73], or panic disorder [56] between the group with probable adult or persistent ADHD and the non-ADHD group. There were no significant differences in family history of anxiety or mood disorders between the group with probable adult ADHD and the non-ADHD group [56]. There were no significant differences between the group with probable adult ADHD and the non-ADHD group on diagnoses of any ED [56], or between the group with probable persistent ADHD and the non-ADHD group on diagnoses of binge ED [65]. Past psychotherapy was significantly higher in the group with probable persistent ADHD [65].

3.4.14. Disordered Eating Differences in ADHD and Non-ADHD Adults with Obesity

Table 8 summarises the differences in disordered eating between ADHD and non-ADHD patients with obesity in the included studies. Regarding the Bulimic Investigatory Test, Edinburgh (BITE) [106], the groups with diagnosed persistent or probable adult ADHD scored significantly higher overall than the non-ADHD group [55,70]. The group with probable adult ADHD also scored higher on the symptom scale, but not on the severity scale [56]. On the Binge Eating Scale (BES) [107], the groups with diagnosed or probable childhood, adult, or persistent ADHD all scored significantly higher than the non-ADHD groups [57,64,70]. On the Eating Attitude Test (EAT-40), which assesses anorexia nervosa symptoms [108], there was no significant difference between the group with probable childhood ADHD and the non-ADHD group [78].

Table 8. Summary of findings regarding differences in disordered eating outcomes between ADHD and non-ADHD participants with obesity.

Study Outcome	Findings
Bulimic behavior	
Bulimic total score (BITE) [106]	↑ADHD [55,70]
Bulimic symptoms (BITE) [106]	↑ADHD [56]
Bulimic severity (BITE) [106]	N.S [56]
Binge-type eating	
Binge eating (BES; EPQ) [107,109]	↑ADHD [57,63,64,70]
Eating large amounts (EPQ) [109]	N.S [63]
Disinhibited eating and loss of control (EI; GFCQ-T) [110,111]	Mostly ↑ADHD [50,60,74]
Emotional cravings and eating (EES; EI; GFCQ-T) [110–112]	Mostly ↑ADHD [50,60,65,74]
Secret eating (EPQ) [109]	↑ADHD [63]

Table 8. *Cont.*

Study Outcome	Findings
Food craving and addiction	
Snacking (EPQ) [109]	↑ADHD [63]
Hunger (EI) [110]	↑ADHD [60,74]
Food cravings (GFCQ-T) [111]	↑ADHD [50,51]
Food addiction (YFAS 2.0) [113]	↑ADHD [57,64]
Nighttime eating	
Nighttime eating overall (EPQ; NEQ) [109,114]	Mostly ↑ADHD [55,56,63]
Morning anorexia (NEQ) [114]	N.S [56]
Evening hyperphagia (NEQ) [114]	N.S [56]
Nocturnal ingestions (NEQ) [114]	N.S [56]
Mood and sleep disturbances (NEQ) [114]	↑ADHD [56]
Restricted eating	
Anorexia nervosa symptoms (EAT-40) [108]	N.S [78]
Cognitive restraint (EI) [110]	↓ADHD [60,74]

↑ADHD = ADHD patients scored higher on the outcome than non-ADHD participants. ↓ADHD = ADHD patients scored lower on the outcome than non-ADHD participants. BES = Binge Eating Scale. BITE = Bulimic Investigatory Test, Edinburgh. EAT-40 = Eating Attitude Test. EES = Emotional Eating Scale. EI = Eating Inventory. EPQ = Eating Pattern Questionnaire. GFCQ-T = General Food Cravings Questionnaire-Trait. N.S = no significant differences between ADHD and non-ADHD participants. NEQ = Nighttime Eating Questionnaire. YFAS 2.0 = Yale Food Addiction Scale.

On the Eating Inventory (EI) [110], there was no significant difference between the group with diagnosed persistent ADHD and the non-ADHD group on the total score nor the disinhibition sub-scale [74]. The group with probable adult ADHD scored significantly higher on the disinhibition sub-scale [60]. Both those with probable adult ADHD and diagnosed persistent ADHD scored significantly higher on the hunger sub-scales and lower on cognitive restraint [60,74]. The group with diagnosed persistent ADHD also scored significantly higher on the emotional eating sub-scale [74]. On the Emotional Eating Scale (EES) [112], the group with probable adult ADHD scored significantly higher than the non-ADHD group [60], but there were no significant differences between the group with diagnosed persistent ADHD and the non-ADHD group [65].

On the Eating Pattern Questionnaire (EPQ) [109], the group with probable adult ADHD scored significantly higher on snacking between meals, binge eating, nighttime eating, and secret eating [63]. There was no significant difference between groups regarding eating large amounts of food [63]. On the Nighttime Eating Questionnaire (NEQ) [114], the group with probable adult ADHD scored significantly higher overall in one study [55], but not in another [56]. The latter study also found no significant differences between the two groups on the following sub-scales: morning anorexia, evening hyperphagia, and nocturnal ingestions. However, the ADHD group scored significantly higher on the mood and sleep sub-scale. On the Yale Food Addiction Scale (YFAS 2.0) [113], the groups of diagnosed childhood and adult ADHD and probable persistent ADHD groups scored significantly higher than the non-ADHD groups [57,64]. On the General Food Cravings Questionnaire-Trait (GFCQ-T) [111], the group with probable adult ADHD scored significantly higher than the non-ADHD group on the total score [50,51], as well as on the sub-scales loss of control and emotional cravings [50].

3.4.15. Operative Complications and Protocol Adherence

Table 9 summarises differences in operative complications and post-surgery weight outcomes between ADHD and non-ADHD patients with obesity in the included studies (see Table S5 for study characteristics and findings for all treatment response papers). Post-operative complications were significantly more common in the diagnosed and medicated ADHD group than in the non-ADHD group, while no significant differences were seen in intra-operative complications, specific post-operative complications, or any serious post-operative complications [77]. The diagnosed ADHD group spent significantly longer in hospital post-operation than the non-ADHD group, but there was no significant difference in rates of reoperation within 30 days between the two groups [67]. After bariatric surgery, the group with probable adult ADHD was also significantly less likely to follow the hospitals' standardised appointments protocol [71].

Table 9. Summary of findings regarding operative complications and BMI outcomes post-surgery between ADHD and non-ADHD participants with obesity.

Outcomes	Findings
Operative complications	
Intra-operative complications	N.S [77]
Any post-operative complications	↑ADHD [77]
Specific post-operative complications	N.S [77]
Any serious post-operative complications	N.S [77]
Length of time in hospital post-operation	↑ADHD [67]
Reoperation within 30 days	N.S [67]
Adherence to hospital appointments	↓ADHD [71]
BMI changes	
BMI loss—3 months	N.S [69]
BMI loss—6 months	↓ADHD [69]
BMI loss—12 months	Mostly N.S [52,61,69]
BMI loss—18 months	N.S [71]
BMI loss—2 years	↑ADHD [61]
BMI loss—3 years	↑ADHD [61]
BMI loss—4 years	↑ADHD [61]
BMI loss—5 years	↑ADHD [61]
Weight changes	
Lost >50% of excess weight—12 months	N.S [69]
Weight loss—12 months	N.S [69,77]
Weight loss—2 years	N.S [77]

↑ADHD = ADHD patients scored higher on the outcome than non-ADHD participants. ↓ADHD = ADHD patients scored lower on the outcome than non-ADHD participants. BMI = Body Mass Index. N.S = no significant differences between ADHD and non-ADHD participants.

3.4.16. Post-Surgery Weight Change Outcomes

Findings regarding weight changes were mixed. One study found that after surgery, the diagnosed ADHD group had significantly higher BMI loss than the non-ADHD group every year for five years [61], whereas another found more mixed results post-RYGB surgery, regarding BMI loss, weight loss, and surgery success (defined as losing more than 50% of excess weight) over 3, 6, and 12 months between the group with probable adult ADHD and the non-ADHD group [69]. Three other studies found no difference in BMI loss one year after RYGB surgery [52] or achieved BMI 18 months after surgery (mostly RYGB) [71] between the group with probable adult ADHD and the non-ADHD group and no difference in weight loss one and two years after surgery for the diagnosed and medicated ADHD group compared to the non-ADHD group [77].

3.4.17. Post-Surgery Health-Related Quality of Life Changes

Table 10 summarises post-surgery differences in health-related quality of life, eating behaviour, and psychopathology between ADHD and non-ADHD patients with obesity in the included studies. Two studies found mixed results for post-surgery differences on the SF-36. In one study [71], the group with probable adult ADHD scored lower on the general health scale than the non-ADHD group. There were no significant differences between the two groups on the mental health, bodily pain, vitality, or social functioning scales. In the other study [77], the group with diagnosed and medicated ADHD scored lower on the physical and mental components of health-related quality of life at one year follow up and on the mental components at two years follow up compared to the non-ADHD group. There were no significant differences in the physical components between the two groups at two-years follow-up [77].

Table 10. Summary of findings regarding differences in post-surgical outcomes between ADHD and non-ADHD participants with obesity.

Outcomes	Findings
Health-related quality of life (SF-36) [92]	
Physical components—1 year	↓ADHD [77]
Mental components—1 year	↓ADHD [77]
General health—1.5 years	↓ADHD [71]
Mental health—1.5 years	N.S [71]
Bodily pain—1.5 years	N.S [71]
Vitality—1.5 years	N.S [71]
Social functioning—1.5 years	N.S [71]
Physical components—2 years	N.S [77]
Mental components—2 years	↓ADHD [77]
Obesity-related problems (OP) [91]	
Obesity-related problems—1 year	↑ADHD [77]
Obesity-related problems—2 years	↑ADHD [77]
Eating behavior	
% lipids intake	↑ADHD [71]
% mono/poly-unsaturated fat intake	↑ADHD [71]
% carbohydrates intake	↓ADHD [71]
% of individuals grazing	↑ADHD [71]
Mealtime length	↓ADHD [71]
% of individuals with positive ED criteria	↑ADHD [71]
Alcohol and substance use	
Alcohol intake	↑ADHD [71]
Problematic alcohol use (AUDIT) [104]	↑ADHD [52]
Substance-user disorders	↑ADHD [77]
Psychopathology	
Anxiety and depression (HADS) [98]	↑ADHD [52]
Depression (BDI) [101]	N.S [71]
Self-harm	↑ADHD [77]

↑ADHD = ADHD patients scored higher on the outcome than non-ADHD participants. ↓ADHD = ADHD patients scored lower on the outcome than non-ADHD participants. AUDIT = Alcohol Use Disorders Identification Test. BDI = Beck's Depression Inventory. ED = eating disorder. HADS = Hospital Anxiety and Depression Scale. N.S = no significant differences between ADHD and non-ADHD participants. OP = Obesity-related Problems scale. SF-36 = Short Form Health Survey.

3.4.18. Post-Surgery Changes in Eating Behaviour

One study looked at eating changes post-surgery [71]. After surgery, percentage lipid intake, percentage mono/poly-unsaturated fat intake, alcohol intake, and percentage of individuals grazing were all significantly higher in the probable adult ADHD group than the non-ADHD group. Percentage carbohydrate intake and mealtime length were significantly lower in the probable ADHD group.

3.4.19. Post-Surgery Changes in Psychopathology

After RYGB surgery, the probable adult ADHD group scored significantly higher on HADS and AUDIT than the non-ADHD group [52]. After surgery (mostly RYGB), the percentage of individuals with positive ED criteria was significantly higher in the probable adult ADHD group than the non-ADHD group [71]. There were no significant differences in the percentage of individuals with positive screening for depression, measured using the BDI, between the two groups [71]. After surgery, the diagnosed and medicated ADHD group had higher rates of self-harm and substance-use disorders compared to the non-ADHD group [77].

3.4.20. Treatment Responses After Non-Surgical Intervention

Table 11 summarises differences in non-surgical intervention outcomes between ADHD and non-ADHD patients with obesity in the included studies. Pagoto and colleagues [73] describe findings from their 16-week clinic-based behavioural weight loss program, which combined dietary modifications, physical activity recommendations, and behavioural strategies such as self-monitoring and goal setting to promote sustainable weight loss. Participants were assessed on their perception of the difficulty of the basic components of the program (e.g., tracking calories, keeping a diet diary, etc.), using the Perceived Difficulty Index (PDI) [73], with the probable adult ADHD group reporting finding these "weight loss skills" significantly more challenging than the non-ADHD group (29.78 ± 6.35 versus 23.02 ± 8.53; $p < 0.05$). Measured using the Weight Lifestyle Self-Efficacy (WEL) [115] and the Weight and Lifestyle Inventory (WALI) [116], this group also reported significantly more emotional eating (19.36 ± 5.31 versus 13.27 ± 6.77; $p < 0.01$), more fast-food meals per week (1.94 ± 1.92 versus 0.81 ± 1.78; $p < 0.05$), and a lower ability to resist eating during negative emotions, availability of food, social pressure, physical discomfort, and positive activities (75.73 ± 42.72 versus 103.87 ± 29.32, $p < 0.05$), compared to the non-ADHD group. There were no significant differences in meals skipped per week (1.57 ± 2.00 versus 1.40 ± 2.17, $p = 0.28$) or days per week of >20 min moderate physical activity (2.50 ± 2.61 versus 3.48 ± 1.79, $p = 1.28$) between the two groups. Percentage weight loss and success (defined as 5% weight loss) were lower in the adult ADHD group (−3.34% ± 3.53 versus −5.59% ± 3.43, 31% versus 61%, $p < 0.05$).

Two other studies looked at weight outcomes for ADHD groups after non-surgical interventions and found them to be worse than those of the non-ADHD group. In one of these studies, BMI loss and weight loss were lowest in the diagnosed ADHD group, middling in the ADHD symptom group, and highest in the non-ADHD group after unspecified treatment [53]. In the other study, BMI loss was consistently significantly lower in the diagnosed ADHD group from one to five years after obesity pharmacotherapy [61].

Table 11. Summary of findings regarding differences in outcomes after non-surgical intervention between ADHD and non-ADHD participants with obesity.

Outcomes	Findings
Behavioral weight loss program	
Perceived difficulty of program (PDI) [73]	↑ADHD [73]
Emotional eating (WALI) [116]	↑ADHD [73]
Fast-food meals per week (WALI) [116]	↑ADHD [73]
Meal skipping (WALI) [116]	N.S [73]
Self-efficacy to resist eating in different situations (WEL) [115]	↓ADHD [73]
Moderate physical activity (WALI) [116]	N.S [73]
% weight loss	↓ADHD [73]
% meeting 5% weight loss goal	↓ADHD [73]
Pharmacotherapy	
BMI loss—1 year	↓ADHD [61]
BMI loss—2 years	↓ADHD [61]
BMI loss—3 years	↓ADHD [61]
BMI loss—4 years	↓ADHD [61]
BMI loss—5 years	↓ADHD [61]
Unspecified treatment	
BMI loss	↓ADHD [53]
Weight loss	↓ADHD [53]

↑ADHD = ADHD patients scored higher on the outcome than non-ADHD participants. ↓ADHD = ADHD patients scored lower on the outcome than non-ADHD participants. BMI = Body Mass Index. N.S = no significant differences between ADHD and non-ADHD participants. PDI = Perceived Difficulty Index. WALI = Weight and Lifestyle Inventory. WEL = Weight Lifestyle Self-Efficacy.

3.4.21. Targeted Interventions for Autistic or ADHD Patients with Obesity

Crowley and colleagues [58] detail case reports of two 19- and 20-year-old female patients with autism and cyclothymic disorder (one with additional mild intellectual disability), who were treated for obesity with Topiramate (BMI > 30). After 1–2 years, both patients no longer had obesity (or overweight; BMI < 25). Azran and colleagues [54] detail a case report of a 52-year-old male whose ADHD medication (oral methylphenidate) had ceased working post-RYGB surgery. The patient was switched to transdermal methylphenidate, and the medication's therapeutic effects were regained.

Levy and colleagues [68] conducted a longitudinal clinical intervention study of the effects of ADHD medication on weight change in 78 participants (72 female, mean age = 41.3) with diagnosed persistent ADHD and severe obesity (mean BMI = 42.7). Sixty-five participants received pharmacotherapy, almost exclusively psychostimulants (including methylphenidate). In several cases, a nonstimulant, atomoxetine, was used due to residual anxiety symptoms. Thirteen patients remained as controls as they elected not to receive medication, had side effects, or obtained no clear benefit from trials of several medications for ADHD. There was a significant difference in weight changes between the two groups. After an average of 466 ± 260 days, weight change in the intervention group was −12.36% of initial weight and in controls +2.78% ($p < 0.001$). Weight loss in treated subjects was 15.05kg (10.35%), and weight gain was 3.26 kg (7.03%) in controls ($p < 0.001$). Table S6 contains further study characteristics and findings for all case reports and intervention studies.

4. Discussion

This scoping review assessed the literature on autism and ADHD in adults with obesity to identify gaps relevant to clinical practice. The findings indicate a lack of research on this topic, especially regarding autism in this population.

4.1. Autism in Obesity

Only two studies, both case reports, considered autism in obesity. These reports described using weight loss drugs to successfully treat three autistic patients with obesity [58,66]. There were no studies exploring rates of autism in patients with obesity; the experiences and perspectives of autistic patients, their clinicians, or their carers; or clinical differences autistic patients may present with.

Research on autistic patients with EDs suggests that autism can affect ED symptoms, presentation, and treatment outcomes [19,117]. It is likely that autistic individuals with obesity also experience distinct challenges linked to sensory, cognitive, and social processing differences [7,8]. Yet, this review found little exploration of these differences, and no adjunct psychotherapies were proposed. Autism is often seen as a complex condition focused on developmental, communication, and social differences, leading obesity researchers to overlook its potential links to obesity. Autistic traits like sensory sensitivities, rigid eating patterns, and social difficulties are rarely prioritised in obesity research or treatment. Additionally, autism in adults, especially those with milder traits, may go unrecognised in patients with obesity, leaving the intersection of autism and obesity underexplored. Overall, there remains a substantive gap in developing autistic-friendly pathways for treating obesity.

4.2. Prevalence of ADHD in Obesity

Compared to autism, there is more literature on ADHD in obesity. Most studies were on patient populations, and there were no large general population cohort studies, limiting conclusions. Furthermore, five of the eight studies did not report or adjust for participants using ADHD medication, which can affect eating and weight.

However, current findings suggested that ADHD may be overrepresented in individuals with obesity [62], regardless of binge eating status [59]. Docet and colleagues [62] reported ADHD prevalence at 20.6% in patients with obesity, compared to 6.8% for individuals without obesity. However, this estimate is significantly higher than a recent meta-analysis [36], which found adult ADHD prevalence in metabolic and bariatric surgery candidates to be 9.9% and persistent ADHD to be 8.9%. Docet and colleagues [62] also found ADHD to be especially overrepresented in women with obesity, at 24%, versus just 9.7% for males [62], although as males made up less than one quarter of this sample, sex-specific conclusions are limited. One study also found that ADHD was more prevalent in severe obesity than in milder obesity [53], but other studies did not find this [76]. There were also mixed findings regarding whether ADHD traits decreased in patients after obesity treatment [52,72]. Overall, it seems likely that a significant proportion of patients presenting for obesity treatment will have ADHD, and so this is something that clinicians should be aware of in their patient population.

4.3. Clinical Profiles of ADHD in Obesity

ADHD patients with obesity experienced unique challenges compared to their non-ADHD counterparts, including reduced income, education, and employment [65,77]. These socioeconomic disparities, consistent with broader ADHD research [118], may exacerbate obesity management difficulties by limiting access to health resources and exposing individuals to obesogenic environments [119]. ADHD patients also report increased obesity-related problems and reduced health-related quality of life [77,120]. This may reflect compounded challenges of living with both ADHD and obesity.

ADHD patients also showed increased ADHD traits and impulsivity [57,60,64,79], as well as reduced cognitive flexibility [75], which may influence their ability to adapt to structured weight-loss programs. Personality traits such as heightened neuroticism and lower agreeableness, conscientiousness, self-directedness, and cooperativeness [56,64] may further hinder goal-oriented behaviours essential for sustained weight management. Interventions focusing on building self-regulation, self-efficacy, and interpersonal support could help mitigate these challenges.

Psychopathology was also more prevalent in ADHD patients with obesity, including higher rates of depressive and anxiety symptoms, emotional dysregulation, alexithymia, and problematic alcohol use [50,51,56,64,65,70,71,74,78,79], and many of these issues continued post-bariatric surgery [52,71,77]. These findings align with broader evidence of poorer mental health in ADHD populations [121], which may complicate obesity treatment by undermining motivation, adherence to lifestyle interventions, and overall functioning. Targeted approaches, such as dialectical behaviour therapy (DBT) for emotional dysregulation [122], could be particularly beneficial. The higher likelihood of past psychotherapy in ADHD patients [65] underscores the need for integrated care addressing both psychological and physical health.

Eating behaviours in ADHD patients with obesity were characterised by increased bulimic symptoms, binge eating, secret eating, snacking, hunger, and food cravings and addiction [50,51,56,57,60,63,64,70,74]. Emotional and nighttime eating may also have been elevated in ADHD patients [50,55,56,60,63,65,74]. ADHD patients also showed decreased cognitive restraint [60,74]. These behaviours may stem from core ADHD symptoms, such as impulsivity and emotional dysregulation, which disrupt eating regulation and drive maladaptive habits. The heightened prevalence of food cravings may reflect dopaminergic dysregulation in ADHD [123], further complicating weight management. Post-bariatric surgery, ADHD patients still had increased percentages of lipid and mono-polyunsaturated fat intake and lower carbohydrate intake. They were more likely to graze, meet ED criteria, and have shorter meal lengths [71]. Integrating interventions such as mindfulness-based eating approaches [124], pharmacological treatments addressing impulsivity [68], or behavioural interventions increasing cognitive restraint [125] may be beneficial. Additionally, ADHD patients reported more weight-loss attempts lasting less than three days [73], highlighting the need for interventions to improve persistence.

Despite these differences, some characteristics were similar between ADHD and non-ADHD patients with obesity, such as sex, age, age of obesity onset, BMI, number of physical comorbidities, rates of type 2 diabetes, weight loss attempts lasting more than three days, and type of obesity surgery received [51,56,57,60,64,65,69–71,73]. Additionally, no differences were found in cognitive inhibition, extraversion, openness, novelty seeking, reward dependence, persistence, or self-transcendence [56,60,64]. Somatization, psychiatric disorders, family history of anxiety or mood disorders, bulimic severity, and eating large amounts did not differ significantly between ADHD and non-ADHD groups [56,63,65,73,78]. These findings suggest that while ADHD may influence specific obesity-related challenges, there are shared characteristics across ADHD and non-ADHD individuals with obesity.

4.4. Post-Surgical Outcomes of ADHD Patients with Obesity Compared to Non-ADHD Patients

Compared to non-ADHD counterparts, ADHD patients with obesity had increased post-operative complications, longer hospital stays post-operation, and reduced adherence to follow-ups, but showed no differences in intra-operative or serious complications, or reoperations within 30 days [67,71,77]. ADHD-related impulsivity and organisational challenges may underlie these issues. Structured follow-ups, appointment reminders, and tailored care coordination could improve adherence and outcomes.

Bariatric surgery may disrupt the therapeutic effects of some oral ADHD medications due to malabsorption, but switching to transdermal administration methods may overcome these issues, as suggested in one case report [54], and could mitigate these challenges. Most studies found no significant differences in BMI or weight changes between ADHD and non-ADHD patients [52,61,69,71,77]. This suggests bariatric surgery may be preferable for this population, as it was the only treatment that did not result in poorer weight outcomes for ADHD patients compared to non-ADHD patients. This aligns with findings by Dickinson and colleagues [61], who highlighted bariatric surgery as a viable but underutilised option for ADHD patients with obesity. Although mixed findings on quality-of-life changes suggest ADHD may hinder sustained improvements [71,77]. Behavioural strategies and integrated support tailored to ADHD patients might enhance long-term quality-of-life outcomes.

4.5. Behavioural Weight Loss Program Outcomes of ADHD Patients with Obesity

ADHD patients found following a behavioural weight loss program [73] more challenging than their non-ADHD counterparts, potentially due to cognitive inflexibility, impulsivity, and difficulties with planning and self-regulation [60,75]. They also reported lower self-efficacy in resisting eating in different situations (i.e., poorer cognitive restraint), as observed in ADHD patients before treatment [60,74]. These challenges may also explain the reported elevated rates of emotional eating and fast-food consumption [73]. Resultantly, ADHD patients had reduced percentage weight loss and were less likely to meet the program's 5% weight loss target [73]. Addressing core ADHD symptoms alongside weight-loss strategies, such as combining behavioural interventions with ADHD medication, could improve outcomes.

4.6. Pharmacotherapy Outcomes of ADHD Patients with Obesity

Compared to non-ADHD patients, ADHD patients showed reduced BMI loss after pharmacotherapy for obesity [61]. Despite this, pharmacotherapy for ADHD may still facilitate weight management. For example, Levy and colleagues [68] demonstrated that ADHD medication, particularly stimulant medications that target core ADHD symptoms like impulsivity and inattention, could improve obesity outcomes by reducing overeating and improving dietary control. Although it is notable that ADHD medication in this study was not suitable for one in every six participants, suggesting alternative interventions may be needed for some patients.

4.7. Psychotherapy Outcomes of ADHD Patients with Obesity

No studies considered specific psychotherapy adaptions to obesity treatments for ADHD patients. Given the unique challenges faced by this group, developing ADHD-specific psychotherapy protocols could address gaps in current care. For instance, integrating executive functioning training, emotion regulation, and motivational enhancement techniques into traditional obesity therapies might improve outcomes. Future research should explore the efficacy of these tailored approaches, ensuring they account for the cognitive, emotional, and behavioural profiles of ADHD patients.

4.8. Summary of Findings from Included Papers

In summary, weight loss drugs can successfully treat autistic patients with obesity. ADHD appears to be overrepresented in individuals with obesity, regardless of binge eating status. ADHD patients had lower socioeconomic status, poorer health-related quality of life, increased impulsivity, cognitive inflexibility, and neuroticism, alongside lower agreeableness, conscientiousness, self-directedness, and cooperativeness. ADHD patients also exhibited higher psychopathology, problematic alcohol use, and disordered eating. They had poorer outcomes from behavioural weight loss programs and obesity pharmacotherapy, though ADHD medication was effective for weight loss. ADHD patients had comparable weight outcomes to non-ADHD patients after bariatric surgery, but they experienced more complications, longer hospital stays, and poorer adherence, potentially also requiring transdermal ADHD medication.

4.9. Summary of Clinical Implications

While further research is needed before clinical recommendations can be made, the findings suggest potential interventions for autistic and ADHD patients with obesity. Autistic individuals likely face distinct challenges in obesity treatment due to sensory, cognitive, and social processing differences, which may require tailored interventions. Case reports suggest obesity medication may also be effective.

ADHD is common in obesity patients, and clinicians should consider ADHD-related challenges, such as lower socioeconomic status, poorer health-related quality of life, cognitive differences, psychopathology, and disordered eating. Bariatric surgery and ADHD medication may offer the best outcomes, but tailored care strategies are needed to address challenges like poor adherence and medication malabsorption. ADHD patients may also benefit from integrated care addressing both physical and psychological health, with adjunct therapies like DBT, motivational interviewing, and mindfulness, potentially improving outcomes. Future research should investigate ADHD-specific psychotherapies and the effectiveness of tailored interventions.

4.10. Limitations

This review focused on adult patients with obesity, limiting generalisability to paediatric and adolescent populations. Additionally, it examined autism and ADHD prevalence and influence on obesity, rather than obesity prevalence or influence on autism or ADHD, making findings more applicable to obesity-focused clinicians and researchers, rather than those specialising in autism or ADHD. Studies on biological or genetic mechanisms were excluded as these were less likely to have imminent clinical utility. Although grey literature was not explicitly excluded, no grey literature-specific databases were searched, meaning some relevant sources may have been missed, potentially introducing publication bias.

For this review, obesity was classified as a BMI ≥ 30, which does not consider variations in body composition such as differences in muscle and fat mass. This limitation is significant as individuals with the same BMI may have very different health risks and obesity-related challenges, especially when additional factors such as physical activity, diet, and medication are not considered.

Reviewed studies largely came from Western Europe. Few studies reported on participants' ethnicity or race, and most participants were women. This presents generalisability challenges as autism, ADHD, and obesity presentations vary across demographics [61,62,126–128]. There is a pressing need for research that (explicitly) includes minoritised and underrepresented groups, including those from the global south, men and other gender minorities, and non-white populations.

4.11. Future Research

Future research should examine the specific needs of autistic and ADHD patients with obesity to improve treatment inclusivity. Developing targeted psychotherapeutic and educational interventions could address the distinct symptoms of these populations, potentially enhancing outcomes. Including more diverse populations in research will ensure findings are culturally relevant and more universally applicable.

5. Conclusions

This review highlights the need for more research on autism and obesity. For ADHD, findings suggest frequent co-occurrence with obesity, accompanied by significant clinical differences. However, lived experiences and tailored interventions remain underexplored.

Supplementary Materials: The following supporting information can be downloaded at: https://www.mdpi.com/article/10.3390/nu17050787/s1, Table S1. Eligibility criteria for papers included in this review. Table S2. Full search strategy for each database. Table S3. Descriptions of studies reporting prevalence of ADHD in adults with Obesity. Table S4. Descriptions of studies reporting differences in clinical profiles of ADHD adults compared to non-ADHD adults with Obesity. Table S5. Descriptions of studies reporting differences in response to Obesity treatment in ADHD adults compared to non-ADHD adults. Table S6. Descriptions of case reports and one intervention study. Descriptions of studies reporting differences in clinical profiles of ADHD adults compared to non-ADHD adults with Obesity. Figure S1. Number of included publications from 2001 to 2024.

Author Contributions: Conceptualization, L.M., K.T., and V.M.; methodology, L.M.; validation, A.M., and E.Z.; formal analysis, L.M., A.M., and E.Z.; data curation, L.M., K.T., and V.M.; writing—original draft preparation, L.M.; writing—review and editing, L.M., A.M., V.M., and K.T.; visualization, L.M.; supervision, K.T. and V.M.; project administration, L.M. and K.T.; funding acquisition, K.T., V.M., and L.M. All authors have read and agreed to the published version of the manuscript.

Funding: This research is funded by the National Institute for Health and Care Research (NIHR) Maudsley Biomedical Research Centre (BRC) and the Psychiatry Research Trust. The views expressed are those of the authors and not necessarily those of the NIHR or the Department of Health and Social Care.

Conflicts of Interest: The authors declare that they have no conflicts of interest related to this study.

Abbreviations

The following abbreviations are used in this manuscript:

AADHDS	Adult ADHD Scale
ADHD	Attention-Deficit/Hyperactivity Disorder
ADHD-SCL-90-R	16 ADHD-relevant items from the Symptom Checklist-90-Revised
ADHD-SR	the German ADHD Rating Scale
APA	American Psychological Association
ASRS-v1.1	Adult ADHD Self-Report Scale
AUDIT	Alcohol Use Disorders Identification Test
BAI	Beck's Anxiety Inventory
BDI	Beck's Depression Inventory
BES	Binge Eating Scale
BFI	Big Five Inventory
BIS-11	Barratt Impulsiveness Scale Version 11
BITE	Bulimic Investigatory Test, Edinburgh
BMI	Body Mass Index, kg/m^2
CAARS-SSV	Self-report Screening Version of the Conners' Adult ADHD Rating Scale
CENTRAL	Cochrane Central Register of Controlled Trials
CLT	Cards and Lottery Task
DBT	Dialectical Behaviour Therapy
DERS-16	Difficulties in Emotion Regulation Scale
DIVA 2.0	2nd version of the Diagnostic Interview for ADHD in adults

DSM-IV	Diagnostic and Statistical Manual of Mental Disorders, Fourth Edition
EAT-40	Eating Attitude Test
ED	eating disorder
EES	Emotional Eating Scale
EHQ-ES	Revised Questionnaire of Eating and Weight patterns
EI	Eating Inventory
EPQ	Eating Pattern Questionnaire
F9.0	ICD-10 code denoting ADHD
GFCQ-T	General Food Cravings Questionnaire-Trait
HADS	Hospital Anxiety and Depression Scale
ICD-10	International Classification of Diseases, 10th Revision
K-SADS-E	Schedule for Affective Disorders and Schizophrenia module f or ADHD, adapted for adults
MINI	Mini-International Neuropsychiatric Interview
n	number of participants
N/a	not applicable
N.S	not significant
N06BA	ICD-10 code denoting Central Nervous System Stimulants
NEQ	Nighttime Eating Questionnaire
OP	Obesity-related Problems
OSF	Open Science Framework
PDI	Perceived Difficulty Index
PEACE	Pathway for Eating Disorders and Autism developed from Clinical Experience
PRISMA	Preferred Reporting Items for Systematic Reviews and Meta-Analyses
PROSPERO	International database of systematic review protocols
RYGB	Roux-en-Y Gastric Bypass
SCID-5	Structured Clinical Interview for DSM-5 Clinician Version
SCL-90	Symptom Checklist-90
SD	standard deviation
SF-36	36-item Short Form Health Survey
ST	Stroop Test
STAI	State-Trait Anxiety Inventory
TAS-20	Toronto Alexithymia Scale-20
TCI	Temperament and Character Inventory
USA	United States of America
WALI	Weight and Lifestyle Inventory
WEL	Weight Lifestyle Self-Efficacy
WURS-25	short-version of the Wender Utah Rating Scale
YFAS 2.0	Yale Food Addiction Scale

References

1. Zwennes, C.T.; Loth, C.A. "Moments of Failure": Coping With Attention Deficit Hyperactivity Disorder, Sleep Deprivation, and Being Overweight: A Qualitative Hermeneutic–Phenomenological Investigation Into Participant Perspectives. *J. Addict. Nurs.* **2019**, *30*, 185–192. [CrossRef] [PubMed]
2. Healy, S.; Pacanowski, C.; Kennedy, L.; Obrusnikova, I. "This cage that I'm stuck inside": Autistic adults' perceptions of weight management, body weight, and body image. *Autism* **2021**, *25*, 1985–1998. [CrossRef] [PubMed]
3. Cortese, S.; Peñalver, C.M. Comorbidity between ADHD and obesity: Exploring shared mechanisms and clinical implications. *Postgrad. Med.* **2010**, *122*, 88–96. [CrossRef] [PubMed]
4. Cortese, S.; Castellanos, F.X. The relationship between ADHD and obesity: Implications for therapy. *Expert Rev. Neurother.* **2014**, *14*, 473–479. [CrossRef]
5. Tchanturia, K.; Dandil, Y.; Li, Z.; Smith, K.; Leslie, M.; Byford, S. A novel approach for autism spectrum condition patients with eating disorders: Analysis of treatment cost-savings. *Eur. Eat. Disord. Rev.* **2021**, *29*, 514–518. [CrossRef]
6. APA. *Diagnostic and Statistical Manual of Mental Disorders: DSM-5*; American Psychiatric Association: Washington, DC, USA, 2013; Volume 5.

7. Kinnaird, E.; Norton, C.; Pimblett, C.; Stewart, C.; Tchanturia, K. Eating as an autistic adult: An exploratory qualitative study. *PLoS ONE* **2019**, *14*, e0221937. [CrossRef]
8. Nimbley, E.; Golds, L.; Sharpe, H.; Gillespie-Smith, K.; Duffy, F. Sensory processing and eating behaviours in autism: A systematic review. *Eur. Eat. Disord. Rev.* **2022**, *30*, 538–559. [CrossRef] [PubMed]
9. Bottema-Beutel, K.; Kapp, S.K.; Lester, J.N.; Sasson, N.J.; Hand, B.N. Avoiding ableist language: Suggestions for autism researchers. *Autism Adulthood* **2021**, *3*, 18–29. [CrossRef]
10. Kenny, L.; Hattersley, C.; Molins, B.; Buckley, C.; Povey, C.; Pellicano, E. Which terms should be used to describe autism? Perspectives from the UK autism community. *Autism* **2016**, *20*, 442–462. [CrossRef] [PubMed]
11. Pineo, E. "But the Bumpies Hurt!": Autism and the Importance of Identity-first Language. *Incl. Disabil.* **2022**. [CrossRef]
12. Crane, L.; Batty, R.; Adeyinka, H.; Goddard, L.; Henry, L.A.; Hill, E.L. Autism diagnosis in the United Kingdom: Perspectives of autistic adults, parents and professionals. *J. Autism Dev. Disord.* **2018**, *48*, 3761–3772. [CrossRef] [PubMed]
13. Lockwood Estrin, G.; Milner, V.; Spain, D.; Happé, F.; Colvert, E. Barriers to autism spectrum disorder diagnosis for young women and girls: A systematic review. *Rev. J. Autism Dev. Disord.* **2021**, *8*, 454–470. [CrossRef]
14. NHS. Autism Statistics, October 2022 to September 2023. Autism Waiting Time Statistics. 2023. Available online: https://digital.nhs.uk/data-and-information/publications/statistical/autism-statistics/october-2022-to-september-2023# (accessed on 8 March 2024).
15. Li, Z.; Halls, D.; Byford, S.; Tchanturia, K. Autistic characteristics in eating disorders: Treatment adaptations and impact on clinical outcomes. *Eur. Eat. Disord. Rev.* **2022**, *30*, 671–690. [CrossRef] [PubMed]
16. Hudson, C.C.; Bajwa, H.E.; Beard, C.; Björgvinsson, T. Psychometric properties of the 10-item Autism Quotient in an acute psychiatric sample. *Res. Autism Spectr. Disord.* **2024**, *110*, 102299. [CrossRef]
17. Babb, C.; Brede, J.; Jones, C.R.; Elliott, M.; Zanker, C.; Tchanturia, K.; Serpell, L.; Mandy, W.; Fox, J.R. "It's not that they don't want to access the support... it's the impact of the autism': The experience of eating disorder services from the perspective of autistic women, parents and healthcare professionals. *Autism* **2021**, *25*, 1409–1421. [CrossRef] [PubMed]
18. Zhang, R.; Birgegård, A.; Fundín, B.; Landén, M.; Thornton, L.M.; Bulik, C.M.; Dinkler, L. Association of autism diagnosis and polygenic scores with eating disorder severity. *Eur. Eat. Disord. Rev.* **2022**, *30*, 442–458. [CrossRef] [PubMed]
19. Babb, C.; Brede, J.; Jones, C.R.; Serpell, L.; Mandy, W.; Fox, J. A comparison of the eating disorder service experiences of autistic and non-autistic women in the UK. *Eur. Eat. Disord. Rev.* **2022**, *30*, 616–627. [CrossRef] [PubMed]
20. Kinnaird, E.; Norton, C.; Stewart, C.; Tchanturia, K. Same behaviours, different reasons: What do patients with co-occurring anorexia and autism want from treatment? *Int. Rev. Psychiatry* **2019**, *31*, 308–317. [CrossRef]
21. Nazar, B.P.; Peynenburg, V.; Rhind, C.; Hibbs, R.; Schmidt, U.; Gowers, S.; Macdonald, P.; Goddard, E.; Todd, G.; Micali, N.; et al. An examination of the clinical outcomes of adolescents and young adults with broad autism spectrum traits and autism spectrum disorder and anorexia nervosa: A multi centre study. *Int. J. Eat. Disord.* **2018**, *51*, 174–179. [CrossRef] [PubMed]
22. Nimbley, E.; Maloney, E.; Sharpe, H.; Gillespie-Smith, K.; Tchanturia, K.; Duffy, F. A mixed method systematic review into the impact of ED treatment in Autistic people and those with high Autistic traits. *Int. J. Eat. Disord.* **2024**, *58*, 117–138. [CrossRef]
23. Li, Y.J.; Xie, X.N.; Lei, X.; Li, Y.M.; Lei, X. Global prevalence of obesity, overweight and underweight in children, adolescents and adults with autism spectrum disorder, attention-deficit hyperactivity disorder: A systematic review and meta-analysis. *Obes. Rev.* **2020**, *21*, e13123. [CrossRef]
24. Zheng, Z.; Zhang, L.; Li, S.; Zhao, F.; Wang, Y.; Huang, L.; Huang, J.; Zou, R.; Qu, Y.; Mu, D. Association among obesity, overweight and autism spectrum disorder: A systematic review and meta-analysis. *Sci. Rep.* **2017**, *7*, 11697. [CrossRef] [PubMed]
25. Sedgewick, F.; Leppanen, J.; Tchanturia, K. Autistic adult outcomes on weight and body mass index: A large-scale online study. *Eat. Weight Disord.-Stud. Anorex. Bulim. Obes.* **2020**, *25*, 795–801. [CrossRef]
26. Gilmore, D.G.; Longo, A.; Hand, B.N. The Association Between Obesity and Key Health or Psychosocial Outcomes Among Autistic Adults: A Systematic Review. *J. Autism Dev. Disord.* **2022**, *52*, 4035–4043. [CrossRef] [PubMed]
27. Cortese, S.; Bernardina, B.D.; Mouren, M.-C. Attention-deficit/hyperactivity disorder (ADHD) and binge eating. *Nutr. Rev.* **2007**, *65*, 404–411. [CrossRef]
28. Ptacek, R.; Stefano, G.B.; Weissenberger, S.; Akotia, D.; Raboch, J.; Papezova, H.; Stepankova, T.; Goetz, M.; Domkarova, L. Attention deficit hyperactivity disorder and disordered eating behaviors: Links, risks, and challenges faced. *Neuropsychiatr. Dis. Treat.* **2016**, *12*, 571–579. [CrossRef] [PubMed]
29. El Archi, S.; Cortese, S.; Ballon, N.; Réveillère, C.; De Luca, A.; Barrault, S.; Brunault, P. Negative affectivity and emotion dysregulation as mediators between ADHD and disordered eating: A systematic review. *Nutrients* **2020**, *12*, 3292. [CrossRef] [PubMed]
30. Cortese, S.; Angriman, M.; Maffeis, C.; Isnard, P.; Konofal, E.; Lecendreux, M.; Purper-Ouakil, D.; Vincenzi, B.; Bernardina, B.D.; Mouren, M.-C. Attention-deficit/hyperactivity disorder (ADHD) and obesity: A systematic review of the literature. *Crit. Rev. Food Sci. Nutr.* **2008**, *48*, 524–537. [CrossRef]

31. Cortese, S.; Vincenzi, B. Obesity and ADHD: Clinical and neurobiological implications. In *Behavioral Neuroscience of Attentio Deficit Hyperactivity Disorder and Its Treatment*; Springer: Berlin/Heidelberg, Germany, 2012; pp. 199–218.
32. Cortese, S.; Angriman, M. Attention-deficit/hyperactivity disorder, iron deficiency, and obesity: Is there a link? *Postgrad. Me* **2014**, *126*, 155–170. [CrossRef]
33. Cortese, S.; Moreira-Maia, C.R.; St Fleur, D.; Morcillo-Peñalver, C.; Rohde, L.A.; Faraone, S.V. Association between ADHD an obesity: A systematic review and meta-analysis. *Am. J. Psychiatry* **2016**, *173*, 34–43. [CrossRef] [PubMed]
34. Cortese, S.; Tessari, L. Attention-deficit/hyperactivity disorder (ADHD) and obesity: Update 2016. *Curr. Psychiatry Rep.* **2017**, *1* 1–15. [CrossRef] [PubMed]
35. Hanć, T.; Cortese, S. Attention deficit/hyperactivity-disorder and obesity: A review and model of current hypotheses explainin their comorbidity. *Neurosci. Biobehav. Rev.* **2018**, *92*, 16–28. [CrossRef] [PubMed]
36. Caci, H.; Chierici, A.; Iannelli, A. Attention-deficit/hyperactivity disorder in adolescent and adult candidates for metabolic an bariatric surgery: A systematic review and meta-analysis. *Obes. Rev.* **2024**, *25*, e13802. [CrossRef]
37. Guner, S.T.; Göker, Z.; Üneri, Ö.Ş. Comorbidity of Attention Deficit and Hyperactivity Disorder and Obesity: A Systemati Review. *Psikiyatr. Guncel Yaklasimlar* **2019**, *11*, 466–482.
38. Racicka, E. Correlations between attention deficit hyperactivity disorder and obesity-a systematic review of the literatur *Psychiatr. Pol.* **2013**, *47*, 89–102. [PubMed]
39. Franco, A.R.; Da Fonseca, I.C.; Ribeiro, N.; Nova, V.V.; Gamito, A. Neurobiological correlation between attentio deficit/hyperactivity disorder and obesity. *Eur. Psychiatry* **2021**, *64*, S238. [CrossRef]
40. de Velasco, R.M.; Barbudo, E.; Perez-Templado, J.; Silveira, B.; Quintero, J. Review of the association between obesity and ADHI *Actas Esp. Psiquiatr.* **2015**, *43*, 16–23.
41. Seymour, K.E.; Reinblatt, S.P.; Benson, L.; Carnell, S. Overlapping neurobehavioral circuits in ADHD, obesity, and binge eatin Evidence from neuroimaging research. *CNS Spectr.* **2015**, *20*, 401–411. [CrossRef] [PubMed]
42. Davis, C. Attention-deficit/hyperactivity disorder: Associations with overeating and obesity. *Curr. Psychiatry Rep.* **2010**, *1* 389–395. [CrossRef] [PubMed]
43. Pagoto, S.; Curtin, C.; Appelhans, B.M.; Alonso-Alonso, M. Attention deficit/hyperactivity disorder and the clinical managemer of obesity. *Curr. Obes. Rep.* **2012**, *1*, 80–86. [CrossRef]
44. Mocanu, V.; Tavakoli, I.; MacDonald, A.; Dang, J.T.; Switzer, N.; Birch, D.W.; Karmali, S. The impact of ADHD on outcome following bariatric surgery: A systematic review and meta-analysis. *Obes. Surg.* **2019**, *29*, 1403–1409. [CrossRef]
45. Aromataris, E.; Munn, Z. JBI Manual for Evidence Synthesis. JBI. 2020. Available online: https://jbi-global-wiki.refined.site space/MANUAL (accessed on 26 January 2025). [CrossRef]
46. Makin, L.; Zesch, E.; Meyer, A.; Mondelli, V.; Tchanturia, K. Autism, ADHD, and Their Traits in Adults with Bulimia Nervosa an Binge Eating Disorder: A Scoping Review. *Eur. Eat. Disord. Rev.* **2025**. [CrossRef] [PubMed]
47. Tricco, A.C.; Lillie, E.; Zarin, W.; O'Brien, K.K.; Colquhoun, H.; Levac, D.; Moher, D.; Peters, M.D.; Horsley, T.; Weeks, L et al. PRISMA extension for scoping reviews (PRISMA-ScR): Checklist and explanation. *Ann. Intern. Med.* **2018**, *169*, 467–47 [CrossRef] [PubMed]
48. Haddaway, N.R.; Page, M.J.; Pritchard, C.C.; McGuinness, L.A. PRISMA2020: An R package and Shiny app for producin PRISMA 2020-compliant flow diagrams, with interactivity for optimised digital transparency and Open Synthesis. *Campbell Sys Rev.* **2022**, *18*, e1230. [CrossRef]
49. Akcan, G.; Uğraş, S.; Cömert, I.T.; Yükseloğlu, H.; İşlek, D.; Tutkun, E. Investigation of the Relationship between Food Addictio and Anxiety, Depression and Attention Deficit/Hyperactivity in Obese and Non-Obese. *Prog. Nutr.* **2021**, *23*. [CrossRef]
50. Alfonsson, S.; Parling, T.; Ghaderi, A. Screening of adult ADHD among patients presenting for bariatric surgery. *Obes. Surg.* **201** *22*, 918–926. [CrossRef]
51. Alfonsson, S.; Parling, T.; Ghaderi, A. Self-reported symptoms of adult attention deficit hyperactivity disorder among obes patients seeking bariatric surgery and its relation to alcohol consumption, disordered eating and gender. *Clin. Obes.* **2013**, 124–131. [CrossRef]
52. Alfonsson, S.; Sundbom, M.; Ghaderi, A. Is age a better predictor of weight loss one year after gastric bypass than symptoms o disordered eating, depression, adult ADHD and alcohol consumption? *Eat. Behav.* **2014**, *15*, 644–647. [CrossRef]
53. Altfas, J.R. Prevalence of attention deficit/hyperactivity disorder among adults in obesity treatment. *BMC Psychiatry* **2002**, *2*, [CrossRef] [PubMed]
54. Azran, C.; Langguth, P.; Dahan, A. Impaired oral absorption of methylphenidate after Roux-en-Y gastric bypass. *Surg. Obes Relat. Dis.* **2017**, *13*, 1245–1247. [CrossRef]
55. Brancati, G.; Barbuti, M.; Weiss, F.; Calderone, A.; Santini, F.; Perugi, G. Attention-deficit/hyperactivity disorder (ADHD) in adul obese patients referred to bariatric surgery. *Eur. Psychiatry* **2022**, *65*, S385. [CrossRef]

56. Brancati, G.E.; Cosentino, V.; Barbuti, M.; Weiss, F.; Calderone, A.; Fierabracci, P.; Salvetti, G.; Santini, F.; Perugi, G. Prevalence and Correlates of Self-Reported ADHD Symptoms in Bariatric Patients: Focus on Mood and Anxiety Comorbidity, Disordered Eating, and Temperamental Traits. *Obes. Surg.* **2024**, *34*, 3335–3347. [CrossRef] [PubMed]
57. Brunault, P.; Frammery, J.; Montaudon, P.; De Luca, A.; Hankard, R.; Ducluzeau, P.H.; Cortese, S.; Ballon, N. Adulthood and childhood ADHD in patients consulting for obesity is associated with food addiction and binge eating, but not sleep apnea syndrome. *Appetite* **2019**, *136*, 25–32. [CrossRef] [PubMed]
58. Crowley, B.; Howe, Y.J.; McDougle, C.J. Topiramate for weight loss in two young adult women with autism spectrum disorder. *J. Child Adolesc. Psychopharmacol.* **2015**, *25*, 183–185. [CrossRef] [PubMed]
59. Davis, C.; Patte, K.; Levitan, R.D.; Carter, J.; Kaplan, A.S.; Zai, C.; Reid, C.; Curtis, C.; Kennedy, J.L. A psycho-genetic study of associations between the symptoms of binge eating disorder and those of attention deficit (hyperactivity) disorder. *J. Psychiatr. Res.* **2009**, *43*, 687–696. [CrossRef] [PubMed]
60. Dempsey, A.; Dyehouse, J.; Schafer, J. The relationship between executive function, AD/HD, overeating, and obesity. *West. J. Nurs. Res.* **2011**, *33*, 609–629. [CrossRef] [PubMed]
61. Dickinson, K.; Parmar, P.; Reyes, A.B.; Hale, E.W. Bariatric Surgery Is Highly Effective and Underutilized in Patients with ADHD: A 5-Year Retrospective Cohort Study. *Obes. Surg.* **2024**, *34*, 2066–2072. [CrossRef]
62. Docet, M.F.; Larranaga, A.; Fernandez Sastre, J.L.; Garcia-Mayor, R.V. High rate of attention deficit hyperactivity disorder in obese adults: A case-control study. *Obes. Metab.* **2010**, *6*, 121–124.
63. Docet, M.; Larranaga, A.; Perez Mendez, L.; Garcia-Mayor, R. Attention deficit hyperactivity disorder increases the risk of having abnormal eating behaviours in obese adults. *Eat. Weight Disord.-Stud. Anorex. Bulim. Obes.* **2012**, *17*, e132–e136. [CrossRef] [PubMed]
64. El Archi, S.; Brunault, P.; De Luca, A.; Cortese, S.; Hankard, R.; Bourbao-Tournois, C.; Ballon, N.; Réveillère, C.; Barrault, S. Do emotion dysregulation, alexithymia and personality dimensions explain the association between attention-deficit/hyperactivity disorder and binge eating among bariatric surgery candidates? *Front. Psychol.* **2021**, *12*, 745857. [CrossRef] [PubMed]
65. Gruss, B.; Mueller, A.; Horbach, T.; Martin, A.; de Zwaan, M. Attention-deficit/hyperactivity disorder in a prebariatric surgery sample. *Eur. Eat. Disord. Rev.* **2012**, *20*, e103–e107. [CrossRef] [PubMed]
66. Järvinen, A.; Laine, M.K.; Tikkanen, R.; Castrén, M.L. Beneficial effects of GLP-1 agonist in a male with compulsive food-related behavior associated with autism. *Front. Psychiatry* **2019**, *10*, 97. [CrossRef]
67. Lagerros, Y.T.; Brandt, L.; Sundbom, M.; Hedberg, J.; Bodén, R. Risk of delayed discharge and reoperation of gastric bypass patients with psychiatric comorbidity—A nationwide cohort study. *Obes. Surg.* **2020**, *30*, 2511–2518. [CrossRef] [PubMed]
68. Levy, L.; Fleming, J.; Klar, D. Treatment of refractory obesity in severely obese adults following management of newly diagnosed attention deficit hyperactivity disorder. *Int. J. Obes.* **2009**, *33*, 326–334. [CrossRef] [PubMed]
69. Marchesi, D.G.; Ciriaco, J.G.M.; Miguel, G.P.S.; Batista, G.A.P.; Cabral, C.P.; Fraga, L.C. Does the Attention Deficit Hyperactivity Disorder interfere with bariatric surgery results? *Rev. Do Colégio Bras. De Cir.* **2017**, *44*, 140–146. [CrossRef] [PubMed]
70. Nazar, B.P.; Pinna, C.M.d.S.; Suwwan, R.; Duchesne, M.; Freitas, S.R.; Sergeant, J.; Mattos, P. ADHD rate in obese women with binge eating and bulimic behaviors from a weight-loss clinic. *J. Atten. Disord.* **2016**, *20*, 610–616. [CrossRef] [PubMed]
71. Nicolau, J.; Ayala, L.; Francés, C.; Sanchís, P.; Zubillaga, I.; Pascual, S.; Fortuny, R.; Masmiquel, L. Are subjects with criteria for adult attention-deficit/hyperactivity disorder doing worse after bariatric surgery? A case-control study. *Nutr. Hosp.* **2015**, *31*, 1052–1058.
72. Nielsen, F.; Georgiadou, E.; Bartsch, M.; Langenberg, S.; Müller, A.; de Zwaan, M. Attention deficit hyperactivity disorder prevalence and correlates pre-and post-bariatric surgery: A comparative cross-sectional study. *Obes. Facts* **2017**, *10*, 1–11. [CrossRef] [PubMed]
73. Pagoto, S.L.; Curtin, C.; Bandini, L.G.; Anderson, S.E.; Schneider, K.L.; Bodenlos, J.S.; Ma, Y. Weight loss following a clinic-based weight loss program among adults with attention deficit/hyperactivity disorder symptoms. *Eat. Weight Disord. -Stud. Anorex. Bulim. Obes.* **2010**, *15*, e166–e172. [CrossRef] [PubMed]
74. Şahan, E.; Zengin Eroğlu, M.; Sertçelik, S. Eating behaviors, depression, and anxiety levels of pre bariatric surgery patients with obesity comorbid with or without Attention deficit and hyperactivity disorder: ADHD or Major Depression? Which is more related with eating behaviors? *Brain Behav.* **2021**, *11*, e01915. [CrossRef]
75. Schäfer, L.; Schmidt, R.; Müller, S.M.; Dietrich, A.; Hilbert, A. The cards and lottery task: Validation of a new paradigm assessing decision making under risk in individuals with severe obesity. *Front. Psychiatry* **2020**, *11*, 690. [CrossRef]
76. Stahel, P.; Nahmias, A.; Sud, S.K.; Lee, S.J.; Pucci, A.; Yousseif, A.; Youseff, A.; Jackson, T.; Urbach, D.R.; Okrainec, A.; et al. EEvaluation of the genetic association between adult obesity and neuropsychiatric disease. *Diabetes* **2019**, *68*, 2235–2246. [CrossRef]
77. Stenberg, E.; Larsson, H.; Marsk, R.; Cao, Y.; Sundbom, M.; Näslund, E. Association between attention deficit hyperactivity disorder and outcomes after metabolic and bariatric surgery: A nationwide propensity-matched cohort study. *Surg. Obes. Relat. Dis.* **2023**, *19*, 92–100. [CrossRef] [PubMed]

78. Taymur, I.; Dilektas, E.; Budak, E.; Gungor, B.B.; Cayci, M.; Akgul, A.I.; Sahin, Z.A.; Askin, R. Relationship between the symptoms of attention deficit hyperactivity disorder in childhood, general psychopathological features, and eating attitudes in patients applying for bariatric surgery. *Bull. Clin. Psychopharmacol.* **2015**, *25*, S90.
79. Taymur, I.; Budak, E.; Onen, S.; Bicer, B.; Dilektaslı, E.; Cayci, M.; Demirci, H.; Gungor, B.B. The Relationship Between Childhood and Adult Attention-Deficit–Hyperactivity Disorder and General Psychopathological Features in Individuals Who Apply for Bariatric Surgery. *Bariatr. Surg. Pract. Patient Care* **2016**, *11*, 116–122. [CrossRef]
80. Ward, M.F. The Wender Utah Rating Scale: An aid in the retrospective diagnosis of childhood attention deficit hyperactivity disorder. *Am. J. Psychiatry* **1993**, *150*, 885. [PubMed]
81. Günay, Ş.; Savran, C.; Aksoy, U.M. Erişkin Dikkat Eksikliği Hiperaktivite Ölçeğinin (Adult ADD/ADHD DSM IV-Based Diagnostic Screening and Rating Scale) Dilsel Eşdeğerlilik, geçerlik güvenirlik ve norm çalişmasi. *Marmara Üniversitesi Atatürk Eğitim Fakültesi Eğitim Bilim. Derg.* **2005**, *21*, 133–150.
82. Abbass, K.; Corbisiero, S.; Stieglitz, R.D. Development and psychometric properties of the ADHD-SCL-90-R screening scale for adult ADHD. *J. Clin. Psychol.* **2021**, *77*, 1428–1442. [CrossRef] [PubMed]
83. Rösler, M. *Homburger ADHS-Skalen für Erwachsene: HASE*; Untersuchungsverfahren zur Syndromalen und Kategorialen Diagnostik der Aufmerksamkeitsdefizit-/Hyperaktivitätsstörung (ADHS); Hogrefe: Göttingen, Germany, 2008.
84. Kessler, R.C.; Adler, L.; Ames, M.; Demler, O.; Faraone, S.; Hiripi, E.; Howes, M.J.; Jin, R.; Secnik, K.; Spencer, T.; et al. The World Health Organization Adult ADHD Self-Report Scale (ASRS): A short screening scale for use in the general population. *Psychol. Med.* **2005**, *35*, 245–256. [CrossRef] [PubMed]
85. Conners, C.; Erhardt, D.; Epstein, J.; Parker, J.; Sitarenios, G.; Sparrow, E. Self-ratings of ADHD symptoms in adults I: Factor structure and normative data. *J. Atten. Disord.* **1999**, *3*, 141–151. [CrossRef]
86. Ramos-Quiroga, J.A.; Nasillo, V.; Richarte, V.; Corrales, M.; Palma, F.; Ibáñez, P.; Michelsen, M.; Van de Glind, G.; Casas, M.; Kooij, J.J.S. Criteria and concurrent validity of DIVA 2.0: A semi-structured diagnostic interview for adult ADHD. *J. Atten. Disord.* **2019**, *23*, 1126–1135. [CrossRef]
87. Endicott, J.; Spitzer, R.L. A diagnostic interview: The schedule for affective disorders and schizophrenia. *Arch. Gen. Psychiatry* **1978**, *35*, 837–844. [CrossRef] [PubMed]
88. Grevet, E.H.; Bau, C.H.; Salgado, C.A.; Ficher, A.; Victor, M.M.; Garcia, C.; Sousa, N.O.; Nerung, L.; Belmonte-de-Abreu, P. Interrater reliability for diagnosis in adults of attention deficit hyperactivity disorder and oppositional defiant disorder using K-SADS-E. *Arq. De Neuro-Psiquiatr.* **2005**, *63*, 307–310. [CrossRef]
89. Sheehan, D.V.; Lecrubier, Y.; Sheehan, K.H.; Amorim, P.; Janavs, J.; Weiller, E.; Hergueta, T.; Balker, R.; Dunbar, G.C. The Mini-International Neuropsychiatric Interview (MINI): The development and validation of a structured diagnostic psychiatric interview for DSM-IV and ICD-10. *J. Clin. Psychiatry* **1998**, *59*, 22–33. [PubMed]
90. First, M.B.; Williams, J.B.; Karg, R.S.; Spitzer, R.L. *User's Guide for the SCID-5-CV Structured Clinical Interview for DSM-5® Disorders: Clinical Version*; American Psychiatric Publishing, Inc.: Washington, DC, USA, 2016.
91. Karlsson, J.; Taft, C.; Sjöström, L.; Torgerson, J.S.; Sullivan, M. Psychosocial functioning in the obese before and after weight reduction: Construct validity and responsiveness of the Obesity-related Problems scale. *Int. J. Obes.* **2003**, *27*, 617–630. [CrossRef] [PubMed]
92. Sullivan, M.; Karlsson, J.; Ware, J.E., Jr. The Swedish SF-36 Health Survey—I. Evaluation of data quality, scaling assumptions, reliability and construct validity across general populations in Sweden. *Soc. Sci. Med.* **1995**, *41*, 1349–1358. [CrossRef]
93. Stanford, M.S.; Mathias, C.W.; Dougherty, D.M.; Lake, S.L.; Anderson, N.E.; Patton, J.H. Fifty years of the Barratt Impulsiveness Scale: An update and review. *Personal. Individ. Differ.* **2009**, *47*, 385–395. [CrossRef]
94. Stroop, J.R. Studies of interference in serial verbal reactions. *J. Exp. Psychol.* **1935**, *18*, 643. [CrossRef]
95. John, O.P.; Donahue, E.M.; Kentle, R.L. Big five inventory. *J. Personal. Soc. Psychol.* **1991**. [CrossRef]
96. Cloninger, C. *The Temperament and Character Inventory (TCI): A Guide to Its Development and Use*; Center for Psychobiology of Personality, Washington University: St. Louis, MI, USA, 1994.
97. Beck, A.T.; Epstein, N.; Brown, G.; Steer, R.A. An inventory for measuring clinical anxiety: Psychometric properties. *J. Consult. Clin. Psychol.* **1988**, *56*, 893. [CrossRef]
98. Zigmond, A.S.; Snaith, R.P. The hospital anxiety and depression scale. *Acta Psychiatr. Scand.* **1983**, *67*, 361–370. [CrossRef] [PubMed]
99. Andrade, L.; Gorenstein, C.; Vieira Filho, A.; Tung, T.C.; Artes, R. Psychometric properties of the Portuguese version of the State-Trait Anxiety Inventory applied to college students: Factor analysis and relation to the Beck Depression Inventory. *Braz. J. Med. Biol. Res.* **2001**, *34*, 367–374. [CrossRef] [PubMed]
100. Derogatis, L.R. *SCL-90-R Revised Manual*; Johns Hopkins University School of Medicine: Baltimore, MA, USA, 1983.
101. Beck, A.; Steer, R.; Hautzinger, M. *Beck-Depressions-Inventar (BDI); Testhandbuch, 1*; Aufl Huber: Bern, Switzerland, 1994.

102. Bjureberg, J.; Ljótsson, B.; Tull, M.; Hedman-Lagerlöf, E.; Sahlin, H.; Lundh, L.-G.; Bjärehed, J.; DiLillo, D.; Messmanmoore, T.L.; Gumpert, C.H.; et al. Development and validation of a brief version of the difficulties in emotion regulation scale: The DERS-16. *J. Psychopathol. Behav. Assess.* **2016**, *38*, 284–296. [CrossRef]
103. Loas, G.; Fremaux, D.; Marchand, M. Étude de la structure factorielle et de la cohérence interne de la version française de l'échelle d'alexithymie de Toronto à 20 items (TAS-20) chez un groupe de 183 sujets sains. *L'Encéphale: Rev. Psychiatr. Clin. Biol. Et Thérapeutique* **1995**, *21*, 117–122.
104. Saunders, J.B.; Aasland, O.G.; Babor, T.F.; de la Fuente, J.R.; Grant, M. Development of the Alcohol Use Disorders Identification Test (AUDIT): WHO Collaborative Project on Early Detection of Persons with Harmful Alcohol Consumption—II. *Addiction* **1993**, *88*, 791–804. [CrossRef] [PubMed]
105. García Díaz, E.; Martín Folgueras, T.; Morcillo Herrera, L.; Jiménez Sosa, A. Valoración diagnóstica y psicopatológica del trastorno por atracón en obesos mórbidos intervenidos de bypass gástrico. *Nutr. Hosp.* **2012**, *27*, 553–557.
106. Henderson, M.; Freeman, C. A self-rating scale for bulimia the 'BITE'. *Br. J. Psychiatry* **1987**, *150*, 18–24. [CrossRef] [PubMed]
107. Greeno, C.G.; Marcus, M.D.; Wing, R.R. Diagnosis of binge eating disorder: Discrepancies between a questionnaire and clinical interview. *Int. J. Eat. Disord.* **1995**, *17*, 153–160. [CrossRef] [PubMed]
108. Garner, D.M.; Garfinkel, P.E. The Eating Attitudes Test: An index of the symptoms of anorexia nervosa. *Psychol. Med.* **1979**, *9*, 273–279. [CrossRef]
109. Larrañaga Vidal, A.; García-Mayor, R. Alta frecuencia de trastornos de la conducta alimentaria inespecíficos en personas obesas. *Nutr. Hosp.* **2009**, *24*, 661–666.
110. Stunkard, A.J.; Messick, S. Eating Inventory [Database Record]. APA PsycTests. 1988. Available online: https://psycnet.apa.org/doiLanding?doi=10.1037/t15085-000 (accessed on 26 January 2025). [CrossRef]
111. Nijs, I.M.; Franken, I.H.; Muris, P. The modified Trait and State Food-Cravings Questionnaires: Development and validation of a general index of food craving. *Appetite* **2007**, *49*, 38–46. [CrossRef] [PubMed]
112. Arnow, B.; Kenardy, J.; Agras, W.S. The Emotional Eating Scale: The development of a measure to assess coping with negative affect by eating. *Int. J. Eat. Disord.* **1995**, *18*, 79–90. [CrossRef]
113. Gearhardt, A.N.; Corbin, W.R.; Brownell, K.D. Development of the Yale Food Addiction Scale Version 2.0. *Psychol. Addict. Behav.* **2016**, *30*, 113. [CrossRef] [PubMed]
114. Allison, K.C.; Lundgren, J.D.; O'Reardon, J.P.; Martino, N.S.; Sarwer, D.B.; Wadden, T.A.; Crosby, R.D.; Engel, S.G.; Stunkard, A.J. The Night Eating Questionnaire (NEQ): Psychometric properties of a measure of severity of the Night Eating Syndrome. *Eat. Behav.* **2008**, *9*, 62–72. [CrossRef]
115. Clark, M.M.; Abrams, D.B.; Niaura, R.S.; Eaton, C.A.; Rossi, J.S. Self-efficacy in weight management. *J. Consult. Clin. Psychol.* **1991**, *59*, 739. [CrossRef]
116. Wadden, T.A.; Foster, G.D. Weight and lifestyle inventory (WALI). *Obes. Res.* **2006**, *14*, 99S. [CrossRef] [PubMed]
117. Nimbley, E.; Gillespie-Smith, K.; Duffy, F.; Maloney, E.; Ballantyne, C.; Sharpe, H. "It's not about wanting to be thin or look small, it's about the way it feels": An IPA analysis of social and sensory differences in autistic and non-autistic individuals with anorexia and their parents. *J. Eat. Disord.* **2023**, *11*, 89. [CrossRef]
118. Russell, A.E.; Ford, T.; Williams, R.; Russell, G. The association between socioeconomic disadvantage and attention deficit/hyperactivity disorder (ADHD): A systematic review. *Child Psychiatry Hum. Dev.* **2016**, *47*, 440–458. [CrossRef]
119. Iguacel, I.; Villanueva, D.N.; Antón-Solanas, I.; Moreno, L.A. Social determinants and obesogenic environment. In *Childhood Obesity*; Elsevier: Amsterdam, The Netherlands, 2025; pp. 157–187.
120. Krauss, A.; Schellenberg, C. ADHD symptoms and health-related quality of life of adolescents and young adults. *Eur. J. Health Psychol.* **2022**, *29*, 165–174. [CrossRef]
121. Agnew-Blais, J.C.; Polanczyk, G.V.; Danese, A.; Wertz, J.; Moffitt, T.E.; Arseneault, L. Young adult mental health and functional outcomes among individuals with remitted, persistent and late-onset ADHD. *Br. J. Psychiatry* **2018**, *213*, 526–534. [CrossRef]
122. Meyer, J.; Zetterqvist, V.; Unenge Hallerbäck, M.; Ramklint, M.; Isaksson, J. Moderators of long-term treatment outcome when comparing two group interventions for adolescents with ADHD: Who benefits more from DBT-based skills training? *BMC Psychiatry* **2022**, *22*, 767. [CrossRef] [PubMed]
123. Mota, N.R.; Poelmans, G.; Klein, M.; Torrico, B.; Fernàndez-Castillo, N.; Cormand, B.; Reif, A.; Franke, B.; Vásquez, A.A. Cross-disorder genetic analyses implicate dopaminergic signaling as a biological link between Attention-Deficit/Hyperactivity Disorder and obesity measures. *Neuropsychopharmacology* **2020**, *45*, 1188–1195. [CrossRef]
124. Kao, T.S.A.; Ling, J.; Alanazi, M.; Atwa, A.; Liu, S. Effects of mindfulness-based interventions on obesogenic eating behaviors: A systematic review and meta-analysis. *Obes. Rev.* **2024**, *26*, e13860. [CrossRef] [PubMed]
125. Kaur, T.; Ranjan, P.; Kaloiya, G.S.; Bhatia, H.; Prakash, B.; Singh, A.; Sarkar, S.; Jadon, R.S.; Jorwal, P.; Baitha, U. Effectiveness of cognitive retraining intervention on weight loss and lifestyle-related behaviours among adults: A systematic review and meta-analysis. *Diabetes Metab. Syndr. Clin. Res. Rev.* **2024**, *18*, 102969. [CrossRef] [PubMed]

126. Faheem, M.; Akram, W.; Akram, H.; Khan, M.A.; Siddiqui, F.A.; Majeed, I. Gender-based differences in prevalence and effects ADHD in adults: A systematic review. *Asian J. Psychiatry* **2022**, *75*, 103205. [CrossRef] [PubMed]
127. Napolitano, A.; Schiavi, S.; La Rosa, P.; Rossi-Espagnet, M.C.; Petrillo, S.; Bottino, F.; Tagliente, E.; Longo, D.; Lupi, E.; Casula, L et al. Sex differences in autism spectrum disorder: Diagnostic, neurobiological, and behavioral features. *Front. Psychiatry* **2022**, 1 889636. [CrossRef]
128. Guagliardo, S.; Lundberg, M.; Schork, A.; Cox, N.; Shuey, M. Evaluating the Impact of Biological Sex on Adhd Presentatio Prevalence, and Genetic Risk. *Eur. Neuropsychopharmacol.* **2024**, *87*, 30. [CrossRef]

nutrients

MDPI

Review

Enteral Tube Nutrition in Anorexia Nervosa and Atypical Anorexia Nervosa and Outcomes: A Systematic Scoping Review

Namrata Dhopatkar [1,*], Johanna L. Keeler [2], Davide Gravina [2,3], Jacinda Gower [1,4], Hiba Mutwalli [2,5], Sevgi Bektas [2,6], Sarah J. Fuller [7,8], Hubertus Himmerich [1,2] and Janet Treasure [2,*]

1 South London and Maudsley NHS Foundation Trust, London SE5 8AZ, UK; hubertus.himmerich@kcl.ac.uk (H.H.)
2 Centre for Research in Eating and Weight Disorders, Institute of Psychiatry, Psychology and Neuroscience, King's College, London SE5 8AF, UK; johanna.keeler@kcl.ac.uk (J.L.K.); davide.gravina@kcl.ac.uk (D.G.); hiba.mutwalli@kcl.ac.uk (H.M.); sevgi.bektas1@kcl.ac.uk (S.B.)
3 Department of Clinical and Experimental Medicine, University of Pisa, 56127 Pisa, Italy
4 South West London and St George's Mental Health NHS Trust, London SW17 0YF, UK; jacinda.gower@swlstg.nhs.uk
5 Department of Clinical Nutrition, College of Applied Medical Sciences, Imam Abdulrahman Bin Faisal University, Dammam 31441, Saudi Arabia
6 Department of Psychology, Hacettepe University, Ankara 06800, Türkiye
7 Northamptonshire Healthcare NHS Foundation Trust, Northampton NN15 7PW, UK; sarah.fuller@nhs.net
8 Department of Brain Sciences, Imperial College London, London SW7 2AZ, UK
* Correspondence: namrata.dhopatkar@slam.nhs.uk (N.D.); janet.treasure@kcl.ac.uk (J.T.)

Abstract: Background: Anorexia nervosa and atypical anorexia nervosa require refeeding as a core part of their treatment, and enteral tube nutrition (ETN) may be needed in some individuals either to supplement or replace oral nutrition. This scoping review aimed to explore outcomes associated with phases of ETN, including initial nutrition, transition from enteral nutrition to oral intake, and to overall nutrition; **Methods**: The Preferred Reporting Items for Systematic Reviews and Meta-Analyses extension for scoping reviews checklist was used. A systematic search was performed using the Ovid and the Web of Science databases, using relevant search terms identifying 37 studies to be included in the review. Quantitative and qualitative data were synthesised and presented; **Results**: ETN resulted in similar or higher weight gain than oral nutrition. Refeeding syndrome parameters were comparable between ETN and oral nutrition with some indication that prophylactic phosphate supported mitigation of hypophosphataemia. Global psychological parameters related to the eating disorder improved with nutrition; however, there was an indication that weight and shape concerns did not improve during this period. There was a lack of evidence related to transition from ETN to oral intake. Qualitative data indicated meanings attached to the tube, suggesting that additional support may be needed for the transition away from the tube. Furthermore, consideration may be required to support individuals in mitigating trauma related to ETN under restraint; **Conclusions**: ETN, when required, is a viable alternative to oral intake. Results indicated the need for further research, especially in the transition from ETN to oral intake with regard to strategies of transition and support, and outcomes related to these strategies.

Keywords: enteral tube nutrition; nasogastric; transition; weaning; anorexia nervosa; atypical anorexia nervosa

1. Introduction

Anorexia nervosa (AN) is an eating disorder characterised by restriction of oral nutrition, resulting in a significantly low weight, along with an associated fear of weight gain and body dysmorphia [1]. It is known to be correlated with significant morbidity and has one of the highest mortality rates among mental health disorders with a standardised mortality ratio of ~5 [2]. Atypical anorexia nervosa (AAN), while characterised by body image fears like AN, does not meet the criteria for significantly low weight. However, AAN is associated with significant weight loss and, like AN, is related to significant medical instability [3]. Nutritional rehabilitation, to reduce risk and promote health, is key in the treatment of AN and AAN, typically through oral nutritional support [4], which would include regular food intake, and oral nutritional supplement (ONS) drinks if needed. However, as food restriction is part of both illnesses, it may be difficult for sufferers to accept oral nutrition; therefore, nutrition via other means, such as enteral tube nutrition (ETN), may be required. ETN may also be used in mitigating the risks of medical instability, especially while reintroducing nutrition, and may be used for those deemed most at risk [5] or as part of a protocol for those needing to be admitted for refeeding [6]. In situations where ETN is refused, there may be a need for its compulsory administration as a way of reducing the risk to life, with the use of appropriate legal means [5].

When required in AN or AAN, ETN is typically administered via a nasogastric (NG) tube that delivers liquid nutrition directly into the stomach. However, other tubes may be used occasionally; for instance, the percutaneous endoscopic gastrostomy (PEG) tube—a more permanently placed tube delivering nutrition to the stomach. NG tubes have the disadvantage of a higher likelihood of displacement, especially with tube tampering (for example, an individual attempting tube removal) or with vomiting. Additionally, the use of a NG tube may encourage the competitive element of an eating disorder as a 'visual' symbol of its severity and of the individual's alliance with the eating disorder. A disadvantage of a PEG tube is that it requires an endoscopic procedure with placement across the stomach wall, making it more invasive. Nutrition, typically polymeric formulas (containing whole proteins, carbohydrates, lipids, and micronutrients) or ONS drinks, may be administered in both these tubes in similar ways; for example, as a continuous feed administered via an enteral pump over a defined time period or as 'boluses' akin to meals or snacks. When indicated, for example, in gastroparesis and with significant compensatory or physiological vomiting [5,7], the feed may be administered via tubes placed into the jejunum, such as nasojejunal tubes and gastrostomy tubes with jejunal extensions.

Refeeding an individual who has been restricting their food intake, with or without compensatory behaviours, be it through oral intake (OI) or ETN, involves a shift in the metabolic status from the 'starved' to a 'fed' state, thus increasing their risk of refeeding syndrome (RFS) [8]. With the increased availability of nutrients, a combination of increased blood glucose with a corresponding increase in insulin secretion, electrolyte, and fluid shifts between the extra- and intra-cellular compartments of the body, and an increased need for vitamins involved in metabolic processes can be seen. This may result in features such as hypophosphataemia, hypokalaemia, and hypomagnesemia. Clinical presentation of RFS can range from a combination of features such as oedema, cardiac arrythmias, and cardiac failure which can, on occasion, be fatal [8]. Refeeding hypophosphataemia (RH) has often been used as an indicator of RFS, both being linked with the severity of malnutrition [8]. Various methods have been trialled to mitigate the risk of RFS and its morbidity, including a graded reintroduction of nutrition [9], reducing energy provision through carbohydrates in the initial phase of nutrition [10], and the use of continuous ETN [11]. In restrictive eating disorders, such as AN and AAN, the effects of undernutrition pose a significant physical health risk to individuals; thus, the risk of managing these while also mitigating

RFS risk needs careful consideration. A recent guidance proposes starting refeeding at least at 10–20 kcal/kg/day (1400 kcal/day for those under 18 years old) in those with a high RFS risk, with a steady increase to 60 kcal/kg/day, and careful monitoring of their physical state, to support safe refeeding [5].

ETN use may be considered inevitable in some cases, such as food refusal and medical severity. However, it is important to explore outcomes associated with ETN, including physical health parameters, potential adverse outcomes, length of stay data, psychological parameters, qualitative data, and long-term outcomes to acquire a broader picture of its effects in AN and AAN.

Resistance to nutrition of any kind, be it oral or ETN, may prolong the time spent in the hospital by service users. Conversely, acceptance of ETN by an individual may increase dependence on medicalised nutrition and impair their capacity to take back responsibility for their own nourishment, potentially prolonging an admission and time away from their community. Thus, exploring the nutritional transition from ETN back to OI is of importance.

The outcomes associated with ETN use, its efficacy, and the risks involved in its administration for eating disorders and AN have been previously reviewed [12,13]. The aim of this systematic scoping review is to add to the evidence base by evaluating ETN outcomes in AN and AAN at various stages, including initial refeeding and transition from ETN to OI, to rationalise transition strategies both initially, while starting nutrition, and when weaning from ETN to OI.

2. Methods

This review was conducted based on the Preferred Reporting Items for Systematic Reviews and Meta-Analyses Extension for Scoping Reviews (PRISMA-ScR) checklist [14]. A systematic search was performed utilising the following databases: Embase (Ovid), MEDLINE (Ovid), APA PsycInfo (Ovid), and the Web of Science (WoS) Core Collection from inception until 5th June 2024. A combination of search terms was used, including 'anorexia nervosa' or 'atypical anorexia nervosa' with 'enteral nutrition' or 'nasogastric' or 'tube feeding' or 'gastrostomy' or 'PEG' or '*jejunal' or 'jejunostomy' or 'transition' or 'weaning' or 'refeeding' or 'nutrition* support' or 'nutrition* supplement' or 'meal support' or 'meal based'.

For inclusion in the scoping review, studies had to be (a) original research presenting outcomes related to ETN and (b) in participants with a diagnosis of AN or AAN. Exclusion criteria were (a) case reports, case series, and conference abstracts, (b) studies published in languages other than English, (c) animal studies, (d) reviews, letters, comments, books, and editorials, and (e) studies whose outcomes could not be related to ETN or to the diagnosis of AN or AAN. References were exported to and de-duplicated in EndNote 20 and Rayyan [15].

The initial screening of titles and abstracts for the inclusion and exclusion criteria was undertaken by two researchers independently (ND and DG). Full texts of possible articles were examined, and any difference in opinion was resolved through discussion with supervising authors (JT and HH) and other co-authors. References from relevant articles were also screened to include all pertinent studies. The protocol for the review was registered prospectively on the Open Science Framework (https://doi.org/10.31219/osf.io/2v6jf). While the registered protocol did not specify the search terms '*jejunal', 'jejunostomy', 'PEG' or 'gastrostomy', it was thought to be important to amend the search by adding these terms of possible routes of ETN administration within these eating disorders for the thoroughness of the search.

Data from quantitative and qualitative studies identified as eligible were extracted (ND) and a third of these data were independently verified (JG). The quality of the studies was examined using the Joanna Briggs Institute Critical Appraisal Tools [16,17]. However, as this was a scoping review, all eligible articles were included to explore the breadth of available research. Data extraction was followed by synthesis of information guided by the objectives of the study and emerging categories based on methodology and outcomes studied.

3. Results

Figure 1 illustrates the flowchart of the search methodology to identify eligible studies as per PRISMA guidelines [14]. The original database search yielded 5262 results, and after removing duplicates, 4355 references remained. Titles and abstracts were screened for eligibility, of which 145 articles were deemed eligible for the full-text examination, which yielded 36 eligible studies. One additional study was included from contact with research authors. Thus, 37 studies were identified as eligible for inclusion in the scoping review.

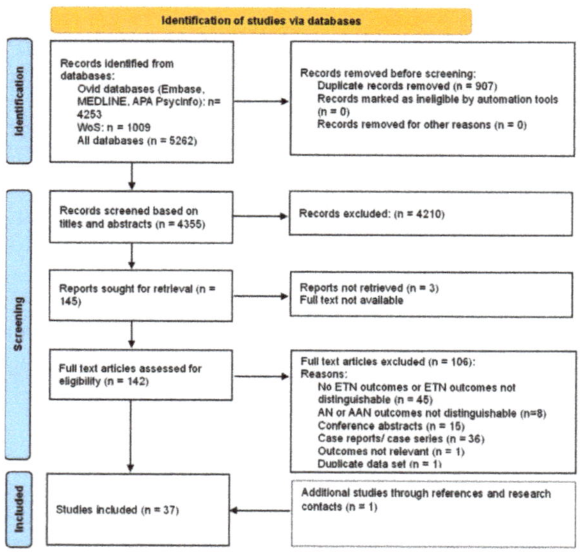

Figure 1. PRISMA flow diagram illustrating the process for study selection.

3.1. Baseline Data and Study Designs

3.1.1. Study and Participant Characteristics

Study and participant characteristics, as well as baseline data from the 37 studies, are presented in Table 1. Study locations included Italy (*n* = 10), Australia (*n* = 8), France (*n* = 8), the USA (*n* = 4), Germany (*n* = 2), the UK (*n* = 2), Canada (*n* = 1), Denmark (*n* =1), and Norway (*n* = 1). Of the 31 quantitative studies, 27 were naturalistic cohorts examining practice within their setting, either as single cohorts with an ETN intervention or multiple cohorts with at least one arm examining an ETN intervention. Four studies followed a randomised controlled trial (RCT) design, of which two compared an ETN arm with an OI arm [18,19], while the other two compared two ETN arms [10,20]. All the quantitative studies except one [19] were conducted in hospital settings. Six studies were of a qualitative design, all of which explored participants' experience of ETN or involuntary treatment with ETN in a hospital setting. Additionally, three studied the views of staff administering ETN [21–23], and two explored carers' views about ETN in their loved ones [22,23].

Of the included studies, 12 were conducted in participants younger than 18 years of age. The combined mean age (SD) of participants (n = 1155) was 14.78 (1.64) years in 10 of these studies. A total of 10 studies were undertaken on those above the age of 18 years. In four of these studies, the combined mean age (SD) of participants (n = 533) was found to be 25.73 (7.8) years. A total of 14 studies were conducted with participants spanning these age categories. In 13 of these studies, the combined mean age (SD) was 22.04 (7.35) years in their participants (n = 1512).

Studies were in predominantly female populations except for one study examining outcomes in male sufferers [24]. All studies included participants diagnosed with AN and four studies included participants with AAN [6,21,25,26]. However, outcomes related to AN and AAN were not reported separately in these studies.

3.1.2. Indications and Methods of ETN

Tables 2–5 provide details of nutritional provision and related outcomes: initially (Table 2), overall (Tables 3 and 4), and during the transition from enteral to oral nutrition in the enteral groups (Table 5), within the quantitative studies. Further details of the initial nutritional protocols and the summary of psychological outcomes are presented in Supplementary Tables S1 and S2, respectively. Methods of ETN administration were heterogeneous. Of the quantitative naturalistic studies, 13 specified administering ETN through continuous feeds, one study reported administration via a bolus method, while 13 did not report a continuous or a bolus method. Three RCTs had ETN arms with a continuous feed [10,18,20], while one did not specify the continuous or bolus method [19]. Of the qualitative studies, two described their participants receiving continuous ETN [21,27]. One study reported a mixture of methods for ETN under restraint [28], two were in participants with lived experience of bolus NG under restraint feeds [22,23] and one did not report on methods of ETN administration [29].

Ten studies [6,10,19,20,30–35], including three RCTs [10,19,20], initially relied on ETN exclusively as part of the protocol in their ETN arms, with the addition of OI over time. One RCT [18] had an ETN arm with some OI from the start. Seven studies, as part of the protocol, encouraged some OI from the start with ETN supplementing nutrition [24,36–41]. Two studies were comparing a protocol change to ETN supplementing OI with a historical protocol with OI only refeeding [24,36]. Nine studies described oral nutritional rehabilitation as first-line, with ONS or ETN used only when required [25,26,42–48].

Nocturnal ETN, as a way of supplementing energy intake while managing gastrointestinal and psychological discomfort, was stated in two studies [24,36]. Nocturnal ETN was also used in studies as a method of transition from exclusive ETN to using ETN as a supplement to OI [10,20,30,31]. Daytime ETN was specified in one study to reduce AN-related hyperactivity [18]. The route of ETN was mainly via a NG tube with one study specifying ETN through a PEG tube [37]. None of the studies specified feeding through a jejunal route.

Six studies examined outcomes related to nutrition administered involuntarily under appropriate legislation in some or all participants [21–23,28,37,42].

Energy prescriptions varied widely in studies. Five studies based in Europe described conservative initial prescriptions with slow increases to the target prescriptions [26,32–35]. Seven had standard initial prescriptions in their ETN arms, between 1200 and 1800 kcal/day, and variable increases during the study to the target prescription, and were mainly based in Europe and North America [6,25,36,38,39,47,49]. Four studies with higher energy prescriptions starting above 1800 kcal/day, with increases to at least 2400 kcal/day, were all based in Australia [10,20,30,31].

Table 1. Study and participant characteristics and baseline data of included studies.

Author, Year *Country*	Objectives	Group Type (Number)	Participant Characteristics				Baseline Anthropometry		Other Baseline Measures/Comments
		Grouping as defined by original study or by route of nutrition	Diagnosis (*tool*), **subtypes**	Gender (%)	Age in years (M ± SD) (*Med ± IQR/range*)	DOI in months (M ± SD) (*Med ± IQR/range*)	Weight (kg, M ± SD) **BMI (kg/m^2, M ± SD)**	% IBW/**EBW**/*mBMI*	(M ± SD) Or (*Med ± IQR/range*)
Randomised trials									
Madden et al., 2015b [20] *Australia*	Comparing outcomes in admissions for med. stab (MS) versus weight restoration (WR)	1. MS w/NG (n = 41) 2. WR w/NG (n = 41)	AN diagnosis (*DSM-4*) **AN-R (n = 57)** **AN-BP (n = 25)**	1. Female/male (95/5%) 2. Female/male (95/5%)	1. 14.89 ± 1.36 2. 14.88 ± 1.56	1. 7.39 ± 5.42 2. 7.85 ± 6.89	NR **NR**	**1. 77.28 ± 6.67** **2. 79.25 ± 5.95**	
Parker et al., 2021 [10] *Australia*	Evaluating refeeding outcomes comparing low vs. standard CHO feed	1. Low CHO feed w/NG (n = 15) 2. Standard CHO feed w/NG (n = 11)	AN diagnosis (*DSM-5*) **NR**	Female (100%)	Overall: 17.5 ± 1.1 1. 17.5 ± 1.3 2. 17.5 ± 0.9	NR	1. 43.7 ± 4.7 2. 45.1 ± 2.8 **1. 16.3 ± 1.7** **2. 16.7 ± 0.9**	*1. 77.8 ± 9.1* *2. 79.3 ± 5.2*	PO4: 1.: 1.18 ± 0.19 mmol/L 2.: 1.11 ± 0.13 mmol/L K: 1.: 3.75 ± 0.44 mmol/L 2.: 3.72 ± 0.32 mmol/L Mg: 1.:0.94 ± 0.09 mmol/L 2.: 0.94 ± 0.05 mmol/L
Rigaud et al., 2007 [18] *France*	Evaluating outcomes comparing NG and oral refeeding	1. NG (n = 41) 2. OI (n = 40)	AN diagnosis (*DSM = 4*) **AN-R (n = 56)** **AN-BP (n = 25)**	1. Female/male (97/3%) 2. Female/male (98/2%)	1. 22.5 ± 4.5 2. 24.2 ± 3.8	*1. 54 ± 22.8* *2. 38.4 ± 24*	1. 34.0 ± 3.9 2. 34.7 ± 4.3 **1. 12.1 ± 1.5** **2. 12.8 ± 2.0**	NR	-
Rigaud et al., 2011b [19] *France*	Comparing binge-purge symptoms in nut rehab with NG nutrition and CBT vs. CBT with OI in BN and AN-BP	1. NG + CBT (n = 52; n AN = 19) 2. OI + CBT (n = 51, n AN = 17)	AN or BN diagnosis (*DSM-IV*) **AN-BP: (n = 36)**	Female (100%)	1. 27.4 ± 8.1 2. 27.9 ± 6.2	1. 117.6 ± 74.4 1. 100.8 ± 64.8	NR **In AN subgroups:** **1. 15.8 ± 1.3** **2. 16.2 ± 1.0**	NR	-
Retrospective cohort studies									
Agostino et al., 2013 [6] *Canada*	Comparing NG versus oral protocols for refeeding	1. NG (n = 31) 2. OI (n = 134)	AN or EDNOS -restrictive form (*DSM IV*) **NR**	1. Female/male (94/6%) 2. Female/male (96/4%)	1. 14.9 ± 2.1 2. 14.9 ± 1.7	NR	NR **1. 16.6 ± 2.2** **2. 16.7 ± 2.3**	1. 82 ± 10 2. 85 ± 13	-
Blikshavn et al., 2020 [42] *Norway*	Evaluating outcomes related to physical restraint in hospital including NG under restraint (NG-R)	1. NG-R (n = 8) 2. No NG-R (n = 30)	AN diagnosis (*DSM-5*) **NR**	Female (89.5%) Male (10.5%)	15.9 ± 1.9	NR	NR **15.2 ± 1.9**	NR	2. No NG-R—study did not specify whether any of this group had NG without restraint
Braude et al., 2020 [46] *Australia*	Evaluating outcomes of a medical stabilisation protocol	1. NG (n = 27) 2. OI (n = 68)	AN diagnosis (*NR*) **AN-R (n = 61)** **AN-BP (n = 34)**	Female (89.5%) Male (10.5%)	*21 (**18–29**)*	NR	NR **17.1 ± 3.8**	-	-

Table 1. *Cont.*

Author, Year *Country*	Objectives	Group Type (Number)	Participant Characteristics				Baseline Anthropometry		Other Baseline Measures/Comments
Bufano et al., 1990 [49] *Italy*	Evaluating outcomes of NG refeeding.	1. NG (n = 9)	AN diagnosis *(DSM III)* **AN-R (n = 9)**	Female (100%)	NR	17.0 ± 14.0	34.51 ± 4.48 **NR**	NR	-
Gentile, 2012 [38] *Italy*	Evaluating outcomes of NG refeeding in BMI ≤ 12	1. NG (n = 10)	AN diagnosis *(DSM-IV-TR)* **NR**	NR	23.9 ± 11.1	56.3 ± 47.7	27.9 ± 3.3 **11.2 ± 0.7**	NR	PO4 ↓- n = 3 (30%)
Gentile et al., 2008 [47] *Italy*	Evaluating outcomes of a refeeding protocol including NG when needed in BMI ≤ 13.5	1. NG (n = 32) 2. OI (n = 67) n = 75 completed study overall, n = 32 (100%) from NG gp, n = 43 (64%) from OI gp	AN diagnosis *(DSM-IV-TR)* **NR**	Female (96%) Male (4%)	1. 21.8 ± 9.1 2. 18.9 ± 6.2	1. 45.6 ± 40.8 2. 36.5 ± 42.0	1. 31.9 ± 4.8 2. 32.7 ± 5.2 **1. 12.3 ± 0.9** **2. 12.8 ± 0.7**	NR	Baseline data from 'completers' of study
Hanachi et al., 2013 [33] *France*	Evaluation of liver function with refeeding including NG	1. ↑ AST/ALT gp w/ETN (n = 54) 2. ↔ AST/ALT gp w/ETN (n = 72)	AN diagnosis *(DSM-IV-TR and 5)* **AN-R (n = 73)** **AN-BP (n = 53)**	Female (93%) Male (7%)	1. 28.0 ± 9.0 2. 32.0 ± 12.0 *	NR	1. 31.5 ± 6.0 2. 33.1 ± 5.0 **1. 11.2 ± 1.7** **2. 12.7 ± 1.7 ***	-	ALT 1.: 174 ± (57–2614) 2.: 49 ± (9–119) * AST: 1.: 133 ± (46–2120) 2.: 27 ± (6–57) * GGT: 1.: 150 ± (17–555) 2. 45 ± (8–233) * ALP: 1.: 128 ± (41–440) 2.: 61 ± (22–122) *
Kells et al., 2022 [25] *USA*	Evaluating factors contributing to RH	1. NG (n = 44) 2. OI (n = 256)	AN or AAN diagnosis *(DSM IV-TR or 5)* **AN-R (n = 255)** **AN-BP (n = 35)** **AAN (n = 6)** **Missing (n = 4)**	Female (88.3%) Male (11.7%)	15.5 ± 2.5	NR	42.8 ± 9.6 **16.3 ± 2.6**	*82 ± 12.1*	
Marchili et al., 2023 [43] *Italy*	Comparing NG nutrition outcomes including those related to the timing of starting NG	1. NG (n = 101) 2. OI (n = 214)	AN diagnosis *(DSM-5)* **NR**	1. Female/male (91/9%) 2. Female/male (88/12%)	Overall: 14.4 ± 1.2 1. 14.6 ± 1.8 2. 14.4 ± 2.3	NR	NR **1. 14.5 ± 1.9** **2. 16.1 ± 2.8 ***	NR	BMI percentile, *median (IQR)*: 1. *0.2 (5.1)* 2. *1.9 (19.5)* *

Table 1. *Cont.*

Author, Year *Country*	Objectives	Group Type (Number)	Participant Characteristics				Baseline Anthropometry		Other Baseline Measures/Comments
Martini et al. 2024 [44] *Italy*	Evaluation of BMI and treatment satisfaction comparing NG and OI	1. NG: (n = 97) 2. OI: (n = 97)	AN diagnosis (DSM 5) **AN-R: (n = 124)** **AN-BP (n = 70)**	Female (100%)	1. NR 2. NR **Overall >18 and <65**	1. 84 ± 108 2. 84 ± 96	1. 37 ± 6 2. 37 ± 5.5 **1. 13.99 ± 1.76** **2. 14.01 ± 1.89**	-	NG and OI group were matched for age, duration of illness, AN subtype, BMI, psychiatric co-morbidities, energy intake, EDE-Q total score and number of hospitalisations via propensity score matching
Nehring et al., 2014 [50] *Germany*	Evaluations of outcomes including longer-term outcomes related to NG nutrition	1. NG (n = 71) 2. OI (n = 137)	AN diagnosis *(ICD 10)* **NR**	Female (100%)	1. 14.3 ± 1.6 2. 15.3 ± 1.6 *	1. 7.9 ± 5.3 2. 12.3 ± 11.3	NR **1. 14.3 ± 1.3** **2. 15.1 ± 1.4 ***	NR	1.: NG during any of their admissions 1. vs. 2. BMI percentiles and BMI s.d scores were comparable
Pruccoli et al., 2021 [51] *Italy*	Evaluating outcomes related to the timing of starting NG and atypical antipsychotics (AAP)	1. Early AAP+ early NG (n = 18) 2. Early AAP + late NG (n = 12) 3. Late AAP + early NG (n = 20) 4. Late AAP + late NG (n = 18) 5. NG only (n = 11)	AN diagnosis *(DSM-5)* **AN-R (n = 78)** **AN-BP (n = 1)**	Female (98.7%) Male (1.3%)	Overall:14.6 ± 2.0 1. 14.7 ± 2.3 2. 14.5 ± 1.8 3. 14.3 ± 1.7 4. 15.2 ± 1.5 5. 14.2 ± 2.0	Overall: 14.8 ± 11.5 1. 15.8 ± 14.3 2. 10.3 ± 6.3 3.12.7 ± 9.3 4. 19.0 ± 13.0 5. 15.0 ± 10.3	NR **Overall:** **13.7 ± 1.7** **1. 14.2 ± 1.9** **2. 13.5 ± 1.6** **3.13.3 ± 1.6** **4. 13.6 ± 1.2** **5. 13.8 ± 1.6**	NR	-
Pruccoli et al., 2022 [52] *Italy*	Comparing 'treatment resistance' (TR-AN) and 'good outcome' (GO-AN) in AN and associations.	1. NG (n = 33) 2. OI (n = 43) Both NG and OI methods used in the TR AN (n = 30) and GO AN (n = 46)	AN diagnosis *(DSM-5)* **AN-R (n = 70)** **AN-BP (n = 6)**	Female (94.7%) Male (5.3%)	14.9 ± 1.9	Overall: 14.2 ± 11 TR AN: 18 ± 14.2 GO AN: 11.7 ± 7.4	NR **Overall:** **14.3 ± 1.7**	NR	EDI 3-EDRC score sig higher in TR-AN than GO-AN
Pruccoli et al., 2024 [26] *Italy*	Evaluating effect of the use of olanzapine on refeeding syndrome (RFS) features	1. NG (n = 44) 2. Other: OI or PN (n = 69) Overall group separated into RFS (n = 46) and no-RFS (n = 67)	AN or AAN diagnosis (DSM-5) **AN-R (n = 103)** **AN-BP (n = 8)** **AAN (n = 2)**	Female (90.3%) Male (9.7%)	*Overall: 15 (3)*	RFS gp: *11 (9)* No RFS gp: *9 (11)*	**RFS gp: *14* (2)** **No RFS gp: *14* (3)**	*RFS gp: 71 ± 10* *No RFS gp: 72 ± 10*	2. PN n = 1 in RFS gp. OI numbers not specified.
Rigaud et al., 2010 [40] *France*	Evaluating the use of low sodium versus standard sodium OI during refeeding	1. Low sodium OI w/NG (n = 176) 2. Standard sodium OI w/NG (n = 42) Both groups—similar NG	AN diagnosis *(DSM-4)* **AN-R (n = 116)** **AN-BP (n = 102)**	Female (98%) Male (2%)	1. 23.3 ± 5.1 2. 22.1 ± 4.2	NR	1. 36 ± 3.8 2. 36.6 ± 4.3 **1. 13.2 ± 1.2** **2. 13.8 ± 1.7**	-	1. vs. 2.: FFM and FM n.s

Table 1. *Cont.*

Author, Year *Country*	Objectives	Group Type (Number)	Participant Characteristics				Baseline Anthropometry		Other Baseline Measures/Comments
Robb et al., 2002 [36] *USA*	Comparing short-term outcomes in NG vs. OI refeeding in female adolescents with AN	1. NG (n = 52) 2. OI (n = 48)	AN diagnosis *(DSM-4)* **NR**	Female (100%)	1. 14.8 ± 1.9 2. 15.0 ± 1.8	NR	1. 41.1 ± 4.7 2. 42.5 ± 7.6 **1. 15.5 ± 1.7** **2. 16.0 ± 1.8**	NR	1. (n = 52/52) + 2. (n = 28/48)—treated in an adolescent. medical unit until medically stable, then psychiatric unit. 2. n = 20/48—treated in the adolescent medical unit with psychiatric. consultation
Silber et al., 2004 [24] *USA*	Comparing outcomes in NG vs. OI refeeding in male adolescents with AN	1. NG (n = 6) 2. OI (n = 8)	AN diagnosis *(DSM-4 male applicable criteria)* **NR**	Male (100%)	1. 13.8 ± 2.0 2. 14.9 ± 1.7	NR	1. 42.9 ± 10.7 2. 46.2 ± 11.0 **1. 15.3 ± 1.7** **2. 17.4 ± 2.3**	NR	
Zuercher et al., 2003 [41] *USA*	Comparing outcomes of NG vs. OI refeeding in AN	1. NG (n = 155) 2. OI (n = 226)	AN diagnosis *(DSM-4)* **AN-R (n = 180)** **AN-BP (n = 201)**	Female (100%)	1. 25.7 ± 9.6 2. 25.2 ± 8.4	1. 105.6 ± 102 2. 104.4 ± 93.6	1. 38.0 ± 5.5 2. 42.1 ± 5.4 **1. 14.2 ± 1.7** **2. 15.7 ± 1.7**	-	Overall cohort recommended NG, but the OI gp declined NG.
Prospective cohort studies									
Born et al., 2015 [37] *Germany*	Evaluating a compulsory refeeding protocol for AN	1. PEG (n = 57) 2. No PEG (n = 11), w/NG (n = 3) and no NG (n = 8)	AN diagnosis *(NR)* **AN-R (n = 32)** **AN-BP (n = 36)**	Female (95.6%) Male (4.4%)	1. 27.2 ± 8.8 2. 22.9 ± 6.1	1. 118.8 ± 84 2. 87.6 ± 66	NR **1. 12.2 ± 1.4** **2. 12.7 ± 1.3**	-	Most participants under 'legal guardianship' during admission
Kezelman et al., 2018 [31] *Australia*	Evaluating anxiety symptoms related to rapid refeeding	1. NG (n = 31)	AN diagnosis *(DSM-5)* **AN-R (n = 24)** **AN-BP (n = 7)**	Female (100%)	16.91 ± 1.1	16.7 ± 21.1	NR **16.31 ± 1.94**	NR	Anxiety disorder comorbidity: n = 20 (64.5%)
Madden et al., 2015a [30] *Australia*	Evaluating outcomes from rapid refeeding in adolescents	1. NG (n = 78)	AN diagnosis *(DSM-4)* **AN-R (n = 53)** **AN-BP (n = 25)**	Female (95%) Male (5%)	14.84 ± 1.46	7.60 ± 6.16	40.99 ± 5.72 **NR**	78.37 ± 6.50	
Minano Garrido et al., 2021 [35] *France*	Evaluating muscle strength and peak expiratory flow (PEF) rate with refeeding in BMI < 13	1. NG (n = 23)	AN diagnosis *(DSM-5)* **AN-R (n = 18)** **AN-BP (n = 5)**	Female (100%)	25.6 ± 6.2	110.4 ± 76.8	NR **11.4 ± 1.3**	-	PEF (L/min): 253.3 ± 60 (N: 418 ± 24.5) Muscle strength Medical Research Council (MRC) score: 37.7 ± 7.7 (N: 60) Axial muscle strength impaired *
Murciano et al., 1994 [39] *France*	Evaluating muscle strength and respiratory and diaphragmatic function with refeeding	1. NG (n = 15)	AN diagnosis *(DSM III revised)* **NR**	Female (100%)	24.9 ± 8.7	NR	37.1 ± 4.7 **13.5 ± 1.1**	63 ± NR	FEV1, % predicted.: 87 ± 17

Table 1. *Cont.*

Author, Year *Country*	**Objectives**	**Group Type (Number)**	**Participant Characteristics**				**Baseline Anthropometry**		**Other Baseline Measures/Comments**
Paccagnella et al., 2006 [32] *Italy*	Evaluating outcomes in NG refeeding when using specific criteria for commencing NG	1. NG (n = 24)	AN diagnosis *(DSM-IV)* **AN-R (n = 19) AN-BP (n = 5)**	Female (100%)	18.5 ± 6.18	NR	33.0 ± NR **12.9 ± NR**	-	Cardiovascular symptoms: n > 60% PO4 and K within range
Rigaud et al., 2011a [48] *France*	Evaluation of long-term outcomes in AN after hospitalisation for refeeding	1. NG (n = 262) 2. OI (n = 222)	AN diagnosis *(DSM-IV)* **AN-R (n = 347) Other (n = 137)**	Female (95.4%) Male (4.6%)	22.8 ± 4.4	42 ± 16.8	NR **12.8 ± 1.6**	-	
Rigaud et al., 2012 [34] *France*	Evaluating outcomes of refeeding in AN with BMIs < 11	1. NG (n = 41)	AN diagnosis *(DSM-IV)* **AN-R (n = 35) Other (n = 6)**	Female (95%) Male (5%)	28.9 ± 5.4	115.2 ± 40.8	25.9 ± 1.4 **10.1 ± 0.57**	-	Low PO4: 17% Low K: 4%
Trovato et al., 2022 [45] *Italy*	Evaluating which refeeding strategy is associated with better outcomes in AN	1. Food only (n = 66) 2. Food + ONS (n = 63) 3. NG + food: (n = 6) 4. NG + food + ONS (n = 51)	AN diagnosis *(DSM-5)* **NR**	Female (89%) Male (11%)	*14 (13–16)*	NR	NR NR	NR	n = 33 (18%)—reasons for admission other than nut. rehab. n = 105 (56.5%)—BMI < 14 kg/m^2; weight loss > 1 kg/week
Qualitative studies									
Fuller et al., 2023 [22] *UK*	Evaluating the impact of NG R for AN treatment	1. Patients (n = 7) 2. Carers (n = 13) 3. Staff (n = 16)	1. AN diagnosis *(NR)* ** **NR**	1. Female (100%) 2. Female (85%), male (15%) 3. Female (69%), male (31%)	*1. NR* ***(19–54)***	*1. NR* ***(36–≥360)***	-	-	1. Lived experience of NG R 2. Carers whose loved ones experienced NG R. 3. Staff involved in NG R decisions and administration.
Fuller et al., 2024 [23] *UK*	Identifying best practice when NG R is needed	1. Patients (n = 7) 2. Carers (n = 13) 3. Staff (n = 16)	1. AN diagnosis *(NR)* ** **NR**	1. Female (100%) 2. Female (85%), male (15%) 3. Female (69%), male (31%)	*1. NR ±* ***19–54***	*1. NR ±* ***36–≥360***	-	-	1. Lived experience of NG R 2. Carers whose loved ones experienced NG R 3. Staff involved in NG R decisions and administration
Halse et al., 2005 [29] *Australia*	Evaluating meanings and perceptions attached to NG	1. Overall (n = 23) n = 17/23 discussed NG	AN diagnosis *(NR)* **NR**	Female (100%)	14.8 ± NR	NR	NS **15.6 ± NS**	-	n = 2: first admission n = 14: 2–5 previous admissions
Kezelman et al., 2016 [27] *Australia*	Evaluating experiences of rapid refeeding	1. NG (n = 10)	AN diagnosis *(DSM-5)* **AN-R (n = 9) AN-BP (n = 1)**	Female (100%)	17.5 ± 0.97	*NR ±* ***1–36***	NS **16.12 ± 1.53**	-	n = 7 had comorbid diagnoses (1 or more) of phobias, anxiety disorders, OCD and depression

Table 1. *Cont.*

Author, Year *Country*	Objectives	Group Type (Number)	Participant Characteristics				Baseline Anthropometry		Other Baseline Measures/Comments
Mac Donald et al., 2023 [28] *Denmark*	Evaluating the impact of multiple IT events in the context of AN treatment	1. Overall (n = 7). Lived experience of 5 or more IT events including NG R	AN diagnosis (NR) **	Female (100%)	>18	-	-	-	n = 4 continued to have AN/AAN. n = 6 current psychiatric co-morbidities.
Matthews Rensch et al., 2023 [21] *Australia*	Acceptability and views of the use of NG nutrition	1. NG (n = 8) 2. Staff (n = 12)	AN, OSFED or AAN diagnosis *(NR)* **AN (n = 6) AAN (n = 1) OSFED (restrictive subtype) (n = 1)**	1. Female (100%) 2. NR	*1. 22* ***(18–27)***	*1. NR ±* ***7.5–168***	-	-	n = 4: first admission: n = 2: second admission n = 2: >2 admissions

↑: high; ↔: normal range; ↓: low; AAN: atypical anorexia; ALP: alkaline phosphatase; ALT: alanine transaminase; AN: anorexia nervosa; AN-BP: anorexia nervosa binge-purge subtype; AN-R: anorexia nervosa restrictive subtype; AST: aspartate transferase; BMI: body mass index; CHO: carbohydrate; DSM: Diagnostic and Statistical Manual; DOI: duration of illness; EBW: expected body weight; EDE- Q: eating disorder examination questionnaire; EDI: eating disorder inventory; EDNOS: eating disorder not otherwise specified; EDRC: eating disorder risk composite score; FEV1: forced expiratory volume 1; FFM: fat-free mass; FM: fat mass; GGT: gamma glutamyl transpeptidase; GO-AN: good outcome anorexia nervosa; IBW: ideal body weight; ICD: International Classification of Diseases; IT: involuntary treatment; K: potassium; mBMI: median body mass index; Mg: magnesium; MS: medical stabilisation; NG: at least some nutrition provided through nasogastric tube feeding; NG R: nasogastric tube feeding under restraint; NR: not reported; NS: not specified; n.s: not significantly different; OCD: obsessive–compulsive disorder; OI: oral intake only; ONS: oral nutritional supplements; OSFED: other specific feeding or eating disorder; PEG: percutaneous endoscopic gastrostomy providing at least some nutrition; PEF: peak expiratory flow; PN: parenteral nutrition; PO4: phosphate; TR-AN: treatment-resistant anorexia nervosa; w/NG: with NG nutrition; WR: weight restoration; * significantly different; ** lived experience of AN treatment.

Table 2. Summary of initial nutrition and related outcomes.

Author, Year	Cohort (s), Specifics, (n)	Initial Nutritional Overview (Within 2 Weeks of Refeeding Initiation)				Outcomes	Adverse Outcomes
		Initial Prescription kcal/d [a] *(Actual Intake)* M ± SD [a]	Kcal Increase per Day [a] (kcal/d [a])	Target kcal/Day [a] *(Actual Intake)* M ± SD [a]	Prophylactic PO4 Given	Weight: kg, BMI: kg/m^2 Weight gain/week: kg M ± SD or *Median (Range)*	M ± SD or *Median (Range)* Occurrence: n, % PO4: Serum Phosphate, K: Serum Potassium, Mg: Serum Magnesium Serum Levels: mmol/L [a]
Studies with participants < 18 years of age							
Agostino et al., 2013 [6]	1. NG (n = 31)	1500–1800 (*1617 ± 276 **)	200	2276 ± 123	Y	1. vs. 2.: - Weight gain week 1: 1.22 ± 1 vs. 0.08 ± 0.9 * - Weight gain of at least 0.5 kg/week: 84% vs. 32% - Patients not gaining weight or losing weight: 6% vs. 51%	1. vs. 2.: - Moderate ↓ PO4: n = 0 vs. n = 3 (1.8%) - ↓ K: n = 1 (3.2%) vs. n = 1 (0.7%)—both h/o laxative abuse - No RFS in either group
	2. OI (n = 134)	1000–1200 (*1069 ± 212 **)	150	2373 ± 220	NR		
Madden et al., 2015a [30]	1. NG (n = 78)	2400	As required	Max 3800	Y	Weight gain: - Week 1: 2.79 ± 1.27 - Week 0–0.5 (NG predominant): 1.78 ± 1.78 * - Week 0.5–1 (OI predominant): 1.01 ± 0.81	No ↓ PO4, hypoglycaemia or RFS

Table 2. *Cont.*

Author, Year	Cohort (s), Specifics, (n)	Initial Nutritional Overview (Within 2 Weeks of Refeeding Initiation)				Outcomes	Adverse Outcomes
		Initial Prescription kcal/d [a] *(Actual Intake)* M ± SD [a]	Kcal Increase per Day [a] (kcal/d [a])	Target kcal/Day [a] *(Actual Intake)* M ± SD [a]	Prophylactic PO4 Given	Weight: kg, BMI: kg/m^2 Weight gain/week: kg M ± SD or *Median (Range)*	M ± SD or *Median (Range)* Occurrence: n, % PO4: Serum Phosphate, K: Serum Potassium, Mg: Serum Magnesium Serum Levels: mmol/L [a]
Pruccoli et al., 2024 [26]	1. NG (n = 44) 2. Other (mainly OI) (n = 69)	15–20 kcal/kg/d (high risk 5–10)	NR (↑ every 2–3 days)	RFS gp: *(1378 ± 289)* No RFS gp: *(1357 ± 231)*	NR	NR	1. vs. 2.: RFS occurrence: n = 18/44 (41% of NG gp) vs. n = 28/69 (41% of 'other' gp) No RFS: n = 26/44 (59% of NG gp) vs. n = 41/69 (59% of 'Other' gp) Of 'RFS' occurrence gp (n = 46): 39% from NG group, 61% from 'Other' gp.
Robb et al., 2002 [36]	1. NG (n = 52) 2. OI (n = 48)	1800 (NG: 600, OI:NG = 2:1) NR	400 (day 2), 200 (day 3) NR	Energy for target weight gain: 1–2 kg/week	N	NR	1: - Anti-anxiety medication given for tube placement: n = 2 (3.8%) - Tube removed, needing replacement: n = 3 (6%) - Epistaxis: n = 6 (12%) - Nasal irritation: n = 15 (29%) - No RFS or aspiration pneumonia
Silber et al., 2004 [24]	1. NG (n = 6) 2. OI (n = 8)	NR	NR	NR	NR	NR	1: - Nasal irritation: n = 1 (17%) - Epistaxis: n = 1 (17%) - No RFS or aspiration pneumonia
Trovato et al., 2022 [45]	4 gps: -NG + food (n = 6) -NG + food + ONS (n = 51) -Food only (n = 66) - Food + ONS (n = 63)	40 kcal/kg/d	NR	At least 40 kcal/kg/d (NG: max 1500)	NR	NR	No RFS, or electrolyte abnormalities in any gp
Studies with participants ≥ 18 years of age							
Braude et al., 2020 [46]	1. NG (n = 27) 2. OI (n = 68)	NR	NR	NR	NR	In the overall cohort: - Weight gain over LOS: 1.4 ± 2.9 - LOS: *9.6 (5.8–19.7) days*	In overall cohort: -Refeeding electrolyte derangement in 26.3% - Hypoglycaemia in 11.1% - NG gp associated with: ↓ K. (OR: 9.4 95% CI: 1.8–50.3) * - NG not associated with ↓ PO4 or ↓ Mg

Table 2. *Cont.*

Author, Year	Cohort (s), Specifics, (n)	Initial Nutritional Overview (Within 2 Weeks of Refeeding Initiation)				Outcomes	Adverse Outcomes
		Initial Prescription kcal/d [a] *(Actual Intake)* M ± SD [a]	Kcal Increase per Day [a] (kcal/d [a])	Target kcal/Day [a] *(Actual Intake)* M ± SD [a]	Prophylactic PO4 Given	Weight: kg, BMI: kg/m^2 Weight gain/week: kg M ± SD or *Median (Range)*	M ± SD or *Median (Range)* Occurrence: n, % PO4: Serum Phosphate, K: Serum Potassium, Mg: Serum Magnesium Serum Levels: mmol/L [a]
Rigaud et al., 2010 [40]	1. Low sodium OI w/NG (n = 176) 2. Std sodium OI w/NG (n = 42)	NR	NR	Week 1: *(1583 ± 207)* Week 1: *(1638 ± 234)*	NR	1. vs. 2.: - Weight gain week 1: 0.73 ± 0.18 vs. 1.42 ± 0.23	Overall cohort: - No NG-related severe adverse effects - No RFS - Sinusitis: n = 12 (6%) 1. vs. 2.: - Oedema: n = 11 (6%) vs. n = 9 (21%) *
Rigaud et al., 2007 [18]	1. NG (n = 41) 2. OI (n = 40)	NR	NR	Energy for target weight gain 1 kg/week (if BMI < 12.5 kg/m^2: week 1: <30 kcal/kg/d)	Y	1. vs. 2.: - OI similar - Overall energy intake higher * (as energy via NG + OI in NG gp) - Hunger rating higher * in first 2 weeks. - BP episode complete cessation in week 1: 80% vs. 50% in AN-BP participants * NG gp: AN-BP vs. AN-R: found NG more 'useful' in week 1 * AN-R vs. AN-BP: anxiety associated. with OI alongside NG higher *	No RFS, severe ↓ K or ↓ PO4 in either group 1.: - Gastro-oesophageal reflux: n = 2 (5%) - Sinusitis: n = 2 (5%)
Rigaud et al., 2011b [19]	1. NG + CBT (n = 52) (AN subgp: n = 19) 2. OI + CBT (n = 51) (AN subgp n = 17)	NR	NR	NR	NR	1. vs. 2.: - BP abstinence at day 8: 79% vs. 16% * - Similar results in AN and BN subgps	NR
Studies with participants across both age categories							
Gentile, 2012 [38]	1. NG (n = 10)	*Median: 1199*	NR	2508	Y	Baseline vs. day 15: - BMI: 11.2 ± 0.7 vs. 12.9 ± 0.9 - Weight: 27.9 ± 3.3 vs. 32.0 ± 3.8 - Weight gain over 15 days: *4.35 kg*	- PO4, Mg, K within range during refeeding - No RFS - No gastrointestinal symptoms reported by participants - No aspiration or tube malposition
Kells et al., 2022 [25]	1. NG (n = 44) 2. OI (n = 256)	1000–3000 *(1714 ± 324)*	250	NR	Y	1. vs. 2.: - Initial prescription higher *. - Formula given over admission higher * - Weight gain similar between groups	1. vs. 2.: - ↓ PO4 risk 3x higher - K and Mg nadir n.s.

Table 2. *Cont.*

Author, Year	Cohort (s), Specifics, (n)	Initial Nutritional Overview (Within 2 Weeks of Refeeding Initiation)				Outcomes	Adverse Outcomes
		Initial Prescription kcal/d [a] *(Actual Intake)* M ± SD [a]	Kcal Increase per Day [a] (kcal/d [a])	Target kcal/Day [a] *(Actual Intake)* M ± SD [a]	Prophylactic PO4 Given	Weight: kg, BMI: kg/m^2 Weight gain/week: kg M ± SD or *Median (Range)*	M ± SD or *Median (Range)* Occurrence: n, % PO4: Serum Phosphate, K: Serum Potassium, Mg: Serum Magnesium Serum Levels: mmol/L [a]
Murciano et al., 1994 [39]	1. NG (n = 15)	NR	NR	Week 1: *(1824 ± 399)*	NR	Day 0 vs. Day 7 of refeeding: - Weight: 37.1 ± 4.7 vs. 39.2 ± 4.3 - Diaphragmatic function improvement at day 7 * - no muscle mass increase at day 7 n.s.	NR
Paccagnella et al., 2006 [32]	1. NG gp (n = 24)	<1000	NR	Day 12: 1455	NR	On starting NG: - Abdominal symptoms ↓ - Cardiovascular symptoms ↓	- Mild RFS features: n = 2 (8%)
Parker et al., 2021 [10]	1. Low CHO feed (n = 15) 2. Standard CHO feed (n = 11)	*1260–1890*	Day 2: 2500	Week 1 median (range): *3350 (3188, 3350)* Week 1 median (range): *3325 (2844, 3350)*	Y—if PO4 ≤ 1 mmol/L pre-refeeding	1. vs. 2. - Weight gain: week 1: 2.7 ± 1.9 vs. 2.7 ± 1.6 - Day when med stab reached: *2.0 (0.0,* 3.3) vs. 2.0 *(0.8, 5.0)*	1. vs. 2.: - lower levels of RH in 1. * (day of RH occurrence: 2.9 ± 1.2) - PO4 at week 1: 1.06 ± 0.15 vs. 0.88 ± 0.12 * - RH not correlated to %mBMI - Requirement for K and Mg supplementation during refeeding: n.s - Hypoglycaemia: 0/14 vs. 1/10 n.s. - No RFS, oedema or admission to the intensive care unit reported in either group
Rigaud et al., 2012 [34]	1. NG (n = 41)	25 kcal/kg/d	10 kcal/kg/d (in 2 days)	Day 6–10: 40 kcal/kg/d	Y	Baseline vs. week 1: - Weight: 25.9 ± 1.4 vs. 27.1 ± 1.0 - BMI: 10.1 ± 0.28 vs. 10.7 ± 0.2 - FFM: 24.1 ± 1.1 vs. 25.3 ± 0.9 - FM: 1.6 ± 0.9 vs. 1.8 ± 0.7 Baseline neuropathy in n = 6 (15%) → improved within 3 weeks of refeeding.	↓ PO4: n = 4 (10%) Refeeding oedema: n = 9 (22%)
Zuercher et al., 2003 [41]	1. NG (n = 155) 2. OI (n = 226)	NR	300 every 3 days NR	Energy for the target weight gain of >1 kg/week	NR	NR	1. vs. 2.: - Oedema: 19% vs. 13% -gastro-oesophageal reflux: 14% vs. 11% No aspiration pneumonia in either gp

Table 2. *Cont.*

Author, Year	Cohort (s), Specifics, (n)	Initial Nutritional Overview (Within 2 Weeks of Refeeding Initiation)				Outcomes	Adverse Outcomes
		Initial Prescription kcal/d [a] *(Actual Intake)* M ± SD [a]	Kcal Increase per Day [a] (kcal/d [a])	Target kcal/Day [a] *(Actual Intake)* M ± SD [a]	Prophylactic PO4 Given	Weight: kg, BMI: kg/m^2 Weight gain/week: kg M ± SD or *Median (Range)*	M ± SD or *Median (Range)* Occurrence: n, % PO4: Serum Phosphate, K: Serum Potassium, Mg: Serum Magnesium Serum Levels: mmol/L [a]
Studies in which age category is unclear							
Bufano et al., 1990 [49]	1. NG (n = 9)	25% estimated req.	25% req	100% req. (2311 ± 607)	N	Early anthropometry: NR n = 3 (33%): Baseline ↓ K normalised after NG	- ↓ PO4 within 2 weeks of NG start: n = 3 (33%) - Other electrolytes within range during refeeding - No gastrointestinal symptoms reported by participants

[a] unless otherwise specified; * significant difference; ↑ increase; ↓ decrease; AN: anorexia nervosa; AN-BP: anorexia nervosa binge-purge subtype; AN-R: anorexia nervosa restrictive subtype; BN: bulimia nervosa; BMI: body mass index; BP: binge-purge episodes; CBT: cognitive behavioural therapy; CHO: carbohydrate content; ETN: enteral tube nutrition; FFM: fat-free mass in kg; FM: fat mass in kg; Gp: group; K: potassium; LOS: length of stay; Mg: magnesium; N: no; NG: nasogastric nutrition group with at least some nutrition via NG; NR: not reported; n.s: no significant difference; OI: oral intake group; ONS: oral nutritional supplements; PO4: phosphate; req: requirements; RFS: refeeding syndrome; RH: refeeding hypophosphataemia; subgp: subgroup; Y: yes.

Table 3. Summary of overall nutrition and outcomes relate to anthropometry and physiology.

Author, Year	Overall Nutrition				Outcomes	
	Cohort (s)	*Target Nutrition:* (kcal/d or kcal/kg/d) Mean ± SD *Median (IQR, Range)*	*Duration of ETN (Days)* Mean ± SD (Range) *Median (IQR)*	*Length of Stay (LOS) (Days)* Mean ± s.d *Median (IQR)*	*Anthropometry* *Weight: kg* *Weight Gain per Week: kg/week* *BMI: kg/m^2* *%EBW/IBW/BMI: %* Mean ± SD *Median (IQR, Range)*	*Physiological*
Studies in participants < 18 years of age						
Agostino et al., 2013 [6]	1. NG 2. OI	1.: 2276 ± 123 2.: 2373 ± 220	NR	1. vs. 2.: 33.8 ± 11 vs. 50.9 ± 24 *	1. vs. 2.: Weight gain over LOS: 4.44 ± 2 vs. 4.81 ± 2.3	-
Blikshavn et al., 2020 [42]	1. NG-R 2. no NG-R	1. and 2.: NR	NR Majority of NG-R episodes in first 8 weeks	Overall: 142 ± 95.9. 1.: LOS NR	Overall: Weight gain over LOS: 7.4 ± 4.5. BMI adm vs. d/c: 15.2 ± 1.9 vs. 18.3 ± 1.7. 1. vs. 2.: weight gain, BMI, BMI percentile change n.s.	-
Madden et al., 2015a [30]	1. NG	1.: 2400–3000	Aiming for max.: 15	28.62 ± 15.28	Overall weight gain over LOS: 5.12 ± 2.96 % EBW baseline vs. at 2.5 weeks: 78.37% ± 6.5 vs. 85.58% ± 6.46 * Gain of 7.21% ± 3.70 over 2.5 week	-No hypoglycaemia seen during treatment. -Refeeding electrolyte results as per initial nutrition outcomes.

Table 3. *Cont.*

Author, Year	Overall Nutrition			Outcomes		
	Cohort (s)	*Target Nutrition:* (kcal/d or kcal/kg/d) Mean ± SD *Median (IQR, Range)*	*Duration of ETN (Days)* Mean ± SD (Range) *Median (IQR)*	*Length of Stay (LOS) (Days)* Mean ± s.d *Median (IQR)*	*Anthropometry Weight: kg Weight Gain per Week: kg/week BMI: kg/m²* *%EBW/IBW/BMI: %* Mean ± SD *Median (IQR, Range)*	*Physiological*
Madden et al., 2015b [20]	1. Medical stabilisation w/NG 2. Weight restoration w/NG	1. and 2.: 2400–3000	Aiming for max.: 15	1. vs. 2.: 21.73 ± 5.92 vs. 36.89 ± 17.06 * 1.: d/c on med stab. 2.: d/c after weight restoration.	1. vs. 2. %EBW at hospital discharge: 84.4% vs. 92% *	-
Marchili et al., 2023 [43]	1. NG 2. OI	1. and 2.: NS	*21 (13)*	1. vs. 2.: 30 ± 11 vs. 16 ± 9 *	BMI adm vs. d/c: 1. 14.5 ± 1.9 vs. 15.5 ± 1.7 2. 16.1 ± 2.8 vs. 16.7 ± 2.8 (1.vs 2. BMI at adm *, BMI at d/c *)	-
Nehring et al., 2014 [50]	1. NG 2. OI	1. and 2.: NS	NR	1. vs. 2.: LOS longer in NG gp *.	-	-
Pruccoli et al., 2021 [51]	1. E AAP + E NG 2. E AAP + L NG 3. L AAP + E NG 4. L AAP + L NG 5. NG only	NS	7 (at least) Early NG start: ≤7 days of adm.	1. vs. 3. and 4.: LOS: 81.3 ± 31.4 vs. 182.6 ± 110.9 * and 155.4 ± 56.4 *, respectively.	Overall BMI: adm vs. d/c: 13.7 ± 1.7 vs. 15.6 ± 1.7 Early vs. late AAP: BMI change. n.s. Early vs. late NG: BMI change n.s.	-
Pruccoli et al., 2022 [52]	1. NG 2. OI	1. and 2.: NS	NR	NR	Overall: BMI adm vs. d/c: 14.3 ± 1.7 vs. 16.0 ± 1.6 6-month FU BMI (for those with available data, i.e., the 'good outcome' group): 17.3 ± 2.3	-
Pruccoli et al., 2024 [26]	1. NG 2. other	RFS gp: 1378 ± 289. No RFS gp: 1357 ± 231	NR	NR	Admission vs. d/c %mBMI: RFS gp: 71 ± 10 vs. *79 (11)* No RFS gp: 72 ± 10 vs. *80 (13)* Admission vs. d/c BMI: RFS gp: *14 (2)* vs. *15 (2)* No RFS gp: *14 (3)* vs. *16 (3)*	-RFS results as specified in the initial nutrition table: -NG use similar in the RFS and No RFS groups
Robb et al., 2002 [36]	1. NG 2. OI	1. and 2.: Target weight gain: 1–2 kg/week 1. max intake: 3255 ± 668 2. max intake: 2508 ± 478	NR	1. vs. 2.: 22.3 ± 13.5 vs. 22.1 ± 9.4.	1. vs. 2.: Weight gain over LOS: 5.4 ± 4.0 vs. 2.4 ± 1.8 * BMI change over LOS: 2.03 ± 1.4 vs. 0.9 ± 0.7 * d/c BMI: 17.5 ± 1.3 vs. 16.8 ± 1.6. n.s.	-
Silber et al., 2004 [24]	1. NG 2. OI	1. max energy intake: 4350 2. max energy intake: 3400	NR	1. vs. 2.: 36 ± 11 vs. 39.9 ± 22	1. vs. 2.: Weight gain over LOS: 10.9 vs. 3. BMI change 3.75 ± 2.3 vs. 1.2 ± 0.8. 1. BMI admission vs. d/c: 15.3 ± 1.7 vs. 19.1 ± NR 2. 17.4 ± 2.3 vs. 18.5 ± NR	-
Trovato et al., 2022 [45]	1. NG + ONS + OI 2. ONS + OI 3. OI 4. NG + OI	All groups: At least **40 kcal/kg/d** If weight loss ↑ to **50 kcal/kg/d**	NR	Overall: 27.5 (14–40) 1. vs. 2. LOS shorter * 1. vs. 4. LOS shorter *	NR d/c when weight restored.	-

Table 3. *Cont.*

Author, Year	Overall Nutrition				Outcomes	
	Cohort (s)	*Target Nutrition:* (kcal/d or kcal/kg/d) Mean ± SD *Median (IQR, Range)*	*Duration of ETN (Days)* Mean ± SD (Range) *Median (IQR)*	*Length of Stay (LOS) (Days)* Mean ± s.d *Median (IQR)*	*Anthropometry* *Weight: kg* *Weight Gain per Week: kg/week* *BMI: kg/m²* *%EBW/IBW/BMI: %* Mean ± SD *Median (IQR, Range)*	*Physiological*
Studies in participants ≥ 18 years of age						
Braude et al., 2020 [46]	1. NG 2. OI	1. and 2.: NR	*6 (2–12)*	Overall: 9.6 (5.8–19.7). BMI < 16 vs. >16: 11.7 (6.7–20.8) vs. 7.8 (5.3–15.9) *	Overall: Weight gain over LOS: 1.4 ± 2.9 1. vs. 2. anthropometry: NR	-
Hanachi et al., 2013 [33]	1. ↑ AST/ALT w/ETN gp 2. ↔ AST/ALT w/ETN gp	1. 1069 ± 350 via NG. Via OI: NS 2. 1763 ± 510 * via NG Via OI: NS	28 (study length)	NR	1. vs. 2.: lower weight gain in group 1 * BMI ↑: 1.5 ± 1.0 vs. 2.0 ± 0.8 *	1. n = 52/54 had normalised LFTs by week 4 of ETN. 2. no development of deranged LFTs during refeeding via ETN.
Martini et al., 2024 [44]	1. NG 2. OI	1. 1501 ± 369 2. 1421 ± 321	25 ± 19	1. vs. 2.: 39 ± 23 vs. 36 ± 20.	BMI adm vs. d/c: 1. 13.99 ± 1.76 vs. 14.80 ± 1.63 2. 14.01 ± 1.89 vs. 14.51 ± 1.69 BMI increase: 1. vs. 2.: 0.81 ± 0.74 vs. 0.55 ± 0.69 *	-
Rigaud et al., 2010 [40]	1. Low sodium gp w/NG 2. Std sodium gp w/NG	1.: 2647 ± 192 (862 ± 92 via NG). 2.: 2684 ± 186 (812 ± 109 via NG).	60 (at least)	1. and 2.: 60 (at least)	Month 1: True weight gain vs. expected weight gain: 1. 3.8 ± 0.3 vs. 4.0 ± 0.4 n.s 2. 6.7 ± 0.5 vs. 3.9 ± 0.3 * Overall, at BMI 15–16: n = 192 (88%)—weight ↔ for 7–10 days despite no change in energy input.	Overall: Urinary sodium output ↑ at 4–6 weeks of refeeding
Rigaud et al., 2007 [18]	1. NG 2. OI	1. and 2.: Prescription to achieve target weight gain: 1 kg/week	60 (at least)	1. and 2.: 67–70	1. vs. 2.: Weight gain in 8 wks: 9.6 vs. 5.9 * Weight gain/week over study period: 1.358 vs. 0.882 * FFM gain and FM gain higher in NG gp * BMI of 18.5 achieved at d/c: n = 16 (39%) vs. n = 3 (8%) *	-
Rigaud et al., 2011b [19]	1. NG + CBT gp (AN subgp) 2. OI + CBT gp (AN subgp)	1. and 2.: In AN subgp: target weight gain: 1.5–2 kg/month.	60 days (at least)	n/a (outpatient study)	In AN subgps: 1. vs. 2.: FFM at 8 weeks higher in NG gp *, remained higher at 6 months FU *. BMI adm vs. 8 wk in AN (both gps): 1. 15.8 ± 1.3 vs. 17.4 ± 1.1 * 2. 16.2 ± 1.0 vs. 16.6 ± 0.9	
Studies in participants across both age categories						
Born et al., 2015 [37]	1. PEG 2. No PEG	1.: Max. 3000 2.: NR	NR	Overall: 150.2 ± 80.8. range: 56–348. 1. vs. 2.: longer *	Overall: Weight gain over LOS: 12 ± 5.1. BMI adm vs. d/c: 12.3 ± 1.4 vs. 16.7 ± 1.7. 1. vs. 2.: weight gain over LOS: 12.2 ± 5.2 vs. 11.3 ± 4.7 n.s	-

Table 3. *Cont.*

Author, Year	Overall Nutrition				Outcomes	
	Cohort (s)	*Target Nutrition:* (kcal/d or kcal/kg/d) **Mean ± SD** *Median (IQR, Range)*	*Duration of ETN (Days)* **Mean ± SD (Range)** *Median (IQR)*	*Length of Stay (LOS) (Days)* **Mean ± s.d** *Median (IQR)*	***Anthropometry Weight: kg Weight Gain per Week: kg/week BMI: kg/m²* *%EBW/IBW/BMI: %*** **Mean ± SD** ***Median (IQR, Range)***	*Physiological*
Gentile, 2012 [38]	1. NG	1.: ~2800	90	NR	Weight gain/week: 1.1 ± NR * Adm vs. day 90: Weight: 27.9 ± 3.3 vs. 43 ± 5.7 * BMI: 11.2 ± 0.72 vs. 17.3 ± 1.6 *	n = 1 (10%)—hypoglycaemia on day 90—after NG cessation
Gentile et al., 2008 [47]	1. NG 2. OI	1.: Energy via NG: 1375 ± 211. Energy via OI NS. 2.: NS	133.8 ± 76	1. vs. 2.: 222 ± 136.9 vs. 164.3 ± 118.6	1. vs. 2.: Weight gain over LOS: 15.9 ± 3.4 vs. 14.0 ± 2.3 Adm and inpatient d/c BMI similar in both gps	-
Kells et al., 2022 [25]	1. NG 2. OI	1. and 2.: 1000–3000	NR	Overall: 7.4 ± 5.9	Overall weight gain over LOS: 1.8 ± 1.5 1. vs. 2.: weight gain similar n.s.	Refeeding electrolyte results as per initial nutrition outcomes.
Kezelman et al., 2018 [31]	1. NG	1.: 2400–3800	NR	24.81 ± 12.51	BMI admission vs. d/c: 16.32 ± 1.94 vs. 19.36 ± 1.15 *	-
Minano Garrido et al., 2021 [35]	1. ETN	1.: **50 kcal/kg/d**	35 (duration of study)	35 (at least)	Baseline vs. end of study: BMI: 11.4 ± 1.3 vs. 12.6 ± 1.02 * Total muscle strength, proximal muscle strength: ↑ with time * Axial muscle strength, distal muscle strength: n.s.	Baseline vs. end of study: Peak expiratory flow ↑ *, although still below normal range.
Murciano et al., 1994 [39]	1. NG	1.: Average ETN: Day 7-day 30: *1841 ± 519*. Day 30–45: *1567 ± 527* OI energy: NR	42 (at least)	56 (at least)	Day 0 vs. Day 30 and day 45 of refeeding: Weight: 37.1 ± 4.7 vs. 41.8 ± 4.8 * and 42.9 ± 4.6 *. Muscle mass (kg): 11.2 ± 4.1 vs. 15.1 ± 4.6 * and 16.6 ± 4.9 *. Fat free mass (kg): 33.3 ± 3.7 vs. 36.1 ± 3.1 * and 36.3 ± 2.9 * Fat mass (kg): 3.5 ± 1.5 vs. 5.7 ± 2.1 * and 6.5 ± 2.3 *	-Diaphragmatic function ↑ at Day 30 * and Day 45 * vs. Day 0 -FEV1 ↑ at Day 30 * vs. Day 0
Paccagnella et al., 2006 [32]	1. NG	1.: ~1450	20.7 ± 7.1	NR.	Weight: early refeeding: 33 ± NR, later refeeding: 40.4 ± NR, FU: 46.1 ± NR. BMI: early refeeding: 12.9 ± NR, late refeeding: 15.8 ± NR. FU: 17.3 ± NR	-
Parker et al., 2021 [10]	1. Low CHO w/NG 2. Standard CHO w/NG	1.: *3350 (3188, 3350)* 2.: *3325 (2844, 3350)*	1. and 2.: 7 (at least)	1. vs. 2.: 24.3 ± 11.3 vs. 24.4 ± 6.5	1. vs. 2.: weight gain by week 3: 6.5 ± 2.3 vs. 6.4 ± 2.0. 1. and 2: %mBMI ↑ over time *	1. vs. 2.: No difference in hypoglycaemia incidence. RFS parameters as per initial outcomes.
Rigaud et al., 2012 [34]	1. NG	1.: Week 3: **45 kcal/kg/d** (maintenance) Week 4: → target weight gain: 0.7–1 kg/week	21 (at least)	NR	Baseline vs. day 28: Weight: 25.9 ± 1.4 vs. 30.5 ± 1.2 BMI: 10.1± 0.28 vs. 12.1 ± 0.2 FFM: 24.1 ± 1.1 vs. 27.4 ± 1.0 FM: 1.6 ± 0.9 vs. 3.1 ± 0.9	-

Table 3. *Cont.*

Author, Year	Overall Nutrition				Outcomes	
	Cohort (s)	*Target Nutrition:* **(kcal/d or kcal/kg/d)** **Mean ± SD** *Median (IQR, Range)*	*Duration of ETN (Days)* **Mean ± SD (Range)** *Median (IQR)*	*Length of Stay (LOS) (Days)* **Mean ± s.d** *Median (IQR)*	*Anthropometry* *Weight: kg* *Weight Gain per Week: kg/week* *BMI: kg/m²* *%EBW/IBW/BMI: %* **Mean ± SD** *Median (IQR, Range)*	*Physiological*
Zuercher et al., 2003 [41]	1. NG 2. OI	1. and 2.: Target weight gain → >1 kg/week	36 ± 21	1. vs. 2.: 60.8 ± 17.3 vs. 48.3 ± 19.4 *	1. vs. 2.: Weight gain mean diff. over LOS: 8.1 vs. 5.7 weight gain/week: 0.91 vs. 0.82 NG > ½ LOS vs. NG < ½ LOS vs. OI: Weight gain/week: 1.0 vs. 0.77 * vs. 0.82 * MUAC higher * if NG > ½ LOS compared with NG < ½ LOS and OI gps.	1. vs. 2.: No difference in medical complications when controlled for severity of illness
Age category unclear						
Bufano et al., 1990 [49]	1. NG	1.: 100% requirements. 2311 ± 607	21 ± 14	NR	Weight gain/month: 8.22 ± 3.43 Tricipital and MUAC. ↑ *	-ALT, AST ↑ with NG: n = 9 (100%) → normalised within 1–2 weeks after stopping NG. -n = 2: 'intense' ↑ in appetite → normalised ~ 1 month post d/c

* significant difference; ↑: increase; ↔: normal range; AAP: atypical anti-psychotics; adm: admission; ALT: alanine transaminase; AN: anorexia nervosa; AST: aspartate transaminase; BMI: body mass index; BMR: basal metabolic rate; CBT: cognitive behavioural therapy; CHO: carbohydrate content; d/c: discharge; diff: difference; E AAP: early atypical antipsychotics start; %EBW: %expected body weight; E NG: early NG start; ETN: enteral tube nutrition; FEV1: forced expiratory volume 1; FFM: fat-free mass; FM: fat mass; FU: follow up; Gp: group; %IBW: % ideal body weight; K: potassium; L AAP: late atypical antipsychotics start; LFTs: liver function tests; L NG: late NG start; LOS: length of stay; %mBMI: % median BMI; Mg: magnesium; MUAC: mid-upper arm circumference; NG: nasogastric nutrition group; NG-R: NG under restraint; n.s: no significant difference; NR: not reported; OI: oral intake group. ONS: oral nutritional supplements; PEG: percutaneous endoscopic gastrostomy nutrition; PO4: phosphate; RH: refeeding hypophosphataemia; w/NG: with NG.

Table 4. Summary of relapses, readmissions, and longer-term outcomes.

Author, Year	Cohort (s)(n).	Readmissions **Mean ± SD** *Median (IQR)*	Longer-Term Outcomes **Mean ± SD** *Median (IQR)* **Occurrence: n (%)**
Studies with participants < 18 years of age			
Agostino et al., 2013 [6]	1. NG (n = 31) 2. OI (n = 134)	1. vs. 2.: readmission rates at 6 months.: n = 4 (12.9%) vs. n = 31 (23%)	-
Blikshavn et al., 2020 [42]	1. NG-R (n = 8) 2. no NG-R (n = 30)	1. vs. 2. at 5-year FU: Readmissions: n = 5 (63%) vs. n = 9 (30%) n.s. (medium effect size)	1. vs. 2. at 5 yr FU: ED diagnosis: n = 6 (75%) vs. n = 10 (33.3%) * BMI: *18.5 (15.6–20.8)* vs. *19.7 (19–20.7)* n.s. (medium effect size)
Madden et al., 2015a [30]	1. NG (n = 78)	-	At 12-month FU: % EBW: 95.33% ± 9.47 *

Table 4. *Cont.*

Author, Year	Cohort (s)(n).	Readmissions Mean ± SD *Median (IQR)*	Longer-Term Outcomes Mean ± SD *Median (IQR)* Occurrence: n (%)
Madden et al., 2015b [20]	1. Medical stabilisation. gp w/NG (n = 41) 2. Weight restoration gp w/NG (n = 41)	1. vs. 2.: Hospital days over 12 months, post initial d/c: 22.78 ± 41.59 vs. 27.51 ± 51.70 Overall hospital days (including initial admission) lower in 1. * Readmission rates: 36.1% vs. 33.3% Reasons for admissions similar in both groups (malnutrition, self-harm)	1. vs. 2.: %EBW change admission to 12-month FU: 17.77 ± 11.36 vs. 15.75 ± 9.24. n.s. Full remission at 12-month FU: 30% vs. 32.5%. n.s.
Marchili et al., 2023 [43]	1. NG (n = 101) 2. OI (n = 214)	1. vs. 2.: Relapse: n = 14 (13.9%) vs. n = 33 (15.4%) Time to recurrence of symptoms median (IQR): 8.2 (9.7) vs. 3.0 (6.0) months *	
Nehring et al., 2014 [50]	1. NG (n = 71) 2. OI (n = 137):	1. vs. 2.: No. of hospital admissions higher in 1. *	1. vs. 2.: At FU (mean 6 years): BMI and height (marker of growth) →no difference
Pruccoli et al., 2022 [52]	1. NG (n = 33): 2. OI (n = 43):	-	Good outcome gp (completed initial admission, available for FU at 6 months and %mBMI > 70% at FU) vs. treatment resistant gp: NG use in admission: n = 23 (50%) vs. n = 10 (33.3%) * Treatment resistance associated with older participants, higher EDI 3 EDRC scores and less NG use *
Studies with participants ≥ 18 years of age			
Braude et al., 2020 [46]	1. NG (n = 27) 2. OI (n = 68)	Overall readmissions rate: 57.9% (timescale NR) Readmissions within 3 months: 30.3% Lower BMI: → longer initial admission * and lower readmissions in 3 months *	-
Rigaud et al., 2007 [18]	1. NG (n = 41) 2. OI (n = 40)	1. vs. 2.: Time before relapse in weeks: 34.3 ± 8.2 vs. 26.8 ± 7.5 * % relapsing patients at year 1: 44% vs. 52% Energy, lipids, CHO, protein intake ↓ with time over 1 year in both gps. *	-
Rigaud et al., 2011b [19]	1. NG + CBT (n = 52, AN subgp: n = 19) 2. OI + CBT (n = 51, AN subgp: n = 17)	-	1. vs. 2. BP episode ↓ of >75%: At 3 months FU: n = 46 (88%) vs. n = 23 (45%) * At 12 months FU: n = 43 (82%) vs. n = 23 (45%) * Similar results in AN and BN.
Studies with participants across the age categories			
Born et al., 2015 [37]	1. PEG (n = 57) 2. No PEG (n = 11)	Overall: Readmissions: n = 7 (10.3%) Duration of follow-up—NR	-
Gentile et al., 2008 [47]	1. NG (n = 32) 2. OI (n = 67)	-	In those completing the study (n = 75): Weight gain rate at outpatient d/c vs. inpatient d/c: 1.4 ± 1.1 kg/month vs. 3.1 ± 1.6 kg/month
Rigaud et al., 2011a [48]	1. NG (n = 262) 2. OI (n = 222)	Overall relapse rate: At year 1: 52.1% At year 2: +16.4% ETN > 2 months–↓ relapse at 2-year FU *.	Overall (13-year FU): n = 292 (60.3%) recovered. n = 125 (25.8%) 'good outcome'. n = 31 (6.4%) 'bad outcome'. n = 31 (6.4%) 'severe outcome'. n = 6 died.
Rigaud et al., 2012 [34]	1. NG (n = 41)	n = 12 (29%): readmitted >4 times	6-year FU: n = 15 (36.6%) recovered; n = 11 (27%) 'good outcome'; n = 6 (14.6%) 'poorer outcome'; n = 6 (14.6%) 'severe outcome'; n = 2 (4.9%) died

* significant difference; ↓ decrease; AN: anorexia nervosa; BMI: body mass index; BN: bulimia nervosa; BP: binge-purge; d/c: discharge; CBT: cognitive behavioural therapy; CHO: carbohydrate; % EBW: percentage expected body weight; ED: eating disorder; EDI: Eating Disorder Inventory; EDRC: Eating Disorder Risk Composite; ETN: enteral tube nutrition; FU: follow up; gp: group; %mBMI: percentage median BMI; NG: nasogastric tube feeding group; NG-R: NG feeding under restraint; NR: not reported; NS: not specified; n.s: not statistically different; OI: oral intake group; subgp: subgroup; w/NG: with NG nutrition.

Table 5. Transition from ETN to OI and outcomes.

Author, Year	Cohort (s)	Transition from ETN Towards Increasing Oral Nutrition				Outcomes During Transition Weight: kg BMI: kg/m^2 Mean ± SD Occurrence: n (%)
		Basis for OI Introduction	When Transition Began	Strategies Used: Energy: kcal/d Median (Range)	Duration of Transition	
Studies in participants < 18 years of age						
Agostino et al., 2013 [6]	1. NG 2. OI	Med stab. + target energy reached, or NG completed for 7 days. NG only: max. 7 days	On day 7 at least	As OI ↑, NG titrated ↓. When NG ceased: NS	Over 3 days	1. vs. 2.: weight gain/week in days 1–14 incorporating transition: 1.06 ± 0.9 vs. 0.69 ± 0.6 1.: NG days 1–7 (mostly NG) vs. NG days 1–14 (incorporating transition): weight gain/week: 1.22 ± 1 vs. 1.06 ± 0.9
Kezelman et al., 2018 [31]	1. NG	When med stab	NS	As OI ↑, NG nocturnal and titrated ↓. OI staged plans from 1800 to 3800 kcal/d as required.	NS d/c when no NG required and BMI ≥ 18.5 kg/m^2	-
Madden et al., 2015a [30]	1. NG	When med stab	Days 1–7 of admission	↑ OI during the day with nocturnal NG. Energy prescription: Days 1–7: NG 1000. OI 1500–1800 Days 8–14: NG 500 OI 2100–2400 Day 15 onwards: aiming for OI only 2400–3000	Aiming: by day 15	Weight gain: Week 0.0–0.5 (NG predominant): 1.78 ± 1.78 Week 0.5–1 (OI predominant): 1.01 ± 0.81 Week 1–1.5 (NG ↓, OI ↑): 0.51 ± 0.59. Week 1.5–2 (NG further ↓, OI ↑): 0.22 ± 0.48 Week 2–2.5 (NG stopped, OI only): 0.22 ± 0.62
Madden et al., 2015b [20]	1. MS w/NG 2. WR w/NG	When med stab at daytime.	NS	↑ OI started with daytime med stab till day 15 when aiming for full OI. 1.: full med stab maintained for 72 hrs—d/c 2.: after full med stab., continue target weight restoration at 1 kg/week until weight restored.	Aiming: by day 15	-
Robb et al., 2002 [36]	1. NG 2. OI	OI from the start. Basis of transition towards ↑ OI and ↓ NG NS.	NS	As OI ↑ NG titrated ↓. by 2 hrs/night (300 kcal). NG cessation: when 95% IBW reached, OI at maintenance req. →d/c after 3–4 days.	NS	-
Silber et al., 2004 [24]	1. NG 2. OI	OI from the start. Basis of transition towards ↑ OI and ↓ NG NS	NS	As OI ↑ NG titrated ↓. NG cessation: when OI → at maintenance req. d/c 1–2 days after.	NS	-
Trovato et al., 2022 [45]	1. NG + ONS + food 2. ONS + food 3. food only 4. NG + food	OI 1st line. If OI < 70% intake ONS introduced. If OI + ONS < 30% intake NG introduced. NG ↓ based on weight ↑.	NS	As weight ↑ NG ↓.	NG ↓ over 6–7 days. 4/5 of NG for 2 days 3/5 of NG for 2 days 2/5 of NG for 2 days.	-
Studies in participants ≥ 18 years of age						
Rigaud et al., 2010 [40]	1.Low sodium w/NG 2. Standard sodium w/NG	OI from the start. Basis of transition towards ↑ OI and ↓ NG: NS	NS	1.: low sodium OI changed to standard sodium OI when urinary sodium clearance improved ~4–6 weeks. NG ↓: NS	NS NG:OI: Month 1: 1:1.7 Month 2: 1:2.2	-
Rigaud et al., 2007 [18]	1. NG (intervention arm) 2. OI (control arm)	OI from the start. Encouraged to ↑ OI.	NS	As OI ↑, NG titrated ↓. Target weight gain: 1 kg/week.	NS NG: OI Month 1: 1:2.7 Month 2: 1:3.3	1. vs. 2.: OI ↑ similar. n.s. 1.: OI ↓ and weight ↓ when NG stopped: n = 4 (9.8%). OI ↑ 1 week after NG stopped: n = 25 (61%)

Table 5. *Cont.*

Author, Year	Cohort (s)	Transition from ETN Towards Increasing Oral Nutrition				Outcomes During Transition Weight: kg BMI: kg/m² Mean ± SD Occurrence: n (%)
		Basis for OI Introduction	When Transition Began	Strategies Used: Energy: kcal/d Median (Range)	Duration of Transition	
Rigaud et al., 2011b [19]	1. NG + CBT (AN subgp: n = 19) 2. OI + CBT (AN subgp: n = 17)	NS	OI introduced in week 4.	OI introduction in steps every 2–3 days: Step 1 breakfast, step 2 lunch, step 3 dinner. As OI ↑, NG titrated ↓	5 weeks (from week 4 to 8) Duration of NG: 8 weeks.	-
Studies in participants across both age categories						
Born et al., 2015 [37]	1. PEG 2. No PEG	OI from the start. Basis of further transition: NS	NS.	OI encouraged. ETN continued until BMI > 17 kg/m² + able to maintain weight with OI for 2 weeks	NS	-
Gentile 2012 [38]	1. NG	NG duration ↓ with weight ↑. Basis of transition towards ↑ OI and ↓ NG: NS.	~Day 30 of refeeding	↑ OI with ↓NG: Energy prescribed: Day 30: NG 1100 OI 1412 Day 60: NG 1000 OI 1819 Day 90: NG 800 OI 2135	~2 months. NG stopped after Day 90	BMI Day 30 vs. Day 90: 14.1 ± 0.9 vs. 17.3 ± 1.6 BMI ↑ mean diff in BMI pts: Day 0 to Day 30 (NG > OI): 2.9 BMI pts in 1 month. Day 30 to Day 90 (OI > NG): 3.2 BMI pts in 2 months. Weight gain: Day 0 to Day 30 (NG > OI): 7 kg in 1 month. Day 30 to Day 90 (OI > NG): 8.1 kg in 2 months. n = 1: severe hypoglycaemia after stopping NG
Gentile et al., 2008 [47]	1. NG 2. OI	OI encouraged from the start. ↑ OI → when past life-threatening stage + agreeing to ↑ OI	NS	OI encouraged.	NS.	-
Paccagnella et al., 2006 [32]	1. NG	OI introduced on days 3–4.	Days 3–4	↑ OI encouraged. When OI >50% energy requirements, NG ↓. At d/c OI only. Average intake at d/c: ~1450 kcal/d	NS. NG duration: 20.7 ± 7.1 days	Abnormal baseline ALT improved in n = 5 (out of n = 7), others (n = 2) improved within 3 weeks of stopping NG.
Parker et al., 2021 [10]	1. Low CHO feed 2. Standard CHO feed	When med stab.	Med stab in both gps: at day 2 On average OI introduced on Day 3.	Staged OI plans between 1800 and 3800 kcal/day. Replacement ONS as needed. As OI ↑, NG, nocturnal and titrated ↓. At week 1: energy via OI vs. total energy: 1.: 2300 (1800, 2300) vs. 3350 (3188, 3350). 2.: 2300 (1800, 2300) vs. 3325 (2844, 3350). NG cessation: NS.	NS NG continued until week 3. NG:OI: Week 2: 1:4 Week 3: 1:6.5	1. vs. 2.: Weight gain by week 1 (NG predominant in 0–0.5 week): 2.7± 1.9 vs. 2.7 ± 1.6 n.s. Weight gain by week 2 (OI predominant 0.5–2.0 week): 4.9 ± 1.9 vs. 4.6 ± 1.5. n.s. Weight gain by week 3 (higher proportion OI): 6.5 ± 2.3 vs. 6.4 ± 2.0 Weight gain/week ↓ with time.
Rigaud et al., 2012 [34]	1. NG	Protocol based	Days 11–21: OI introduced. Timing of NG ↓: NS	OI introduced as small meals (300–400 kcal). From week 4—target weight gain: 0.7–1 kg/week. As OI ↑, NG titrated ↓. NG cessation: NS	NS	BMI ↑ mean diff.: Days 1–2 (NG) vs. Days 13–15 (OI introduced): 1.2 BMI pts Days 13–15 vs. Days 28–32 (NG ↓): 0.8 BMI pts. Weight gain mean diff.: Days 1–2 (NG) to days 13–15 (OI introduced): 2.8 kg Weight gain days 13–15 to days 28–32: 1.8 kg

Table 5. *Cont.*

Author, Year	Cohort (s)	Transition from ETN Towards Increasing Oral Nutrition				Outcomes During Transition Weight: kg BMI: kg/m^2 Mean ± SD Occurrence: n (%)
		Basis for OI Introduction	When Transition Began	Strategies Used: Energy: kcal/d Median (Range)	Duration of Transition	
Zuercher et al., 2003 [41]	1.NG 2. OI	OI from the start. Basis of transition towards ↑ OI and ↓ NG: NS	NS.	NG cessation: with enough OI practice prior to d/c.	NS Duration of NG: 36 ± 21 days	-
Age category unclear						
Bufano et al., 1990 [49]	1. NG	When participant asked for OI to start.	NS	NG stopped when OI > (BMR +30%) for ≥3 consecutive days	NS	n = 2: spontaneous ↑ in OI to >3000 kcal/d, ↑ number of meals & ↑ CHO: P intake. Lasted for ~1 month post d/c

↑: increase; ↓: decrease; ALT: alanine transaminase; BMI: body mass index; BMR: basal metabolic rate; CBT: cognitive behavioural therapy; CHO: carbohydrate content; d/c: discharge; diff: difference; ETN: enteral tube nutrition; Gp: group; hrs: hours; %IBW: % ideal body weight; med. stab.: medical stabilisation. MS: medical stabilisation group; NG: nasogastric tube nutrition; NS: not specified; n.s: no significant difference; OI: oral intake; ONS: oral nutritional supplements; P: protein; PEG: percutaneous endoscopic gastrostomy nutrition; pts: points; req: requirement; subgp: subgroup; w/NG: with nasogastric tube nutrition; WR: weight restoration group.

3.2. Outcomes Related to ETN During Initial Nutrition

3.2.1. Anthropometric Outcomes

Reported weight gain in the initial refeeding phase of ETN (Table 2) was between 0.73 and 2.79 kg/week [6,10,25,30,34,38–40]. Weight gain with a conservative energy prescription in a study (1.2 kg in week one) [34] was comparable with a standard prescription in another study (1.22 kg in week one) [6]. Other studies with standard energy prescriptions reported weight gains of 2.0 kg [38] and 2.1 kg [39] in week one. Studies prescribing higher energy intakes reported gains of 2.7 kg [10] and 2.79 kg [30] in the first week of refeeding. Studies comparing ETN and OI cohorts found contrasting results with one reporting higher weight gain with the former group [6], while the other reporting similar weight gain in both groups [25], despite a significantly higher energy prescription in the ETN cohorts of both studies. Studies with higher energy prescriptions were in adolescent or young adult populations.

Overall, ETN and OI appeared to be comparable in achieving weight gain in this phase of refeeding. Furthermore, results suggested factors in addition to energy prescription affecting weight increase during this phase. A study comparing a standard sodium cohort with a low sodium intake group found a higher weight gain associated with the former, indicating that fluid balance related to sodium retention may be one such factor [40].

3.2.2. Physiological and Psychological Outcomes

Results indicated improvement in function in this early phase of refeeding in studies across age categories. Diaphragmatic function improved within week one in one study [39], and neurological function by week three in another [34]. However, early refeeding was not associated with structural changes, such as muscle mass increases [39]. Hunger ratings improved in the first two weeks in one study [18]. In two RCTs in adults, binge-purge episodes improved in the ETN cohorts compared with the OI groups [18,19]. The ETN group reported increased anxiety in the first week of refeeding compared with the OI group in one study [18]. However, the anorexia nervosa binge-purge subgroup (AN-BP) in this cohort reflected on ETN being 'useful' which may have been related to a reduction in binge-purge episodes [18].

3.2.3. RFS Parameters

Studies with Conservative Energy Prescriptions

The results regarding RFS parameters were heterogeneous (Table 2). Signs of mild RFS [32], refeeding oedema, and phosphate level reduction despite phosphate prophylaxis [34], were reported in two studies in participants across age categories. In contrast, an RCT in adults with an ETN and an OI arm supplemented with prophylactic phosphate reported no RFS, RH, or reduction in potassium levels during refeeding in either group [18]. A recent study in adolescents comparing groups presenting with or without RFS found that both groups had similar BMIs (mean BMIs: 14 kg/m^2), a similar average energy intake, and similar ETN usage [26]. Overall, conservative energy prescription did not appear to mitigate RFS risk fully. ETN and OI routes appeared to have similar risks related to RFS. There appeared no differences in results based on age categories.

Studies with Standard Energy Prescriptions

Results from studies with the standard refeeding energy prescriptions were also heterogeneous. One study reported a lower incidence of RH in its ETN arm compared with its OI cohort [6]. However, most participants in the ETN arm had been given prophylactic phosphate which may have influenced the results. Additionally, a single ETN cohort, also given prophylactic phosphate, reported no reduction in phosphate levels during refeeding [38]. Both these studies used ETN as part of their refeeding protocol. Contrastingly, one study reported a three times higher risk of phosphate reduction in their ETN cohort compared with their OI group despite prophylactic phosphate being given [25]. In this study, ETN was administered as a replacement bolus when OI was refused (food and ONS). Baseline anthropometry was not significantly different between the ETN and OI groups; however, the ETN cohort had a higher energy provision overall [25]. Furthermore, another study, without prophylactic phosphate administration, reported that 33% of its participants required phosphate supplementation two weeks after starting refeeding [49]. These studies were conducted in adolescents [6], across the age categories [25,38] or where the age category was unclear [49] and no differentiation could be made in results based on age.

Studies with Higher Energy Prescriptions

A NG cohort (mean % Expected Body Weight (% EBW) 78%) starting refeeding at 2400 kcal/day, and an increasing energy prescription as required, with prophylactic phosphate given, reported no incidence of phosphate reduction in its participants [30].

An RCT with a rapid increase in energy prescription, comparing arms with a low-carbohydrate feed and a standard carbohydrate feed, reported a significantly lower incidence of phosphate reduction in the low-carbohydrate feed arm. Requirements for potassium and magnesium supplementation due to lowering levels were not significantly different between the groups [10]. This study only provided prophylactic phosphate if levels were $\leq$1 mmol/L prior to refeeding.

These studies were conducted in adolescents [30], or in adolescents and young adults [10], with no studies in an exclusively adult population.

RFS—Other Parameters

With regard to other RFS parameters, a study in adults in which ETN was provided when participants were unable to comply with OI or were unwell and at a higher risk reported a higher incidence of hypokalaemia but not RH or hypomagnesaemia [46]. ETN use and electrolyte derangements were not associated with BMI (mean 17.1 kg/m^2) in this study [46]. Contrastingly, another study in participants across age categories with a mean BMI of 16.3 kg/m^2, in which ETN was provided with OI refusal, found no difference in potassium or magnesium levels between ETN and OI cohorts [25].

RFS Parameters Summary

In summary, RFS-related derangements occurred in various contexts, including in studies with conservative or standard refeeding rates designed to mitigate RFS risk. While a lower BMI is said to increase RFS risk, studies with participants with a relatively higher BMI [25,46] given ETN were also associated with a reduction in phosphate and potassium levels, suggesting the need for a broader exploration of factors increasing RFS risk. Both these studies had ETN administered if OI was refused, or participants were more severely ill. Phosphate prophylaxis, in general, seemed to reduce the risk of RH. However, some studies highlighted that RH may be seen despite prophylaxis and that careful monitoring for the occurrence of RFS and supplementation of electrolytes when needed is of importance. Overall, ETN, as a nutritional route, did not appear to influence RFS risk. The use of low carbohydrate refeeding may support RFS risk reduction. However, more research is needed in this regard. No particular patterns were seen in age categories with RFS risk regarding energy prescription or route of nutrition. However, studies with higher ETN energy prescriptions had been conducted in adolescents or young adults only.

3.3. Overall Outcomes Related to ETN

3.3.1. Anthropometric Outcomes

Weight gain outcomes were presented variably, although all ETN arms across studies showed weight gain from admission to discharge (Table 3). Some studies reported weight changes over the length of the study, ranging from a mean difference of 4.44 kg to 15.9 kg over a varied treatment period [6,10,24,30,36,47], approximating to a range of 0.5–2.2 kg/week. Other studies reported weight gain per week of treatment or study, ranging from 0.91 kg to 1.35 kg/week [18,38,41]. Two studies comparing ETN arms within each study found similar weight gain when both arms had feeds with equivalent energy prescriptions [10] and greater weight increases when one arm had a higher energy prescription than the other [33], as expected.

Cohort studies comparing ETN and OI arms showed either a similar weight gain [25,46,47] or a higher weight gain in the ETN arm compared with the OI arm [18,36,41]. Furthermore, in a cohort study, those given ETN for longer than half their stay had a higher weight gain per week compared with those with ETN for less than half their stay or those in the OI arm [41]. Additionally, a recent cohort study found a significantly higher BMI increase in its ETN group compared with the OI group [44]. This study matched participants who had received ETN with those who had continued with just OI through propensity scoring for confounders such as BMI, duration of illness, other psychiatric co-morbidities, Eating Disorders Examination Questionnaire (EDE-Q) scores, and number of hospitalisations, thus attempting to match the two groups as closely as possible.

Results were heterogeneous when comparing weight gain in ETN and OI arms in regard to energy prescriptions. Higher energy prescriptions in the ETN arms compared with OI arms either resulted in a higher weight gain in the ETN arm as expected [18,24,36] or similar weight gain in the ETN arm despite the higher energy prescription [25]. Contrastingly, one study reported a higher increase in BMI in the ETN arm despite similar energy prescriptions in both the ETN and OI arms [44].

In summary, included studies have shown consistent weight restoration in ETN arms, this being either higher or comparable with the OI arms. Studies have not shown a pattern related to the age of included participants. The heterogeneity of results suggests that factors, other than the mode of nutrition and energy prescription, such as acceptance of nutrition, presence of compensatory behaviours, and types of support provided, may also influence weight gain and need exploration within these contexts.

Studies reporting on fat-free mass changes described improvement over time in the ETN arms [18,19,39]. Mid-upper arm circumference (MUAC) and tricipital skinfold thickness increased significantly in a single cohort study [49]. MUAC was significantly increased in a group given ETN for more than half of their inpatient stay compared with those given ETN for less than half of their stay and those in the OI arm [41]. A study with a single ETN cohort reported increased muscle mass, fat-free mass, and fat mass at days 30 and 45 of admission compared with these measures at baseline [39]. A study comparing an ETN arm with an OI arm reported a significantly higher gain in fat-free mass and fat mass through two months of treatment in the ETN arm [18]. Structural changes were seen at the end of the study duration in these studies, lasting between 21 days and 60 days. Both fat mass and fat-free mass improvement correlated with weight restoration suggesting structural changes were driving these findings. Studies were predominantly in adults or across age populations.

3.3.2. Physiological Outcomes

Physiological outcomes are presented in Table 3. Studies were predominantly in adults or across age populations. Liver function outcomes showed contradictory results. Two studies with abnormal baseline results, given ETN with a conservative prescription, had an improvement in liver function [33,35]. Two studies with normal baseline liver function showed contrasting results. One study reported normal results after ETN with a standard energy prescription [38], while another, also with a standard energy prescription, showed a worsening of liver function in participants, which improved on cessation of ETN [49].

Lung function was investigated in two studies. Peak expiratory flow improved at the end of one single cohort study [35], as did diaphragmatic function and forced expiratory volume 1 in another [39]. The former study also assessed muscle strength, which improved in patients given ETN, even with only partial weight recovery [35].

3.3.3. Outcomes Related to Eating Disorder Symptoms and Other Psychological Outcomes

Eating Disorder Psychopathology

Psychological outcomes are presented in Supplementary Table S2. In terms of eating disorder symptoms, two RCTs in adults reported a significant reduction in binge-purge episodes in the ETN arms compared with the OI arms [18,19]. One study reported a continued significant reduction in these symptoms in its ETN arm in comparison with the OI arm at three- and 12-month follow-ups [19].

Eating disorder psychopathological overall scores showed improvement in both ETN and OI cohorts in studies across the age categories [18–20,41,44]. However, in a study using a rapid refeeding protocol in adolescents with AN, while global EDE-Q scores and Eating Concern and Restraint subscales improved with treatment, the Weight and Shape Concern subscales did not show a significant difference [31]. EDE-Q improvement was significantly related to treatment satisfaction in a study of adult participants [44]. Depression, anxiety, and self-esteem symptoms did not moderate the occurrence of full remission in adolescents in one study [20].

In summary, symptoms related to the eating disorder, for example, eating concern, restraint, and binge-purge episodes, appeared to improve with ETN. However, those specifically related to body image disturbance, such as weight and shape concerns, did not seem to change with nutritional treatment and weight restoration. Treatment satisfaction was associated with EDE-Q reduction, suggesting that participants associated the usefulness of AN treatment with psychological improvement.

General Psychopathology

Regarding broader psychopathology, a rapid refeeding protocol with ETN in an adolescent cohort was associated with improved measures of anxiety and depression. However, these measures were not significantly associated with BMI change over time [31]. One study in adults reported greater increases in Quality of Life scores in patients given ETN compared to OI over the course of treatment [19].

3.3.4. Length of Stay Outcomes

Length of Stay When Comparing ETN and OI Cohorts

Results on length of stay were heterogeneous (Table 3). Some studies found that ETN was associated with a significantly longer admission compared with the OI group [41,43,50]. Other studies reported similar lengths of stays in the ETN and OI arms [24,36]. However, one study reported a significantly longer stay in the OI arm compared to the ETN arm [6]. This study provided a significantly higher energy prescription from the start for the ETN arm in comparison with the OI arm, which may have influenced the results. All studies were in adolescents [6,24,36,43,50] except for one study in participants across the ages [41].

Other Factors Influencing Length of Stay in ETN—Timing of Initiation and Adjunctive Treatment

A study comparing the use and timing of atypical antipsychotics (AAP) and of NG nutrition initiation, found that those who were given AAP and NG early had a significantly shorter stay than those with a late AAP and a late NG start [51]. Furthermore, a study reported a longer admission if NG, when required, was started more than 10 days after admission [43]. Regarding adjunctive nutrition, a study reported a shorter stay in a cohort given ONS alongside NG nutrition and food when compared with the cohort given NG nutrition and food only [45]. All these studies were in adolescent populations.

In summary, factors such as ETN use, the timing of ETN initiation, and whether ETN is used alongside ONS or combined with treatments such as AAPs, may influence the duration of admission. Most of this evidence was in adolescent populations.

3.3.5. Readmissions, Relapses, and Remission

Variable results were reported regarding readmissions and relapses (Table 4). Two studies reported a longer time period before the recurrence of symptoms in the ETN cohort compared with the OI group [18,43]. Furthermore, another study reported lower relapse rates at the two-year follow-up in the cohort given ETN for two months compared with the OI group [48]. Readmission rates were reported as similar in the ETN and OI cohorts in one study [6]. Contrastingly, another retrospective study reported a higher number of admissions in the cohort that needed ETN in at least one admission [50]. Studies were heterogeneous in regard to age groups.

An RCT with both arms receiving ETN initially, testing the hypothesis that inpatient treatment until weight restoration would reduce readmission days, found that both cohorts—one with participants discharged after medical stabilisation and the other when participants were weight restored—had a similar number of readmission days, disproving their hypothesis [20]. Both cohorts had similar eating disorder remission rates at the one-year follow-up. Furthermore, a study with a 5.5-year follow-up found similar rates of remission in the ETN and OI cohorts [50]. Both these studies were conducted in adolescent populations.

In summary, when ETN was part of the protocol, either initially [6] or when specific OI parameters were not met [43] or were provided for at least two months [18,48], studies had better readmission and relapse outcomes associated with the ETN arms compared with OI cohorts. However, when ETN was required because of food refusal, the number of hospitalisations were higher [50], which may be indicative of the severity of the illness. The RCT by Madden et al. (2015b) [20] in medically unstable adolescents with AN suggested that longer admissions for weight restoration may not result in higher remission rates at the one-year follow-up.

3.4. *Strategies Used for Transition from ETN to OI and Related Outcomes*

Methods of transition from ETN towards more OI and outcomes are presented in Table 5. The protocols for the transition from ETN to OI were heterogeneous. OI in the ETN cohorts varied from being present from the start to being introduced with parameters of medical stabilisation. The duration of the transition phase varied from three days to three months. Indications for stopping ETN were based on acceptance of OI [6,24,41,49], anthropometric criteria [36], combinations of criteria [37], and cessation of ETN as part of the protocol for nutrition [10,20,30,38].

Anthropometric outcomes related to the transition phase were not compared with other phases, such as the ETN-only, predominantly ETN, or OI-only phases. However, trends in studies in adolescent [6,30] and mixed-age populations [38] indicated a deceleration of weight restoration during this phase compared with the ETN-only and the predominantly ETN phases. A study in adults described some participants (n = 5, 12%) in its ETN arm having a decrease in OI and showing weight loss following ETN cessation [18]. Difficulties in weight restoration may reflect barriers encountered in the acceptance of OI during the transition process. Factors influencing these outcomes within transition protocols need to be explored.

One cohort study in adolescents reported that the use of ONS alongside ETN and food intake resulted in a shorter length of stay compared with ETN and food intake alone [45]. This suggests that the use of ONS may support the transition process and hence the reduction in length of admission.

3.5. *Qualitative Data and Their Synthesis*

Six studies, two in adolescents or young adults [27,29] and four in adults [21–23,28], investigated qualitative data in ETN (Supplementary Table S3). The following areas were explored.

3.5.1. Initiation of ETN

A theme emerging in participants starting ETN was the physical, undeniable presence of the tube with associated descriptors, such as 'unpleasant', 'scary', 'feeling petrified', or 'traumatised' [21,22,29], with these feelings intensified if participants were anxious or staff inexperienced [29]. Alienation from the decision-making process of ETN initiation [21] and the tube being associated with unfairness, punishment and a fight for control were described [22,28,29]. Conversely, clear communication about the rationale and the process of ETN and weight and discharge targets was described as helpful [27].

Benefits described were the tube as a means of recognising illness severity [27,29], a way of communicating their thoughts and feelings to their family [29], the relief of not having the responsibility for nutrition [28,29] and not having to taste or smell food [28], and, for some, a motivator to start OI [29].

3.5.2. The Presence of Feed with or Without OI

In a study (participants aged 16–19 years) with a faster refeeding protocol with the expectation that daytime OI would be combined with nocturnal ETN, the participants reported that while the mechanics of eating became more manageable, the sensation of fullness, especially towards the end of the day, continued to be pronounced [27]. Conversely, in a study in adults, with NG nutrition only, participants felt that OI alongside ETN would have been beneficial in continuing the 'habit of eating' [21].

3.5.3. Resisting ETN

In studies exploring the lived experience of NG under restraint, participants described alignment with the eating disorder, with physical restraint being a new standard, feelings of isolation from peers, feeling 'stuck' [22], experiencing internal coercion from the eating disorder and external coercion through involuntary treatment, and feeling trapped, hunted, and dehumanised [28]. Self-harm or purging after a feed could result in further restraint [28]. Resistance at the start subsiding through the admission with acceptance or learned helplessness was described by some [28]. Covert resistance was also expressed, such as tampering with feeds, negotiating ETN reduction with staff, and recruiting carers for ETN cessation [29].

3.5.4. Transition Towards More OI

In one study, in which the protocol began with NG nutrition only, participants expressed worries about losing the habit of regular eating, with related difficulties transitioning back to OI [21]. Moreover, they compared themselves to those who were given food and expressed distress with exposure to food smells and not being allowed to eat [21]. Participants in a study with OI concomitant with ETN expressed the helpfulness of supported meals, with staff interacting with them rather than being 'stared at', during the transition to OI [27]. In this protocol, some described developing food aversions when expected to eat while needing NG nutrition. However, for those with a shorter duration of illness, the same protocol improved their enjoyment of food [27]. In one study of lived experience of NG nutrition under restraint, participants expressed feeling stuck and unable to move back to oral nutrition [22]. In some participants in another study, the tube was recognised as a part of their 'self' or as part of their eating disorder identity [29].

3.5.5. A Life-Saving Measure

Participants acknowledged the need for ETN and its life-saving nature [21,22,28,29]. Upon reflection, knowing that NG under restraint would be administered if one did not comply with refeeding treatment, was seen as supportive of the battle against the eating disorder [28]. In retrospect, they were grateful for the life they were able to have afterwards [22,28]. Clinicians described meeting grateful patients who had been physically restrained for ETN in the past [22]. Looking back, participants described how they had lacked care towards themselves at the time, identifying that this had now changed, and they were not 'self-destructive' anymore [28].

3.5.6. Trauma

Tube insertion and feeding were articulated as traumatic in the studies exploring NG under restraint [21,22,28]. Words used to describe this were 'petrified', 'intrusive', 'haunted (by it)', 'smell. . .taste it', and 'an assault' [22,28]. Hearing someone else being restrained for NG nutrition, carried them back to the time they had similar experiences [22]. Participants recalled being sensitive to sounds and receding into feeling like an animal hunted, leaving a lasting imprint on them [28]. Participants described re-experiencing the physical sensation of the tube insertion when they watched a NG insertion as part of their job or feeling retraumatised when needing to be tested for Coronavirus disease via nasal swabs. Some were diagnosed with post-traumatic stress disorder related to their experience [22]. Involuntary treatment was seen as a motivator, in retrospect, to never be in that situation again [28]. Parents and carers also described the trauma of hearing screams on the ward and imagining that it is their child being restrained for feeding. They, however, also expressed empathy for staff having to restrain patients as a life-saving measure [22].

3.5.7. Ways of Improving the Experience of ETN

An explanation of the rationale, clear communication, and goal-setting for ETN cessation and for discharge were described as important parts of a collaborative treatment plan [21,23,27]. Individualised treatment plans, even within protocol-based treatment, were emphasised [23,27]. The importance of a safe space for the service users and carers to communicate their views and feelings was thought of as critical [23]. Establishing trust between the treatment team, service users, and carers was seen as a central part of this process [23].

4. Discussion

ETN is used in AN and AAN as a supportive measure needed in the context of food refusal and markers of medical compromise, such as those outlined in the Medical Emergencies in Eating Disorders guidance [5]. This systematic scoping review explored the use of ETN and associated outcomes in AN and AAN with a particular focus on transitions between ETN and OI.

The following questions were explored:

4.1. Is ETN a Viable and Safe Method of Providing Nutrition in AN and AAN?

This review found consistent improvement in anthropometry associated with ETN with conservative, standard, and higher energy prescriptions in this population. Both conservative and standard energy prescriptions produced similar weight gain initially, possibly influenced by fluid retention and sodium homeostasis. Studies with higher initial energy prescriptions followed by rapid increases in provided energy, all in adolescents or young people, showed higher weight gain per week and overall weight gain [10,20,30], part of which may have been related to fluid shifts, especially in early refeeding. Early and overall weight gain results seen here are in keeping with previous reviews, which found significant weight gain in the initial period with ETN in AN and an overall weight gain of 1 kg/week with NG nutrition [13,53]. When comparing ETN with OI, this review found either similar or higher weight gain in the ETN cohorts and is aligned with the findings of a previous review [12].

Regarding RFS parameters, most studies given prophylactic phosphate showed protection against hypophosphataemia. Overall, there was no evidence that ETN, when compared with OI, was associated with an increased RFS risk. Risks appeared similar in the different age categories. This largely aligns with evidence from previous reviews [12,53].

In summary, ETN, when required, is a viable alternative for supporting physical health improvement and does not appear to increase the risk of refeeding syndrome.

4.2. Does ETN Affect the Length of Admissions in AN and AAN?

The length of stay in ETN cohorts showed heterogeneous results in this review, with some studies showing a tendency towards longer admissions in ETN cohorts compared to OI cohorts. A previous review similarly reported that NG feeding was associated with a longer stay if ETN was in response to medical severity [54]. However, when ETN was part of a routine protocol, the length of stay was shorter than in OI-only cohorts [54]. The duration of ETN, and thus the length of stay, may be dependent on the severity of the illness and complexities in management. Additionally, if NG under restraint is required for a service user, this will likely mean a longer admission. Furthermore, decisions regarding discharge may be based on multiple factors, including discharge criteria of an eating disorder service, service user factors such as age, duration of illness, engagement with treatment, and preference to continue admission, as well as logistical factors such as the need for hospital beds, social care needs of the service user, and available follow-up support. These factors also need to be considered while analysing length-of-stay data. Regarding ETN, Pruccoli et al. (2021) [51] and Marchili et al. (2023) [43] highlighted the importance of clear decision-making in ETN initiation and the usefulness of adjunctive treatment in influencing admission length. Thus, a protocol or pathway for when ETN is indicated, including the process of initiation and cessation with some flexibility to personalise the pathway, with the involvement of the multidisciplinary team, service users, and carers [55], is indicated in supporting shorter inpatient stays.

4.3. What Are the Psychological Outcomes and Qualitative Data Related to ETN?

Overall, outcomes of the eating disorder and quality of life scores improved with treatment regardless of the route of nutrition [18–20,31,41,44]. Service users associated better quality of life and the perception of the usefulness of treatment with the reduction in eating disorder symptomatology [19,44]. Although eating concerns were reduced, weight concerns did not improve with nutritional treatment [31], suggesting the need for focused psychological support, such as body image work, in this context.

Qualitative data highlighted meanings attached by some service users to ETN, including being further aligned to AN with a firmer 'AN identity'. Work to externalise the AN identity may be needed to mitigate these effects [56].

With regard to NG under restraint, a few service users may experience multiple episodes over long periods of time [42], indicating the need to explore risk factors associated with this intervention. The severity of illness and the need for NG under restraint may influence outcomes, such as the persistence of an eating disorder diagnosis during follow-up [42]. NG under restraint has been shown to be associated with long-term trauma. More research is needed for less restrictive supportive measures of nutrition, even when the eating disorder is severe [55]. Furthermore, research is also needed to proactively support service users in mitigating the effects of trauma.

4.4. How Is the Transition from ETN to OI Managed?

This review did not find any studies exploring the transition from ETN in AN and AAN. However, weight restoration slowed down during the transition period, which may indicate difficulties faced during this phase of refeeding. One study found that the cohort using ONS alongside NG nutrition and OI was associated with a reduced length of stay compared with NG and OI [45]. This may indicate the usefulness of ONS in the transition process.

A study of participants admitted to a medical ward for the treatment of restrictive eating disorders reported on the importance participants placed on having OI alongside NG nutrition [57], suggesting that this would be considered supportive of transition by service users. Another study found that the incidence of NG nutrition reduced from 67% to 11% when a protocolised meal support system was introduced in their unit [58]. It is possible that methods, such as changing from continuous to bolus ETN and reducing ETN for a few days, may also be helpful strategies, as described in a review exploring weaning from tube dependency in a paediatric population [59].

Qualitative data in this review indicate that the feeding tube could become a part of the 'self' and a signifier of illness [22,29]. This may inadvertently perpetuate the sick role and isolation of sufferers from their community. A planned exit strategy from ETN to OI may be indicated, with support provided to sufferers in finding their own identity outside of the eating disorder [56].

4.5. Strengths and Limitations of the Review

This scoping review explored outcomes in AN and AAN associated with ETN with a focus on transitions to and from ETN to OI. The study followed PRISMA guidance for scoping reviews and search strategies. Included studies were identified independently by two researchers, and any disagreements were resolved through discussion with co-authors and supervisors. The results were categorised according to study objectives.

However, the heterogeneity between studies in terms of a limited number of baseline characteristics, the content of nutritional protocols, and duration of ETN within them, and the outcomes measured made comparisons between studies difficult. This review only included studies published in English. Most studies were observational, and therefore, had associated biases. ETN may be used only when needed for medical stabilisation and food refusal, making outcome comparisons with cohorts that accept and continue with OI difficult. Studies researching ETN under restraint, by baseline characteristics and severity of illness, may affect outcomes and may have introduced further bias. However, as a scoping review, it was thought important to explore all avenues of investigating outcomes in ETN. Although this review included studies with participants diagnosed with AAN, evidence related to AAN could not be differentiated from that associated with AN. Most participants were female, with only one study conducted in an exclusively male population. Therefore, results may not be generalisable to male sufferers. Differentiation of outcomes related to the age of participants could not be made. Furthermore, most studies came from Europe, North America, and Australia, and results may not be generalisable to populations from other continents.

4.6. Future Research Recommendations

Research suggestions in areas that have gaps in the evidence base are presented in Figure 2. Populations in which more research would be beneficial would be those presenting with AAN. Furthermore, those with AN or AAN and co-morbidities or conditions that have the potential to prolong ETN use; for example, personality disorders, mood and anxiety disorders, and autism, require more research. Comparing those with a recent onset eating disorder with those who have had a long-standing eating disorder would be important. Additionally, research is needed in AN and AAN in male and gender-diverse populations. Furthermore, research comparing outcomes based on age categories would support differentiating strategies in paediatric and adult populations.

Interventions that would benefit from more evidence include the use of ETN as bolus feeds and bolus replacement feeds, as this method is commonly used in eating disorders treatment, and most of the current evidence relates to continuous ETN. The use of propensity scoring, such as used in Martini et al. (2024) [44], matching characteristics, including severity, of participants in the ETN and OI naturalistic cohorts, may support making comparisons more meaningful.

More details on the methods of ETN feeding procedures followed, including the proportion of nutrition through ETN and OI and relating these with pre-treatment OI, would be important. Additionally, methods of transition from ETN and the outcomes need to be explored. Psychological support strategies, to reduce distress and ambivalence about recovery, with a personalised approach, need further research.

Comparing outcomes between ETN-predominant, OI predominant, and OI-only phases during the nutritional transition from ETN to OI, would enhance knowledge and guide supportive strategies. Additionally, connecting quantitative and qualitative data within individuals in a study to co-produce care pathways may be helpful. Furthermore, exploring a wider range of potential recovery-related biomarkers, such as the gut microbiome, metabolic, and immunological parameters, may be of value.

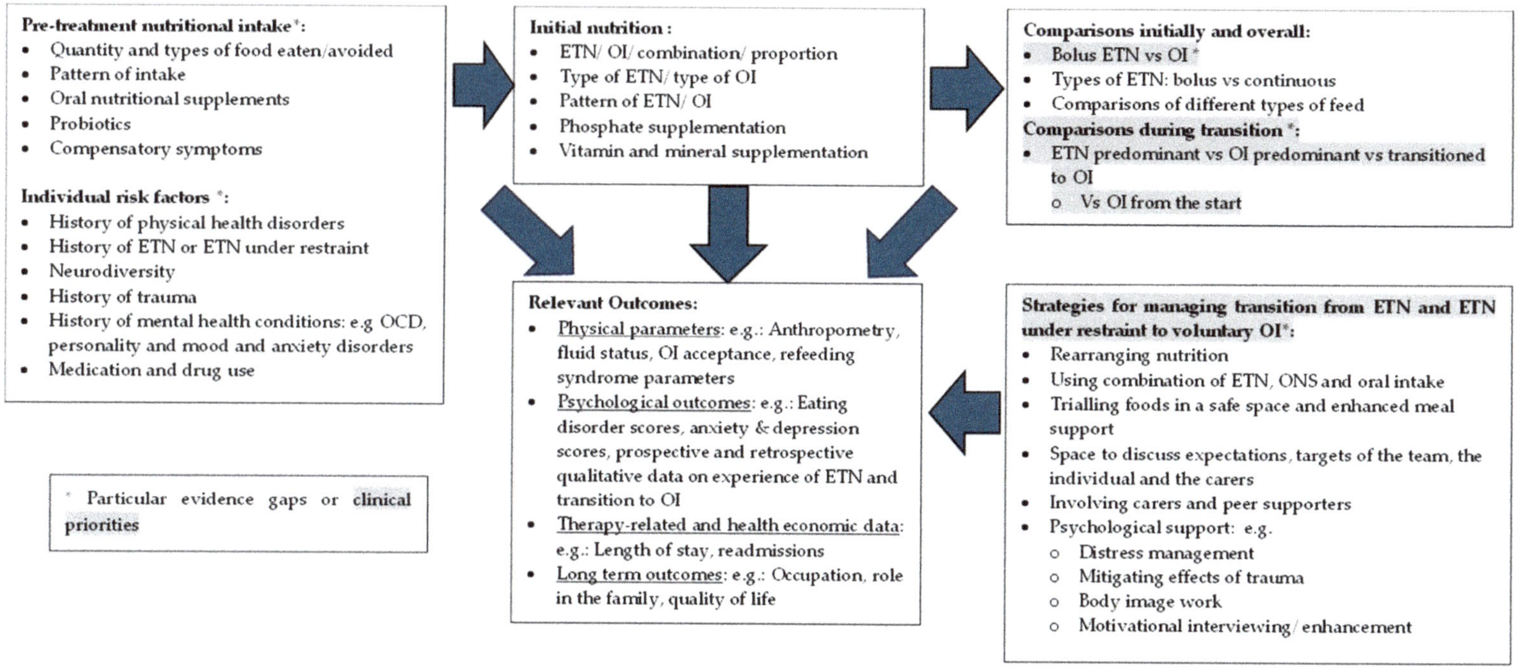

Figure 2. Examples of future research recommendations in the field of enteral nutrition for underweight people with eating disorders.

5. Conclusions

ETN is a viable option for improvement in physical health when this route of nutrition is needed. The evidence so far shows that it can support weight restoration without increasing the risk of RFS or the risk of readmissions. ETN may increase the length of stay, and the reasons for this need to be explored. The evidence so far indicates an overall improvement in eating disorder related scores with nutritional treatment; however, more research on psychological outcomes and exploring strategies to support recovery in the context of ETN is required. More research is needed in exploring methods of transition that are effective and supportive of service users' ability to accept responsibility for their nutrition. Research into mitigating trauma associated with NG under restraint is also needed.

Supplementary Materials: The following supporting information can be downloaded at: https://www.mdpi.com/article/10.3390/nu17030425/s1, Table S1: Summary of initial nutritional protocols, Table S2: Summary of psychological outcomes and Table S3: Summary of qualitative data.

Author Contributions: Conceptualization: N.D., J.T. and H.H.; methodology, N.D., J.T., H.H. and J.L.K.; investigation, N.D., J.L.K. and J.G.; data curation, N.D., D.G., H.M., S.B. and J.G.; writing—original draft preparation, N.D.; writing—review and editing; N.D., J.T., H.H., J.L.K., S.J.F., J.G., H.M., S.B. and D.G.; visualisation, N.D., J.T., H.H. and J.L.K.; supervision, J.T., H.H. and J.L.K.; project administration, N.D., J.T. and H.H. All authors have read and agreed to the published version of the manuscript.

Funding: This research did not receive any direct external funding. J.T. and H.H. receive salary support from the National Institute for Health Research (NIHR) Biomedical Research Centre (BRC) at the South London and Maudsley NHS Foundation Trust (SLaM) and Kings College London. H.M. acknowledges the financial support from the Royal Embassy of Saudi Arabia Cultural Bureau for her PhD training. J.L.K. received a PhD stipend from the Medical Research Council (Reference Number: MR/N013700/1). For the purpose of open access, the author has applied a Creative Commons Attribution (CC BY) licence to any Author Accepted Manuscript version arising. S.B. acknowledges financial support from the Ministry of National Education of Türkiye for funding her postgraduate studentship.

Data Availability Statement: No new data were created or analysed in this study. Data sharing is not applicable to this article.

Conflicts of Interest: The funders had no role in the design of the study; in the collection, analyses, or interpretation of data; in the writing of the manuscript; or in the decision to publish the results. The views expressed in this review are those of the authors and not necessarily those of the National Health Service, NIHR or the Department of Health and Social Care.

References

1. American Psychiatric Association. *Diagnostic and Statistical Manual of Mental Disorders*, 5th ed.; American Psychiatric Association: Arlington, VA, USA, 2013.
2. Himmerich, H.; Hotopf, M.; Shetty, H.; Schmidt, U.; Treasure, J.; Hayes, R.D.; Stewart, R.; Chang, C.K. Psychiatric comorbidity as a risk factor for mortality in people with anorexia nervosa. *Eur. Arch. Psychiatry Clin. Neurosci.* **2019**, *269*, 351–359. [CrossRef] [PubMed]
3. Brennan, C.; Illingworth, S.; Cini, E.; Bhakta, D. Medical instability in typical and atypical adolescent anorexia nervosa: A systematic review and meta-analysis. *J. Eat. Disord.* **2023**, *11*, 58. [CrossRef] [PubMed]
4. National Institute for Health and Care Excellence. *Eating Disorders: Recognition and Treatment*; NG69; National Institute for Health and Care Excellence: London, UK, 2017.
5. Royal College of Psychiatrists. Medical Emergencies in Eating Disorders: Guidance on Recognition and Management. Available online: https://www.rcpsych.ac.uk/docs/default-source/improving-care/better-mh-policy/college-reports/college-report-cr233-medical-emergencies-in-eating-disorders-(meed)-guidance.pdf?sfvrsn=2d327483_63 (accessed on 7 July 2024).

6. Agostino, H.; Erdstein, J.; Di Meglio, G. Shifting Paradigms: Continuous Nasogastric Feeding With High Caloric Intakes i Anorexia Nervosa. *J. Adolesc. Health* **2013**, *53*, 590–594. [CrossRef] [PubMed]
7. Watters, A.; Gibson, D.; Dee, E.; Mascolo, M.; Mehler, P.S. Superior mesenteric artery syndrome in severe anorexia nervosa: case series. *Clin. Case Rep.* **2020**, *8*, 185–189. [CrossRef] [PubMed]
8. Reber, E.; Friedli, N.; Vasiloglou, M.F.; Schuetz, P.; Stanga, Z. Management of Refeeding Syndrome in Medical Inpatients. *J. Cli Med.* **2019**, *8*, 2202. [CrossRef]
9. National Institute for Health and Care Excellence. *Nutrition Support for Adults: Oral Nutrition Support, Enteral Tube Feeding an Parenteral Nutrition*; CG32; National Institute for Health and Care Excellence: London, UK, 2006.
10. Parker, E.K.; Flood, V.; Halaki, M.; Wearne, C.; Anderson, G.; Gomes, L.; Clarke, S.; Wilson, F.; Russell, J.; Frig, E.; et al. A standar enteral formula versus an iso-caloric lower carbohydrate/high fat enteral formula in the hospital management of adolescent an young adults admitted with anorexia nervosa: A randomised controlled trial. *J. Eat. Disord.* **2021**, *9*, 1–12. [CrossRef]
11. Kohn, M.R.; Madden, S.; Clarke, S.D. Refeeding in anorexia nervosa: Increased safety and efficiency through understanding th pathophysiology of protein calorie malnutrition. *Curr. Opin. Pediatr.* **2011**, *23*, 390–394. [CrossRef]
12. Bendall, C.; Taylor, N.F. The effect of oral refeeding compared with nasogastric refeeding on the quality of care for patien hospitalised with an eating disorder: A systematic review. *Nutr. Diet. J. Dietit. Assoc. Aust.* **2023**, *80*, 44–54. [CrossRef]
13. Rizzo, S.M.; Douglas, J.W.; Lawrence, J.C. Enteral Nutrition via Nasogastric Tube for Refeeding Patients With Anorexia Nervos A Systematic Review. *Nutr. Clin. Pract.* **2019**, *34*, 359–370. [CrossRef]
14. Tricco, A.C.; Lillie, E.; Zarin, W.; O'Brien, K.K.; Colquhoun, H.; Levac, D.; Moher, D.; Peters, M.D.J.; Horsley, T.; Weeks, L et al. PRISMA Extension for Scoping Reviews (PRISMA-ScR): Checklist and Explanation. *Ann. Intern. Med.* **2018**, *169*, 467–47 [CrossRef]
15. Ouzzani, M.; Hammady, H.; Fedorowicz, Z.; Elmagarmid, A. Rayyan—A web and mobile app for systematic reviews. *Syst. Re* **2016**, *5*, 210. [CrossRef] [PubMed]
16. Moola, S.M.Z.; Tufanaru, C.; Aromataris, E.; Sears, K.; Sfetcu, R.; Currie, M.; Qureshi, R.; Mattis, P.; Lisy, K.; Mu, P.-F. Systemati reviews of etiology and risk. In *JBI Manual for Evidence Synthesis*; Aromataris, E.M.Z., Ed.; JBI: Adelaide, Australia, 2020.
17. Barker, T.H.; Habibi, N.; Aromataris, E.; Stone, J.C.; Leonardi-Bee, J.; Sears, K.; Hasanoff, S.; Klugar, M.; Tufanaru, C.; Moola, S et al. The revised JBI critical appraisal tool for the assessment of risk of bias for quasi-experimental studies. *JBI Evid. Synth.* **202** *22*, 378–388. [CrossRef] [PubMed]
18. Rigaud, D.; Brondel, L.; Poupard, A.T.; Talonneau, I.; Brun, J.M. A randomized trial on the efficacy of a 2-month tube feedin regimen in anorexia nervosa: A 1-year follow-up study. *Clin. Nutr.* **2007**, *26*, 421–429. [CrossRef] [PubMed]
19. Rigaud, D.J.; Brayer, V.; Roblot, A.; Brindisi, M.C.; Verges, B. Efficacy of tube feeding in binge-eating/vomiting patients: A 2-month randomized trial with 1-year follow-up. *J. Parenter. Enter. Nutr.* **2011**, *35*, 356–364. [CrossRef] [PubMed]
20. Madden, S.; Miskovic-Wheatley, J.; Wallis, A.; Kohn, M.; Lock, J.; Le Grange, D.; Jo, B.; Clarke, S.; Rhodes, P.; Hay, P.; et al. A randomized controlled trial of in-patient treatment for anorexia nervosa in medically unstable adolescents. *Psychol. Med.* **2015**, *4* 415–427. [CrossRef]
21. Matthews-Rensch, K.; Young, A.; Cutmore, C.; Davis, A.; Jeffrey, S.; Patterson, S. Acceptability of using a nasogastric refeedin protocol with adult patients with medically unstable eating disorders. *J. Eval. Clin. Pract.* **2023**, *29*, 49–58. [CrossRef]
22. Fuller, S.J.; Tan, J.C.T.; Nicholls, D. Nasogastric tube feeding under restraint: Understanding the impact and improving car *BJPsych Bull.* **2023**, *48*, 163–167. [CrossRef]
23. Fuller, S.J.; Tan, J.C.T.; Nicholls, D. The importance of individualised care, good communication and trust for reducing nasogastri tube feeding under physical restraint: Qualitative multi-informant study. *BJPsych Open* **2024**, *10*, e86. [CrossRef]
24. Silber, T.J.; Robb, A.S.; Orrell-Valente, J.K.; Ellis, N.; Valadez-Meltzer, A.; Dadson, M.J. Nocturnal nasogastric refeeding fo hospitalized adolescent boys with anorexia nervosa. *J. Dev. Behav. Pediatr. JDBP* **2004**, *25*, 415–418. [CrossRef]
25. Kells, M.; Gregas, M.; Wolfe, B.E.; Garber, A.K.; Kelly-Weeder, S. Factors associated with refeeding hypophosphatemia ir adolescents and young adults hospitalized with anorexia nervosa. *Nutr. Clin. Pract.* **2022**, *37*, 470–478. [CrossRef]
26. Pruccoli, J.; Barbieri, E.; Visconti, C.; Pranzetti, B.; Pettenuzzo, I.; Moscano, F.; Malaspina, E.; Marino, M.; Valeriani, B.; Parmeggian A. Refeeding syndrome and psychopharmacological interventions in children and adolescents with Anorexia Nervosa: A focu on olanzapine-related modifications of electrolyte balance. *Eur. J. Pediatr.* **2024**, *183*, 1935–1941. [CrossRef] [PubMed]
27. Kezelman, S.; Rhodes, P.; Hunt, C.; Anderson, G.; Clarke, S.; Crosby, R.D.; Touyz, S. Adolescent patients' perspectives or rapid-refeeding: A prospective qualitative study of an inpatient population. *Adv. Eat. Disord.* **2016**, *4*, 277–292. [CrossRef]
28. Mac Donald, B.; Gustafsson, S.A.; Bulik, C.M.; Clausen, L. Living and leaving a life of coercion: A qualitative interview study o patients with anorexia nervosa and multiple involuntary treatment events. *J. Eat. Disord.* **2023**, *11*, 40. [CrossRef]
29. Halse, C.; Boughtwood, D.; Clarke, S.; Honey, A.; Kohn, M.; Madden, S. Illuminating multiple perspectives: Meanings o nasogastric feeding in anorexia nervosa. *Eur. Eat. Disord. Rev.* **2005**, *13*, 264–272. [CrossRef]
30. Madden, S.; Miskovic-Wheatley, J.; Clarke, S.; Touyz, S.; Hay, P.; Kohn, M.R. Outcomes of a rapid refeeding protocol in Adolescen Anorexia Nervosa. *J. Eat. Disord.* **2015**, *3*, 8. [CrossRef]

31. Kezelman, S.; Crosby, R.D.; Rhodes, P.; Hunt, C.; Anderson, G.; Clarke, S.; Touyz, S. Anorexia nervosa, anxiety, and the clinical implications of rapid refeeding. *Front. Psychol.* **2018**, *9*, 1097. [CrossRef]
32. Paccagnella, A.; Mauri, A.; Baruffi, C.; Berto, R.; Zago, R.; Marcon, M.L.; Pizzolato, D.; Fontana, F.; Rizzo, L.; Bisetto, M.; et al. Application criteria of enteral nutrition in patients with anorexia nervosa: Correlation between clinical and psychological data in a "lifesaving" treatment. *JPEN J. Parenter. Enter. Nutr.* **2006**, *30*, 231–239. [CrossRef]
33. Hanachi, M.; Melchior, J.C.; Crenn, P. Hypertransaminasemia in severely malnourished adult anorexia nervosa patients: Risk factors and evolution under enteral nutrition. *Clin. Nutr.* **2013**, *32*, 391–395. [CrossRef]
34. Rigaud, D.; Tallonneau, I.; Brindisi, M.C.; Verges, B. Prognosis in 41 severely malnourished anorexia nervosa patients. *Clin. Nutr.* **2012**, *31*, 693–698. [CrossRef]
35. Minano Garrido, E.; Di Lodovico, L.; Dicembre, M.; Duquesnoy, M.; Ohanyan, H.; Melchior, J.C.; Hanachi, M. Evaluation of muscle-skeletal strength and peak expiratory flow in severely malnourished inpatients with anorexia nervosa: A pilot study. *Nutrition* **2021**, *85*, 111133. [CrossRef]
36. Robb, A.S.; Silber, T.J.; Orrell-Valente, J.K.; Valadez-Meltzer, A.; Ellis, N.; Dadson, M.J.; Chatoor, I. Supplemental nocturnal nasogastric refeeding for better short-term outcome in hospitalized adolescent girls with anorexia nervosa. *Am. J. Psychiatry* **2002**, *159*, 1347–1353. [CrossRef] [PubMed]
37. Born, C.; de la Fontaine, L.; Winter, B.; Muller, N.; Schaub, A.; Frustuck, C.; Schule, C.; Voderholzer, U.; Cuntz, U.; Falkai, P.; et al. First results of a refeeding program in a psychiatric intensive care unit for patients with extreme anorexia nervosa. *BMC Psychiatry* **2015**, *15*, 57. [CrossRef] [PubMed]
38. Gentile, M.G. Enteral nutrition for feeding severely underfed patients with anorexia nervosa. *Nutrients* **2012**, *4*, 1293–1303. [CrossRef] [PubMed]
39. Murciano, D.; Rigaud, D.; Pingleton, S.; Armengaud, M.H.; Melchior, J.C.; Aubier, M. Diaphragmatic function in severely malnourished patients with anorexia nervosa: Effects of renutrition. *Am. J. Respir. Crit. Care Med.* **1994**, *150*, 1569–1574. [CrossRef]
40. Rigaud, D.; Boulier, A.; Tallonneau, I.; Brindisi, M.C.; Rozen, R. Body fluid retention and body weight change in anorexia nervosa patients during refeeding. *Clin. Nutr.* **2010**, *29*, 749–755. [CrossRef]
41. Zuercher, J.N.; Cumella, E.J.; Woods, B.K.; Eberly, M.; Carr, J.K. Efficacy of voluntary nasogastric tube feeding in female inpatients with anorexia nervosa. *J. Parenter. Enter. Nutr.* **2003**, *27*, 268–276. [CrossRef]
42. Blikshavn, T.; Halvorsen, I.; Ro, O. Physical restraint during inpatient treatment of adolescent anorexia nervosa: Frequency, clinical correlates, and associations with outcome at five-year follow-up. *J. Eat. Disord.* **2020**, *8*, 20. [CrossRef]
43. Marchili, M.R.; Diamanti, A.; Zanna, V.; Spina, G.; Mascolo, C.; Roversi, M.; Guarnieri, B.; Mirra, G.; Testa, G.; Raucci, U.; et al. Early Naso-Gastric Feeding and Outcomes of Anorexia Nervosa Patients. *Nutrients* **2023**, *15*, 490. [CrossRef]
44. Martini, M.; Longo, P.; Di Benedetto, C.; Delsedime, N.; Panero, M.; Abbate-Daga, G.; Toppino, F. Nasogastric Tube Feeding in Anorexia Nervosa: A Propensity Score-Matched Analysis on Clinical Efficacy and Treatment Satisfaction. *Nutrients* **2024**, *16*, 1664. [CrossRef]
45. Trovato, C.M.; Capriati, T.; Bolasco, G.; Campana, C.; Papa, V.; Mazzoli, B.; Zanna, V.; Marchili, M.R.; Basso, M.S.; Maggiore, G.; et al. Five-Year Inpatient Management of Teenagers With Anorexia Nervosa: Focus on Nutritional Issues. *J. Pediatr. Gastroenterol. Nutr.* **2022**, *74*, 674–680. [CrossRef]
46. Braude, M.R.; Con, D.; Clayton-Chubb, D.; Nandurkar, R.; Chua, L.E.; Newnham, E.D. Acute medical stabilisation of adults with anorexia nervosa: Experience of a defined interdisciplinary model of care. *Intern. Med. J.* **2020**, *50*, 77–85. [CrossRef] [PubMed]
47. Gentile, M.G.; Manna, G.M.; Ciceri, R.; Rodeschini, E. Efficacy of inpatient treatment in severely malnourished anorexia nervosa patients. *Eat. Weight. Disord.* **2008**, *13*, 191–197. [CrossRef] [PubMed]
48. Rigaud, D.; Pennacchio, H.; Bizeul, C.; Reveillard, V.; Verges, B. Outcome in AN adult patients: A 13-year follow-up in 484 patients. *Diabetes Metab.* **2011**, *37*, 305–311. [CrossRef] [PubMed]
49. Bufano, G.; Bellini, C.; Cervellin, G.; Coscelli, C. Enteral nutrition in anorexia nervosa. *JPEN J. Parenter. Enteral. Nutr.* **1990**, *14*, 404–407. [CrossRef]
50. Nehring, I.; Kewitz, K.; von Kries, R.; Thyen, U. Long-term effects of enteral feeding on growth and mental health in adolescents with anorexia nervosa--results of a retrospective German cohort study. *Eur. J. Clin. Nutr.* **2014**, *68*, 171–177. [CrossRef]
51. Pruccoli, J.; Pelusi, M.; Romagnoli, G.; Malaspina, E.; Moscano, F.; Parmeggiani, A. Timing of psychopharmacological and nutritional interventions in the inpatient treatment of anorexia nervosa: An observational study. *Brain Sci.* **2021**, *11*, 1242. [CrossRef]
52. Pruccoli, J.; Pettenuzzo, I.; Parmeggiani, A. Treatment response in children and adolescents with anorexia nervosa: A naturalistic, case-control study. *Eat. Weight. Disord. EWD* **2022**, *27*, 2879–2887. [CrossRef]
53. Hale, M.D.; Logomarsino, J.V. The use of enteral nutrition in the treatment of eating disorders: A systematic review. *Eat. Weight. Disord.* **2019**, *24*, 179–198. [CrossRef]
54. Hindley, K.; Fenton, C.; McIntosh, J. A systematic review of enteral feeding by nasogastric tube in young people with eating disorders. *J. Eat. Disord.* **2021**, *9*, 90. [CrossRef]

55. Fuller, S.J.; Tan, J.; Nicholls, D. Decision-making and best practice when nasogastric tube feeding under restraint: Multi-informant qualitative study. *BJPsych Open* **2023**, *9*, e28. [CrossRef]
56. Conti, J.E.; Joyce, C.; Hay, P.; Meade, T. "Finding my own identity": A qualitative metasynthesis of adult anorexia nervosa treatment experiences. *BMC Psychol.* **2020**, *8*, 110. [CrossRef] [PubMed]
57. Morgan, K.; Cutmore, C.; Matthews-Rensch, K. Adding mini meals to a nasogastric refeeding protocol for patients with eating disorders can be achieved on general hospital wards. *J. Hum. Nutr. Diet. Off. J. Br. Diet. Assoc.* **2023**, *36*, 1207–1213. [CrossRef] [PubMed]
58. Couturier, J.; Mahmood, A. Meal support therapy reduces the use of nasogastric feeding for adolescents hospitalized with anorexia nervosa. *Eat. Disord.* **2009**, *17*, 327–332. [CrossRef] [PubMed]
59. Krom, H.; de Winter, J.P.; Kindermann, A. Development, prevention, and treatment of feeding tube dependency. *Eur. J. Pediatr.* **2017**, *176*, 683–688. [CrossRef]

nutrients

MDPI

ystematic Review

Potomania and Beer Potomania: A Systematic Review of Published Case Reports

Keila S. Micoanski [1,2], Jose M. Soriano [1,3,*] and Monica M. Gozalbo [1,2,3]

[1] Unit of Psychology and Applied Nutrition, Food & Health Lab, Institute of Materials Science, University of Valencia, 46980 Paterna, Spain; keilamicoanski@outlook.com (K.S.M.); monica.gozalbo@uv.es (M.M.G.)
[2] Department of Medicine and Public Health, Food Science, Toxicology and Legal Medicine, University of Valencia, 46010 Burjassot, Spain
[3] Joint Research Unit on Endocrinology, Nutrition and Clinical Dietetics, Health Research Institute La Fe, University of Valencia, 46026 Valencia, Spain
* Correspondence: jose.soriano@uv.es

Abstract: Background/Objectives: Potomania and beer potomania are rare but important causes of dilutional hyponatremia, resulting from excessive fluid intake combined with low solute consumption. This systematic review aimed to identify and describe the clinical presentations, underlying causes, complications, and management approaches in published case reports of these conditions. **Methods**: A systematic search was conducted in PubMed, Embase, Web of Science, and Scopus. Inclusion criteria were case reports and letters to the editor with confirmed diagnoses of potomania or beer potomania. The Joanna Briggs Institute (JBI) checklist was used to evaluate study quality. The SPIDER framework guided the selection process. A qualitative, narrative synthesis was performed. **Results**: Forty-four cases were included. Hyponatremia was the most frequent finding, commonly accompanied by neurological symptoms such as confusion and seizures. Beer potomania was more prevalent among male patients and associated with alcohol consumption and poor nutrition. Potomania was linked to restrictive diets, psychiatric disorders, or excessive intake of various non-alcoholic fluids. Management typically involved fluid restriction, correction of electrolytes, nutritional support, and psychiatric care. Five cases developed osmotic demyelination syndrome due to rapid sodium correction. **Conclusions**: Increased clinical awareness of potomania and beer potomania is essential to prevent severe outcomes. Early identification, individualized management, and cautious correction of serum sodium are crucial. Despite the limitations of case report evidence, this review provides meaningful insights into diagnosis and treatment.

Keywords: excessive liquid intake; hyponatremia; osmotic demyelination syndrome; potomania

1. Introduction

Potomania is a disorder characterized by the excessive intake of fluids without an underlying physical disorder. It can manifest as polydipsia when it refers to drinking excessive water, psychogenic polydipsia (when it is associated with mental disorders), and beer potomania when this excessive consumption is of beer [1,2]. An adult under normal physiological conditions drinks an average of 2 L of water daily, and symptoms are generally rare when fluid consumption is less than 10 L per day [3]. However, when an excess of water intake exceeds the kidneys' elimination capacity, hypotonic hyponatremia can occur, with a reduction in plasma osmolality [4,5].

Potomania is defined as a clinical condition characterized by excessive fluid intake, particularly of liquids with low solute content, in the context of insufficient dietary protein and electrolyte consumption. This imbalance reduces renal solute availability, limiting the kidneys' capacity to excrete free water and predisposing individuals to dilutional hyponatremia. The condition often arises from a combination of contributing factors, including maladaptive social behaviors (e.g., detox practices, competitive drinking), nutritional deficiencies, and underlying psychiatric disorders such as schizophrenia, obsessive-compulsive disorder (OCD), and bipolar disorder, which are frequently associated with psychogenic polydipsia [6,7].

Beer potomania is a specific subtype of potomania characterized by the chronic ingestion of large volumes of beer alongside a diet low in protein and electrolytes. Unlike general potomania, which may involve excessive intake of any hypo-osmolar liquid, beer potomania involves a unique combination of a solute-poor beverage and restricted solute intake from food. Since beer contains minimal electrolytes and negligible protein, it provides insufficient solute to facilitate water excretion, impairing free water clearance and leading to hyponatremia. Although both conditions share the mechanism of dilutional hyponatremia secondary to fluid overload, their etiologies, clinical contexts, and treatment approaches differ substantially [8].

The clinical importance of potomania lies in its potential to cause life-threatening hyponatremia, which can present with neurological symptoms such as seizures, altered mental status, and even osmotic demyelination syndrome if not carefully managed. Despite its severity, potomania is often underdiagnosed or misattributed to other causes of hyponatremia due to its rarity and overlapping clinical presentations. Diagnosis is further complicated by the lack of standardized criteria and reliance on patient history, which may be incomplete or unreliable, especially in those with psychiatric conditions or substance use disorders. Timely recognition and tailored interventions are critical to prevent complications and guide appropriate treatment [9,10].

In this review, cases were classified as potomania or beer potomania based on the following diagnostic criteria: (1) documented excessive intake of fluids—typically water or beer—with volumes generally exceeding 4–10 L per day; (2) presence of hypotonic hyponatremia (serum sodium < 135 mmO/L); (3) low urine osmolality (<100 mOsm/kg in most cases); (4) absence of alternative causes of hyponatremia such as renal failure, syndrome of inappropriate antidiuretic hormone secretion (SIADH), or adrenal insufficiency; and (5) dietary patterns indicating low solute or protein intake. For beer potomania, additional criteria included a reported history of chronic beer consumption with limited nutritional intake [10,11].

While individual case reports have highlighted unique presentations of potomania and beer potomania, there is a lack of synthesized evidence offering a comprehensive overview of their clinical characteristics, risk factors, and outcomes. No prior systematic review has compiled these cases to identify common patterns or to inform clinical decision-making. Given the growing recognition of fluid-induced hyponatremia and the need for awareness among clinicians, particularly in emergency and psychiatric settings, this systematic review aims to bridge the existing gap by analyzing and summarizing available evidence from case reports [12,13]. This synthesis will provide insights into diagnostic strategies, therapeutic interventions, and potential complications, supporting the development of clinical guidelines and future research directions.

2. Materials and Methods

To evaluate the conduct of this study and increase transparency and reproducibility, this review was registered in the PROSPERO systematic review registry database

(ID: CRD42024528002). This systematic review was conducted by the Preferred Reporting Items for Systematic Reviews and Meta-Analyses (PRISMA 2020) guidelines [14]. A completed PRISMA checklist is provided as Supplementary Materials.

Using a standardized search strategy, the databases searched for the most current data were PubMed, Embase, Web of Science, and Scopus. Boolean search strings included the following: (Potomania) OR (Beer) AND (Potomania) OR (Cider Potomania), (Potomania) AND (Anorexia), (Potomania) AND (Schizophrenia), (Potomania) AND (Exercise), (Potomania) AND (Excessive water intake), (Hyponatremia) AND (Potomania). The search included studies published up to January 2025.

Since all included studies were case reports, the SPIDER framework was used instead of PICO. The Sample included individuals with potomania or beer potomania; the Phenomenon of Interest was the clinical presentation and outcomes; the Design consisted of case reports and letters to the editor; the Evaluation involved descriptive clinical data; and the Research type was qualitative and observational.

Table 1 describes the SPIDER framework (Sample, Phenomenon of Interest, Design, Evaluation, Research type).

Table 1. SPIDER Framework Used for Eligibility Criteria.

S (Sample)	Individuals diagnosed with potomania or beer potomania in published case reports.
PI (Phenomenon of Interest)	Clinical presentation, diagnostic process, treatment approaches, and outcomes related to potomania.
D (Design)	Case reports and letters to the editor describing individual or multiple clinical cases.
E (Evaluation)	Descriptive data on clinical features, laboratory findings, diagnostic tools, therapies, and patient outcomes.
R (Research Type)	Qualitative, observational evidence (non-comparative).

Inclusion criteria: (i) case reports/letters to the editor with potomania diagnosis; (ii) all age groups; (iii) clear diagnostic markers or characteristics; and (iv) reported treatment outcomes.

Exclusion criteria: (i) reviews, meta-analyses, observational or experimental studies; (ii) animal studies; (iii) irrelevant or incomplete data; (iv) languages other than English, Spanish, and French; and (v) inaccessible full texts.

Duplicates were removed with Rayyan QCR®. Two reviewers (K.S.M. and M.G.) independently screened records and extracted data. J.M.S resolved disagreements.

Quality was assessed with the JBI Case Report Checklist. Results are in Supplementary Table S1. No studies were excluded for low quality.

Due to descriptive data, a narrative synthesis was performed, focusing on clinical profiles, diagnostic criteria, treatments, and outcomes.

Quality assessment of the included case reports was conducted using the Joanna Briggs Institute (JBI) Critical Appraisal Checklist for Case Reports. The results of this appraisal are summarized in Supplementary Table S1 and were used to guide the interpretation of findings. No cases were excluded based on low quality alone.

Because of the descriptive nature of the data, the findings were synthesized narratively. The synthesis focused on clinical characteristics, diagnostic markers, therapeutic approaches, and outcomes reported in the included case reports.

Descriptive statistics such as means, ranges, and proportions were used to summarize clinical and laboratory data reported in the case studies.

3. Results

A total of 44 individual cases were included in this systematic review. The mean age of patients was 45 years. Key demographic features are summarized in Table 2. Approximately 70% of the cases involved male patients. The cases were geographically diverse, with reports from Europe, North America, Asia, and South America. The detailed process of search results and selection is shown in Figure 1.

Table 2. The description of the case reports included author and year, gender, and main diagnosis.

Author and Year	Age (Years)	Gender	Diagnosis
Lodhi et al. (2017) [15]	59 and 60	Male	Beer Potomania
Yu ZL and Fisher (2022) [16]	53	Male	Beer Potomania
Bhattarai et al. (2010) [7]	52	Male	Beer Potomania
Kujubu et al. (2015) [17]	84	Male	Beer Potomania
Senanayake et al. (2023) [10]	41	Female	Beer Potomania
Dodoo et al. (2022) [18]	56	Male	Beer Potomania
Stasishin et al. (2021) [19]	A middle-aged	Male	Beer Potomania
Laubner et al. (2020) [20]	55	Male	Beer Potomania
Mifsud et al. (2018) [21]	68	Male	Beer Potomania
So BYF and Chan GCW (2023) [22]	51	Male	Potomania
Perez Gomez et al. (2022) [8]	45	Male	Beer Potomania
Macías Robles et al. (2009) [5]	42	Male	Potomania
Soliman et al. (2018) [12]	67	Male	Potomania
Sterns et al. (2010) [23]	45	Male	Beer Potomania
Lum G. (2013) [24]	63	Male	Beer Potomania
Windpessl et al. (2017) [9]	61	Female	Potomania
Rafei et al. (2016) [25]	66	Male	Beer Potomania
Pallavi, R. (2015) [26]	68	Female	Beer Potomania
Srisung et al. (2015) [27]	69	Male	Potomania
Patel et al. (2012) [28]	56	Female	Beer Potomania
McGraw et al. (2012) [2]	Mid-30s	Male	Beer Potomania
Haran et al. (2010) [29]	41	Male	Beer Potomania
Fox BD (2002) [30]	51	Female	Potomania
Lord (2000) [11]	26	Male	Cider Potomania
Sharif et al. (2023) [31]	42	Male	Beer Potomania
Akatsuka et al. (2023) [32]	32	Male	Beer Potomania
Campeão (2013) [33]	48	Male	Potomania
Chaudhary et al. (2012) [13]	40	Female	Potomania
Axelrod et al. (2011) [34]	39	Female	Beer Potomania
Pizzini et al. (2011) [35]	76	Male	Potomania
Caron et al. (1977) [36]	Case 1: 59 Case 2: 25 Case 3: 18	Female Male Female	Potomania
Goëb et al. (2003) [37]	20	Female	Potomania

Table 2. *Cont.*

Author and Year	Age (Years)	Gender	Diagnosis
Hirel and Thobois. (2014) [38]	61	Female	Potomania
Couillard et al. (2021) [39]	54	Female	Potomania
Haymann (2014) [40]	45	Female	Potomania
Tejedor et al. (2014) [41]	41	Male	Potomania
Domínguez et al. (2013) [6]	72	Female	Potomania
Alda et al. (2007) [42]	18	Male	Potomania
Benítez-Mejía et al. (2021) [43]	52	Female	Potomania
Milisenda et al. (2012) [44]	60	Male	Beer Potomania
Campbell (2010) [45]	33	Male	Beer Potomania

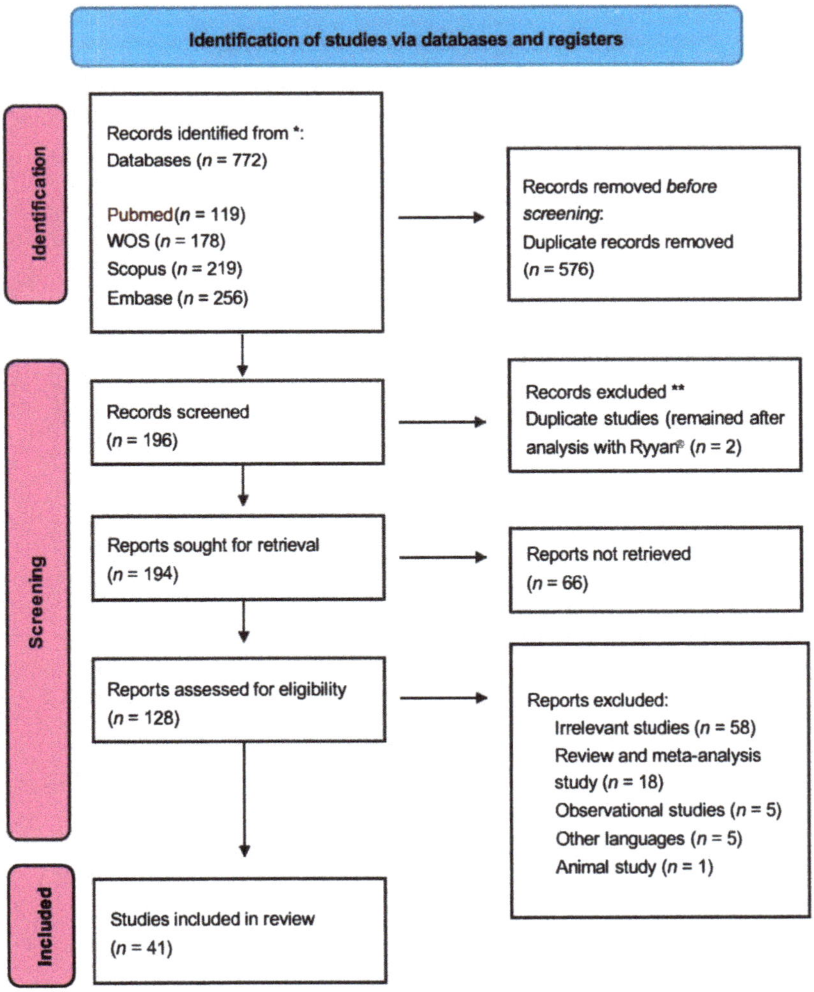

Figure 1. PRISMA flow diagram adapted from Page et al. [14] of the study selection process. * A total of 772 records were identified through database searching. ** After removing duplicates and applying eligibility criteria, 41 studies were included in the final review.

Hyponatremia was the primary clinical manifestation, with serum sodium levels ranging from 102 to 129 mmO/L. Most cases presented with severe hyponatremia (<120 mmO/L), and the most common symptoms were nausea, confusion, headache, altered mental status, seizures, and, in some cases, coma. Symptoms such as seizures and altered mental status were common, as previously described by Musch et al. [46] and Sailer et al. [47]. Fluid intake and psychiatric comorbidities are described in Table 3.

Urine osmolality was reported in 36 cases and was consistently low (around <100 mOsm/kg, referring to the average of the values found) in most patients, consistent with impaired renal capacity to excrete excess water due to low solute intake. Laboratory findings are detailed in Table 4.

Psychiatric comorbidities were present in over half of the patients, including schizophrenia, bipolar disorder, and depression. Many of these patients also had a history of psychogenic polydipsia or compulsive water intake.

Beer potomania was described in 26 of the 44 cases, predominantly affecting middle-aged males with a history of chronic alcohol consumption and poor nutritional intake. In contrast, potomania was often associated with excessive intake of other fluids (e.g., water, soda, sports drinks). It was linked to restrictive diets, eating disorders, or excessive hydration due to exercise.

Management strategies included the following:

- Fluid restriction (n = 40);
- Intravenous saline or hypertonic saline (n = 28);
- Electrolyte correction (e.g., potassium, magnesium, thiamine);
- Nutritional support;
- Psychiatric evaluation and intervention, where applicable.

Osmotic demyelination syndrome (ODS) was reported in five cases, all of which involved overcorrection of sodium (>10 mmO/L in 24 h). These cases emphasize the importance of cautious correction and close monitoring. Biochemical reference values used for interpretation appear in Table 5.

Outcomes were generally favorable with appropriate treatment but delayed diagnosis or overly aggressive sodium correction led to complications in a subset of patients. Mortality was reported in two cases.

The methodological quality of the included case reports was assessed using the Joanna Briggs Institute (JBI) checklist. Most cases scored well in domains such as clarity of clinical history and diagnostic reasoning. However, several reports lacked long-term follow-up or detailed outcome descriptions. These limitations were considered when interpreting the findings and drawing conclusions.

Although case reports and series are considered lower levels of evidence due to their uncontrolled nature, they play an important role in advancing medical knowledge, especially in rare disorders such as potomania. They help inform clinical decision-making when higher-level evidence is lacking. In this review, all included case reports were critically appraised using the Joanna Briggs Institute (JBI) checklist. Most studies demonstrated acceptable methodological quality, particularly in reporting clinical history and diagnostic reasoning. However, some lacked detail on treatment outcomes or long-term follow-up, and these limitations were considered in the interpretation of findings [48,49].

All included case reports listed in Tables 2–4 are cited either in the main text or referenced within the tables themselves to ensure transparency and traceability of data sources.

Table 3. Demographic and clinical characteristics of potomania participants.

Demographic and Clinical Characteristics of Potomania Participants											
					Biochemical Analysis						
Author and Year	Age	Gender	Type of Drink Consumed	Body Mass Index	Serum Sodium (mmO/L)	Serum Potassium (mmO/L)	Serum Chloride (mmO/L)	Creatinine mg/dL	Serum Osmolarity mOsm/kg	Urine Osmolality mOsm/kg	Urine Sodium (mmO/L)
So BYF and Chan GCW (2023) [22]	51 years old	Male	Malted soybean milk drink	NR	118 mmO/L	3.4 mmO/L	NR	1.76 mg/dL	NR	120 mOsm/kg	21 mmO/L
Macías Robles et al. (2009) [5]	42 years old	Male	Water	NR	98 mmO/L	1.67 mmO/L	NR	0.42 mg/dL	200 mOsm/kg	270 mOsm/kg	10 mmO/L
Soliman et al. (2018) [12]	67 years old	Male	Herbal tea (detox)	NR	111 mmol/	NR	NR	NR	NR	NR	NR
Srisung et al. (2015) [27]	69 years old	Male	Liquids	NR	117 mmOl/	NR	NR	0.7 mg/dL	250 mOsm/kg	132 mOsm /kg	NR
Campeão (2013) [33]	48-year-old male	Male	Water	NR	NR	NR	NR	NR	NR	NR	NR
Pizzini et al. (2011) [35]	76 years old	Male	Water	NR	161 mmO/L	NR	NR	4.2 mg/dL	NR	NR	NR
Caron et al. (1977) [36]	25 years old 59 years old 18 years	Male Female Female	Water	NR	139.5 mmO/L 138.5 mmO/L 142 mmO/L	4.5 mmO/L 4.5 mmO/L 4 mmO/L	NR	0.86 mg/dL 1.0 mg/dL 0.6 mg/dL	NR	NR	NR
Tejedor et al. (2014) [41]	41 years old	Male	Isotonic drinks	NR	111 mmO/L	3.1 mmO/L	79 mmO/L	NR	227 mOsm/kg	64.88 mOsm/kg	NR
Alda et al. (2007) [42]	18 years old	Male	Water	NR	NR	NR	NR	NR	NR	NR	NR
Lord (2000) [11]	26 years old	Male	Cider Potomania	NR	106 mmOl/	2.9 mmO/L	NR	0.55 mg/dL	239 mOsm/kg	NR	NR
Windpessl et al. (2017) [9]	61 years old	Female	Water and tea	19.9 kg/m^2	122 mmO/L	3.1 mmO/L	87 mmO/L	1.1 mg/dL	251 mOsm/kg	NR	NR
Fox BD (2002) [30]	51 years old	Female	Water	33.2 kg/m^2	108 mmO/L	2.6 mmO/L	NR	0.71 mg/dL	226 mOsm/kg	147 mOsm/kg	20 mmO/L
Chaudhary et al. (2012) [13]	40 years old	Female	Tea	NR	97 mmO/L	2 mmO/L	55 mmO/L	NR	NR	40 mOsm/kg	<10 mmO/L
Goëb et al. (2003) [37]	20 years old	Female	Water	Reported as obese	NR	NR	NR	NR	NR	NR	NR
Hirel and Thobois. (2014) [38]	61 years old	Female	Water	NR	123 mmO/L	NR	NR	NR	NR	NR	NR
Couillard et al. (2021) [39]	54 years old	Female	Coca-Cola Zero	21 kg/m^2	147 mmol	1.26 mmO/L	NR	0.61 mg/dL	NR	NR	NR
Haymann (2014) [40]	45 years old	Female	Water	NR	103 mmO/L	4.7 mmO/L	NR	3.87 mg/dL	NR	NR	55 mmO/L
Domínguez et al. (2013) [6]	72 years old	Female	Water	NR	111 mmO/L	2.2 mmO/L	NR	NR	NR	NR	NR
Benítez-Mejía et al. (2021) [43]	52 years old	Female	Water	NR	108 mEq/L	NR	74 mmO/L	0.32 mg/dL	224 mOsm/kg	90 mOsm/kg	NR

NR: not reported.

Table 4. Demographic and clinical characteristics of participants with beer potomania.

Demographic and Clinical Characteristics of Participants with Beer Potomania										
				Biochemical Analysis						
Author and Year	Age	Gender	Body Mass Index kg/m²	Serum Sodium mmO/L	Serum Potassium mmO/L	Serum Chloride mmO/L	Creatinine mg/dL	Serum Osmolarity mOsm/kg	Urine Osmolality mOsm/kg	Urine Sodium mOsm/kg
Lodhi et al. (2017) [15]	Case 1: 59 years old Case 2: 60 years old	Male	Case 1: 16 Case 2: 17.5 kg/m²	Case 1: 118 Case 2: 106 mmO/L	Case 1: 4 Case 2: 4.6 mmO/L	Case 1: 90 Case 2: 74 mmO/L	Case 1: 0.56 Case 2: 0.4 mg/dL	Case 1: 259 Case 2: 232 mOsm/kg	Case 1: - Case 2: 159 mOsm/kg	Case 1: 19 Case 2: 19 mmO/L/mEq/L
Yu ZL and Fisher (2022) [16]	53 years old	Male	Reported as thin and cachectic	113 mmO/L	4 mmO/L	70 mmO/L	0.43 mg/dL	258 mOsm/kg	94 mOsm/kg	<15 mmO/L
Bhattarai et al. (2010) [7]	52 years old	Male	NR	107 mmO/L	4 mmO/L	69 mmO/L	0.40 mg/dL	284 mOsm/kg	383 mOsm	6 mmO/L
Kujubu et al. (2015) [17]	84 years old	Male	NR	116 mmO/L	4.1 mmO/L	85 mmO/L	0.58 mg/dL	250 mOsm/kg	182 mOsm/kg	35 mEq/L
Dodoo et al. (2022) [18]	56 years old	Male	NR	102 mmO/L	4.2 mmO/L	73 mmO/L	0.3 mg/dL	245 mOsm/L	44 mOsm/L	7 mmO/L
Stasishin et al. (2021) [19]	Middle-aged	Male	NR	110 mmO/L	NR	NR	NR	NR	261 mOsm/kg	<20 mmO/L
Laubner et al. (2020) [20]	55 years old	Male	NR	105 mmO/L	4.1 mmO/L	66.9 mmO/L	0.57 mg/dL	219 mOsm/kg	NR	NR
Mifsud et al. (2018) [21]	68 years old	Male	NR	98 mmO/L	3.36 mmO/L	59 mmO/L	Reported as normal limits	218 mOsm/kg	NR	12 mmO/L
Perez Gomez et al. (2022) [8]	45 years old	Male	NR	122 ** mmO/L	NR	NR	NR	NR	NR	NR
Sterns et al. (2010) [23]	45 years old	Male	NR	96 mmO/L	3.5 mmO/L	56 mmO/L	1.0 mg/dL	203 mOsm/kg	732 mOsm/kg	7 mmO/L
Lum G. (2013) [24]	63 years old	Male	NR	106 mmO/L	4.8 mmO/L	73 mmO/L	0.8 mg/dL	245 mOsm/kg	227 mOsm/kg	<20 mmO/L
Rafei et al. (2016) [25]	66 years old	Male	NR	122 mmO/L	5 mmO/L	88 mmO/L	1 mg/dL	268 mOsm/kg	223 mOsm/kg	20 mmO/L
McGraw et al. (2012) [2]	Mid-30s	Male	16 kg/m²	105 mmO/L	NR	NR	NR	225 mOsm/kg	75 mOsm/kg	16 mEq/L
Haran et al. (2010) [29]	41 years old	Male	NR	94 mmO/L	3.2 mmO/L	59 mmO/L	NR	NR	NR	NR
Sharif et al. (2023) [31]	42 years old	Male	NR	97 mmO/L	NR	NR	NR	208 mOsm/kg	90 mOsm/kg	<5 mmO/L
Akatsuka et al. (2023) [32]	32 years old	Male	NR	104 mEq/L	NR	NR	17.1 mg/dL	NR	NR	NR
Milisenda et al. (2012) [44]	60 years old	Male	NR	95 mmO/L	1.7 mmO/L	NR	NR	280 mOsml	NR	NR
Campbell (2010) [45]	33 years old	Male	NR	95 mmO/L	NR	NR	NR	NR	NR	NR
Senanayake et al. (2023) [10]	41 years old	Female	18.2 kg/m²	121 mmO/L	5.2 mmO/L	88 mmO/L	1.02 mg/dL	265 mOsmol/kg	309 mOsmol/kg	60 mEq/day
Pallavi, R. (2015) [26]	68 years old	Female	17.5 kg/m²	119 mmO/L	2.8 mmO/L	NR	NR	277 mOsm/kg	79 mOsm/kg	8 mmO/L
Patel et al. (2012) [28]	56 years old	Female	NR	97 mmO/L	NR	NR	NR	NR	NR	NR
Axelrod et al. (2011) [34]	39 years old	Female	NR	NR	NR	NR	NR	NR	NR	NR

NR: not reported; ** based on estimated calculations.

Table 5. Reference Ranges for Relevant Biochemical Parameters.

Biochemistry References Range	
Serum sodium	133–146 mmO/L
Serum potassium	3.5–5.3 mmO/L
Serum chloride	95–108 mmO/L
Creatinine	0.6–1.2 mg/dL
Serum osmolarity	275–295 mOsmol/kg
Urine osmolality	Normal early morning urine > 600 mmol/kg
Urine sodium	40–220 mmol/24 h

References ranges were taken from Fuggle and Munro [50].

4. Discussion

The results of this review provide a broad overview of the clinical characteristics, manifestations, and outcomes associated with potomania and beer potomania. Across the 44 cases analyzed, distinct patterns of excessive fluid consumption, consistent clinical symptoms, and the development of hypotonic hyponatremia were observed in both conditions.

Excessive fluid intake increases total body water, dilutes plasma osmolality, and suppresses vasopressin secretion, reducing urine concentration and promoting diuresis [51]. However, when fluid intake is not accompanied by sufficient solute intake, urinary osmolality drops to around 100 mOsm/kg, limiting renal water excretion and leading to dilutional hyponatremia [52,53]. This mechanism is particularly evident in beer potomania, a condition resulting from high-volume beer consumption combined with low dietary solute and protein intake. A low urine osmolality reflects intact renal dilution capacity, but hyponatremia occurs when solute excretion is insufficient to eliminate excess water [15,54]. This dissociation between urine dilution capacity and solute-dependent water clearance has also been explored by Wilke et al. [55], who demonstrated vasopressin-independent regulation of aquaporin-2 under conditions of food deprivation.

Beer potomania was first described in the 1970s [56,57] and remains a reference for current understanding [58]. Excessive fluid intake increases total body water, dilutes plasma osmolality, and suppresses vasopressin secretion.

Additionally, very low-sodium diets prompt the kidneys to retain more sodium and water, decreasing delivery of filtrate to diluting nephron segments and further limiting water excretion—even in the absence of vasopressin [55,59]. Examples include extreme weight loss diets [23], beer potomania [54], and intake of carbohydrate-rich but sodium-poor beverages such as malted soy drinks [22], which can exacerbate hyponatremia compared to complete starvation [60].

Dietary solute intake, particularly protein and sodium, is essential for the renal excretion of free water. In patients with severely restricted diets, the low solute load impairs the kidneys' ability to eliminate excess water, even when the capacity to dilute urine is preserved [58].

Patterns of fluid consumption and etiological context differ significantly between potomania and beer potomania. Potomania involved varied liquids, including water [61], cider [11], tea [12,13], Coca-Cola Zero® [39], isotonic drinks [41], and soy-based drinks [22], while beer potomania was specifically linked to high beer consumption [62,63]. These differences reflect broader social and dietary influences, including the predominance of beer potomania in males (19 out of 23 cases), potentially due to cultural norms around alcohol consumption [60].

Symptomatically, patients with both forms of potomania presented similar clinical features: fatigue, nausea, vomiting, confusion, seizures, and altered consciousness [46,47,64].

Symptoms such as seizures and altered mental status were common, as previously described by Musch et al. [46] and Sailer et al. [47]. Potomania, schizophrenia, bipolar disorder, OCD, and substance use disorders were frequently reported [5,24,33,35], as was psychogenic polydipsia, which affects approximately 6% to 20% of patients with schizophrenia and is also prevalent in individuals with intellectual disabilities or autism spectrum disorders [65].

Diagnosis of beer potomania is based on a history of excessive beer intake, poor diet, and the exclusion of other causes of hyponatremia. It typically presents with low urine sodium and osmolality [57,58,63]. Potomania due to other fluids is diagnosed by identifying excessive intake and ruling out other etiologies of hyponatremia. Laboratory criteria for diagnosis include serum sodium < 135 mEq/L, serum osmolality < 280 mOsm/kg, and urine osmolality < 100 mOsm/kg [1].

Treatment involves fluid restriction, correction of electrolyte imbalances, and cautious use of intravenous fluids to avoid rapid sodium correction [66]. Some case reports, such as that by Yu and Fisher [16], emphasize the risks of initial fluid resuscitation in beer potomania, which may exacerbate hyponatremia if not properly monitored.

In beer potomania, alcohol cessation and nutritional support are also essential [2]. Sodium correction should not exceed 10–12 mmO/L in 24 h or 18–25 mmO/L in 48 h [54,66]. In cases of overcorrection, 5% dextrose or desmopressin may be administered [66,67]. Some case reports, such as that by Yu and Fisher [16], emphasize the risks of initial fluid resuscitation in patients with beer potomania, which may exacerbate hyponatremia if not properly monitored.

Osmotic demyelination syndrome (ODS) is a severe complication of rapid sodium correction and is characterized by symptoms such as paralysis, dysarthria, and dysphagia. Risk factors include alcoholism, malnutrition, liver disease, and correction rates > 25 mmO/L over 24–48 h [44,46,54]. Three cases in this review reported ODS [6,13,28], highlighting the need for careful management. When ODS occurs, lowering sodium using hypotonic solutions and dextrose infusions is recommended [68].

Psychiatric management also poses challenges, as several medications (e.g., lithium, carbamazepine, oxcarbazepine, valproate) may contribute to or exacerbate hyponatremia [66]. Conversely, some antipsychotics, such as risperidone and olanzapine, may reduce compulsive fluid intake behaviors [1].

Despite offering a comprehensive clinical synthesis, this study has limitations. Case reports may be subject to publication bias, with more severe or unusual presentations more likely to be reported. Additionally, the limited sample size and absence of control groups reduce the generalizability of findings. Diagnostic methods and interventions varied considerably across cases, making standardization difficult. Furthermore, sociocultural factors such as dietary habits and patterns of alcohol use may limit applicability to broader populations.

5. Conclusions

Potomania and beer potomania are uncommon but potentially life-threatening causes of hyponatremia, often overlooked in clinical practice. This systematic review highlights the importance of recognizing distinct fluid consumption patterns, psychiatric comorbidities, and nutritional deficiencies associated with both conditions. While potomania encompasses a broader range of liquid intakes, beer potomania is specifically linked to excessive beer consumption and low dietary solute intake.

Timely diagnosis relies on thorough patient history and laboratory evaluation, including assessment of serum sodium and serum and urine osmolality. Effective treatment includes fluid restriction, correction of electrolyte imbalances, nutritional support, and careful monitoring to prevent osmotic demyelination syndrome. Special attention should be given to psychiatric assessment and management, especially in patients with psychogenic polydipsia or other mental health conditions.

Although this review is based on case reports, which limits generalizability, it provides clinically relevant insights that can inform diagnosis and management in settings where higher-level evidence is lacking. Further research with standardized methodologies is necessary to better understand the epidemiology, outcomes, and optimal treatment approaches for these rare conditions.

Supplementary Materials: The following supporting information can be downloaded at: https://www.mdpi.com/article/10.3390/nu17122012/s1, Table S1: JBI critical appraisal checklist for case reports; Table S2: PRISMA 2020 Checklist.

Author Contributions: K.S.M.: conceptualization, data curation, formal analysis, investigation, methodology, project administration, writing—original draft preparation, and writing—review and editing. M.M.G.: conceptualization, data curation, formal analysis, investigation, methodology, project administration, supervision, validation, writing—original draft preparation, and writing—review and editing. J.M.S.: corresponding author, conceptualization, data curation, formal analysis, investigation, methodology, project administration, supervision, and writing—review and editing. All authors have read and agreed to the published version of the manuscript.

Funding: This research received no external funding.

Institutional Review Board Statement: This review was registered in the Prospero systematic review registry database on 9 April 2024. ID: CRD42024528002. This systematic review was conducted based on the Preferred Reporting Items for Systematic Reviews and Meta-Analyses (PRISMA).

Data Availability Statement: This review was registered in the Prospero systematic review registry database. ID: CRD42024528002.

Conflicts of Interest: The authors declare no conflicts of interest.

Abbreviations

ADH	Antidiuretic Hormone
JBI	Joanna Briggs Institute
mOsm	Milliosmoles
mOsm/kg	Milliosmoles per kilogram
PMCID	PubMed Central Identifier
PMID	PubMed Identifier
PICO	Participants, Intervention, Comparison, and Outcomes
PRISMA	Preferred Reporting Items for Systematic Reviews and Meta-Analyses
QCR	Query and Collection Review
WOS	Web of Science

References

1. Dundas, B.; Harris, M.; Narasimhan, M. Psychogenic polydipsia review: Etiology, differential, and treatment. *Curr. Psychiatry Rep.* **2007**, *9*, 236–241. [CrossRef] [PubMed]
2. McGraw, M. Beer potomania: Drink in this atypical cause of hyponatremia. *Nursing* **2012**, *42*, 24–30. [CrossRef] [PubMed]
3. de Leon, J.; Verghese, C.; Tracy, J.I.; Josiassen, R.C.; Simpson, G.M. Polydipsia and water intoxication in psychiatric patients: A review of the epidemiological literature. *Biol. Psychiatry* **1994**, *35*, 408–419. [CrossRef] [PubMed]
4. Gillum, D.M.; Linas, S.L. Water intoxication in a psychotic patient with normal renal water excretion. *Am. J. Med.* **1984**, *77*, 773–774. [CrossRef] [PubMed]
5. Macías Robles, M.D.; López Fonticiella, M.P.; Maciá Bobes, C.; Fernández San Martín, A. Hiponatremia aguda grave en un paciente esquizofrénico potomano. *An. Sist. Sanit. Navarra* **2009**, *32*, 117–120. [CrossRef]

6. Domínguez, R.O.; Laguarde, N.; Pinkala, E.; González, S.E. Potomanía y desequilibrio osmótico: Ceguera cortical definitiva po[r] mielinólisis extrapontina. *Neurologia* **2013**, *28*, 449–450. [CrossRef]
7. Bhattarai, N.; Kafle, P.; Panda, M. Beer potomania: A case report. *BMJ Case Rep.* **2010**, *2010*, bcr10.2009.2414. [CrossRef] [PubMed] [PubMed Central]
8. Perez-Gomez, M.V.; Sanchez-Ospina, D.; Tejedor, A.; Ortiz, A. The mysterious death of the beer drinking champ: Potential role for hyperacute water loading and acute hyponatremia. *Clin. Kidney J.* **2022**, *15*, 1196–1201. [CrossRef]
9. Windpessl, M.; Schwarz, C.; Wallner, M. "Bowel prep hyponatremia"—A state of acute water intoxication facilitated by low dietary solute intake: Case report and literature review. *BMC Nephrol.* **2017**, *18*, 54. [CrossRef]
10. Senanayake, J.; Haji Rahman, R.; Boucher, B.; Ali, M.Z.; Madanat, S.; Hammell, C.; Chuy, F. Multi-etiological hyponatremia in association with suspected beer potomania. *Cureus* **2023**, *15*, e36407. [CrossRef] [PubMed] [PubMed Central]
11. Lord, R.C.C. Cider potomania. *Ann. Clin. Biochem.* **2000**, *37*, 729–730. [CrossRef] [PubMed]
12. Soliman, M.; Fuller, W.; Usmani, N.; Akanbi, O. Acute severe hyponatremia as a serious health implication of herbal detox regimens. *Cureus* **2018**, *10*, e3697. [CrossRef] [PubMed]
13. Chaudhary, S.; Kashani, K.; Prasad, S. 1194: "iced tea potomania" complicated by early osmotic demyelination. *Crit. Care Med* **2012**, *40*, 1–328. [CrossRef]
14. Page, M.J.; McKenzie, J.E.; Bossuyt, P.M.; Boutron, I.; Hoffmann, T.C.; Mulrow, C.D.; Shamseer, L.; Tetzlaff, J.M.; Akl, E.A. Brennan, S.E.; et al. The PRISMA 2020 statement: An updated guideline for reporting systematic reviews. *BMJ* **2021**, *372*, n71 [CrossRef]
15. Lodhi, M.U.; Saleem, T.S.; Kuzel, A.R.; Khan, D.; Syed, I.A.; Rahim, U.; Iqbal, H.I.; Rahim, M. "Beer potomania"—A syndrome of severe hyponatremia with unique pathophysiology: Case studies and literature review. *Cureus* **2017**, *9*, e2000. [CrossRef] [PubMed] [PubMed Central]
16. Yu, Z.L.; Fisher, L. Beer potomania: Why initial fluid resuscitation may be harmful. *Case Rep. Nephrol.* **2022**, *2022*, 8778304 [CrossRef] [PubMed] [PubMed Central]
17. Kujubu, D.A.; Khosraviani, A. Beer potomania—An unusual cause of hyponatremia. *Perm. J.* **2015**, *19*, 74–76. [CrossRef] [PubMed] [PubMed Central]
18. Dodoo, S.N.; Agyemang-Sarpong, A.; Taka, N.; Akatue, R.A.; Williams, M.L. Takotsubo cardiomyopathy in the setting of severe hyponatremia and beer potomania: A case report. *Clin. Case Rep.* **2022**, *10*, e6717. [CrossRef] [PubMed] [PubMed Central]
19. Stasishin, D.; Schaffer, P.; Khan, Z.; Murphy, C. Severe metabolic derangement: A case of concomitant diabetic ketoacidosis and beer potomania. *BMJ Case Rep.* **2021**, *14*, e243486. [CrossRef] [PubMed] [PubMed Central]
20. Laubner, G.; Gintautaitė, G.; Badaras, R. Challenges in the diagnostics and management of hydrochlorothiazide-induced severe hyponatremia in a habitual beer drinker. *Acta Med. Litu.* **2020**, *27*, 39–44. [CrossRef] [PubMed] [PubMed Central]
21. Mifsud, S.; Schembri, E.L.; Mercieca Balbi, M.; Gruppetta, M.; Clark, J. Beer, hyponatraemia and cardiac conduction defects. *BMJ Case Rep.* **2018**, *2018*, bcr-2018-224260. [CrossRef] [PubMed] [PubMed Central]
22. So, B.Y.F.; Chan, G.C.W. Low-solute hyponatremia in a kidney transplant recipient. *Clin. Nephrol.* **2023**, *99*, 307–310. [CrossRef] [PubMed]
23. Sterns, R.H.; Hix, J.K.; Silver, S. Treating profound hyponatremia: A strategy for controlled correction. *Am. J. Kidney Dis.* **2010**, *56*, 774–779. [CrossRef] [PubMed]
24. Lum, G. Severe hyponatremia in a schizophrenic patient. *Clin. Chem.* **2013**, *59*, 887–889. [CrossRef] [PubMed]
25. Rafei, H.; Yunus, R.; Khurana, P. Beer potomania: A challenging case of hyponatremia. *J. Endocrinol. Metab.* **2016**, *6*, 123–126. [CrossRef]
26. Pallavi, R. An unsuspected cause of hyponatremia: Beer potomania. *J. Am. Geriatr. Soc.* **2015**, *63*, 1714–1715. [CrossRef] [PubMed]
27. Srisung, W.; Mankongpaisarnrung, C.; Anaele, C.; Dumrongmongcolgul, N.; Ahmed, V. A rare case of low-solute hyponatremia in a nonalcoholic person. *Case Rep. Nephrol. Dial.* **2014**, *5*, 49–53. [CrossRef] [PubMed] [PubMed Central]
28. Patel, N.; Sacks, A. True beer potomania causing critical hyponatremia. *Chest* **2012**, *142*, 414A. [CrossRef]
29. Haran, M.; Shtern, Y.; Lodha, A.; Kupfer, Y. Severe hyponatremia: A novel approach to treatment. *Chest* **2010**, *138*, 135A. [CrossRef]
30. Fox, B.D. Crash diet potomania. *Lancet* **2002**, *359*, 942. [CrossRef] [PubMed]
31. Sharif, M.W.; Singh, A.; Enabi, J.; Karkee, R.; Sanivarapu, R. Delayed presentation of osmotic demyelination syndrome treated with plasmapheresis. *Cureus* **2023**, *15*, e47399. [CrossRef] [PubMed] [PubMed Central]
32. Akatsuka, M.; Tatsumi, H.; Osanami, A.; Yamashita, T.; Masuda, Y. A case of hyponatremia due to beer potomania followed by acute kidney injury [abstract]. *Crit. Care Med.* **2023**, *51* (Suppl. S1), 320. [CrossRef]
33. Campeão, N. Neuropsychiatric symptoms in acute porphyria—A case report. *Psychother. Psychosom.* **2013**, *82* (Suppl. S1), 134. [CrossRef]
34. Axelrod, A.F.; Angles, C.; Siu, G. Rehabilitation after central pontine myelinolysis induced from beer potomania: A case report. *PMR* **2011**, *3* (Suppl. S1), S276. [CrossRef]

35. Pizzini, M.C.; Leone, D.; Favali, L.; Morini, M.; Silingardi, I.; Iori, M. The "Healthy" Psychogenic Potomania [Internet]. 2011. Available online: https://www.researchgate.net/publication/307731686_Abstract_Book_of_the_XVI_Congresso_Nazionale_FADOI_-_Firenze_15-18_Maggio_2011/fulltext/57d848ac08ae6399a39921f1/Abstract-Book-of-the-XVI-Congresso-Nazionale-FADOI-Firenze-15-18-Maggio-2011.pdf?__cf_chl_tk=MJFaqxgPmqM_LzJooItO9VXhGsUgqKZEzC_9LcTacdk-1749726033-1.0.1.1-PI7KntuEgwUTTmlVZIy5phaAXAsIx.9wy8t8cobeEII (accessed on 2 March 2024).
36. Caron, C.; Montambault, P.; Nawar, T.; Plante, G.E.; Kandalaft, N. La potomanie: Réévaluation des épreuves d'investigation et présentation inhabituelle avec hydronéphrose et méqavessie. *CMAJ* **1977**, *116*, 1359–1363. [PubMed] [PubMed Central]
37. Goëb, J.L.; Vercruysse, D.; Duverger, P.; Pettenati, H.; Rannou-Dubas, K.; Gohier, B. Crossed glances on a potomaniac patient. *Ann. Med. Psychol.* **2003**, *161*, 296–302. [CrossRef]
38. Hirel, C.; Thobois, S. Une potomanie révélatrice d'une maladie de Huntington [Potomania revealing Huntington's disease]. *Rev. Neurol.* **2014**, *170*, 141–142. [CrossRef] [PubMed]
39. Couillard, F.; Ayroulet, C.; Roussin, C.; Vanhecke, C.; Goossens, J.; Combres, H.; Ly, K.H.; Francois, C. Une hypokaliémie symptomatique induite par une consommation excessive de Coca-Cola zéro®. *Nutr. Clin. Métabol.* **2021**, *35*, 317–320. [CrossRef]
40. Haymann, J.P. Diagnostic d'une polyurie par un physiologiste: Discussion de cas cliniques. *Med. Intensive Reanim.* **2014**, *23*, 370–377. [CrossRef]
41. Cruz Tejedor, M.; Zubillaga Muñoz, S.; De Pablo Hermida, A.M.; Nevado Losada, E.; García Sánchez, E.; Hernández Sánchez, E.M.; Albert de la Cruz, P. Hiponatremia grave secundaria a potomanía de bebidas isotónicas en un paciente esquizofrénico. *Emergencias* **2014**, *26*, 239–240.
42. Alda, M.; Campayo, J.G.; Cerdán, C.; Laguna, C. Potomanía secundaria a topiramato. *Med. Clin.* **2007**, *128*, 397–398. [CrossRef]
43. Benítez-Mejía, J.F.; Morales-Cuellar, J.; Restrepo-López, J.S.; Giraldo-Carmona, E.M.; Cabrera-Gómez, E. Psychogenic polydipsia and severe hyponatremia in bipolar affective disorder. *Actas Esp. Psiquiatr.* **2021**, *49*, 288–290. [PubMed] [PubMed Central]
44. Milisenda, J.C.; Coloma, E.; Grau, J.M. Potomanía de cerveza. Una causa poco conocida de hiponatremia grave. *Med. Clin.* **2012**, *138*, 410–411. [CrossRef] [PubMed]
45. Campbell, M.C. Hyponatremia and central pontine myelinolysis as a result of beer potomania: A case report. *Prim. Care Companion J. Clin. Psychiatry* **2010**, *12*, PCC.09100936. [CrossRef] [PubMed] [PubMed Central]
46. Musch, W.; Xhaet, O.; Decaux, G. Solute loss plays a major role in polydipsia-related hyponatraemia of both water drinkers and beer drinkers. *QJM* **2003**, *96*, 421–426. [CrossRef] [PubMed]
47. Sailer, C.O.; Winzeler, B.; Nigro, N.; Suter-Widmer, I.; Arici, B.; Bally, M.; Schuetz, P.; Mueller, B.; Christ-Crain, M. Characteristics and outcomes of patients with profound hyponatraemia due to primary polydipsia. *Clin. Endocrinol.* **2017**, *87*, 492–499. [CrossRef] [PubMed]
48. Murad, M.H.; Sultan, S.; Haffar, S.; Bazerbachi, F. Methodological quality and synthesis of case series and case reports. *BMJ Evid.-Based Med.* **2018**, *23*, 60–63. [CrossRef] [PubMed] [PubMed Central]
49. Moola, S.; Munn, Z.; Tufanaru, C.; Aromataris, E.; Sears, K.; Sfetcu, R.; Currie, M.; Lisy, K.; Qureshi, R.; Mattis, P.; et al. Systematic reviews of etiology and risk. In *JBI Manual for Evidence Synthesis*; Aromataris, E., Lockwood, C., Porritt, K., Eds.; JBI: Adelaide, Austrialia, 2024. Available online: https://synthesismanual.jbi.global (accessed on 2 March 2024). [CrossRef]
50. Fuggle, S.; Munro, J. *Clinical Biochemistry Protocol*; Version: Issue 14 V2.2; Eastbourne District General Hospital & Conquest Hospital, Hastings, Clinical Biochemistry Team: Eastbourne, UK, 2020.
51. Robertson, G.L. Antidiuretic hormone: Normal and disordered function. *Endocrinol. Metab. Clin. N. Am.* **2001**, *30*, 671–694. [CrossRef] [PubMed]
52. Pedersen, E.B.; Thomsen, I.M.; Lauridsen, T.G. Abnormal function of the vasopressin–cyclic-AMP–aquaporin-2 axis during urine concentrating and diluting in patients with reduced renal function: A case-control study. *BMC Nephrol.* **2010**, *11*, 26. [CrossRef] [PubMed] [PubMed Central]
53. Berl, T. Impact of solute intake on urine flow and water excretion. *J. Am. Soc. Nephrol.* **2008**, *19*, 1076–1078. [CrossRef] [PubMed]
54. Sanghvi, S.R.; Kellerman, P.S.; Nanovic, L. Beer potomania: An unusual cause of hyponatremia at high risk of complications from rapid correction. *Am. J. Kidney Dis.* **2007**, *50*, 673–680. [CrossRef] [PubMed]
55. Wilke, C.; Sheriff, S.; Soleimani, M.; Amlal, H. Vasopressin-independent regulation of collecting duct aquaporin-2 in food deprivation. *Kidney Int.* **2005**, *67*, 201–216. [CrossRef] [PubMed]
56. Demanet, J.C.; Bonnyns, M.; Bleiberg, H.; Stevens-Rocmans, C. Coma due to water intoxication in beer drinkers. *Lancet* **1971**, *2*, 1115–1117. [CrossRef] [PubMed]
57. Hilden, T.; Svendsen, T.L. Electrolyte disturbances in beer drinkers: A specific hypo-osmolality syndrome. *Lancet* **1975**, *2*, 245–246. [CrossRef] [PubMed]
58. Fenves, A.Z.; Thomas, S.; Knochel, J.P. Beer potomania: Two cases and review of the literature. *Clin. Nephrol.* **1996**, *45*, 61–64. [PubMed]
59. Blaustein, D.A.; Schwenk, M.H. "Beer potomania" in a non-beer drinker. *Clin. Nephrol.* **1997**, *48*, 203–204. [PubMed]

60. Sudhinaraset, M.; Wigglesworth, C.; Takeuchi, D.T. Social and cultural contexts of alcohol use: Influences in a social-ecologic framework. *Alcohol Res.* **2016**, *38*, 35–45. [PubMed] [PubMed Central]
61. Fernandes, C.F.; Gouveia, C.; Gouveia, P.; Camacho, B.; Borges, M.J. Potomania in pediatric age? The diagnostic challeng *Pediatr. Oncall J.* **2024**, *21*, 118–120. [CrossRef]
62. Ouellette, L.; Michel, K.; Riley, B.; Jones, J. Beer potomania: Atypical cause of severe hyponatremia in older alcoholics. *Am. Emerg. Med.* **2018**, *36*, 1303. [CrossRef] [PubMed]
63. Liamis, G.L.; Milionis, H.J.; Rizos, E.C.; Siamopoulos, K.C.; Elisaf, M.S. Mechanisms of hyponatraemia in alcohol patien *Alcohol Alcohol.* **2000**, *35*, 612–616. [CrossRef] [PubMed]
64. Musch, W.; Decaux, G. Utility and limitations of biochemical parameters in the evaluation of hyponatremia in the elder *Int. Urol. Nephrol.* **2001**, *32*, 475–483. [CrossRef] [PubMed]
65. Komatsu, H.; Ono, T.; Onouchi, Y.; Onoguchi, G.; Maita, Y.; Ishida, Y.; Maki, T.; Oba, A.; Tomita, H.; Kakuto, Y. Polydipsi and autistic traits in patients with schizophrenia spectrum disorders. *Front. Psychiatry* **2023**, *14*, 1205138. [CrossRef] [PubMed [PubMed Central]
66. Spasovski, G.; Vanholder, R.; Allolio, B.; Annane, D.; Ball, S.; Bichet, D.; Decaux, G.; Fenske, W.; Hoorn, E.J.; Ichai, C.; et a Clinical practice guideline on diagnosis and treatment of hyponatraemia. *Nephrol. Dial. Transplant.* **2014**, *29* (Suppl. S2), i1–i3 [CrossRef] [PubMed]
67. Malhotra, K.; Ortega, L. Central pontine myelinolysis with meticulous correction of hyponatraemia in chronic alcoholic *BMJ Case Rep.* **2013**, *2013*, bcr2013009970. [CrossRef] [PubMed] [PubMed Central]
68. Yun, G.; Baek, S.H.; Kim, S. Evaluation and management of hypernatremia in adults: Clinical perspectives. *Korean J. Intern. Me* **2023**, *38*, 290–302. [CrossRef] [PubMed] [PubMed Central]

MDPI AG
Grosspeteranlage 5
4052 Basel
Switzerland
Tel.: +41 61 683 77 34

Nutrients Editorial Office
E-mail: nutrients@mdpi.com
www.mdpi.com/journal/nutrients

www.ingramcontent.com/pod-product-compliance
Lightning Source LLC
Chambersburg PA
CBHW061620220926
51850CB00005B/553
9783725878017